VENUSES
PENUSES

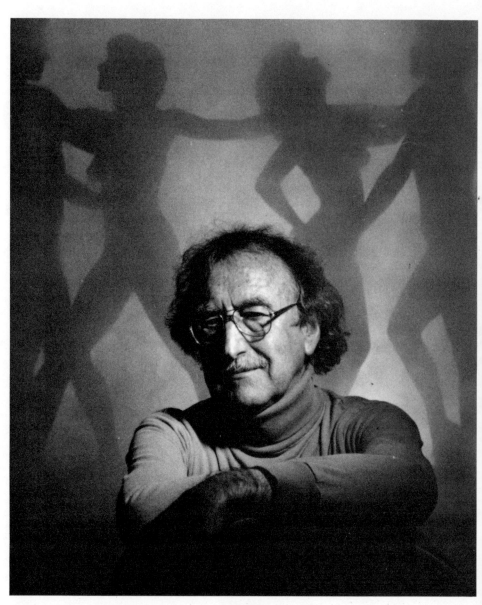

JOHN MONEY

VENUSES PENUSES

SEXOLOGY
SEXOSOPHY
AND
EXIGENCY
THEORY

JOHN MONEY

PROMETHEUS BOOKS
Buffalo, New York

Library of Congress Cataloging-in-Publication Data

Money, John, 1921-
    Venuses penuses.

    Bibliography: p.
    Includes index.
    1. Psychosexual disorders. 2. Gender identity
disorders. 3. Sexual disorders. 4. Sex (Psychology).
5. Sex—Research. I. Title.
RC556.M68 1986   616.85'83   85-46047
ISBN: 0-87975-327-7

Contents

PART II: GENDER-IDENTITY/ROLE [G-I/R] DIFFERENTIATION

**11   Hermaphroditism: Recommendations Concerning
Assignment of Sex, Change of Sex, and Psychologic Management**

**12   An Examination of Some Basic Sexual Concepts:
The Evidence of Human Hermaphroditism**

PART IV: TRANSEXUALISM AND PARAPHILIA

Foreword

The preliminary title of this book, *A Personal Portfolio of Essential Writings in Sexology, Sexosophy, and Exigency Theory*, was too prosaic to alert the attention of its potential readers. It needed not only a scholarly title to ensure proper bibliographic indexing and cataloguing but also a short, eye-catching one, by which to remember it.

The first short title, *Venus's Penises*, had its origin in March 1953, very early in my career as a clinical psychoendocrinologist and sexologist. There was at that time a young boy admitted for pediatric surgery because he had been born with two penises. One was cosmetically more perfect and larger than the other. It was the lesser and malformed one that communicated with the bladder. Surgically it was risky to attempt to connect the well-formed organ to the bladder. Its surgical removal was, therefore, a foregone conclusion, because it was taken as axiomatic that a male should not have two penises. The erotic capability of the two organs was not given priority in the decision-making. The boy himself was too young to be consulted or to give informed consent. Had he been old enough to evaluate the options, it would have been his prerogative not to take for granted the axiom of one man, one penis, and to exercise his right to keep both his penises. The decision of patients and professionals do not necessarily coincide. In recognition of the rights of those too young to exercise them, I wrote what has now become, more than thirty years later, the title piece of this volume:

> The favorite lover of Venus
> Was born with a duplicate penis
> When he tried to evolve her
> A duplicate vulva
> The mayhem made Venus quite heinous
>
> This lover was not to be daunted
> His fabulous organs oft' flaunted
> Found a goddess in China
> With a double vagina
> Which thenceforth he plurally haunted
>
> This sexuological story
> Was crowned with libidinal glory
> When Siamese twins
> With intersex limbs
> Were born ambicopulatory

The publisher and his advisers had some misgivings about being able to market the book under its poetic new title. A search of books in print revealed no listing of a book in the English language that included either the word *penis* or the word *vagina* in the title. Here was a challenge! It was surmounted by means of invoking an artifice of medieval Latin orthography, by which the title was transmogrified into *Venuses Penuses* (correctly pronounced as Venoos'es Penoos'es).

Acknowledgments

Nine people worked assiduously in preparing copy for editing and printing, and in proofing the typeset pages: Sandra Aamodt, Charles Annecillo, Sally Hopkins, Margaret Lamacz, Jeff Leal, Viola Lewis, Elisabeth Money, Hap Morrow, and Bernard Norman. Sally Hopkins designed the dust-jacket, and the photograph of John Money is by Mike Mitchell.

Since the inception of the Johns Hopkins Psychohormonal Research Unit in 1951, the research and writings represented in this volume have been supported by public and private funding agencies as follows: National Institutes of Health, United States Public Health Service Research Grant, 1957 to present; William T. Grant Foundation, 1983 to present; and 1972 to 1977; National Institutes of Health, United States Public Health Service Training Grant, 1977 to 1982; The Upjohn Company, 1973; The Erickson Educational Foundation, 1967 to 1972; National Institutes of Health, United States Public Health Service Research Career Development Award, 1962 to 1967; Josiah Macy Jr. Foundation, 1951 to 1960.

VENUSES
PENUSES

Introduction

In 1982 I made a collation of journal articles from my own bibliography and had three sets of them bound and titled *Principia Theoretica*. This volume became the forerunner of the present publication. Each paper has been selected for inclusion on the criterion of its theoretical significance. The development of theoretical concepts in my writing has been progressive since the publication in 1948 of the first item in my bibliography. The progression is not always apparent, however, partly because it has been saltational, and partly because it has been recorded in a wide variety of periodicals and books, not all of which are readily accessible.

Just as range animals need to be herded periodically, these theoretical concepts needed to be herded together and sorted out both chronologically and categorically. What they share in common is that they all pertain to human clinical and longitudinal research; and to sexology and sexosophy, the empirical and the doctrinal concepts of sex, respectively. Theoretical concepts in those items of my bibliography that pertain to dyslexia, intelligence, specific cognitional disability, and nonsexual psychoendocrine syndromes are not included in the present collection.

One of my satisfactions in organizing this book derives from the familiar rule that the whole is more than the sum of its parts. For me personally, there is utility in having the continuity of my theoretical thinking housed between two covers. For students, other scholars and critics, there is not only utility, but also necessity, for it has long been difficult or impossible to locate some of the papers collected in this one volume. With this impediment removed, exigency theory may soon, perhaps, receive the scholarly attention it deserves; and gender theory, though it has not suffered from neglect, will attain more scholarly consensus and consistency in its application.

The collection of papers in Part V address several extremely vexacious issues in sexual ethics, politics, and the law. It will be good, and much to my satisfation, if the bringing together of these papers generates a more scholarly and rational approach to forensic and moral issues of sex in the body politic. Otherwise we could drift, sooner than we know, toward the brink of a social catastrophe, namely a national inquisition and a secret police of antisexualism.

Prologue
Professional Biography

Becoming a Psychologist

I am American by citizenship, New Zealandic by birth (July 8, 1921), and British and Welsh by ancestry. My father was Australian, and my mother English. My education in New Zealand ended with a trained Teacher's Certificate and a double M.A. from Victoria University of Wellington, one in Philosophy/Psychology, and one in Education. I then became a junior member of the psychology faculty at the University of Otago in Dunedin, New Zealand's southern Scottish Presbyterian city.

It was more or less fortuitous that I took up psychology, a profession I had not even heard of in my high school years. When I graduated, the poverty of the era of the Great Depression made it necessary for me to earn a living rather than to be a full-time university student. The compromise was to continue my education at the Wellington Teachers' Training College, which paid a cost of living stipend, and to attend university lectures after 4 p.m. Evening students were excluded from the basic sciences, but not from psychology which, in those days, still belonged to the department of philosophy. I majored in psychology as well as education.

Getting into Psychohormonal Research

In 1948, I became a graduate student in the Psychological Clinic and the Department of Social Relations at Harvard University. A year earlier, I had left New Zealand. I had chosen America for Ph.D. study rather than England, which was where almost all New Zealand students did graduate work. There was no Ph.D. in Psychology in New Zealand at the time.

My orientation toward the United States was stimulated by American scholarly publications, and by the fact that Ernest Beaglehole was one of my teachers at Victoria University. Ernest Beaglehole was a New Zealander who had a Ph.D. in Social Anthropology from Yale. He was in the generation of Ruth Benedict, Margaret Mead, Robert Linton, and others who were formulating the relationship of personality and culture. It was he who sparked the fire and direction of my future interests in psychology.

During my first year in the United States, I was a psychology resident under Saul Rosenzweig, a Harvard graduate, at the Western Psychiatric Institute affiliated with the University of Pittsburgh. I then moved to Boston and Harvard University. There I studied under Henry Murray, Talcott Parsons, Clyde

5

Kluckohn, Gordon Allport, Richard Solomon, Leo Postman, Jerome Bruner, Robert White, George Gardner, Stanley Cobb, Samuel Stauffer, and others.

At Harvard, I probably would have gone down the mainstream of clinical psychology of the time except for the coincidence of a case presentation in the Fall of 1949 by George Gardner, M.D. for Social Relations course 281A, Clinical Problems of Child Guidance, at the Judge Baker Guidance Center in Boston. The case was one of hermaphroditism in a child who had grown up always as a boy despite having been born with, instead of a penis, an organ the size and form of a clitoris. At puberty, he feminized in physique. It is now known in retrospect that his case was one of the androgen-insensitivity syndrome. Psychologically he was a boy and could not entertain the idea of reassignment as a girl. Even though not too much could be achieved by way of surgery and hormone treatments, he was permitted to continue living as a boy. He has since married and become a father by adoption, and has achieved professional recognition in the world of medicine.

At the time this case was presented, I had begun work on a term paper which would be a complete review of psychosexual theory from Freud and his predecessors to the present. Already it had become clear to me that this review would be of book length, if done properly, and that I did not have the time for such an ambitious undertaking. I decided to move from the general to the extremely specific. I would write a paper that had as its departure the first of Freud's three essays on sexuality. This is the essay in which he briefly mentions hermaphroditism in connection with his theory of innate bisexuality.

In my paper, I reviewed the recent literature on the psychology of hermaphroditism, and presented four case reports. The evidence was sufficient to show that neither anatomy alone, nor genetics, nor hormones would dictate the status of psychosexual differentiation and identity. The theoretical implications of hermaphroditism were sufficiently important that I decided to present a dissertation proposal for a complete review of the literature, and a presentation of ten cases studied in person. That was in June 1950, and I graduated in February 1952.

Operationism

My scientific orientation toward psychology was at the outset of my undergraduate career traceable from Sir Thomas Hunter, the Professor of Psychology at Wellington, through E. B. Titchener, his teacher at Cornell, to Wilhelm Wundt, Titchener's teacher at Leipzig. Through courses in education at the university and at the Wellington Teachers' Training College, I became influenced also by the pragmatism of John Dewey.

When I became a member of the junior faculty in the Department of Psychology at the University of Otago, I got to know a young member of the Philosophy faculty, Ron Reilly, whose office was near my own. He was heavily into logical positivism and introduced me to the thinking of Ludwig Wittgenstein and Karl Popper, who at that time was a refugee at Canterbury University in New Zealand. I got involved in reading Karl Mannheim on the sociology of knowledge, and Felix Kaufmann's *Methodology of the Social Sciences* (Oxford University Press, 1944). Reilly introduced me also to Franz Kafka, but the most important outcome of our acquaintance was my encounter with Percy Bridgeman's book, *The Logic of Modern Physics* (Macmillan, 1960). Bridgeman's operationism has influenced every part of my research life, all of my writings, and I think it correct to say, my entire approach to life.

In the Spring of 1951, while I was still a graduate student at Harvard, Bridgeman offered an interdepartmental seminar, open to students of the Department of Social Relations, on the logic of agreement (one member of that small group, coincidentally, was Henry Kissinger). Bridgeman used the occasion of this seminar to hammer out problems of the logic of verbal operations. His ideas eventually were published in *The Way Things Are* (Harvard University Press, 1959).

There was no big, new influence on my thought as a result of this seminar, but rather a consolidation of what had first begun with my reading of *The Logic of Modern Physics*. Bridgeman and I did not get to know one another over and beyond the teacher-student relationship. I did not meet him again, and the last I heard of him was from his obituary. An operationist to the end, he blew his own brains out when he had had enough of dying with cancer.

Sex Research and Sex Taboo

Kinsey had not been a hot subject of study or debate at Harvard while I was there, though he had already made the first great assault on the sex taboo in America with publication of *Sexual Behavior in the Human Male* (Saunders, 1948). I suppose, in retrospect, that I was influenced by the effects of this assault, but it was after I graduated, rather than before, that I had time to find out what was going on in the wider world around me. It was after the publication of the Female volume in 1953 that I became more attuned to what affect the Kinsey studies were having on loosening the American sexual taboo.

I began my dissertation more under the influence of what earlier writers, psychoanalytical and sexological, had done to break the sexual taboo in the study of sex and eroticism. From them, I assumed I had the right to study sexual matters if I wanted to. I knew that there would be limitations on what could be said and where it could be published and publicly disseminated. I knew, also, that things that are banned in one age become public property in another. I was willing to wait if need be.

It was twenty years later, in connection with expert testimony in pornography trials, that I learned how extraordinarily effective are the social institutions for maintaining the sexual taboo in full force. It has not been as easy for society to change as it had been for me to find my own emancipation from the twentieth century legacy of fundamentalism and victorianism in rural New Zealand. Emancipation is a product of what in psychodynamic language would be called a counterphobic reaction to an excess of the taboo. The alternative is an excess of inhibition, with sexual apathy and inertia replacing sexual curiosity and exploration.

Blending curiosity with caution, I was well aware of the safety, in the society of the time, of studying sex under the umbrella of medicine. Hermaphroditism was an ideal topic in that respect. I found an ally in Stanley Cobb, Professor of Psychiatry at the Massachusetts General Hospital and at Harvard Medical School. He gave me an appointment in his department, whereby I had access to medical libraries and to the clinics in which actual hermaphroditic patients were seen.

Lawson Wilkins and the Pediatric Endocrine Clinic at Johns Hopkins

In Boston, I soon felt accepted as a colleague by those endocrinologists, pediatricians, gynecologists and urologists who were interested in the diagnosis and treatment of hermaphroditism. Through them, I learned of Lawson Wilkins who had established the first pediatric endocrine clinic at Johns Hopkins a few years earlier, and of its reputation for being the largest medical center for hermaphroditism in the world.

I was able to meet him for the first time when he came to conduct an all-day seminar at a pediatrics meeting in Boston. He established the fact that I could speak pediatric English, not losing him in the thickets of psychoanalytic English. He established with me a relationship of trust, trusting me to come to Baltimore, as I requested, to spend two weeks in his clinic. There I would be able to read the unpublished case histories of some of his hermaphroditic patients. I would also have access to the records of some of the older patients, kept in an earlier era in the department of urology by the renowned Hugh Hampton Young before his retirement. There was also the promise of the probability of being able to see and interview two or three patients, so that I would fill the promised quota of ten case studies for my dissertation.

The year 1950, the year in which I began my dissertation, was a great landmark for Lawson Wilkins. It was the year in which he showed that the hormone, cortisol, then newly synthesized, was the substance that he had been looking for to correct the abnormality of adrenocortical functioning in the commonest form of female hermaphroditism, the adrenogenital syndrome, also known as virilizing adrenal hyperplasia. The discovery had actually been made in December, 1949, and it was made concurrently by Fuller Albright and Fred Bartter at Massachusetts General Hospital and Lawson Wilkins at Johns Hopkins. They were friendly rivals working neck and neck in competition. History decreed that it would be Lawson Wilkins whose work on the syndrome became the more extensive and more well known. History also decreed that it would be Lawson Wilkins who, from his background as a well known general pediatrician, would be the person who perceived the practical, as well as the theoretical value, of incorporating medical, psychological, and psychiatric studies in his pediatric endocrine clinic, at this time when the lives of female hermaphrodites could be completely transformed by a treatment which would arrest their extreme degree of body masculinization and allow them to develop feminine body functions for the first time.

He had developed a special working relationship with Dr. Joan G. Hampson, a young psychiatrist at Johns Hopkins. After my visit to his clinic, he saw an opportunity to establish a dual team, with me as a full-time member. So, assuming that he already had my agreement, he wrote the necessary fundraising letters and got the verbal agreement of John C. Whitehorn, the professor of psychiatry, for the establishment of a new research enterprise, which subsequently would become known as the psychohormonal unit.

For a short time, I had some difficulty in deciding whether to commit myself to the Johns Hopkins University, for I had already nearly committed myself to a junior faculty position at Bryn Mawr College. My uncertainty lay partly in the fact that the position at Bryn Mawr College was financially more secure. At Johns Hopkins, there would be the insecurity of depending on grants and their renewal. In addition, the department of psychiatry at the Johns Hopkins Medical School had been formerly virtually unknown to me, and seemed in some ways to be rather lack-luster. Moreover, I was still at that stage in my career of thinking in terms of what an institution had to offer me rather than of thinking more adventurously in terms of what I would be able to create if given the opportunity. It is one of my sayings regarding the laws of chance that there are people who look toward Hartford for insurance, and people who look toward the casinos at Las Vegas. I am not by inclination a gambler, but I have on occasion made big gambles with decisions pertaining to career. I had, for example, gambled on leaving New Zealand and on being accepted for graduate work at Harvard. So now, I decided to take another gamble—that of a career in research. Should it amount to nothing, then I would have to look elsewhere and start all over again.

Upon arrival at Johns Hopkins, I founded the office of psychohormonal research, of which I am still the director. With Howard W. Jones, Jr., Milton T. Edgerton, Claude J. Migeon, and others, I was in 1966 a founding member of the gender identity clinic, the first U.S. clinic to specialize in sex reassignment and transexualism. Later, I served for a year as chairman of its committee. In 1966, also with Migeon, assisted by Marco Rivarola, I founded the research program for the psychohormonal treatment of the paraphilias and sex-offender syndromes. In 1978, the program gained official status as a clinic in the department of psychiatry under Fred Berlin. I became a codirector of the clinic.

My gamble paid off, but, in a way, I have been gambling ever since, allowing security to take second or third place. Had I remained married, and had I had children, perhaps I would not have been able to maintain that attitude.

It was in September, 1951, that I came to Baltimore. I knew that I wanted to study not only the adrenogenital syndrome, but all the different types of hermaphroditism in order to discover all the principles of psychosexual differentiation and development that they would illuminate. I knew, also, that from the outset, I wanted to study the behavioral and psychologic correlates of all the other endocrine disorders of childhood and adolescence. I wanted to learn everything I could about the influence of hormones on behavior. I knew that many textbooks paid lip service to this influence, but that there was scarcely a paragraph of solid, reliable data. I was ready to gamble on trying to fill in the gaps.

Experiments of Nature versus Contrived Experiments

Some people are color blind, some have absolute pitch, some have a photographic memory, some have congenital absence of pain, and some undoubtedly have special gifts or talents in mental functioning that are not yet catalogued in psychology. For the most part, children and teenagers are left to discover their own talents and abilities, or perhaps to fail to do so in an educational and examination system that puts a premium on uniformity.

In childhood, the first formulated vocational ambition I had was for a career in music. Because it was the era of the Great Depression, and there were formidable obstacles to be overcome to finance music lessons and to buy a piano, as a high school student, I worked as a gardener on weekends, and used all the spare time I could find as a music student. By the time I was in my twenties and a student of psychology, I began to investigate my relative lack of success in comparison with that of other music students. I made some comparisons, and found that the accomplished musicians were able to memorize a musical score with a speed and durability of retention that was alien to me. I found that a pianist may not be able to write down a score from memory, but that given the key signature and the first bar, he could begin playing it, and then his finger memory or kinetic memory would take over. It was difficult for me to have to admit that, irrespective of effort, I could never achieve in music the goal that I wanted to set for myself. I would not even be a good amateur.

In 1943, I wrote a masters thesis on creative endeavor in musical composition. With the use of biographical and autobiographical quotations concerning creativity in musicians, I made an examination of the creative process. Using the information I found for self-reference, I was able eventually to reach some conclusions about myself. In particular, I found that I do not have an inventory memory, or as I sometimes call it, an encyclopedic memory. I do, however, have a good ability to formulate categories of relationship, and so I am able to keep a good indexing system. For example, I have an extensive bibliographic reference file, in which I keep a note of all the journal articles and books I read that carry information useful to my research or to possible future directions of research. In this way, I maximize what I have come to consider my chief intellectual asset, namely, an ability to put conceptual order into informational chaos, and an ability to relate concepts to one another to form systems or hierarchies of order. This type of ability needs constant, empirical monitoring, for without it, it can run wild into paranoid, delusional systems. Before the empirical checking is done, I have found that a new hypothesis or theory can be somewhat frightening, for there is no guarantee that it will not be considered crazy by other people, especially if it is unorthodox and against the current climate of one's discipline.

My interest in ordering things into a pattern and my enjoyment in doing so manifested itself early in my life, as early as the age of four to five years. My paternal grandmother, who died when I was young, is said to have remarked on the fact that as a toddler, I liked to arrange toys and blocks by shape or size, and always to pack them neatly away at the end of playing with them. Until I was five, we lived rurally, in the township of Morrinsville, in the Waikato region of the North Island of New Zealand. Household water was run off the roof and stored in a tank. The crossbeams of the tank stand became, for me, a kind of sculpture gallery on which I collected, because of their interesting shapes, worm casts of garden soil, and the casts of bird droppings tinted with the color of fruit and berries the birds had been eating. I was younger than five when we left this place of residence for Lower Hutt, in the metropolitan area of Wellington, the capital city.

I have continued to be a collector of artifacts, as well as of research data. One of my hobbies with art and artifacts is to relocate them, or to mount and display them, with materials or in a context for which they were not originally designed. In this way, an object can often acquire a new significance. A thought or concept can also undergo the same transformation by being taken out of its familiar context. A simple example, and an extraordinarily useful one, is to reverse a conventionally accepted statement of cause and effect. I frequently find myself toying with concepts, and working out potential hypotheses. It is like playing a game of science fiction. There is no better way of getting good, new hypotheses. The creation of new hypotheses is an art form. It is as much an art as the creative process in painting, music, drama, or literature. Only in applied science are hypotheses derived from stated propositions or laws. In original, or creative, science, new hypotheses are subject to a goodly amount of caprice as to whether they will be generated at all in the mind of the scientist. I have not heard of any graduate school that offers a course on creativity in science. Creativity is where science and art coalesce. It has been valuable to me in my work to have this understanding.

In my experience, it has been rare to encounter an individual who had a highly developed inventory memory, and along with it, a highly developed conceptual and theoretical creativity. Not having this joint ability in my own case has meant that I am not at home with numerals and numerical calculations. I am profoundly grateful for desk calculators, for I have experienced, also, the time when it was necessary to do all statistics by hand. Statistics interest me as problems in logic and the systematics of investigative design, not as exercises in applied mathematics. The applied statistics that I have needed to use in my research over the years are actually of the simplest type. That is because the problems I deal with in live, clinical research typically involve multivariate interaction. There are ethical restraints on how many variables one can manipulate in dealing with living human beings. These restraints, and the complexity of human behavior, make it all the more imperative to understand statistics as part of the logic of scientific methodology. I have been greatly interested in the logic of methodology and the philosophy of science. Especially in the earlier part of my career, I devoted considerable attention to these matters in four journal articles, culminating in the book, *The Psychologic Study of Man* (Charles C. Thomas, 1957). If I had not worked out my own philosophy of the study of behavior, as applied to clinical research, then I think my work would have come to a standstill. In order to develop a body of knowledge in psychoendocrinology and sexology, it was imperative for me to have a formulated set of principles and a basic theory on how to proceed. Ironically, other people have been interested only in the findings, and not in the theoretical principles that made it possible to collect data, systematize them and present them.

It goes without saying that I am not against the contrived experiment done at the bench, nor am I against the true-false or multiple choice opinion survey. It is rather that my inclination to collect things and arrange them in an orderly way according to original principles of classification, makes it more congenial for me to work with the so-called experiments of nature. Astronomy and archeology were the two sciences that interested me most as a high school student before I made my acquaintance with psychology. The only sport that ever claimed my wholehearted attention was mountain climbing. Intellectually, I am an explorer, rather than a constructor. I have a curiosity to find out what's there, where it came from, and where it goes. Thus, despite the countless daily irritations and frustrations, I really like the kind of clinical work I do in behavioral endocrinology, behavioral cytogenetics, and behavioral sexology.

Longitudinal Clinical Research

At Harvard, I did courses with people who had great names as founders of the department of social relations. I came strongly under the influence of Henry Murray, and the comprehensive case study method which he had developed. I used this method in the ten case studies of hermaphroditism presented in my dissertation. I learned more about the case study method from my initial contacts with Lawson Wilkins in Baltimore. The medical charts of his patients in the pediatric endocrine clinic were, in fact, longitudinal case studies. They were meticulously kept and often the findings were transformed into graphic representations showing changes over time. They were more systematic than anything I had yet encountered in psychology. They kept a better record of factual findings by clearly separating them from clinical impressions and prognostications. I could not borrow their format in toto for my work, but I became strongly influenced by their empircism and precision.

In those days, the mind-body problem was supposed to have been laid to rest, but of course it hadn't been. What had happened was that psychologists respectfully paid homage to the body, and then respectfully disregarded it. There was an excess of social environmental determinism, and an excess of psychic determinism. In more recent years, I have expressed my criticism by saying that psychologists and psychiatrists may as well be dealing with the astral body, so much do they neglect the corporeal body. The principle I prefer is one of conjoint action, or interaction; thus one may speak of interaction between mind and body, or between heredity and environment, or between hormones and behavior, and so on. Simple dualism is not enough, however. Interposed between the two terms must be the time factor, the critical period. Development cannot, in many instances, take place before the critical period has been reached. Afterwards, it is too late. Development that failed to take place at the appropriate critical period may be permanently impaired.

Another source of my misgivings about personality theory was the very core, I almost want to say the sacred core of this theory, namely, motivation. Eventually, I decided that I could live very well without motivation theory, without having to do any injustice whatsoever to the study of personality or the psychodynamics of behavior. It would not entail my becoming a mechanistic behaviorist. I took the position that the personality, or the ego, is a going concern long before I arrived on the scene to study it. It is like the solar system, kinetic or dynamic by definition. It is not necessary to put instincts, drives, needs, or urges into the personality. All that is necessary is to find relationships between different segments or samples of behavior, which entails the none too easy task of expediently segmenting behavior into what I have referred to as phylisms.

Motivation theory lends itself all too well to the perpetuation of a venerable tradition in clinical psychology, namely, to make predictions in the form of prophecies instead of actuarial probabilities. This tradition dates back to the astrologers of ancient Babylon and no doubt earlier than that. Its use is still widespread in general medicine. Clinical psychologists and psychiatrists are the worst offenders. There is scarcely a psychologic report written today in which predictions are not made in the form of prophecies instead of actuarial probabilities. Likewise, there is scarcely a psychologic report written in which the device of listing the differential diagnosis is resorted to. Prophecy is incompatible with the uncertainty implicit in a list of possible diagnoses, which need to be either ruled out or confirmed. Predictive prophesying seems to me to have been transmitted to us historically from phrenology and handwriting analysis through Rorschach inkblot analysis and other projective tests.

Predictions that are prophetic instead of actuarial probability statements must be stated rather imprecisely if the prophet is not to lose face by having been proved in error. Thus, in psychologic reports today, there is an excess of abstractions, abstruse references to states of being, the conditional and subjunctive mood of verbs, statements qualified with probable or possible, incorrect use of the present for the past tense, and use of the passive voice in order to evade personal commitment to an inference or opinion. There is a dearth of operational statements and definitions, and of saying things literally and empirically. The argot of psychology obfuscates the meaning.

I had an experience in writing my dissertation which left a deep impression on me with respect to psychologic writing. In 1951, I wrote to a gynecologist in England, Professor W.I.C. Morris of Manchester, for a follow-up report on an hermaphroditic baby girl. Her case was of great importance to me because she was one of only six known cases in which a daughter fetus had been masculinized because of an ovarian, or other masculinizing tumor in the mother during the pregnancy. The gynecologist replied by first apologizing that he could not provide me with a psychologic report of the sort he presumed I would need. Then, in short and simple sentences, he proceeded to describe, on the occasion of the girl's most recent check-up at age nine, her appearance, poise, manner, and conversation. She had a ragdoll. It wore winter clothing, which she had sewn onto it herself. This letter left me in no doubt about what I wanted to know. The child appeared socially as a girl and not as either a tomboy or a child wanting to be changed to a boy. A report of psychologic testing alone almost certainly would not have given me that information.

My resolve to avoid jargon talk was strengthened after I began to work in the pediatric endocrine clinic at Johns Hopkins. The pediatricians in the clinic made psychologic referrals because they knew they needed them. They wanted pragmatic reports that they could understand and that they could put to use in case management. There was nothing here of being tolerated or condescended to.

My resolve to use with pediatricians the same English language as they used with me did not need further strengthening, but it got it anyway at the APA annual meeting in 1952. At a crowded plenary session, half a dozen famous psychologists, each associated with a particular test, gave a blind interpretation of the results of that test administered to a man, always the same man, whom they knew only by age and sex. In reading their reports, the various psychologists made reference to dependency, anxiety, depression, paranoia and suicide. Not one, however, even posed a question as to the man's actual health status. They did not think in terms of a differential diagnosis, and they missed entirely the fact that the man quite literally was dying. The moderator of the panel supplied the information that he had had one lung surgically removed because of tuberculosis and, prior to the testing, had been told that his other lung was now affected.

That meeting had a pretty profound effect on me, requiring me to be more critical of psychologic tests and of what they could be expected to do. I was sure that I would never rely on test results alone, no matter how objective they claimed to be, but that I would always, in addition, talk to the patient. I would also look for corroborative or contradictory information from other informants, especially close relatives, and also from written records.

Over the years, I have formulated a system of tests and interview schedules to use in getting data for a case study. An example, suitably modified for use with transexual patients, is published in Chapter 6 of *Transexualism and Sex Reassignment* (Johns Hopkins Press, 1969). Interviews, or summaries of them made with the patient, are tape-recorded and transcribed so that verbatim authenticity is preserved.

When a particular patient's file is one of a sample that will be used for a published report, then all the information appropriate to the topics and sub-topics of that report is extracted from the typed pages onto specially prepared summary sheets. Two or three people check one another in making these summaries. The next stage is to prepare tables, numerically summarizing the findings for all the patients in the sample. As compared with the standard true-false or multiple choice checklist that is administered to a patient, this method puts the responsibility of making the true-false or multiple choice judgment or evaluation on the professional investigator. The raw data are more extensive than he will need, but they are on record. By contrast, when a patient takes an inventory or checklist test, no record is kept of the pertinent extra information he has, even though it would modify the way in which he actually answered the questions. To illustrate, it would be possible to ask a patient to check a list of questions regarding erotic dreaming. It is much safer, however, to have a tape-recorded interview of what he said in response to an inquiry on the topics of those questions and then, from the information given, to make the appropriate evaluations and mark the ratings oneself. By using a jury of two or three raters, it is then possible to get a higher degree of objectivity, as well as of validity and authenticity, than if the entire task of checking over the list was handed over to the patient himself.

There is a weakness in clinical research in medicine that relates to in-adequate specification of how the sample was drawn. All too often, only the number of cases in the sample is specified. There is no statement to indicate how biased the sample might be and for what reasons. Hospital recording often does not allow the relevant information to be readily retrieved. Without the necessary information, many otherwise perfectly good research studies cannot be undertaken.

In clinical research using small groups of rare patients, there is widespread misunderstanding as to what constitutes a control group. In the strict and proper sense, a control group is a random probability sample. Its size will depend on how many potentially significant variables can be identified and held constant. In most behavioral research, the size of a genuine, random probability sample for a control group is too unwieldy for the time, personnel, and finances available. Therefore, one relies instead on a matched contrast or comparison group. For example, a group of 20 men in clinical follow-up because of an extra Y chromosome can be matched with 20 men in clinical follow-up because of an extra X chromosome. The nature and specifications of the comparison group will depend on the variable under study.

So as to maintain a full-time commitment to longitudinal, outcome research, following children from birth to maturity, I strove for academic permanence. Thus, I have remained continuously at The Johns Hopkins Hospital and School of Medicine. I have been completely supported by grants from both the public and the private sector. My current research awards are from the National Institute of Child Health and Human Development (30th year) and from the William T. Grant Foundation.

In my research unit, we study syndromes as well as patients. The number of syndromes is limited according to the criterion that they must be endocrine, cytogenetic, or sexologic. Within these limitations, patients are seen and kept in follow-up regardless of diagnosis. At any one time, there are between five and ten research projects actively under way. Each is usually related to its own specific diagnosis, and may take from one to three years to complete for publication. Each diagnostic group is eventually surveyed, and some are surveyed a second or third time for new research projects. New and more precise techniques for hormone measurement and chromosome identification make new psychoendocrine, or psychocytogenetic studies possible. One may not even guess at what the possibilities might be a year or two years from now. Meantime, there are other subjects on the long-term schedule awaiting their turn.

The Spread of Knowledge

I have become internationally known for my work in both psychoendocrinology and the new and growing science of developmental sexology. In sexology, I am the person who, in 1955 (see Section II, below), first formulated and defined the concept of gender role, later expanded to include identity, as in gender-identity/role (G-I/R). I am by reputation an expert in gender science, research, and clinical care, ranging from neonatal sex assignment in cases of birth defect and ambiguity of the sex organs to the syndromes of erotosexual pathology in adulthood. My expertise covers also the theory of homosexuality, bisexuality, and heterosexuality. In 1961, I proposed the hypothesis that androgen is the libido hormone for both sexes (in *Sex and Internal Secretions,* W.C. Young, ed., Baltimore, Williams and Wilkins).

Not surprisingly, my research in sex attracts more public attention, and also more criticism, than does my research in the wider range of hormones and behavior in human beings. My sex research has related the differentiation and development of gender status to chromosomal genetics, prenatal hormones, postnatal sensory and social experience, juvenile sexual rehearsal play, and the hormones of puberty. Extending psychoendocrinology to include cognitive and intellectual development in many endocrine syndromes of infancy, childhood, and adolescence, I have done research also on learning disability and dyslexia. Examining the effects of child abuse on failure to develop, I have published definitive papers on the psychoendocrinology of the syndrome of abuse dwarfism, which is characterized by child abuse, hormonal insufficiency, statural dwarfism, mental retardation, and social immaturity, all of which are reversible by the simple expedient of early rescue from abuse and change of domicile.

I have always considered that the discovery of new knowledge is an obligation that all medical professionals owe to their patients, so as to avoid the perpetuation of ignorance and harmful treatment. In working on behalf of human beings, however, I have always held it an article of faith that research must be accompanied by the delivery of the best possible in health care—for me, psychological and sexological health care—regardless of people's ability to pay. Since, one way or another, the public pays for research, I have accepted the obligation to pay back this investment by telling the public what I have discovered. Therefore, I have extended my teaching to the public via the popular media, despite the contempt and attempted censorship of ultra-conservatives. I have testified as an expert witness in sex-offender and pornography trials and governmental commissions. I have also engaged actively in scholarly meetings at home and abroad and have published in many scientific and medical journals. In addition, I have followed a very active policy of training young people in research, on a person-to-person basis, and of rewarding their achievements by giving them the privilege of being first author when their research is published. Their greatest difficulty has been in learning the logic of scientific investigation and reporting, free from academic banality and platitude.

In 1969, I designed the first curriculum in sexual medicine for Johns Hopkins medical students, and taught the course until the curriculum was rescinded in 1984. In 1974, I designed a full semester course, Sexology, Biosocial and Human, in the Johns Hopkins Evening College. With assistant and guest lecturers participating, it attracted a large enrollment of undergraduate and graduate students annually until, with a change of administration in 1985, it was cancelled without explanation.

In the last few years, I have expanded my writing interest from the clinic to clinical history. I wrote about the 18th century origins and present consequences of antisexualism and degeneracy theory in *The Destroying Angel* (Prometheus, 1985). In its title, my most recent book presents the original concept, *Lovemaps* (Irvington, 1986). It examines the adverse effects of antisexualism on child development and the genesis of paraphilias.

The combined demands of research, clinical care, and teaching are magnified by the demands of fund-raising, writing and finding a publisher. They require as much dedication as does a monastic career. Sometimes I say, jokingly, that I left the religion of my childhood in New Zealand to become a missionary of psychoendocrinology and sexology in the United States. The sacrifices of monastic life, as some perceive them, are rewards for others. It has been my fate to experience a career in research and authorship as rewarding—which, perhaps, is in itself an accident of fate, upon which the existence of my research unit has depended.

Note

Most of this professional biography was dictated and transcribed in November, 1974, in response to a request made by Dr. James W. Kalat, Assistant Professor, Department of Psychology, Duke University. He was teaching a course in biological psychology by using role models, each of whom supplied statements and representative reprints. Publication plans did not materialize. Thus, my professional biography is here in print for the first time. It is supplemented with a few paragraphs recently written for a biographical listing of authors. [Bibliog. #9.3]

PART I
Research Theory and Design

ONE

Delusion, Belief, and Fact

Absolutist and Non-Absolutist Thinking

Human thinking has formulated the concept which, in the history of philosophy, has been called absolutism or idealism—the *a priori* acceptance of certain assertions or beliefs. Foremost among these are beliefs about the absolute existence of truth, good and right, beauty, and God.[1] The validity of these beliefs cannot be argued satisfactorily in the same way as can the validity of a scientific hypothesis.[2] They are products of thinking which cannot be related to the realm of non-thought. In this respect they are like the product of the thinking of the patient suffering from paranoia, which is promptly labelled a delusion. The problem therefore arises as to whether they are only delusions.

For some people they are little better than delusions,[3] but such a viewpoint cannot be discussed with the absolutists, whose final answer will be that they know because they believe. Like the paranoic their "voices have spoken." Such finality and conviction can be harmless so long as both sides can agree to differ, but becomes difficult when, for example, a politician with immense power behind him has a belief of such a destructive delusionary nature that it requires him to throw the world into a prolonged war. The homicidal impulses of one's neighbor likewise precipitate difficult situations. History has seen also such ugly episodes as the Inquisition and the hunt for witches carried out under the excuse—which we today look upon as delusionary—of an absolutist belief about the will of God.[4]

In the face of such situations, an indifference to such beliefs is impossible, or at least undesirable. Nor is the answer a thorough-going philosophy of relativism which gives license to every man for himself. That also ends in chaos. The problem is to avoid the dilemma of either complete absolutism or total relativism. The solution will require some place for beliefs or standards so that we can avoid the chaos of relativism, and yet at the same time avoid the dangers inherent in standards which, because of their absolutism, are static and unchangeable and at times pernicious.

A Psychological Viewpoint

The psychologist will bring to this problem his knowledge of human beings, their drives and motivations, and he will know that it is necessary to consider their need both for stability on the one hand, and change on the other. Thus he will see certain advantages in both absolutist and relativistic beliefs. Is it possible for him to find a way of combining the virtues of both?

In seeking an answer let us first consider the fact that a perfect pattern of personality adjustment for any single individual or group of individuals is a virtual impossibility. In the first place there are frustrations imposed by the physical environment, the healthy reaction to which is a certain amount of fear. Then there are frustrations imposed by the fact of man's being a social animal: he must give some consideration to the demands and needs of others without whom he cannot develop into full humanity. A possible alternative to growing up in human society is to be reared by wolves,[5] but even then one has to consider the other wolves; otherwise one could not exist even as a wolf-human. Finally there are other frustrations which are due to inefficiencies in the interpersonal relationships with other significant human beings amongst whom one has grown up and lived.[6] These latter frustrations are liable to breed abnormal fear and anxiety and to manifest themselves in patterns of behavior called neurotic,[7] the remedies for which are the concern of the psychotherapist and the social engineer whose techniques, however, are still young and not at all widespread. The fact is that mankind experiences frustration and resultant fear and anxiety, some of which is avoidable, and some not. But in order to deal with this, certain patterns of response have been developed. These patterns may be classified into three broad types:

1. Activities which, in general, do not interfere with interpersonal relations, but rather facilitate them, and which are based on man's capacity to be creative and are manifested in work and work-like activities, recreational activities, religious and humanitarian activities, or aesthetic and scientific activities.[8]

2. Psychosomatic responses which make a person appear physically incapacitated in some way. On the surface they seem to have no relation to interpersonal relations, but they do so in a disguised symbolic way.

3. Manifest disturbance of the capacity for interpersonal relations, traditionally called neuroses and psychoses. It is in this last group of responses that one finds the psychological process the end product of which is a delusionary belief. The patient accepts certain assertions, is convinced of their validity, and proceeds to elaborate further thought and action on them as a basis.

Amongst the first group one also finds people who accept certain assertions as valid with such conviction that they base all further thought and action on them. It is more difficult, however, to label these as delusions, and to leave it at that; for under the more dignified name of beliefs they are held by many people, and not by a single individual who is obviously mentally deranged. In the ultimate analysis they may be classified into four categories—beliefs about the existence and nature of: good and right—the domain of ethics; truth—the domain of logic and scientific method; beauty—the domain of aesthetics; and God—the domain of religion.

These beliefs, accepted as absolutes, have played a very important role in human history. They have been very useful tools which mankind has evolved to facilitate his continued psychosomatic existence. Let us look at them in more detail.

Beliefs about Good and Right

These are given primary place because ultimately they stem from our very existence as human beings.[9] In the final analysis they derive from the fact that man is neither a solitary nor an hermaphroditic animal. A new individual is conceived only when two individuals meet together. His growth until birth is impossible without the mother, and after birth he is again dependent on others for survival. Social development and maturity into full human stature, physical and psychological, are again dependent on human contacts, as, for instance, in the wolf children. Thus by his own biological necessities, man is obliged to be a social creature in order to be human at all. Such a necessity demands that there be some cooperation with at least a few other human beings. Hence arise problems about good and right. The necessity for such concepts or beliefs is an inevitable consequence of being human.

Beliefs about Truth

Thinking or cognitive awareness is a psychological activity which is unique amongst all human activities, for the very fact that one thinks is proof of the existence of thought. It is the one thing about the existence of which we can be certain. However, to be certain about the existence of thinking is of no help whatsoever concerning the existence of anything which is non-thought. There is a gap which can never be completely closed. The great difficulty which philosophers have always met has been how to relate thought or subjective experience to the things of the outside world which to common sense seem so obvious. In other words, it is the problem of determining when a belief becomes a fact. To meet the difficulty, some have postulated truth as an absolute or ideal, more ultimate and real than the things of the outside world. Actually the existence of truth is an assumption we all make; but an absolutist view of truth carries with it many corollaries, for example, the merging of the individual welfare into the welfare of the state. It is the aim of this paper to be able to find a way out of this dilemma; to be able to maintain the value and usefulness of the concept of truth—and the other three absolutes under discussion—without attributing to it all the qualities of an absolute.

Beliefs about Beauty

In the history of human thinking, beliefs about beauty and its standards have not been upheld with quite the same acrimonious dispute as have those about truth and morality. Perhaps this is partly because of the fact that men have felt that they do not matter so much. Then there have been many examples of the changeability of aesthetic standards—artists who lived and died in poverty because it was only a later generation which was psychologically prepared to appreciate their work. It is relatively easy to see the sociological factor in aesthetic standards: that to a large degree what is beautiful depends on the time and place of the person perceiving.[10]

Beliefs about God

That there is a sociological factor underlying beliefs about God has become increasingly clear since the Reformation, both in the increasing freedom as to whether one shall believe in God or not, and as to how one shall conceptualize and worship him. In spite of this freedom, however, there has been great bitterness between believers and non-believers, and believers of differing convictions. The psychologist should be able to look at the matter impartially. He has tended to lay himself open to the criticism that he has been concerned too much with debunking religion. It is necessary for him, however, especially if he is a therapist, to understand that religion plays an important function as a kind of safety valve in the lives of many people. To take it away and leave an emptiness is not wise.

It is now necessary to discuss the relation of these absolutist beliefs to scientific beliefs which are usually called hypotheses or facts. Are they essentially different and irreconcilable, or do they have something in common?

One thing which they have in common is that they are both products of the psychological process we call thinking. This process can be analysed for the sake of greater clarity. It progresses through several stages:[11]

1. The accumulation of experience, extending possibly over years, some of which will be relevant to one type of problem, some to another.

2. The presentation of a problem, either by oneself or some one else, for solution.

3. A seeking for the answer, which, if it is difficult to find, may cause frustration. Meanwhile there is a process of mental "incubation" probably involving mental activity beyond the level of awareness. Sometimes, of course, this stage is almost elided.

4. A sudden insight in which the answer is more or less dramatically and suddenly hit upon.

5. An attempted verification of the insight obtained.

A momentary reflection will show that scientific beliefs and absolutist beliefs have the first four stages, culminating in insight, in common.[12] The difference lies in the final stage, the degree to which verification is possible, a difference which is not so great as may at first appear, for in actuality all verification is a matter of agreement by convention. Scientific hypotheses can be convincingly verified because of the highly developed conventions upon which agreement is reached, namely, the observation, experiment and logical procedures of scientific method, the refined unequivocal symbol language adopted, and the use of measurement. Since the conventions of science are precisely defined and widely accepted, scientific hypotheses may be verified by different people and on different occasions, the same conclusion each time being reached. Personal prejudice and private meanings are excluded.

Not all scientific hypotheses are capable of immediate verification which in some cases has been delayed for want of a suitable intellect,[13] or of improved technical equipment. Further, the hypotheses in some fields of science are, at the present time, more easily verified than those in other fields. If they are accepted without having been convincingly and finally proved, it is because, like the verified hypotheses, they work well, allowing a certain orderliness amongst an otherwise chaotic miscellany of data, and facilitating further thinking and problem-solving. It is still agreement by convention which is the basis of their acceptance, in spite of the fact that they have not been adequately verified according to the strictly defined conventions of science.

Those absolutist beliefs, including the four discussed above, which are widely held and which have played an important part in the history of human thinking, are somewhat similiar to scientific hypotheses which are at the stage of being accepted, but not adequately proved. Here again it is agreed by convention that they be accepted because they work and because they are necessary in the solution of otherwise unresolvable problems.[14] For example, it appears necessary in the light of present day events, that a code for regulating social interaction be accepted by universal consensus of opinion, or, in other words, that it be sociologically validated.

There are some absolutist beliefs, the extreme opposites of scientific hypotheses, which are delusionary. They are purely private and often symbolic in meaning, quite incapable of verification by conventional agreement—the clearest and most exaggerated examples being those found in sufferers from paranoid schizophrenia.

The question now arises as to when a sociological validation is adequate.[15] Does it mean than any hypothesis is valid provided its originator can get a large enough crowd to follow him; and if so how large a crowd? Such a criterion is often actually used today. So long as the hypothesis or belief is not designed to injure the persons, property or beliefs of too many others, it is usually tolerated. But it is a different question when injury is involved, as was seen when the Nazi beliefs were translated into action. The following criterion is offered: an hypothesis, not scientifically verifiable, may be said to be sociologically validated, that is, by convention or agreement, when it appears necessary for the facilitation of continued human psychosomatic existence. This criterion is based on the welfare of the other fellow as well as oneself, a justifiable basis as it is an inevitable consequence of being human, as was pointed out above in discussing beliefs about good and right. Obviously there will be difficulties in deciding specific issues, but this is unavoidable. Indeed it is inherent in the problem of the necessity of agreement by convention.

Relevance of the Argument

Delusion, belief, and fact are not in different logical genera, but are species within the same genus, exhibiting many points of similarity. Any particular proposition, therefore, may quite easily be mistakenly identified according to species, as frequently happens when delusions are held as firm beliefs.

The issue of delusion versus valid belief is one which is of considerable importance in psychotherapy, for the therapist is instrumental in altering a patient's attempts to get control over his problems by such pathological solutions as delusionary beliefs, false interpretations of events or situations, and private meanings of words. They cannot, therefore, be taken away by a simple process of subtraction, but must be replaced. There are only two ways in which the replacement may be made: either the patient is left to the mercies of chance;[16] or he is given systematic guidance by the therapist to whom he will most certainly turn for aid.[17] A therapist should be capable of giving guidance to the patient in his reformulation of a philosophy of life, for all human beings need some such philosophy,[18] and if they are balked by the difficulty of working it out alone, they will accept a ready-made one.

Ready-made philosophies of life need not necessarily be inadequate, but the chances are that, within our cultural pattern at least, they will be, witness the frequency of personality maladjustment and widespread interpersonal and inter-group conflict. The therapist, therefore, is forced into the position of concept-ualizing a philosophy of life which will work better than the one under the strain of which his patient broke down. Fingerposts to such a philosophy have been outlined in this paper, allowing for variations according to time and place, but avoiding complete relativism by having certain fairly stable standards without, however, a rigid dogmatism.

When the psychotherapist aids his patients in the reformulation of a phi-losophy of life, he is not only facilitating the cure of the person, but is also contributing to a changed cultural pattern. Albeit unwittingly, he is becoming a social engineer, a role which it is perfectly fitting for him to adopt since break-downs in personality are the result of conflicting interpersonal demands.[19]

It is illogical, and in actual fact not possible, for a therapist to fit people only to return to the milieu which caused their breakdown. He who did so would be living in an ivory tower of unreality, a dwelling place, unfortunately, favored by many specialists. Such men, it is today commonly agreed, have a measure of responsibility in determining how their findings are used, in which task they also need a new philosophy of life. This paper offers a suitable basis on which to discuss the problems of truth, beauty, and goodness in relation to the question of social change—a question which needs the co-operation of specialists from all disciplines.

Summary

The end products of the psychological process of creative thought, whether they be private delusions, widely accepted beliefs, or scientifically validated facts, are not essentially different one from the other. Rather, they are due to differences in the degree of actual or possible validation of hypotheses. Some hypotheses about truth, good and right, beauty and God have in the past shown themselves to facilitate continued psychosomatic existence, and have had the quality of absolutes attributed to them. These would be better called axioms, accepted on the basis of conventional agreement, and able to change by conventional agreement. Thus would be satisfied the human psychological need for some degree of stability as well as for change. Philosophical stagnation would be avoided, and philosophy would not be at cross purposes with science.

References

1. For a brief exposition on this topic see C.E.M. Joad, *Guide to the Philosophy of Morals and Politics;* London, Victor Gollancz, Ltd., 1938; chapter 12.

2. See Roland Dalbiez, *Psychoanalytical Method and the Doctrine of Freud,* New York, Longmans, Green & Co., 1941, Vol. 2, pp. 1-18. His argument is that idealism postulates the identity of being and knowing. This being so, error at once becomes impossible. "In short," says Dalbiez, "idealism implies the negation of error; but this negation is contradictory; therefore idealism is contradictory" (p. 3). Idealism is still further an unsatisfactory philosophy because its identification of being and knowing makes "criticism of our own beliefs, systematic doubt, and the revision of our opinions impossible" (p. 3). In other words, there is no possibility of distinguishing between delusion, belief, and fact.

3. The pragmatism of John Dewey, for instance, is a rejection of idealism.

4. G. Zilborg and G. Henry, in *A History of Medical Psychology* (New York, W. W. Norton, 1941) give an outline of the history of witch-hunting after the fifteenth century. See especially chapter 6.

5. See Arnold Gesell, *Wolf Child and Human Child,* New York, Scientific Book Club, 1942.

6. See Harry Stack Sullivan's *Conceptions of Modern Psychiatry* (Washington, D.C., The William Alanson White Psychiatric Foundation, 1947) for an exposition of interpersonal factors in personality adjustment.

7. Karen Horney, *Neurotic Personality of Our Time* (New York, W. W. Norton, 1937) defines neurosis in terms of the presence of anxiety and guilt. See pp. 23-29.

8. Karl Menninger in *Love Against Hate* (New York, Harcourt Brace and Co., 1942) devotes several chapters to these activities.

9. Consider in this respect the important place given to ethics in the philosophy of Kant.

10. See L. L. Schücking, *Sociology of Literary Taste;* London, Kegan Paul, 1944.

11. This analysis of thinking was first made by John Dewey in *How We Think* (Boston, D. C. Heath and Co., 1910; revised edition 1933). It has been elaborated by Eliot Dole Hutchinson in Varieties of Insight in Humans, *Psychiatry* (1939) 2:323-332.

12. This viewpoint is taken by Eliot Dole Hutchinson in The Phenomenon of Insight in Relation to Religion, *Psychiatry* (1943) 6:347-357.

13. An example is provided by Freud in his short article, My Contact with Josef Popper-Lynkeus, *Internat. J. of Psychoanal.* (1942) 23:85-87 (also cited in *The Interpretation of Dreams*). In a short story, "Dreaming Is Like Waking," apparently a product of self-analysis, Popper points out that his unusual character had undistorted dreams because there was no conflict: "Order and harmony reign both in my thoughts and in my feelings, nor do the two struggle with each other. . . ." The interpretation of dreams for other people was difficult precisely because they were the disguised product of conflict: "In you other people there seems always to be something

that lies concealed in your dreams, something unchaste in a curious way, a certain secret quality in your being which it is hard to express." It is obvious as Freud points out that this insight of Popper is identical with Freud's own hypothesis concerning dreams. But it was of practically no scientific use as it stood, because it had not the degree of verification which Freud's had.

14. Of relevance here is J. N. Findlay's Morality by Convention, *Mind* (1944) 53: 142-169.

15. George W. Hartmann has offered some criteria for the determination of the validity of hypotheses which are value judgments in Pacificism in the Light of Value Theory, *J. Abnormal and Social Psychol.* (1941) 36:151-174. See particularly p. 165. "As a first approximation of greater 'accuracy' in our value-scales," he writes, "we may tentatively adhere to the basic criterion that a good which moves toward a universal involving all people as an upper limit is higher than one that approaches a particular as a lower limit. From this fundamental theorem, six corollary criteria may be derived:

1.) Inclusiveness—a value that affects *all* men rather than *some* is, other things being equal, superior;

2.) Permanence—a value that lasts is higher than an ephemeral one;

3.) Irrevocability—a value that is not replaceable or readily created by human effort is higher than one that can be produced easily;

4.) Congruency—a value that harmonizes with one's total pattern of beliefs is superior to one that is inconsistent with the entire structure of integrated behaviour;

5.) Cognitive completeness—a value that is based on full information and broad experience is higher than one resting on partial and fragmentary knowledge;

6.) Survival—a value that conduces to the maintenance of the individual or the human race is superior to one that leads to the extinction of either."

16. For example, Anna Freud writes, "At the end of the analysis of an adult, we do not force any patient to cure himself. What he will do with the new possibility open to him, depends upon himself. He may either return to the way of his neurosis, or, if the development of his ego permits, follow the opposite road, which leads to the full satisfaction of his inclinations, or even, if he can contrive to do so, follow the *via media,* i.e. make a syntheiss of the two potentialities within him." Quoted from Roland Dalbiez, p. 262 (reference footnote 2).

17. For a discussion of the problem of free will and determinism, which naturally presents itself here, see Robert P. Knight, Determinism, "Freedom," and Psychotherapy, *Psychiatry,* (1946) 9:251-262.

18. Andras Angyal in *Foundations for a Science of Personality* (New York, Commonwealth Fund, 1941) expresses this viewpoint. He says that the individual, having a tendency toward autonomy, is also "seeking to achieve a state in which he can experience himself as a part of super-individual units, most commonly reaching such a state in esthetic, ethical, social, and religious behaviour. The latter are individualized expressions of the trend toward homonomy. . . . The course of life is, in a way, comparable to a work of art which one creates, shapes, and perfects by living it. . . ."

19. The significance of conflict in determining personality maladjustment is elaborated by John Money, Basic Concepts in the Study of Personality, *Transactions and Proceedings of the Royal Society of New Zealand,* volume containing papers of the Sixth New Zealand Science Congress, 1947.

Note

Originally published in Psychiatry, 11: 33-38, 1948. [Bibliog. #2.1]

Author's Comment: Genesis of Exigency Theory

This, the first paper I wrote for publication, represented the fulfillment of an intellectual obligation, for it marked my scientific emancipation from the tightly sealed, evangelical religious dogma of my childhood and youth. The last sentence of the section on Beliefs about Good and Right contains the concept of "an inevitable consequence of being human." Six basic inevitables of being human were enumerated in the next paper I wrote (reference note 19) and which I read at the Sixth New Zealand Science Congress a few weeks before I left for the United States in 1947. In 1949, the same six inevitables were included in the second of my published papers, "Unanimity in the Social Sciences," which immediately follows in this volume. Reduced to five by telescoping the first two, the inevitables appeared, renamed, in a 1956 publication, "Mind-body Dualism and the Unity of Body-mind" [*Behavioral Science* 1:212-217]—a paper which became the first chapter of *The Psychologic Study of Man* [Springfield, Ill., Charles C. Thomas, 1957]. In their most recent reemergence the five inevitables appear, again renamed, in Chapter 9 of this volume.

Exigency theory represents a fundamental departure from each of the two competing philosophical premises on which most of contemporary psychologic theory is built, namely, teleology construed as motivation; and mechanistic determinism construed as behaviorism or behavior modification. Motivational explanations all too easily can be reduced to tautological exercises in semantics. Mechanism in the form of behaviorism is theoretically restricted to stimulus-response explanations. Exigency theory does not preclude either motivational or stimulus-response explanations, but it does not rely on either as all-encompassing. It brings system to the science of psychology not in terms of forces that drive us, nor in terms of how we perform, but in terms of the imperatives or inevitables that universally confront us as the exigencies of our being what we are. Exigency theory allows the issue of causality not to intrude prematurely into the very language used to describe and record phenomena, which is what motivational theory does do. At the same time, it does not presume a simplistic, reductionistic explanation, as behavioral theory does. Exigency theory is compatible with phenomenology and empiricism. It allows time for the meticulous hard work of science that is necessary to establish a causal relationship. It is particularly valuable in the present era of neuroscience when new and unexpected causal relationships between brain and behavior, mind and behavior, are being discovered.

TWO

Unanimity in the Social Sciences with Reference to Epistemology, Ontology, and Scientific Method

Semantic Confusion

Social scientists frequently assert that there is more unity than disunity amongst them and attribute the appearance of disunity to semantic difficulties. Since, however, they have not yet succeeded in elucidating and avoiding these semantic difficulties, confusion still exists. Even though intending to, social scientists are not always communicating undeniably within the same universe of discourse. Much of this semantic confusion derives from the fact that the epistemological and ontological assumptions are not made explicit. Any attempt to clear the confusion must resort, therefore, in the first place, to a consideration of these assumptions.

Epistemological Considerations

Throughout the ages philosophers have been interested in the problem of how man obtains knowledge and how that knowledge is related to so-called reality. Some have been primarily impressed by what seems to be the evidence of common sense, namely, that things have an existence independent of the mind which perceives them; while others have emphasized the indisputable role of the mind in organizing and interpreting the sensory impressions which it receives, claiming that nothing exists apart from the mind which perceives it. Some of the latter group even go so far as to postulate a concept of a universal mind which knows all and therefore is the ultimate reality. With philosophical speculation alone, it is impossible to decide the issue between these rival points of view which caused so much bitter controversy and incrimination in medieval philosophy when fundamental religious dogma was involved. But if the scientist is to work logically and systematically in his attack on problems, it is necessary to have the philosophical basis of his thinking explicit in his awareness. A suitable basis is provided by the concept that reality as recognized by mankind is a kind of social convention which men agree upon because their perceptual experiences have certain basic similarities. These similarities owe their existence, no doubt, to the fact that perception is mediated through the central nervous system which is more or less similar in all mankind. Thereby it permits people to act as if things have an existence independent of the mind perceiving them, and with certain intrinsic qualities of their own. For science-making, this epistemological viewpoint is one which, while being adequate, makes no ontological assumptions which occasion acrimonious and partisan controversy and disagreement. It recognizes both the "objective" and "subjective" factors in perception, stating them in such a way as to give priority to neither and as to avoid the pitfalls of both the absolutist and relativistic interpretations of the nature of reality.

Agreement by Convention

Essential to the epistemological viewpoint just presented is the concept of agreement by convention, which needs further elaboration. To require just agreement, without further qualification, leads obviously to the position that the majority can't be wrong. The procedure, operation, or convention whereby it is achieved is the crucial matter. Those perceptions with which the human central nervous system is particularly suited to deal, by reason of the specialization of the sense organs, seldom occasion much controversy and there is ready agreement in everyday experience. Thus, the majority agree that chairs are chairs and houses are houses. It is only after philosophical and reflective thinking that doubts rise. But when the phenomena of perception are not so readily mediated by the sensory nervous system, and so are not accessible to immediate sensory experience—as is the case in quantum physics and the biological and the social sciences, for example—then the problem concerning the nature of the reality of the phenomena immediately arises, for it appears in large measure to be a function of the perceiving organism. A way out of this quandary is provided by the theory of operationism which states that such phenomena can be described and defined only in terms of the operations whereby one becomes aware of them. Now, of course, one's awareness of the phenomena may have been in terms of operations which are not shared but are idiosyncratic, in which case the experience will be of a delusional character. Or, the operations may be shared, in which case the experience will be a belief. The experience may be called a fact only if the operations belong to the set of conventions which constitute scientific methodology. The distinguishing characteristic of scientific procedure, in comparison with that of delusional and belief experiences, is that it requires that all apparent perceptual phenomena, in order to achieve factual status, must be demonstrated according to methods which have been found serviceable for the basic scientific goal of problem-solving and the articulation of knowledge.[1] Because they have been found serviceable, these methods of procedure have been conventionally agreed upon, in the course of history, by scientists.

Discrete Entities

When a perceptual experience is one which is readily mediated by the central nervous system, there is in one's awareness knowledge of an apparently discrete entity about which protocol statements can be made. When, however, a perceptual experience is not readily mediated by the central nervous system so that the apparent perceptual stimulus does not enter one's awareness as a discrete entity, but must be defined operationally, then it enters one's awareness as a system of relationships among perceptual stimuli which do appear discrete and about which protocol statements can be made. In everyday language one might say that it is an abstraction derived obliquely, as it were, from more concrete perceptual experiences. The so-called facts of science are abstractions derived from protocol statements about perceptual experiences (observations). Abstractions, let it be emphasized again, are scientific and factual only if they are reached by means of the rigorous operations of science. Otherwise they remain hypotheses. An hypothesis may, of course, be very useful even though it cannot be, or has not yet been, completely demonstrated operationally. However, it should not be confused with a scientifically demonstrated abstraction. Either a scientifically established abstraction or an hypothesis may be used as the initial proposition of a system of deductive reasoning. If an hypothesis is so used, the system may be an organized delusion, more or less. If, however, the hypothesis is potentially scientifically demonstrable, then the system will be genuinely serviceable to science.

Contemporary social science includes instances in which systems of thinking are deduced from initial hypotheses which are assumed to be scientifically demonstrable. Such systems claim, as scientific facts, propositions which actually are derived hypotheses, tenable only if the initial hypothesis is potentially scientifically demonstrable. Clearer recognition of this situation would clear much of the confusion in contemporary social science.

Feed-Back Systems

If perceptual experiences appear to give one immediate knowledge of discrete items or entities, it is possible to follow the scientific procedures characteristic of classical physics and to formulate uniformities of variability in the language of cause and effect relationships. But when perceptual experiences are of the type which must be investigated obliquely and formulated, in operational terms, as relationships among perceptual experiences about which protocol statements can be made, then a different situation exists. There is now no clear differentiation in one's awareness between the "subjective" perceptual process, on the one hand, and the "objective" perceptual stimulus which can be formulated only as a system of cognitively apprehended relationships, on the other. Instead, there is a reciprocal interplay between stimuli and responses; or, as one might say, a *feed-back system* exists.[2] As the perceptual process progresses, the apparent stimulus affects the response, and the response affects what appears to be the stimulus.

If the totality of such an intrinsically dynamic feed-back process in time is to be dealt with scientifically, it is necessary that it be broken up into samples—amongst which the reciprocal relationships may be discovered—by means of procedures which provide one with perceptual experiences about which protocol statements can be made. The samples will be foci in the feed-back system, as it were, and will henceforth be called *operators.* Now, obviously, the choosing of operators may be arbitrary. Many different hypotheses as to what constitutes an operator and a set of operators may be proposed. Once again the test will be whether or not the hypothesis can be put to the test of the rigorous, conventionally accepted procedures of science. Once operators are determined in this way, then a feed-back system can become in itself a phenomenon of scientific investigation and can be treated *as if* it exists independently of the perceiving organism. Only in this way can complete solipsism be avoided.

Although operators are treated, within a given universe of discourse, as partially discrete variables, they may, within another universe or discourse, be analyzable into yet another feed-back system, and so on down a hierarchy of such systems. Within a given feed-back system, however, it will be in their *reciprocal interaction* that uniformities are sought. Because they are not isolated variables, traditional procedures for unidirectional, cause-and-effect variability will be out of place.

The problem of discovering adequate scientific procedures for dealing with feed-back systems is one of the frontier problems of contemporary science-making. It affects quantum physics, the biological and the social sciences. The task is to demonstrate the influence of contributing operators, preferably by directly demonstrating the intensity with which they contribute to the feed-back process; but if such precision is not possible to achieve, then an alternative approach is that of statistical generalization.

Feed-Back in Social Science

With regard to the phenomena studied by social science, it is often said that the "subjective" factors in the perceptual process are so dominant as to make communication and repetition of the experience difficult, if not impossible. Let us examine this statement more closely. In essence it is trying to say that the more or less contemporary operators in the perceptual feed-back process may be in interaction with other operators of much longer duration. The latter have been recalled as memories, a possibility which exists because of the human ability to store up experiences, conscious or unconscious, through the mediation of language or other symbol images. The activity of these memory or stored operators is not unique to the social sciences, but it seems to be especially significant for them. In general it may be said that the physical and biological sciences endeavor to find techniques of procedure which enable their influence to be standardized, and minimized. In some instances the social sciences may be similarly concerned; but in others memory operators are of major interest, witness life history studies; while in still others they must be taken into account simply because they cannot be standardized, as in the so-called effect of situational relativity.

Let us now turn to a detailed consideration of the implications of feedback in the three types of procedure from which the protocol statements of social science are made, taking first of all the method of hidden, or nonparticipant, observer and one subject. I shall omit meanwhile the possibility of a plurality of subjects which introduces additional factors of interpersonal interaction to be considered under type two. It is difficult to arrange the hidden observer technique so that the subject is quite oblivious to the fact that scientific observation is taking place, and at the same time so that behavior relevant to a particular problem, under circumstances which can be reproduced for other subjects and observers, can be elicited. However, the case is interesting because of the analogy with procedure in the physical and biological sciences: perceptual stimuli are demonstrably disparate from perceptual process, and there is no communication between stimulus and observer. The analogy with biology and quantum physics is closer than with classical physics, because the stimulus is in the nature of a process. It cannot be dealt with as a discrete, isolated, single variable. Thus, as has been pointed out in the previous argument, perceptually it will be experienced as a feed-back process, and the scientific task is to develop procedures for breaking up this feed-back process into operators amongst which the reciprocal relationships—that is, the feed-back relationships—can be determined. Success in this scientific task is as yet minimal in the social sciences.

Second, let us take the most usual situations in which the observations of social science are made, namely, participant observation, first of all with one subject. In this case everything which was said concerning nonparticipant observation continues to hold, with some complexities added. In nonparticipant observation, since the observer is hidden, his perceptual reactions do not become part of the perceptual awareness of the subject. But when each is aware of the other, then the manifest perceptual reactions of each one becomes part of the perceptual experience of the other, reciprocally, so that in the feed-back perceptual process of each one there are operators which would not be there except for the mutual interaction. There are also, of course, memory operators in the perceptual feed-back process of each person and, by and large, they will be different for each of them, depending on their respective interpersonal history. Thus, memory operators will influence the perceptual processes—including the manifest perceptual responses—of each person, and these in turn will influence the perceptual process and responses of the other, and so on reciprocally. One cannot, therefore, properly say simply that an observer is regarding a subject, but that he is regarding him in a specific interpersonal context of which he as observer is part. The role of the observer cannot be overlooked or disregarded. Rather, for scientific purposes, the attempt to estimate its influence as precisely as possible must be made. Either the observer's role can be standardized to a certain extent, or, perhaps in addition, he may be trained to be alert to his own reactions so as to take account of their significance. Insufficient attention has been given by social science in general to techniques for scientifically dealing with the role of the observer.

It remains to be added that when there are more than two people in interaction, the situation differs from a two-person interaction only in the complexity of feed-back interlinking, making either for greater diversity because of additional people, or perhaps for overlap and uniformities.

If two or more people in interaction are studied by the hidden-observer technique, then the remarks in this section are, of course, relevant in aiding the non-participant observer to formulate his perceptual experiences.

Third, let us take the case of self-observation, one which has occasioned much scientific controversy. Protocol statements arrived at through self-observation are peculiar to the social sciences, especially psychology. They are often considered as belonging to a completely different category from the hidden-observation type considered above, and frequently there is the derogatory implication that they refer to perceptual phenomena which are "intangible" and have at least a partial "subjective existence" in the "mind." In contrast, it is assumed that the "truly" scientific protocol statements deal with "tangible" phenomena which have an "objective existence" in the "outside" world. This dichotomy, so frequently encountered, rests on the ontological assumption, usually not made explicit, of the traditional sensationalist epistemology, namely, that reality exists *sui generis,* and that it is possible for human beings to have immediate knowledge of it. If one does not make this assumption, but follows the epistemological argument which leads to the concept of perceptual experience as a feed-back process, then it is evident that self-observation is not the only occasion on which perceptual experience is a feed-back process, witness quantum physics and the biological sciences. It is only a different manifestation of it and one in which—judging by the history of science—it is particularly difficult to develop scientific procedures whereby the process can be broken up into operators about which protocol statements can be made and among which reciprocal relationships can be discovered. One factor making for this difficulty is the need to take into consideration the memory or stored operators, mentioned above, which of course greatly increase the complexity of the feed-back process.

Having examined the main features of procedures in the social sciences, one is now able to say that, in spite of superficial evidence to the contrary, these procedures are not fundamentally dissimilar amongst themselves nor from the procedures of the physical and biological sciences. Apparent dissimiliarity can be traced to differences in the complexity of the feed-back systems with which they are involved.

It may be remarked in passing that more than one type of procedure may be used in connection with any given problem area, probably with great benefit. This point is developed at greater length in the section on individual and group.

Unanimity in Social Science

Contemporary social science uses chiefly the method of participant observation in one form or another, whether participation be limited or unrestricted, whether there be single or multiple observers and subjects, whether the subjects be represented directly or only indirectly through some recorded medium of communication, and so on. As pointed out above, when this method is used, protocol statements are, in the strictest sense, about interpersonal relationships, not about persons in isolation.

When the method of self-observation is used, it may appear at first glance that protocol statements are about a single person in isolation, but the influence of memory operators once again introduces interpersonal interaction, which none has completely escaped, man being a social animal. Of course, protocol statements may be of such a nature that the influence of interpersonal memory operators is minimal, but such statements would not be indisputably within the realm of social science.

When the method of nonparticipant observer and only one subject is employed, it is again possible for protocol statements to be of such a nature that interpersonal influences are minimal; for contemporary interpersonal interaction is eliminated if there has been absolutely no communication with the subject, not even indirectly. Further, there is the possibility of developing techniques to minimize or standardize the influence of interpersonal memory operators in the perceptual feed-back processes of the observer; and, finally, it is possible that the subject will manifest no indications of the influence of interpersonal memory operators in his own feed-back processes. However, it is unlikely that all of these conditions would be fulfilled concurrently in a situation indisputably within the realm of social science.

Whatever the procedure employed, then, in situations indisputably within the realm of social science, interpersonal interaction, and not isolated individuals or some such entity as group behavior, will be the process under investigation. In this respect the social sciences are all working within the same universe of discourse, even though in different corners of it. All protocol statements, since interpersonal interaction is a feed-back system, will be about operators in that system.[3] All other scientific propositions will be abstractions derived from such protocol statements. In the ultimate analysis, therefore, the conceptual framework of each of the different branches of social science is built up from protocol statement which are qualitatively similar. From these protocol statements generalized propositions are derived, and from these propositions further second-order generalizations, and so on through the hierarchy of generalization. If any generalized proposition is to be operationally demonstrated, it must be traceable to the ultimate protocol statements from which it may be derived according to the procedures of science. Any generalized proposition which cannot be so traced and demonstrated is in the nature of an hypothesis which may or may not be demonstrable in the near or distant future; and all other propositions hierarchically articulated with it are hypotheses which can be demonstrated only on the condition that the initial hypothesis can be demonstrated. In social science an hypothesis which has not been demonstrated is given sometimes as a demonstrated proposition, and an entire conceptual system built upon it. If the initial hypothesis is incapable of being demonstrated, or if it may be demonstrated only after making allowances and limitations, then the system is not a scientific but a belief system, in the form in which it is presented. For example, social scientists may imply that social phenomena have an existence *sui generis,* and proceed on the basis of this assumption by implication to construct a logically consistent, well-articulated conceptual scheme. Further analysis of the assumption, however, reveals that it is actually an undemonstrated hypothesis, not a demonstrable proposition nor a protocol statement about perceptual experiences; for, as I pointed out above, all protocol statements about social phenomena are about interpersonal interaction.

From what has been said it follows that there should be complete unanimity amongst social scientists whenever they make protocol statements. Similarly, there should be unanimity whenever they present demonstrable, generalized propositions derived from these statements, but not of course when they formulate possible hypotheses. It is not denied that workers in the different branches of social science will, by reason of their specialization, be more interested in some statements and propositions than others. But whenever areas of specialization overlap, the language should invariably be shared in common.

With so much emphasis on a single universe of discourse for the various branches of social science it is not intended to deny that for each one there may sometimes be different universes of discourse, in which case its protocol statements will not be about interpersonal interaction. This is what happens, for instance, when consideration is given to physiology by psychologists, to material artifacts and physiological traits by anthropologists, and to problems of ecology and demography—in which individuals are treated as units-human—by sociologists. Yet, even in these instances, propositions derived from protocol statements may lead back to interpersonal interaction.

Individual and Group

It may easily appear in social science that individual and group are two distinct genera, and that their scientific study requires different methods which, although having something in common, are fundamentally disparate. Or, it may be said that the phenomena are the same, but are approached from different levels of abstraction. Such viewpoints do not expedite unanimity in the social sciences, so let us examine the relationship between individual and group more fully.

Let us commence our examination by recalling that I have pointed out that if perceptual experience is conceptualized as a feed-back system, it is possible to avoid the epistemological and ontological difficulties which are established by the acceptance of a dichotomy between perceptual stimulus and perceptual process, between "outside" and "inside." I have pointed out also that social science is interested in discovering uniformities in the reciprocal interaction of operators, including memory operators, in feed-back systems which always incorporate interpersonal interaction as a subsidiary, if not the chief, feature of concern.

Now, the phenomena of interpersonal interaction may be viewed from two different vantage points, as it were, depending partly on one's chief interest and partly on the procedure employed.

In the first case, the focus of interest is a single individual. More or less contemporary interpersonal interaction will be viewed from his point of view, and ordinarily there will be only the observer and this subject in the scientific situation; or possibly it may be a case of self-observation. As far as other interpersonal influences are relevant, they will be mediated by memory operators which will play a very important role, because the current situation will not be of exclusive interest. After the initial step of making protocol statements, the scientist will be concerned with finding uniformities of feed-back phenomena viewed with the focus of interest on a single individual. One might say that he is interested in discovering patterns which emerge from a study of an individual's cumulative experience over a period of time, say a life history. Going one step further, he may also be interested in the interrelationships amongst these patterns, and their reciprocal interaction and change over a period of time.

In the second case, the focus of interest is the interpersonal interaction of a group of individuals, and the method will usually be that of participant observation. As in the case of the individual approach, the observer's perceptual experience and protocol statements concern an individual in interaction with other individuals. The difference is that all the individuals are interacting contemporaneously and reciprocally. The emphasis will, therefore, be on current, not memory operators in the feed-back systems of interaction. Sometimes it may be necessary to focus on memory operators in order to understand the current situation, and sometimes, indeed, it may be necessary to apply the individual approach to each person participating in order to understand better their interaction as a group. On the whole, however, the observer's orientation is toward the current situation, because his interest, when he passes beyond the stage of making protocol statements, is in finding uniformities in the reciprocal interaction of each individual with the others, regardless of the idiosyncrasies of the several individuals. One might say that he is interested in discovering patterns which emerge from a study of current interpersonal interaction. Going one step further, he may also be interested in the inter-relationships amongst these patterns, and their reciprocal interaction and change over a period of time.

In comparing these two approaches, one should note that in both instances, protocol statements are about interpersonal interaction; but, in the individual approach, the operators in the feed-back process are frequently mediated by memory; whereas in the group approach they are contemporary. The next step in science-making is that of formulating generalizations. In the individual approach the first stage in generalization is the formulation of propositions relating to uniformities in the feed-back relationships of memory and current operators; whereas in the group approach the first stage in generalization is the formulation of propositions relating to uniformities in the feed-back relationships of current operators alone. But, since both current and memory operators pertain to interpersonal feed-back systems, there is no clear disparity between the first-step propositions formulated in these two approaches.

The third step in science-making is the formulation of second stage generalizations, namely, uniformities concerning the inter-relationship of first stage propositions. Thus, in the individual approach these uniformities will appear as recurrent patterns typical of the individual. In the group approach they will appear as recurrent patterns typical of the group. These patterns may or may not be disparate. In some instances an individual pattern may be idiosyncratic, whereas in others it may be regularly shared by an entire group of individuals. The patterns arrived at, through either approach, by further stages of generalization may also be either disparate or correlative, it being a matter of much importance in the interest of scientific clarity to determine which.

It follows that the individual and group approaches are neither completely disparate nor completely complementary. Especially as far as the most generalized propositions are concerned, the problem contexts may be quite disparate; but there are some contexts in which the propositions may be exactly complementary, the one being, point for point, the counterpart of the other. Thus, for some problems either of the two approaches may be equally suitable. For example, a given hypothesis, that certain aspects of interpersonal interaction (the operators) are a feed-back process which has certain recognizable, distinguishing characteristics, may be tested in either of two ways. First, one may use a cross-cultural survey, testing the hypothesis by comparing an adequately selected sample of groups. In each group in which it is possible to demonstrate the operators—if the hypothesis holds—there should also be the feed-back process with its distinguishing characeristics.[4] Second, one may use a comparative case history index, testing the hypothesis by comparing an adequately selected sample of individuals. Once again, if the hypothesis holds, in each individual in which it is possible to demonstrate the operators, there should also be the feed-back process with its distinguishing characteristics.

Operators in Interpersonal Feed-Back

Whatever approach an investigator uses, he is, in the last analysis, dealing with a feed-back system of interpersonal interaction in so far as he is in the realm of social science. Confronted with such a feed-back system, he will be immobilized, as far as scientific investigation is concerned, unless it is possible to demonstrate some foci of reference, that is, some operators. It is to this problem that I now turn, in the attempt to provide a frame of reference which will be a common denominator, as it were, for the study of interpersonal interaction. First, let me review some considerations relevant to all feed-back systems.

Since the operators of a feed-back system are not experienced in perceptual awareness as more or less discrete entities, they are in the nature of generalizations from perceptual experiences about which protocol statements can be made. Thus, the operator in a feed-back system is a proposition which is demonstrated either fully, partially, or not at all. It is highly probable that a single operator can itself, under certain circumstances, be conceputalized as a feed-back system. Thus, sexual role is considered an operator in the interpersonal feed-back system, but with a change to the physiological and biochemical universe of discourse, then sexual role itself becomes a feed-back system.

Just as each operator is initially an hypothesis which must be demonstrated, so also the implicit proposition that a given feed-back system can be broken up into a given set of operators is initially an hypothesis which must be demonstrated scientifically.

Now let us turn to the analysis of interpersonal feed-back systems about to be presented. Each of the six operators is a proposition which can be demonstrated from perceptual experiences about which protocol statements can be made. The implicit proposition that interpersonal interaction can be adequately analysed in terms of these six operators is an hypothesis which is believed demonstrable, but which will be demonstrated only as it is put to the test on different types of research problem. It should be a useful frame of reference for investigating the dynamics of personality in clinical psychological problems, for formulating the dynamics of cultural patterns, and for understanding the dynamics of the various types of cultural and social change. In fact, its tentative applications in these areas have already indicated its value.

The six operators proposed are inevitables of being human, and they are considered the focus point around which interpersonal processes take place. It is believed that they are as disparate as it is possible for operators in a feed-back system to be, but the subsidiary focus points, presented as corollaries, already reflect feed-back relationships between the six operators.

At first glance the six operators and their subsidiaries may appear to be arbitrarily selected from incomparable logical categories, to be a fortuitous assemblage of primary and derived motivations and their respective stimuli and responses. However, they cohere in so far as they are all inevitables of being human and, since they are conceived as the foci of interpersonal interaction, they permit a methodological escape from the dilemma posed by making a dichotomy of motivation and behavior.

The Inevitables

Aggregation

A minimum of human aggregation is inevitable if human beings exist at all, because the conception and birth of a baby is preceded by the meeting together of two people. Once born, the human baby cannot survive without being fed by someone else, being tended in connection with elimination, and receiving sufficient tactile and kinaesthetic stimulation as an aid to efficient respiratory and circulatory functioning. Other situations than child care also tend to favor aggregation.

Corollaries. Although it is conceivable that at a later age the human organism can exist completely isolated from all members of the species, the initial compulsory social experience seems to leave an indelible imprint, so that loneliness or its possibility is threatening.

Since the inevitability of man's social role is closely associated with the birth and biological helplessness of the human infant, the group concerned with child rearing, usually the family, has a special position in the total pattern of culture. Birth and sex order of siblings and the generation difference between parents and children are also significant factors.

Since social life is essential to existence, and since the process of social participation is not unlearned, as appears to be the case with the ants, termites, and bees, human beings must work out some conventions about living together. These conventions become accepted as regulatory patterns of behavior—sometimes called institutions—which tend to change but slowly. They usually become associated with differentiation of function and superiority-inferiority relationships amongst individuals.

Since the process of social participation is for the most part learned, the conventions about living together must be transmitted to new participants.

Autonomy

The process of growth and development may be viewed as the progressive acquisition of autonomy, based on the human capacity to learn, which, although general, apparently varies in intensity from individual to individual.

Corollaries. Each individual must learn some degree of control of his neuro-muscular system in various types of motor activity, some of which, like work, appear as unambiguously purposeful, while others, such as some forms of play, appear expressive and of intrinsic value in their own right.

Each individual must exercise his ability to manipulate symbols in speaking and thinking, without which he cannot come to terms with certain types of problem.

Because of his ability to use symbols and thus remember experiences, some significant life experiences will, either wittingly or unconsciously, have permanent or long-lasting effects on an individual. The most frequently encountered indication of unconscious content, dreaming, appears to be universal. Unconscious content may be symbolically manifested in other ways, as in sublimatory and creative activity; and in the symptoms of neurotic or psychotic quality. In such cases, as in dreams, the so-called unconscious mechanisms of condensation, displacement, and dramatization are at work.

Role as Male or Female

With the exception of a few hermaphrodites, human beings are suited by reason of their genital physiology for either the male or the female role in the process of reproduction.

Corollaries. Men and women, because of the different reproductive role, are differentially suited to the roles connected with subsistence, at least during the period when a woman is bearing children.

In the course of growing up, males and females must learn to integrate their genital roles with their more general masculine or feminine roles if they are to be reproductively useful.

The woman's role in reproduction and infant care and nurture brings a baby into closer tactile and kinaesthetic contact with her than with a man, for the earliest part of its socialization.

Body Metabolism

Some of the physiological requirements associated with metabolic processes are self-regulatory, but some require witting, purposive activity on the part of the individual, in varying degrees. They include: hunger, thirst, oxygen and carbon dioxide balance, mineral balance, temperature control, humidity control, elimination, and sleep.

Corollary. Existence is not possible without the ability to come to terms with the nonpersonal environment whether it be geographical, geological, climatic, botanical, zoological, or in the form of other regular or unpredictable natural phenomena. In particular, food, shelter, and usually clothing are necessary.

Bodily Features

Human beings have bodily characteristics such as height, weight, skin color, age, organ inferiorities and the effects of disease, by reason of which individuals may either resemble or differ from those amongst whom they exist.

Corollary. In the same way that some of an individual's activities are affected by his bodily features, so the activities of the human race are limited by human biology. Although the limit of man's achievements is not known, the implications of such a limitation are an interesting speculation.

Injury, Disease, and Death

Human beings are capable of being injured either physically or psychically, by either the nonpersonal environment or other human beings. They are also capable of suffering disease, and finally they die.

Corollaries. Actual or threatened injury or disease, and the anticipation of death, may be accompanied by a variety of reactions involving the psyche and the soma in varying degrees, in which unconscious factors may play a prominent role. In the most general sense, these reactions may be called fear and aggression and their derivatives.

Contemplation of death and an attempt to come to terms with the sources of threatening injury or disease are associated with mankind's general attempt to come to terms with imponderables as in myth, magic, religion, philosophy, ideology, and science. The resulting delusions, beliefs, or facts may continue to exist after the individuals who formulated them, and to influence other human beings, by means of man's use of symbols.

The language of a group may embody certain features of vocabulary and syntax—probably as a function of cultural history—which predispose its users to contemplate the universe in a particular fashion.

Summary

When an apparent perceptual stimulus is not experienced in awareness as a discrete, isolated entity, it is not possible to make protocol statements about it. It can be dealt with only by conceptualizing the perceptual process as a feed-back system of interaction between the apparent stimulus, on the one hand, and awareness of perceptual experience, on the other. But, since no protocol statements can be made about a feed-back system as such, it becomes necessary to break it up into operators which reciprocally interact. Complete arbitrariness in the selection of operators is avoided if one follows the conventionally accepted procedures of science when making observations—and correlative protocol statements—from which the operators are derived as abstractions. By so doing solipsism can be avoided and a feed-back system treated *as if* independent of the perceiving organism.

Whether one uses the method of non-participant observation, participant observation, or self-observation, the phenomena which are indisputably in the realm of social science are interpersonal feed-back processes in which there may be either current or memory operators. The problem of demonstrating a significant set of operators for such a feed-back system is one which has not yet been solved. The set of inevitables is put forward as an hypothesis.

References

1. For further treatment of ths topic see Felix Kaufmann, *Methodology of the Social Sciences;* New York, Oxford University Press, 1944; especially chapters 4 and 5.

2. See Norbert Wiener, "Cybernetics," *Scientific American* (1948) 36:536-544.

3. Protocol statements in social science are most commonly about communications, direct or indirect, as in speech, writing, or other symbolic form; and about bodily activity, neuro-muscular, as in gesture, and neuro-glandular. Other foci of protocol statements are suggested later in the article.

4. For an example of the cross cultural approach see D. Horton, "The Functions of Alcohol in Primitive Societies," in *Personality in Nature, Society, and Culture* [C. Kluckhohn and H. A. Murray (eds.); New York, Alfred A. Knopf, 1948; pp. 540-550]. There are no analogous studies with large scale comparisons of case history material, no doubt because there is no comparative index like the Cross Cultural Survey.

Note

Originally published in *Psychiatry*, 12:211–221, 1949. [Bibliog. #2.2]

THREE

Observations Concerning the Clinical Method of Research, Ego Theory, and Psychopathology

Introduction: Clinical Procedure and Research

The scientist who follows the rigorous methods and procedures of science implicitly makes certain axiomatic philosophical assumptions. Among them is the belief, accepted as a kind of credo, that the traditionally defined methods and procedures of science will not fail him in his attempt to find answers to the problems to which he devotes himself. Second is the belief that these problems are worth solving; that in some way, direct or indirect, their solution will benefit the whole or a section of mankind. Third is the belief that the above two beliefs can be telescoped: the traditionally defined method of science will permit the solving of worth-while problems. The assumption of this last belief is obscured by the fact that the most rigorous of the sciences, the physical sciences, have reached such a state of development that the pursuit of pure science, with no apparent concern for the immediate utility or applicability of discoveries, is feasible. Historically, however, the search for solutions to problems of immediate practical importance was antecedent to the appearance of pure science.

In the present day there are still many challenging problems which have not yielded to attack by the rigorous scientific method. Many of the research problems in psychology and the social disciplines belong in this category. It is a matter of opinion as to whether these problems should be approached patiently with exclusive use of the rigorous scientific method, or whether the approach should be as scientific as possible without too much emphasis on a scientifically precise and rigorous procedure. The two approaches are not mutually exclusive, although it is a common misunderstanding that they are.

Although the advocate of the rigorous approach in psychology and the social disciplines may have difficulty in finding problems which will yield to his method so that findings will not be obtuse, equivocal, or trivial, once he succeeds in finding such problems, he will have no difficulty in evaluating his results. He evaluates and defines them operationally, which is possible by virtue of the fact that he has adhered to a method or series of operations which has been agreed upon by convention. The advocate of the less rigorous method will, without search, be confronted by problems to which he would like to find a solution. His difficulty will lie in the evalution and definition of his findings, since an operational definition, like the operation whereby it was arrived at, is open to question. At best he can evaluate his findings against his empirical success in solving the problem by which he was initially confronted. To do so involves a logical tautology which will best be exposed by an examination of the implicit beliefs assumed by this type of investigator who, in actual fact, is most usually working in the applied field, for example, in the clinical field in psychiatry and psychology. First, he accepts the belief that the traditionally defined method of science will guide and direct him—while not being his exclusive method of procedure—in his attempt to solve the problems to which he devotes himself. Second, he also believes, like the rigorous scientist, that these problems are worth solving; that in some way or another their solution will benefit all or a section of mankind. At this point comes the dilemma, for, unlike the rigorous scientist, he cannot telescope his two beliefs. He cannot accept implicitly the belief that the method he uses guarantees, *ipso facto,* the value of his findings and theories. He is caught in a tautology: his procedures and the findings and theories derived from them are evaluated according to their empirical success; there must, therefore, be some criterion whereby to evaluate empirical success. It becomes imperative to establish some standards of evaluation, appraisal, and assessment. In practice such standards are used, albeit in a rule-of-thumb way, without explicit formulation. For example, the clinician dealing with personality assesses a given mode of personality functioning as likely to lead to serious pathology and recommends treatment with the prediction of producing another mode of functioning which is considered more efficient. It is only by making such predictive assertions, which are essentially value judgments, that the investigator can advance his discipline toward greater precison and predictive potentiality. The need is for a greater refinement of the assessment and appraisal of values on an empirical basis, along with a greater refinement of empirical analysis of concepts. These standards of value are the counterpart of the units of measurement in rigorous scientific method, the precision of which they may conceivably approach eventually. The important thing is that they are the appropriate standards with which to appraise the phenomena comprising the problems which the discipline sets itself to solve. It is a contemporary fashion to avoid such appraisal, or at best to use only the standards of statistical normality or typicalness, a procedure which is open to question. It is questionable because statistical procedure is vindicated when the measures of central tendency and dispersion are obtained from a sample which is randomly selected from a theoretically infinite population. The samples investigated by psychology and the social disciplines rarely satisfy this condition, for, since they often manifest feed-back interaction, their characteristics and processes are specific to a given occasion and may be quite changed after an interval. Under such circumstances a sample becomes a finite population specific to the occasion, and not a random selection from an infinite population.

Measurement and enumeration are the methods of assessment in rigorous science. In the less rigorous psychological and social disciplines, measurement is rarely possible. Somewhat more frequently enumeration, and subsequent statistical evaluation, are applicable. On many occasions, however, two other principles of assessment and appraisal are appropriate. They are the principles of saliency and of convergence of indices.[1] According to the type of problem and the technique used, the indices will vary, being established empirically in each case. Of a different order, and more open to the criticism of solipsistic usage, is the principle of similarity, used in the psychological interpretation of symbols as substitutes and disguises for other images and concepts. Actually, use of this principle is a short-cut method of arriving at a hypothesis which may be more fully corroborated according to the principles of enumeration (frequency), saliency, and convergence.

Implications of the Repetition Compulsion

The foregoing introduction serves as a warrant for the theoretical considerations, based on clinical observations, which follow.

It is possible empirically to differentiate the manifestations of psychopathology into two types on the basis of onset. The first type is etiologically associated with a more or less discrete event which may or may not remain within awareness. The so-called traumatic neuroses of war—precipitated suddenly and dramatically by a specific disaster overtaking a person who was otherwise withstanding the stresses and strains of warfare without incapacitating symptoms—are a good example.[2] The second type is related etiologically with what the person experienced as a sequence of diffuse relationships between equivocal meanings and his reactions to them. Since these relationships are cognitively unstructured, ordinarily originate in childhood, and are cumulative, they do not remain clearly within awareness. A large proportion of therapeutic practice is with cases of this type.

Each of these types poses distinctive problems in the formulation of a theory of psychopathology, and it has not proved easy to accommodate them both within a single theoretical scheme. In the revisions of Freudian theory, for example, one observes the effects of the attempt to do so.

Freud's initial work with hypnosis and conversion hysteria revealed the importance of events no longer within awareness in the formation of specific symptoms, albeit not of the entire syndrome. Accordingly he formulated a theory in terms of psychical traumas, blockage of discharge, catharsis, and abreaction.[3] Dissatisfied with the hypnotic method as removing only symptoms without having therapeutic effect on the entire syndrome, Freud turned to the method of free association which, along with the study of dreams and parapraxes, revealed the second type of etiology. A revision of theory accompanied the increase in empirical experience and was formulated in terms of wish-fulfilment and the pleasure principle; instinct, libido, and the Oedipus complex; repression and the ego. The nice polarity of this theory was disturbed by the application of the libido theory to the repressing ego, namely, in the concept of narcissistic libido and in connection with the narcissistic disorders, dementia praecox, paranoia, and melancholia.

The most radical theoretical revision, however, was occasioned by a consideration of a phenomenon of the traumatic neuroses of war, namely, the reproduction and re-enactment in hallucinatory or dream imagery of the original traumatic event. "In the light of such observations," wrote Freud, "we may venture to make the assumption that there really exists in psychic life a repetition compulsion, which goes beyond the pleasure principle . . . which is displaced by it."[4] The repetition compulsion is said to come into action when the individual experiences fright, that is, when danger is encountered without warning and preparation, and when the psychic apparatus becomes flooded by external excitations which become strong enough to break through the protective barrier which screens and protects against stimuli.

It is of considerable significance, in connection with the theory of neurosis, to note that, although the pleasure principle was subordinated to the repetition compulsion in the revised theory, Freud at that time considered that it was "only in rare cases that one could recognize the latter in pure form without the cooperation of other motives."[5] This viewpoint was reiterated six years later in *The Problem of Anxiety* where he expresses much more doubt than he had previously concerning the role of external danger in the etiology of the traumatic neuroses of war. "It is very improbable,' he states, "that a neurosis should come about only by reason of the objective fact of exposure to danger without the participation of the deeper unconscious strata of the mental appartus."[6] These deeper strata are described as being essentially libidinal. In other words, instinctual dangers, especially those which are libidinal in nature, are considered more salient than external dangers in the etiology of symptoms. The significance of this conclusion will become clearer in the discussion of aggression and instinct, below.

Although the pleasure principle and the repetition compulsion are comparable in relation to some of their characteristics, they are not strictly speaking cognate concepts. Thus the repetition compulsion may be brought into action by excessive intensity of external excitation, it is a sensory motor defensive reaction closely allied to aggressive mastery and destructiveness, and it bears a special relationship to ego functioning. The pleasure principle, on the other hand, is a function of intrapsychic impulses which are considered instinctual and independent of external excitation, is postulated as a regulatory mode or principle characteristic of the instincts, especially the libido, and bears a special relationship to the id. It is evident that the disparateness of the two concepts may be reduced to three features: the nature of aggression, the concept of instinct, and the function of the ego, all three of which have been the points of departure for dissenters from Freudian doctrine and for modification of the doctrine within the ranks of orthodoxy. Freud attempted to obviate the disparateness with the hypothesis of the death instinct; but in doing so he changed his conception of instinct and raised some questions concerning the nature of aggression and the functions of the ego. The problem of aggression will be taken up first.

Aggression

In his early writings Freud broached the topic of aggression in connection with libidinal sadism, but the concept was theoretically subordinate to libido.[7] Later, in discussing the vicissitudes of instinct, he considered the relationship between love and hate, coming to the conclusion that hate was to be regarded as a nonlibidinal reaction of the ego. Although hatred is not synonymous with aggression, the one implies the other; yet still only a subsidiary role was given to aggressiveness and destructiveness. Their role became more ill-defined as the theoretical scheme was revised and refined with the differentiation of ego, id, and superego. Since the id was considered the repository of instinctual energy, it became illogical to ascribe libido instincts to the id, and aggressiveness, as a component of the ego instincts, to the ego. Escape from the dilemma was sought by discarding the old polarity of libido and ego instincts, for which was substituted a new polarity of life and death instincts. The life instinct incorporates the libidinal instincts and bears a special relationship to the pleasure principle. Analogously, the death instinct bears a special relationship to the repetition compulsion. As first presented, it was clear that the death instinct, being an innate tendency in living organic matter impelling it towards the reinstatement of an earlier condition, was a convenient biological model for the phenomena of destructiveness directed toward the self. It was not so clear that it was a biological model for aggressive destructiveness directed toward the defence and maintenance of the self. A concise statement appeared, however, in one of Freud's last writings,[8] making it clear that the death instinct could be diverted outwards as an instinct of destruction, necessary for the preservation of the individual. Further, in biological functions the life and death instincts work either antagonistically or in combination. Thus eating is the destruction of the object with the final aim of incorporating it.

According to Freud's conception, the life and death instincts provide a duality from which all human motivation can be derived. The empirical utility of such a dualism is a moot point. For example, aggressive destructiveness which can be directed toward the defence or maintenance of the ego seems to be more than a derivative of an innate tendency in living organic matter impelling it towards the reinstatement of an earlier condition which is ultimately an inorganic state. As Gardner[9] has pointed out, it seems to have a clear biological paradigm of its own, namely, the destructive metabolic processes essential to life. The phenomenon which inaugurated this inquiry—the compulsive repetition of a disastrous or traumatic experience—is more easily explained by such a theory, for it is more in the nature of an attempt aggressively to master a threat to the ego by returning to it in imagery rather than an attempt to return to an inorganic state.

The Concept of Instinct

So much, then, for destructiveness and aggression. The next problem is the metamorphosis of the concept of instinct occasioned by the revisions of *Beyond the Pleasure Principle.* Bibring points out that instinct was originally regarded "as an energic tension arising from organic sources and directed towards an inherently determined aim; that aim was attained circuitously via an object and consisted ultimately in a modification in the organ of origin—in a return of the organ to the state in which it was before stimulation."[10] According to this conception, the source of the instinct was the suitable criterion of classification, the aims and objects being variable. Since it was not always possible to locate definite sources, aim became substituted as the criterion, but no great change in the concept of instinct was necessitated. However, a radical change was introduced with the formulation of the death instinct, for instinct was no longer a tension of energy impinging on the mental sphere, "but a directive or directed 'something' which guided the life processes in a certain direction."[11] The accent was on determining tendency. Such a radical change carries with it important implications concerning motivation and the ego.

Ego Functions

The notion of a more or less autonomous tension seeking discharge regardless of the compliance or antagonism of the ego, appropriate to the concept of instinct as an energy-laden tension, is no longer pertinent. More fitting is the notion that the ego must function within boundaries delineated by the directive principles; or, to use a concept which I have presented elsewhere,[12] there are inevitables of being human within the boundaries of which the ego must function. Six inevitables were identified: aggregation in groups; autonomy and individual separateness; sexual status and reproductive role as male or female; bodily functions associated with metabolism; bodily features; and the potentiality of injury, disease, and death. Three of these inevitables are of special concern in this paper. The third is the focus point under which libidinal phenomena as identified by Freud are chiefly subsumed. The fourth provides the biological paradigm for aggressive destructiveness; and the sixth the biological paradigm for what Freud identified as the self-destructive tendencies of the death instinct.

None of the inevitables can be considered in isolation, however, for they are focus points in a reciprocally interacting feed-back system, each reverberating on the other. Since a feed-back system is by definition dynamic, it is not necessary to search for a theoretical basis for motivation in order to provide a dynamic psychology of personality. Of course it is not denied that human beings have the subjective experiences which they identify as needs or drives. That is an empirically observed phenomenon; but it is not essential that it become a construct and cornerstone of a theory of personality. The advantage of the theory of the inevitables is that it accommodates motivation without involvement in controversial theories of biological inheritance and constitutional predisposition, while at the same time not swinging to the opposite extreme of an environmentalist and relativistic theory of personality. It permits acknowledgement of constitutional and biological factors without being vitiated by an inability to identify them operationally. Nor is it vitiated by speculative theory about phylogenetic inheritance which was essential to Freud's theory of the instincts; it places emphasis on ontogenetic development which yields more auspiciously to empirical operations and procedures. Incidentally, it also demonstrates that sociology, cultural anthropology, and the psychology of personality are in much closer theoretical proximity than is commonly conceded, since the study of the individual cannot be divorced from the study of interpersonal relations.

With motivation theoretically accommodated as above, attention becomes directed to the ego and its functions as being of salient interest in the study of personality and its disorders. Developmentally the ego is responsive to its interpersonal milieu, and its characteristics will vary according to the time and place in which the individual grows up.[13] Nonetheless, regardless of interpersonal milieu, the threefold functions of the ego remain constant. The first is the function of mastery, experienced as the capacity to maintain and defend oneself. The second is an executive and controlling function, representing the ego in its directive capacity, experienced as the ability to make choices and decisions. The third is the spectatorship function, very closely related to cognition, and experienced as a capacity to perceive oneself as object.

The ego functions against a background of sequential experiences which commence with the apprehension of awareness and readiness cues derived from either proprioceptive or exteroceptive stimulation. Next in the sequence is the experience of significates and of doing. Significates are any kind of mental processes such as thinking, imagining, fantasying, dreaming, and hallucinating; and doing is some kind of bodily process, gestural or vegetative. Each sequence expires when the awareness and readiness cues become eventually abolished.

Personality malfunction or dysfunction ensues when the ego functions become disrupted. Disruption of the ego functions ensues whenever awareness and readiness cues associated with any one of the inevitables of being human become accentuated and so affect the whole feed-back system, as well as the significates and doing which the ego experiences. Very often one finds that such an accentuation has been a function of interpersonal relations and experiences; and that it may be so well reinforced and of such long standing that it has the appearance of being virtually ineradicable, exercising constant demands on the ego. Subjectively the accentuation is experienced variously as tension, conflict, anxiety, panic, and feelings of guilt.

When ego functioning is disrupted in this fashion, defensive modes of ego functioning are called into play. They are in the nature of emergency measures, and supplant and interfere with the ordinary modes of ego functioning, thereby presenting a picture of personality disorder. The baffling problem of the differential utilization of defence modes remains as yet unsolved, as does also the problem of the differential strength or stamina of the ego. It is scarcely possible to do more than enumerate and describe the defence modes. They are classified into three groups.

Acting Out

The most easily comprehended defence modes are those in which the ego's mastery function is intensified in an attempt to cope with the disrupting process. Most of the ensuing manifestations do not appear "crazy," so that they are frequently judged and evaluated on a legal and moral basis, rather than a psychiatric one. Psychiatrically they may appear as character disorders.

1. Legitimately described as a defence mode is the attempt at a reasoned, intentional re-examination of the disruption with a view to taking some kind of remedial action. Successful mastery is limited by the complexity of the disruption and the person's skill in exploring all the ramifications with sufficient penetration. The fact that only relatively few people suffer severe breakdown as the sequel to a bereavement is an indication that many use this mode successfully in some situations.

2. Often the above defence mode is used with partial success only. The ramifications of the disruption are too deep for complete exploration and mastery, but a compromise can be reached in the form of a sublimatory reformulation. The disruption continues to exert its influence, but is affiliated with a special skill, talent, or work activity so that the modes of acting out and substitutive reformulation (see below) are combined. The success of this defence is dependent on the indelibility of the sublimation which in turn seems to be dependent on the perplexing ego quality of stamina or cohesiveness.

3. Akin to sublimation is that acting out mode of defence in which an attempt is made to gain mastery of the disruption not directly but through displacement on to a surrogate. The sexual anomalies as means of avoiding full-fledged heterosexuality are examples. Frequently aggressiveness and destructiveness are conspicuous, as in the so-called psychopathic personality and in some forms of criminality and delinquency. Conspicuous also is the frequency with which the acting out of this mode of defence becomes compulsively repetitive, for example, in compulsive housebreaking, lying, firesetting, stealing, and the like. Moreover, the compulsively repeated act may be contrived in such a way that the mastery will be achieved with the external aid of discovery and punishment. The criminal returns to the scene of his crime in order to be apprehended and restrained.

4. Acting out in an attempt to gain mastery of a disruptive situation need not necessarily involve the utilization of a substitute or surrogate, but may be

more directly expressed as escaping, aggressiveness, destructiveness, or a kind of purposeless agitation. Such direct expression is especially observed in the child-hood manifestations of running away, negativism, and temper tantrums.

5. A common sequel to the initial fear, panic, and immobility produced by a sudden and intense traumatic disaster of the type occasioned by fire, earth-quake, battle, and the like, is a persistent but futile attempt at mastery through acting out. Although never mastered, the disastrous experience is repeatedly re-enacted in imagery and gesture or, to use the terminology presented above, in significates and doing. Often the reliving of the experience is stimulated by an external stimulus suggestive of its original occurrence, but it may also have the apparent autonomy of a nightmare. As a sidelight on this defence mode it is interesting to note that during the last war it was often the practice of airmen to return to the air as quickly as possible after being shot down so as to regain the feeling of confidence and mastery.

Amnesic-Type Processes

The ascendency of the mastery function of the ego is the characteristic which gives a certain unity to the first group of defence modes. The unity of this second group derives from the ascendency of the executive and controlling function of the ego which is intensified in an attempt to keep the disrupting process repressed. The inadequacy of repression is that the repressed does not suffer exile easily but continuously presses its claims. An uneasy truce may ensue in which the executive and controlling function partially capitulates.

6. When most successful, repression is evidenced only by panic or anxiety states in which some experience unexpectedly evokes and stimulates the re-pressed disruptive processes.

7. The successful maintenance of repression may not be possible without the contributory compliance of bodily functioning, namely, the so-called hysterical conversions such as blindness, paralysis, anesthesia, deafness, and impotence, which may be considered amnesias for partial somatic functioning.

8. It sometimes appears that the cohesiveness of ego functioning in its entirety is such that the partial amnesia of repression is inadmissible. Amnesia must be all or none, and the manifestation is a fugue state or condition of multiple personality. The ego changes allegiance, as it were, and functions in the service of the disruptive processes, temporarily at least.

9. The thorough amnesia of repression may not always be possible, in which case there is a persistent caution to maintain the amnesia as successfully as possible by compulsive, ritual avoidance of possible evocative stimuli which may activate the disruptive processes. This type of defence is another of those in which symbolic reformulation may also appear, for the avoided stimuli are often symbolic substitutes for other stimuli. Phobias and phobic-like reactions fall into such a pattern.

10. The amnesic task may reach proportions of such magnitude and seem so hopeless and futile that the person enters a state of depressive apathy and inertia, perhaps with suicidal tendency. Unable to keep the disruptive processes in oblivion, he sinks into a state of oblivious disregard. The obliteration achieved by means of alcoholism and drug addiction is a quite similar type of defence.

Substitutive, Symbolic Reformulations

The unity of this third group of defence modes derives from the ascendency of the spectatorship function of the ego. It is as if the ego endeavours to cope with the contradictions and confusions posed by the disruptive processes by elaborating a meaning whereby they are explained, even at the cost of confabulation and magical thinking. This kind of defence mode is related to repression in so far as it functions when repression does not entirely succeed, or breaks down partially or wholly. It is also characterized by regression or the return to more archaic developmental periods and modes of functioning. Its manifestations are those which often appear indisputably "crazy" to the layman.

11. The symbolic use of one verbal or sensory image as a substitute for another is a universal human experience in dreams and verbal fantasy. Hallucinatory imagery is closely allied.

12. Imagery may be superseded by gestures as symbolic substitutes, as is the case in obsessive, apparently autonomous partial somatic functioning. Tics and habit spasms are classic examples.

13. Symbolic gestures do not always appear autonomous but may be complex obsessive-compulsive rituals and ceremonials. They serve the purpose of attempting to preserve the status quo and keep the disruptive process in abeyance; and of denying, isolating, or ritualistically undoing the influence of the disruption.

14. Somewhat related to symbolic gestures, but somatically more incapacitating, are the psychosomatic dysfunctions which appear at first glance as organic diseases.

15. The attribution of causality to external sources (projection) and its reciprocal, the attribution of special virtues to the self (introjection or identification), form an ego defence which is very common especially when symbolic reformulation is at a minimum. With symbolism more intensively utilized it appears in classic form as paranoid delusional thinking.

The Schizophrenic Processes

Each of the fifteen modes of ego defence may be utilized by people who by common consent are regarded as normal. It is only with the intensification of their pervasiveness and saliency that the personality appears manifestly disordered. The grossest manifestations of disorder are the schizophrenic processes, in which the defensive modes of ego functioning become all-pervasive, with the appearance of autonomy.

When symbolic reformulations assimilate into schizophrenic processes they bestow a characteristic bizarrerie of thought and action. The classic example of bizarrerie of thought is the systematized paranoic delusion, the corresponding example for action being the compulsive ritual or ceremonial, which is usually combined with the delusion. In both instances the person has lost the ability to be an impartial spectator of himself.

The amnesic modes of defence assimilate into the schizophrenic process when repression is partially or wholly ineffectual. For example, the condition known as catatonic schizophrenia represents a partial ineffectualness of repression with widespread diffusion of somatic compliance, not necessarily accompanied by symbolic reformulation. The depressive apathy and inertia which may ensue when repression is totally ineffectual is frequently a component of the schizophrenic processes, as when melancholy is combined with bizarrerie of thought and action.

When the acting-out modes of defence assimilate into the schizophrenic processes, the attempt at mastery becomes a travesty of the ego's mastery function. Acting out becomes either turbulently impetuous or compulsively repetitious. It may become all the more bizarre and incomprehensible if, in addition, it is affiliated with symbolic reformulations. Repetitive acting out may be chiefly in the form of repetitive imagery, as in hallucinations, or chiefly in the form of repetitive gestures, as in the activity of the manic state.

The etiology of the schizophrenic processes is puzzling in so far as the intensity and all-pervasiveness of the defence modes seems frequently to be disproportionate to the intensity and pervasiveness of the disruptive processes which can be identified. In the face of ignorance, it is not unreasonable to postulate a psychological quality of ego strength or stamina which differs quantitatively from person to person. It may well be that ignorance in these matters will give way to understanding when the somatic contribution to the disruptive processes is elucidated. Elucidation of the role of somatic functioning may also reveal why any given modes of ego defence dominate, or are alternating and cyclic, in the diverse manifestations of the schizophrenic processes; and why manifestations may be episodic or chronic, and acute or insidious in onset.

Psychotherapeutic Functions

The threefold functions of psychotherapy parallel the three functions of the ego, namely, mastery, control, and spectatorship, and their associated modes of defence. Corresponding to the ego function of mastery is the therapeutic function of providing the patient with the opportunity in the transference relationship of returning to the archaic origins of the disruptive process so that he may re-enact them and find a different kind of resolution of them. In so far as the origins of the disruptive process have been subject to repression, it is necessary that the repression be lifted. This is the second therapeutic function, corresponding to the control function of the ego, and is provided for by such diverse means as the instruction to free associate, the use of hypnosis, or the administration of certain narcotics and intoxicants. Recollection and re-enactment of the archaic origins of the disruptive process by themselves are insufficient, for it is necessary that the patient gain insight into the relationship between the origins and later manifestations of the disruptive process. This is the third therapeutic function, corresponding to the spectatorship function of the ego. It is provided for, when the patient does not educe the relationship spontaneously, by interpretation from the therapist. The patient is more likely to educe the relation spontaneously when the source of the disruptive process was a fairly discrete event, or when there had been only a brief time interval between onset and therapy.

Psychotherapy may be aimed either at a fairly discrete disruptive process and the ego's mode of defence against it, or at a generalized proneness to utilize the mastery, control, or spectatorship modes of defence. It goes scarcely without saying that the latter is by far the more difficult task, and amounts in effect to a complete change of the personality, or character as it is sometimes called.

Psychopathology of Childhood

Although the psychopathology of childhood is not intrinsically different from that of adulthood, the differences which do exist are a function of chronology. First, capacity to utilize each of the ego's three functions and their associated modes of defence is itself a function of chronology. The ego's mastery function is able to be utilized from birth, but manifests itself initially as rather diffuse bodily activity. The control function of the ego is scarcely recognizable in the early months, for the only amnesic mode of defence applicable corresponds to depressive apathy and inertia which is also a rather diffuse bodily manifestation initially. The spectatorshp function of the ego appears later than the others and not until awareness of autonomy and ability to use imagery and linguistic symbols develops. Because the ego functions and defence modes change chronologically, the later manifestation of a disruptive process may be expected to possess certain qualities by virtue of its chronological origins. It may also be expected that the earlier the chronological origins, the more ineradicable and diffuse their influence in shaping the personality.

Second, it is not only ego function which changes chronologically, but also the person's vulnerability to potential disruptive processes. In earliest infancy disruptive processes appear to center exclusively around one of the inevitables of being human, namely, bodily functioning and metabolism. As the spectatorship function develops, the five other inevitables become potential focal points of disruption.

Third, the psychopathology of childhood is a function of chronology in so far as the manifestations of disruptive processes are separated from their origins by a shorter interval than is the case in adulthood. Therefore, childhood psychopathology, especially in the early years, resembles those adult disorders the onset of which is associated with a fairly discrete event which, it will be remembered, were differentiated from the disorders etiologically associated with diffuse relationships. This circumstance renders intelligible a peculiarity of childhood psychotherapy, namely, that it is often sufficient to provide the younger children with an opportunity for acting out. There has been no repression, most likely because the child has not yet achieved the ability to use it, so there is no repression to be lifted. Since the origins of the disruptive process are contemporary and since it is likely that the use of symbolic reformulation has not yet been achieved, in all probability interpretation will not be necessary. The therapist's chief function is to provide the relevant cues which will enable the patient to succeed in his attempt at acting out, and thus to gain the mastery.

Disruptive Processes of Childhood

The potential vulnerabilities of childhood are shared in common by all children. Whether or not they issue in disruptive processes is to a large extent a function of the pattern of interpersonal relationships in which a child participates, and the way in which this pattern is geared to an accentuation or underemphasis of potentially disruptive processes associated with each of the inevitables of being human. Belongingness and affection or loneliness and rejection, indulgence and blandishment or subjugation and compliance may be differentially combined and emphasized in diverse contexts. Naturally enough, parents, siblings, and others in close proximity to the child will exert the most significant influences initially.

Not only the patterns of intimate interpersonal relationship, but also those cultural and social patterns which have become a group's traditional response to the inevitables of being human, and which are influential within both intimate groups and general community, must be taken into account. The culturally defined traditions of interpersonal relationship aggravate the potential disruptions of childhood, if at all, rather homogeneously throughout the group, so that the disruptions are shared in common by the majority of the children. Within our own cultural traditions the disruptions associated with sexual status and role as male or female are a familiar example. The nature and significance of sex differences, menstruation, intercourse, and pregnancy, therefore, become imponderables of childhood and widespread correlates of psychopathology.

Experimental Animal Psychopathology

The so-called animal neuroses, like the human ones, may be either sudden in onset, as when an animal has been subjected to a sudden and intense shock; or cumulative in onset, as when it has been subjected to increasing difficulty of discrimination. Of course, the comparative study of human and animal psychopathology is open to objection in view of the fact that it is not possible to ascertain the mental content of an animal experimentally subjected to conflict. Thus the entire problem of symbolic reformulation remains obscure, or at best speculative. However, it is possible exhaustively to classify the neurotic reactions of animals as counterparts of the ego functions and modes of defence analysed above.

Within the acting-out group of defence modes there are two which have animal counterparts. One of the most common reactions corresponds to type 4: the animal directly expresses behavior indicative of escape, aggressiveness, destructiveness, or agitation.[14] Sometimes there is some degree of substitution or displacement on to a surrogate, the reaction then corresponding to type 3. Thus Liddell has described "a neurotic pig, which, despite prolonged starvation, would balance an apple on its snout for an hour or longer, growl, and then thrust its head into the food box, moving the snout rapidly to and fro, then as rapidly withdraw it, sometimes leaving the apple behind. . . . The pig keeps away from other pigs, but frequently fights with them and occasionally attacks the attendant when he enters the pig pen."[15]

Of the amnesic group of defence modes there are also two which appear to have their counterparts in animal neuroses. Corresponding to type 10 is a reaction of lethargy and inertia reported by several investigators. Wendt, for example, reported that monkeys which were prevented from making substitutive movements by mechanical restraint responded with an inertia resembling partial hypnosis;[16] and Masserman describes two of his cats as "lying passive and immobile between feeding signals in any portion of the cage in which they were placed," and another as lying so still as to appear to be asleep, in which state "he could be placed in various cataleptic postures for periods of from ten to twenty minutes."[17] Corresponding to type 9 is a kind of phobic response of which an instance is recorded by Gantt regarding the dog, Nick. The dog showed a marked degree of antipathy to people formerly associated with him in the laboratory and, when the investigator met him at the station upon his arrival in the country, he paid absolutely no attention to his calling and to other friendly gestures, even turning his head and attempting to pull away.[18]

The defence modes belonging to the substitutive, symbolic group appear to have only one counterpart in the animal neuroses, namely, the psychosomatic disturbances. All observers have reported somatic disturbances in their animals, but only those which become stable and stereotyped may be regarded as corresponding to human psychosomatic disturbance. A good illustration is given by Gantt who reports of dogs that "even after four years' rest without intervening practice a repetition of the original food signal or of the environment produces a stereotyped symptom-complex characterized by defence reactions—negativism, refusal of food, whining, barking, agitated movements, increased respiration, raucous forced breathing, frequent uncontrolled micturition and sexual erections. . . . The neurosis had a marked and constant effect upon the latent period, duration and type of induced erections and ejaculations; a condition resembling premature ejaculation resulted. Outside the experimental camera these sexual functions were normal."[19]

The above five modes of defence are those which have been observed regularly in animal experiments. It is feasible that modes 5, 6, 7, and 12 could also be observed reactions of animals, but the existence of any of the others is a matter more for speculation than observation.

Summary

The paper opened with a discussion of the relationship between clinical procedure and rigorous scientific procedure in relation to research. Then followed a discussion of the theory of psychopathology based on empirical clinical observations. Instigated by an observation of war neurosis, it launched into an investigation of Freudian theory in relation to aggression, instinct, and ego functioning. Thence it proceeded to a presentation of some views on the functioning of the ego and its modes of defence; and concluded with some remarks on psychotherapy and the psychopathology of childhood and animals.

References

1. For a pertinent discussion of principles of assessment and appraisal in relation to dream interpretation, see Roland Dalbiez, *Psychoanalytical Method and the Doctrine of Freud;* London, Longman, Green, 1941; vol. 2, pp. 110-113.

2. See Roy R. Grinker and John P. Spiegel, *Men Under Stress;* Philadelphia, Blakiston, 1945. Also, Abram Kardiner and Herbert Spiegel, *War Stress and Neurotic Illness;* New York, Paul B. Hoeber, 1947.

3. Sigmund Freud, "Psychoanalysis," in *Collected Papers,* 5:107-130; London, Hogarth Press, 1950.

4. Sigmund Freud, *Beyond the Pleasure Principle;* London, International Psychoanalytical Press, 1922; pp. 24-25.

5. Sigmund Freud, *The Problem of Anxiety;* New York, W. W. Norton, 1936; p. 66.

6. Reference footnote 5; p. 26.

7. For an outline of Freudian theory of instinct and aggression see Edward Bibring, "The Development and Problems of the Theory of the Instincts," *Internat. J. Psychoanal.* (1941) 22:102-131.

8. Sigmund Freud, *An Outline of Psychoanalysis;* New York, W. W. Norton, 1949; pp. 20-23.

9. George E. Gardner, in tutorial discussion.

10. Reference footnote 7; p. 127.

11. Reference footnote 7; p. 128.

12. John Money, "Unanimity in the Social Sciences with References to Epistemology, Ontology, and Scientific Method," Psychiatry (1949) 12:211-221.

13. For an illuminating account of the ego's response to its interpersonal milieu see Bruno Bettelheim, "Individual and Mass Behavior in Extreme Situations," in *Readings in Social Psychology,* T. M. Newcomb, E. L. Hartley *et al.* (eds.); New York, Henry Holt, 1947; pp. 628-638.

14. Illustrations will be found in J. H. Masserman, *Behavior and Neurosis;* Chicago, University of Chicago Press, 1943; chapters 4 and 8.

15. Reference footnote 14; p. 170. For convenience all examples have been quoted from the one book.

16. Reference footnote 14; p. 162.

17. Reference footnote 14; p. 67.

18. Reference footnote 14; p. 175.

19. Reference footnote 14; p. 178.

Note

Originally published in *Psychiatry,* 14:55-66, 1951. [Bibliog. #2.3]

FOUR

An Examination of the Concept of Psychodynamics

Three Postulates

Some psychodynamic propositions are so readily understood that the concept of psychodynamics seems self-explanatory. Thus one can say that the teacher's mood affects the pupil's ability to learn, or that a child's character is influenced by a parent's nagging. In the light of such lay examples, the term psychodynamics signifies that sequential psychological phenomena may bear more than a fortuitous relationship to one another—in other words, that one psychological phenomenon may be called the cause or the effect of another. Despite such apparent simplicity, dynamic relationships of cause and effect as propounded in the formal and technical propositions of psychological and psychiatric theory often evoke debate and disagreement. In appears worthwhile, therefore, to examine the concept of psychodynamics more closely.

An examination of current dynamic psychological theories reveals that three essential postulates have been used in order to establish cause-effect relationships and thereby to establish the theories as dynamic. In unembellished form, the three postulates are as follows: (1) behavioral acts and verbal reports are the result of biological driving forces termed instincts, drives, or needs; (2) they are the result of unconscious impulses and motives; and (3) they are the result of the driving force generated by information or messages engendered perceptually-cognitively. These three postulates have not generally been considered mutually inimicable, but as more or less supplementary to one another. They have been combined in diverse ways and proportions, especially with reference to the modifiability of pristine driving forces through learning. It may be asked if all three postulates are equally useful scientifically. Their scientific utility hinges on the kinds of operational test to which they may be put. Each postulate requires an incisive and unambiguous operational test if it is to be given an incisive and unambiguous operational definition and to become more than a linguistic artifact.

Biological Driving Forces

An operational definition requires three terms, one of them an indication that some sort of operation has been carried out—that is, that something has been said or done:

$$z = x + operation\ y$$

Thus:

Sex drive (*z*) is a term used to signify a person's behavioral acts and verbal reports which pertain to genital functioning (*x*) after but not before the administration (*y*) of a specified sex hormone for a given period.

This is one, but not the only, operational definition of sex drive. For certain purposes, especially in animal experiments, it may be useful to substitute an alternative operation for *y,* for example:

. . . after enforced mating deprivation for *n* hours.

Hunger drive is commonly operationally defined in a similar way.

Usually sex drive is not defined as in the foregoing, but inferred as the entity or attributive antecedent to certain behavioral acts and verbal reports. An inference of this type can be formulated into an operational definition as follows:

Sex drive (*z*) is a term used to signify a *selection* (*x*) of a person's behavioral acts and verbal reports after competent specialists have agreed that such behavioral acts and verbal reports should be so signified. (*y*).

This definition is of the unincisive kind tacitly used by many psychologists and psychiatrists. The trouble with it is that the specialists disagree notoriously on the method for the selection of the behavioral acts and verbal reports, which exclusively constitute the raw data of psychology. Different specialists use different criteria for selecting significant behavior and reports.

It is commonly agreed that sex drive has something to do with sex hormone secretion. Thereafter consensus disintegrates into a welter of speculative opinion. The manifestation of human sex drive has been attributed to various ages, stages, and zones of the body. There have been arguments concerning the specificity or generality of its influence, and disputes about the degree to which its detailed expression is innately prescribed or modified by experience. The Oedipus complex, for example, has been described as racially acquired but individually inherited or, by contrast, as a culture-pattern phenomenon individually acquired by members of a given society. It has also been described as literally an incestual impulse or, more generally, as an alignment of interpersonal relationships within the family.

With so many hypotheses, and so many of them refractory to operational test, one may well ask if the postulation of a sex drive, or any other generalized biological drive, is not scientifically more an embarrassment than a support. Without incisive operational demonstrations whereby drive is defined, the term signifies only that an inference has been made from observed behavior and speech. Such an inference may have its utility, but it has proved highly vulnerable to the fallacy of misplaced concreteness: instead of an inference from behavior and report, a drive becomes a concrete entity used to explain that behavior and report. In itself an inference carries no guarantee that it will prove to be an hypothesis capable of empirical verification; it may be, but it also may always remain a linguistic artifact.

As yet, biological experimentation has not been able to provide an operational definition of any drive which combines precision with sufficient generality to be useful in clinical practice and research in human psychology. Rather the reverse holds true: the more biological research expands, the more a definition of a drive is limited to very specific conditions and circumstances. For example, it is no longer sufficient to relate sex drive to sex hormone, but it must be related specifically to adrenal cortical steroids and to androgenic and estrogenic gonadal steroids, each of which differs functionally in a manner by no means completely understood.

The time has come when people scientifically concerned with human psychology should examine carefully the usefulness of drive concepts. It must be decided whether inferred drives should be postulated as a cornerstone of psychodynamic theory; or whether, more modestly, the term drive should be reserved for those occasions when an incisive operational definition can be given. The latter alternative is likely to produce a greater scientific yield.

Unconscious Motives and Impulses

The second psychodynamic hypothesis is that motives and impulses may be unconscious. The corollary is that if these motives and impulses can by some technique be made conscious, then it is in some measure possible to control and direct them.

There is an important difference between saying that a motive or impulse is unconscious and that a drive is unconscious, but the difference is usually glossed over. If a drive is unconscious, then it may not manifest itself directly and may not be recognized without becoming conscious. Thus, so far as the ordinary person is concerned, it would be foolish to say that the sex drive is unconscious. But it would not be so foolish to say that a drive to maintain electrolyte balance in the cell structure is unconscious; yet if it remain unconscious, nothing is added to psychodynamic theory over and above its postulation simply as a drive.

The terms, motive and impulse, thus add a nuance, a twist, to the more general conception of drive. As commonly used, these terms imply a segmentation of a more general drive—its pushing power on this occasion or in that direction; for example, a sexual impulse toward a particular person or type of person. The specificity may be postulated as learned or unlearned.

There is yet another nuance that may be implied in the terms, motive and impulse—namely, that they represent only a partial and disguised manifestation of a more general drive. This is the psychodynamic signification par excellence of the term, unconscious motive or impulse—the signification that opens up an entire realm of psychodynamics. It is the theoretical basis of interpretation: of inferring the whole drive from its partial expression, especially if its partial expression is in gesture only and not communicable in words, and of inferring the whole drive from its disguised or symbolic expression, whether in gesture or word.

At the risk of pedantry, let it be repeated that driving, motivating, or impulsive forces are never observed but always inferred. Only behavioral acts and verbal reports are observed and recorded. The definition of an unconscious motive or impulse is as problematical and as likely to be a linguistic artifact as is the definition of drive itself. As in the case of drive, an unconscious motive or impulse is commonly not defined but inferred as the antecedent to a pattern of behavioral acts and verbal reports. This inference may be spelled out into an operational definition:

An unconscious motive or impulse (z) is a term used to signify a selection of a person's behavioral acts and verbal reports (x) after competent specialists have agreed that such acts and reports should be so signified (y).

As yet, the specialists do not agree; one is left at the mercy of the winds of doctrine. Yet, despite the difficulties, one cannot lightly dismiss the hypothesis of the unconscious as useless. There is a good accumulation of evidence to vindicate the hypothesis of unconscious processes. The most cogent, though not the only evidence, is of the type encountered in traumatic experiences of war. An episode in a person's experience cannot under the ordinary circumstances of life be recalled and communicated. Under the special circumstances of free association, hypnosis, narcoanalysis, or ether abreaction, the episode can be communicated. It may then be verified from independent sources. In addition, its recall and communication is followed by a radical change in the information communicated in the person's subsequent behavior and speech—namely, the disappearance of symptoms of psychopathology. This change alone is testimony in favor of unconscious processes, a kind of verification in itself.

Such an example does not require use of the terms, motive and impulse. It is sufficient to say that a message was incommunicable, except in disguised or symbolic form, or that the message was repressed, or that unconscious processes were at work. Regardless of the origin of messages—in perception, apperception, confabulation, or dream—unconscious processes may be defined operationally, thus:

Unconscious process (z) is a term used to signify that a person displays gestural or verbal anomalies and pathologies of communication (x) at the same time that he is unable to recall and to communicate literally certain messages with which he was formerly acquainted, and that these anomalies and pathologies disappear after recall and literal communication are effected, notably with the aid of such techniques as free association, hypnosis, and the administration of narcotics or ether (y).

Unconscious processes cannot always be associated with amnesia for a specific message and a specific information-bearing episode. Commonly, a person recalls and communicates a diffuse sequence of messages, such as those transmitted between infant and parents. Authentication from an external source is impossible; for the more diffuse the sources of messages, the less the possibility of differentiating the part played by perceptual stimuli from that contributed by cognitive elaboration. The only authentication possible is that anomalies of communication, transmitted by way of general behavior and verbal report, disappear after diffuse messages and their sources are recalled and communicated.

One may, of course, argue that motives and impulses, not messages, are the furnishings of the unconscious. Logical hazards of the language of motivation have already been pointed out, however. An hypothesis formulated in terms of messages and communication may well prove more amenable to operational demonstration, psychologically and neurologically, than one in terms of impulse and motive. One may note that successful psychotherapy appears to be intimately associated with transmission of messages and exchange of information.

Perceptual-Cognitive Information and Messages

The two psychodynamic postulates already discussed are unreservedly teleological; they are concerned with behavior and speech from the point of view of biological purpose and unconscious purpose. But they are not concerned with voluntary purpose. Paradoxically, they may therefore be characterized as deterministic also, representing biological determinism and psychical determinism respectively.

Determinism is commonly regarded as a necessary assumption, for it implies that sequences of events can be formulated in terms of regularity and predictability. Voluntariness, if it implies absolute unpredictability, is a useless assumption for a scientist to make. Absolute unpredictability is not, however, an inevitable correlate of voluntariness. The term, voluntariness, may be utilized to signify that the determinants of some, but not all, aspects of human behavior and speech cannot yet be demonstrated scientifically. In other words, it is a term signifying the scientist's ignorance at times of why people act and talk as they do. And it is safer to signify one's ignorance than to disregard it.

Recent psychological thinking has banned the term, voluntary, and denied that it has any scientific signification whatsoever. Association of the concept of voluntariness with that of free will has doubtless been responsible for this banning since the doctrine of free will implies absolute unpredictability of behavior and speech. It is not surprising, therefore, that when psychodynamic theory has postulated the importance of social and environmental influences in shaping psychological development, it has avoided all implication of voluntary teleology, and determinism has reigned supreme. Thus there have been postulates that attitudes are imprinted like writing on a clean slate; that the superego is a kind of microfilm copy of parental injunctions; or that the ego is an automatic switchboard animated by messages to and fro.

In all such postulates there has been the tacit implication that life's experiences are mediated as perceptual-cognitive information before they shape behavioral acts and verbal reports. But the emphasis has been on perceptual reception and on the influence of remembered perceptual impressions. There has been little place theoretically for the possibility that perceptual stimuli alone are not sufficient to explain behavioral acts and verbal reports, and that they may be transformed by cognitive discrimination and organization, selection and synthesis—that the outcome may be novel or contrary to routine expectation.

If one allows a theoretical place for cognitive processes, despite the difficulty of their operational demonstration, then environmental and social determinism in its pure form is abandoned. An element of unpredictabilty is admitted, and part of this unpredictability may be ascribed to voluntariness which manifests itself as an ability to make choices and selections and to decide on courses of action.

The postulation of voluntariness instead of determinism does not require adoption of the doctrine of free will. Nor does it claim that all behavioral acts and verbal reports are voluntary. It simply asserts that sometimes perceptual-cognitive information is the driving force or so-called cause of human behavior and verbal report in such a way that the things said or done appear to be voluntarily purposeful. The following operational definition of voluntariness is offered:

Voluntary process (z) is a term used to signify that some of a person's communicative signs, gestural and verbal, change or disappear (x) after he becomes acquainted with more information than he had formerly assimilated, whether by filling a void of ignorance or by adding one or more propositions to a pattern of information already possessed (y).

The practice of successful psychotherapy provides many examples of the operations used in this definition, notably the adding of propositions to a pattern of information already held. The physician appraises a given pattern of information as incomplete, unserviceable, or bizarre and uses his psychotherapeutic art to induce its modification, which requires that the patient gain new knowledge or insight. Yet psychodynamic theory has eschewed the concept of voluntariness. More correctly, perhaps, one should say that psychodynamic theory has been primarily concerned with the when and why of failure of voluntariness in cases where organic brain damage cannot be demonstrated. In this respect it has broadened the frontiers of scientific understanding. So limited, however, psychodynamic theory has not been a general theory of human behavior and verbal report, though commonly misrepresented as such.

The weakness of psychodynamic theory occasioned by its failure to grapple with the concept of voluntariness has not wholly escaped notice. Current and growing concern with ego theory, especially with reference to ego control, is evidence of an attempt to reintroduce voluntariness under a new name. But the implications of an expanded ego theory have not, to date, been thoroughly worked out.

To summarize this section: It has been argued that a postulate of environmental and social determinism should be supplanted by a postulate that perceptual-cognitive information has its own dynamic or driving power. This driving power, though characterized as teleological and voluntary, should not be envisaged as an explanatory principle, but as a descriptive one—an admission that there is much in human behavior and report which has not yet yielded to deterministic demonstration and explanation. It is considered worthwhile to admit and signpost regions of ignorance, because research is then more likely to be directed toward them.

An outstanding research challenge is the baffling problem of why individuals react differently to similar perceptual-cognitive messages or sequences of messages. Psychologists and psychiatrists fall back on the assumption that, though similar, the stimulus signs and signals were sufficiently different in nuance to account for differences in reaction—for example, in symptomatology. The time has come to examine the scientific yield stemming from this hypothesis. One suspects that the hypothesis will prove incapable of precise operational demonstration and verification.

Psychologists and psychiatrists also fall back on the assumption of individual differences as an explanation of differences of reaction to similar perceptual-cognitive messages. But the nature of such individual differences has seldom been specified and put to operational test. It is here suggested that individual differences may be, at least in part, differences in perception-cognition and decipherment of messages: from which it follows that psychodynamic research, in both the laboratory and the clinic, might well be oriented toward perception-cognition and the decipherment and communication of information. The approach may be in terms of information and communication and their impairment, and also in terms of neurophysiology and its disturbances.

Summary

Three postulates which are used in psychodynamic theories to provide a basis for psychological cause-effect relationships have been examined in this paper. These postulates are that behavioral acts and verbal reports are the result of (1) biological driving forces, (2) unconscious impulses and motives, and (3) the driving force generated by perceptual-cognitive information. The first two are frankly teleological, though they are simultaneously deterministic in the sense of excluding voluntariness. If voluntariness is excluded from the third postulate, then it signifies strict social and environmental determinism to the total exclusion of teleology. This paper suggests that it is scientifically useful to extend current trends in ego theory by postulating voluntariness rather than attempting to disregard it. This argument has been developed with reference to perceptual-cognitive information and messages, and with reference to the extent to which such information and messages can be recalled and communicated or are unconscious and incommunicable. The terminology of drives and impulses is considered as too refractory for incisive operational definition to justify the use of such concepts as a cornerstone of psychodynamic theory.

Note

Originally published in *Psychiatry*, 17:325-330, 1954. [Bibliog. #2.4]

FIVE

Linguistic Resources and Psychodynamic Theory

Designative and Dynamic Words

Present-day psychological vocabulary includes new word forms, like aggressivity and compulsivity, which are not listed in the 1951 edition of *Webster's New International Dictionary,* nor in the *Oxford English Dictionary.* It also includes similar words, for example creativity and impulsivity, perceptual and instinctual, which, according to the historical illustrations of the *O.E.D.,* were first used in a psychological context and are of recent origin, or which were not listed until as recently as the 1937 edition of *Webster.*

Some people denounce these word forms as perverse technical jargon, debased duplications of more traditional forms such as aggressiveness and creativeness, instinctive and perceptive. In point of fact, they are not debasements for they conform to linguistic precedent. Nor, and this is one of the arguments of this study, are they duplications.

In an attempt to circumvent a tedious exposition, several designative words and their derivatives have been tabulated. It is postulated that close scrutiny of Table I will permit agreement with the following two statements:

(1) -ive
    -iveness
    } are suffixes which imply *illustrating* or *being an example of* the process or source designated by the root.

(2) -ivity
    -uality
    -ual
    -(a/e)nce
    -(a/e)nt
    } are suffixes which imply *manifesting* or *being operated by* powers or capacities characteristic of the process or source designated by the root.

Words of the first type may be called designative, those of the second type, dynamic. Productiveness and productivity are a good example of the difference between the two types of word. Aggressiveness and aggressivity also exemplify the difference. One may say that a person's aggressivity was evident in his Rorschach responses, but this is not synonymous with saying that his aggressiveness was evident—unless he carried out acts of aggression on the inkblot prints or the examiner. It is more nearly synonymous with saying that his aggressive impulses or drives were evident, so much so that there is no obvious error if aggressivity is defined as: a condition of manifesting powers or capacities designated by the term aggress. Presumably impulses or drives are the powers

69

or capacities which give the term aggressivity this dynamic nuance. If this presuming is conceded, then aggressivity embodies an element of the dynamic theory of drives in a word form which sufficiently dissembles its semantic history to be acceptable even to the opponents of the drive theory itself. In this repect, the new derivation incidentally throws light on schizophrenic neologisms.

It is possible that the opponents of new word forms, like aggressivity, inchoately sense its dynamic implication and rebel against yet another animistic endowment for the human organism. Their rebellion is scarcely justified in the case of words like conductivity and resistivity, as used in physics. These words are clearly useful and unequivocal hypothetical constructs. But it may be debated whether psychologists are yet able to demonstrate, in an unambiguous, operational way, that their -ivity words are both useful and unequivocal hypothetical constructs. It is an open question whether it is more useful to attribute certain samples of human behaviour and speech to aggressivity, than to attribute certain samples of psychopathology to *demonivity*.

The linguistic irony of aggressivity is that the older derivatives formed from the root aggress (*gressus,* past participle of *gradi,* to step, go) do not pertain to physical or mental states at all, but to acts. Aggression is defined in *Webster* as: 'a first or unprovoked attack, or act of hostility; also the practice of attack or encroachment.' The corresponding states, physical and mental, are anger, wrath, ire, rage, fury, hostility. Hostility is no stranger to dynamic theory, for it is ready-made with an -ity ending, but it would never do to have *angruality* or *wrathivity.* The short words carry too strongly the connotation of being stimulus provoked and limited in duration, not of enduring potential.

Further, the short words denoting acts or physical and mental states are seldom derived from Latin or Greek. By contrast, all the words listed in Table I are of Latin stock. In contemporary English, dynamic derivatives cannot be formed from Nordic roots, Anglo-Saxon included. There is no *attackivity* (etymologically attack means almost literally 'to stick tacks into') and no *fearance.* There is also no *thinkuality, dreamance, knowivity,* or *choosivity.* Perhaps this is why in contemporary psychology thinking, dreaming, knowing, and choosing are virtually disregarded as dynamic determinants. Motivation is patrician! It requires Latin origins as well as endings.

Is it conceivable that, by a stroke of arch-irony, the dynamic theory of unconscious determinism is itself being unconsciously determined—by our Latin heritage?

Summary

Derivative word forms of recent appearance in psychological vocabulary have been considered in their relationship to dynamic psychological theory. A question has been raised, in view of the observation that the new words are derived from classical and not Nordic roots, as to whether dynamic theory is contingent on linguistic resources, and limited by our verbal habits.

TABLE I

Table of Psychological Vocabulary Showing Recent Derivatives

(Words capitalized and underlined are in current psychological use but have not yet been listed in standard dictionaries; words capitalized without underline have been recently listed.)

Designative words		Designative derivatives			Dynamic derivatives	
Verb	Noun	Adjective	Noun	Noun	Adjective	Noun
sex	sex	—	—	—	sexual	sexuality
—	intellect	intellective	—	—	intellectual	intellectuality
act	act	active	activeness	activity	actual	actuality
sense	sense(s)	sensitive	sensitiveness	sensitivity	sensual	sensuality
					sentient	sentience
perceive	percept	perceptive	perceptiveness	perceptivity	percipient	percipience
					PERCEPTUAL	
	instinct	instinctive	—	instinctivity	INSTINCTUAL	INSTINCTUALITY
conflict	conflict	conflictive	—		CONFLICTUAL	
create		creative	creativeness	CREATIVITY		
impel	impulse	impulsive	impulsiveness	IMPULSIVITY		
aggress		aggressive	aggressiveness	AGGRESSIVITY		
compel		compulsive	COMPULSIVENESS	COMPULSIVITY		
obsess		obsessive	OBSESSIVENESS			
resist		resistive	RESISTIVENESS	resistivity	resistant	resistance
cognize		cognitive			cognizant	cognizance

Note

Originally published in the *British Journal of Medical Psychology,* 28:264-266, 1955; and re-published as an appendix in *The Psychologic Study of Man* (1957). [Bibliog. #2.9]

SIX

Behavior Genetics: Principles, Methods, and Examples from XO, XXY, and XYY Syndromes

Introduction

Behavior genetics is not so much a new field of study as a new concept to supplant the outmoded nature-nurture dichotomy. The term itself indicates a concern with the genetics of behavior. Yet no modern geneticist is so naive as to believe that any given sample of behavior has exclusively genetic origins. Behavioral and social scientists are not always so up to date; some of them still dichotomize the inherited versus the acquired. The fact is that the genotype cannot express itself except in interaction with the environment, whether it be the environment created by neighboring cells in the embryo, the environment provided by the mother in the uterus, the perinatal environment, or the environment encountered in the home and community. Behavior genetics is, therefore, in a sense the science of ascertaining the environmental limits within which the genetic code can operate and unfold itself into a normal phenotype; and the limits which environmental extremes may impose on the genetic code, without destroying it, but obligating it to unfold into a defective or abnormal but viable phenotype.

Since one cannot design experiments to test these limits for the human as for other species, it is necessary to extract all possible information from clinical studies or the so-called experiments of nature. For this reason I turn to examples from behavioral cytogenetics.

Turner's Syndrome

There is considerable accumulated evidence that some behavioral traits associated with Turner's syndrome are related to the chromosomal anomaly that produces the syndrome: 45 chromosomes instead of the normal 46, with only one X chromosome. Usually, individuals with Turner's syndrome have an XO sex chromosome count (45,X). Sometimes, however, they are mosaics (45, X/46, XX): some cells will have an XO, some an XX chromosome constitution, and there are other anomalies of the sex chromosomes which allow the same condition to develop morphologically.

The syndrome is characterized by a number of physical stigmata, among which are cubitus valgus, a low posterior hairline margin, and webbed neck. In a classic case of Turner's syndrome, the webbed neck alone is sufficient for diagnosis.

Short stature is also associated with the syndrome. Patients always develop into short adults, hardly ever more than five feet tall, and often only four and one-half feet. In the pure form of the syndrome, the ovaries are always lacking. In their place are vestigial streaks, instead of the proper gonadal structures; hence, these patients do not undergo teenage sexual development and are sterile.

In evaluating these patients in terms of intelligence, it is necessary to distinguish verbal intelligence from performance (nonverbal) intelligence. No deficit in verbal intelligence has been demonstrated in association with Turner's syndrome. In fact, in some of the girls studied, verbal IQ was quite high. In terms of nonverbal intelligence, however, test results confirm that individuals with Turner's syndrome suffer a neurocognitional deficit in space-form perception—particularly visuoconstructional recognition and performance.

For example, the simple task of copying a hexagon can present a serious problem to an individual with Turner's syndrome.The hexagon is one of the items in the Benton Visual Retention Test. On this test, and on the Bender Visual Motor Gestalt test, Turner patients demonstrate what can be called a degree of space-form blindness, or a partial congenital agnosia. In the Benton test, geometric designs are exposed for ten seconds; then they are withdrawn, and the patient attempts to reproduce them from memory. People with Turner's syndrome generally encounter considerable difficulty in copying these designs with any degree of fidelity.

That this is not simply a case of poor visual memory can be shown by the Bender Visual Motor Gestalt Test, a test similar to, but older than, the Benton, in which the patient is permitted to continue looking at the stimulus figure. Individuals with Turner's syndrome have as great difficulty in copying a design in front of them as they do a design that has been withdrawn. Hence, it is clear that the locus of the problem is the visual perception process itself, not in motor coordination.

Patients with the syndrome who are asked to draw a human person (the Draw-A-Person Test) produce a figure often grossly distorted and defective. That they do so, one might wrongly ascribe to distortion of the body image in view of the morphological defects of the syndrome. Knowing of the parallel difficulty with geometric figures, however, one correctly attributes human-figure distortion to the same source, namely, spaceform disorientation. A few girls with Turner's syndrome escape this particular difficulty, but not more than twenty percent, more or less.

A nonverbal IQ substantially lower than a verbal IQ is, correspondingly, a widespread trait among patients with Turner's syndrome. Difficulty in auditory discrimination has also been demonstrated among a few Turner patients, possibly affecting adversely also their verbal learning and achievement, both at home and at school, insofar as this is reflected in some of the questions on the intelligence test. This hearing deficit, when present, is more likely due to middle ear involvement than to so-called nerve deafness.

Klinefelter's Syndrome

In contrast to Turner's syndrome, Klinefelter's syndrome, which occurs in phenotypic males, is characterized cytogenetically by an extra X chromosome. These individuals have a 47,XXY chromosome constitution.

Boys with Klinefelter's syndrome usually are not diagnosed until later in life. After puberty, they tend to be tall and eunuchoid in their body proportions (long arms and legs); many of them are thin, though a few become mildly obese. They have small testicles, which are often the basis for the detection of these cases in physical examination, and in almost every instance they are sterile, with atrophy of the spermatic tubules. Sometimes they develop breasts like those of an adolescent girl and require surgery for flattening of the chest. Very frequently their condition goes undetected, and it is not known how many of them are in the general population, unrecognized. The prevalence at birth is 1:500 boy babies.

Judging from samples studied, there is a strong tendency for XXY men to be unstable in personality and psychological development. One infers, therefore, instability of the central nervous system, which underlies and mediates psychological development and personality. It may show itself even in mental deficiency. An unusual amount of mental deficiency is associated with the syndrome, although exactly how much is difficult to determine. There is good evidence, however, to prove that the condition, not invariably associated with mental retardation, is also compatible with superior IQ.

When the individual is mentally retarded (and sometimes extremely so), it is both the verbal and nonverbal intelligence which are affected, in contrast to Turner's syndrome, where the deficit lies in the area of nonverbal intelligence specifically.

Testicular Feminization Syndrome

The syndrome of testicular feminization has recently become known as the syndrome of androgen insensitivity. In simplest terms, this syndrome represents an extreme form of male pseudohermaphroditism in which the external sexual differentiation is feminine, but accompanied by the presence of testes and the absence (or, at best, the vestigial remains) of uterus and tubes.

Genetically, affected individuals are males, with the XY chromosome count of a male. Gonadally, they are males, too, since the gonads that exist in the groin or abdomen can be seen, under the microscope, to be testicular in structure. Otherwise, there is nothing masculine about the external sexual differentiation of these people; it is the internal differentiation that is contradictory and ambiguous.

The paradox is usually not discovered until middle adolescence, when a gynecologist is consulted because the girl has not begun to menstruate. Despite her amenorrhea, however, she does grow breasts and develops her own female body configuration at the normal age of puberty. The reason for this development is that the cells of the body, presumably all of them, are androgen-insensitive and therefore unable to respond to male sex hormone. In some cases, this insensitivity is so complete that it is not possible for the body to grow either sexual or axillary hair. Blood measurements that have been made of sex-hormone production have shown that the testicular gonads produce normal amounts of male sex hormone and of female sex hormone, for a male. But the body responds, in these individuals, to only the female part of the hormonal ratio, which it finds sufficient for very good feminization.

Embryologically, it can be understood why, with the testes present as the initial part of sexual differentiation, it is possible for the internal organs to develop as male while the external organs develop exclusively as female. In brief, the explanation is as follows:

The embryonic testis secretes, in due course, not only an androgenic substance, but also a mullerian-inhibiting substance that atrophies the mullerian ducts, preventing their becoming the uterus and tubes and causing them to become vestigial in the normal male. This process of vestigiation continues to quite some degree in XY girls, and usually they are born with, at most, a cord-like structure for a uterus, through which it would be physiologically impossible for menstruation to occur.

In terms of genetics, this syndrome is doubly interesting because affected individuals are genetic males and because the defect which allows this strange differentiation to occur is genetically transmitted. One may find the condition in several generations in a family tree. Since the individuals are sterile, of course, it is in aunts and nieces that one finds it. The exact nature of the genetic transmission is still open to question, as in the exact nature of the presumed enzymatic defect which allows the cells not to utilize male hormone.

What about behavior in people with testicular feminization syndrome? The question can be answered simply. If you were to meet one of them; it would not cross your mind to ask a single question. You would automatically accept the person as a young teenaged girl, a married women, or—if she had adopted children—a mother. There would not be a single clue to make you suspect otherwise.

This interesting paradox shows how, as far as dictation of sexual behavior by the sex chromosomes is concerned, the Y chromosome is completely defeated by the intervention, in this instance, of an embryonic sequence of events, itself under genetic regulation.

Environmental Regulation of Genetics of Behavioral Traits

Individuals with Turner's syndrome are able to differentiate as females in the same way as are girls with testicular feminizing syndrome because an androgenic substance is either missing or is not effective. Herein lies a basic rule, as far as the expression of genetic maleness in the embryo is concerned. For instance, if an animal embryo is castrated in the uterus before the critical period of the morphological development of its external sex organs, it will always differentiate as a female regardless of its XX or XY chromosomal structure. It then becomes possible, by using the proper substitution hormones, to regulate the subsequent behavioral development of that animal so that it will behave like a female even if it has the XY chromosome structure. This example is very interesting because, at this early stage of embryonic morphological development, it demonstrates the principle that androgen is the substance necessary in differentiating the male. One finds the same principle coming to the fore again at puberty, insofar as failures of puberty are more common in the male than in the female (menstrual problems excluded). Here again, nature has her difficulties in carrying through with that extra step required for masculinity.

The same process appears to be in operation with regard to psychosexual differentiation, because all available evidence so far indicates that psychosexual disorders—the bizarre and exotic kinds of sex (or, as they are often called, the perversions)—are more common in males than in females, sometimes to such an extent that they are as yet unheard of in females. For instance, coprophilia, necrophilia, or being "turned on" by urine, or possibly drinking urine (urophilia)— such extraordinary and bizarre things to which the sex drive can become linked—are virtually not heard of in women. If you search the newspapers for an example of a female peeping Tom, you will not find one. If you look for examples of a female exhibitionist who can reach her orgasm only by displaying herself to someone who is startled by the display in public, you will not find that in the newspaper either, but it will not take very long to find a report of a male with such a psychosexual disorder.

Antiandrogenization of the XY Genotype

Experimental counterparts of individuals with testicular feminizing syndrome are rats produced by Friedmund Neumann[8,9] in the laboratories of the Schering Corporation in West Berlin. These rats illustrate in reverse the principle of adding androgen to make maleness. Genetic males, they have normal female external genitalia, as a result of injecting the pregnant mother with the anti-androgen cyproterone acetate. If the feminized male offspring is prevented from having masculinizing puberty by earlier having its testes removed, and then is given female hormone substitution at puberty, it develops as a female and behaves as a female, as is evident, for example, in copulation, when it assumes the position typical of the female. Normal genetic males (the hormonally normal ones) respond to these experimental rats as if they were females. They do not detect the difference. Here again one sees that the expression of genetic traits is defeated, in this case by the intervention of an intra-uterine hormonal phenomenon.

Androgenization of the XX Genotype

The counterpart of antiandrogenization of the XY genotype, as seen in the example of the German rats, is androgenization of the XX genotype, which has been carried out at the Oregon Regional Primate Center, at Beaverton.[15] A female rhesus monkey was masculinized by administering androgen to its mother at a critical stage in fetal development. This female monkey then was born with a normal penis and empty scrotum. Inasmuch as the oldest of these experimental animals are only now entering adolescence, a full report on their adolescent behavior is not yet available, and there is, of course, no report on their adult behavior. However, reports on their childhood behavior indicate that their scores on such activities as aggressive behavior, initiating play and fighting play, rough-and-tumble play, mounting in sexual play and masturbation were closer to the scores of the normal male controls than those of the normal female controls. Those monkeys that have reached adolescence have normal menstrual cycles.

It is presumed that there is a change in the organization of the central nervous system as it applies to the regulation of sexual behavior, presumably localized in the hypothalamus, if one judges from experiments on other animals, using a technique of radioactive hormone uptake in brain cells. Here, then, is another example of a way in which, to a partial extent, at least, the normal expression of genetic traits has been defeated.

Alteration of the Genotype

To modify the expression of genetic traits by introducing hormones at the critical period of fetal development (a point to be stressed again) is a relatively simple matter. A newer group of experiments indicates that it is actually possible environmentally to manipulate heredity so as to modify not only the phenotype (as in the example of the rats or the monkeys, whose genetic type remained the same), but the genotype itself and, with it, the genetic program for behavior. This new concept upsets completely the nineteenth-century point of view which assigned durability and validity only to heredity, and dismissed environmental influences as being relatively unimportant.

One line of experiments comes from the Basel laboratory of Emil Witschi,[13] formerly from the University of Iowa. Using amphibians and regulating the ripeness of the egg, Witschi was able to reverse the morphological sex of males and females, so that they would be able to breed in the reverse sex, completely contradictory of their genetic sex. In other words, it was a case of having an XX female morphologically reversed into a male and then able to breed as a male—but an XX male. A new species!

The most complex example of experimental sex reversal is that achieved by Yamamoto[14] in the small killifish, *Oryzias latipes*. Yamamoto exposed XY (genetic male) larvae of this fish to female sex hormone. Unexposed, they would have differentiated as males. Exposed, they differentiated as XY females. An XY female was then able to breed with a normal XY male and produce young. Twenty-five per cent of the second-generation larvae were then chromosomally XX (female); 50 per cent were XY (male); and 25 per cent were YY, which, if left untreated, would differentiate as males, but, if exposed to estrogen, would become YY females. In the succeeding generation, it was then possible to breed YY females with YY males, the resultant progeny all being YY and, if left unexposed to hormone experimental treatment, differentiating as males. Yamamoto was also able to produce XX males by treating XX larvae with male sex hormone.

These experiments offer an excellent lesson in how not to make genetics theoretically too final and absolute, as did too many nineteenth-century investigators. The fact is, one can experimentally interfere with, and change, the genetic code itself. Hamilton and his colleagues,[5] at the Downstate Medical Center in New York, are using YY males of *Oryzias latipes* to investigate the effect of the Y chromosome on behavior. They tested YY and XY males, in 14 matched pairs, in competitive mating for single XX females; the YY males were clearly dominant. They induced 137 of 155 spawnings. They gained higher scores for: number of contacts with females; quivers, including those at spawning; moving in quick circles around the female; and number of seconds spent alone with females. YY males spent more time chasing XY males, than vice versa, and made more quick circling movements around XY males. When a male of *Oryzias latipes* chases another male, he bites the pursued if he catches up with him. Biting was done almost exclusively by the YY males, and several XY males had their fins lacerated as a result. XY males tended to avoid YY males by remaining at one corner of the tank, near the bottom. One may presume, as Hamilton did, that the presence of an extra Y chromosome, rather than the loss of an X, was responsible for the increased mating dominance of the YY males. Be that as it may; the chief significance of increased dominance, in the present context, is that it was produced by environmental alteration of the genotype itself.

Case Illustrations: XYY Syndrome

Case 1: A 15-year-old boy was brought to me for interviewing and psychological testing, one year after he had been identified as having a chromosomal constitution of XYY. He had first come into the hospital at age 11, and had been seen continuously as an out-patient since that time.

He was a very thin, tall boy, six feet, five inches in height, shy and withdrawn, laconic but not unfriendly. He replied to questions in as few words as possible, and contributed little to the conversation voluntarily. He had recently come out of a special class at school and was about ready to enter the ordinary grade, pretty much suited to his age, in junior high school. This prospect was a bit threatening to him, but even more so to his parents, who were concerned as to whether he would be able to cope with this experience of being thrown into the hurly-burly of a big school and a regular-size class.

In this particular case, it is perhaps more rewarding to begin at the end and move backward through the case history. At the end of 1968, after the first few months of his attendance at the new school, his mother reported that he was making a satisfactory adjustment. She said, however, that the first few weeks had been very difficult for him, for the parents, and, I gathered, for the school as well. Apparently, during that period of time, the teachers were forced to reprimand loudly all of the students in what was a rough class of children who were not very highly achieved. The boy had been assigned to this class because of his own underachievement, as well as his prior difficult background. He took personally the teachers' reprimands of the entire class, with the result that he had difficulty sleeping at night, and his behavior began to deteriorate.

The situation cleared up, the mother reported, after she had conferred with the counselor, who in turn spoke to the teachers. The important point that I learned from her account was that this boy very easily went to pieces emotionally under the slightest pressure. He tended to personalize things, rather than to view himself as part of a group, all members of which were being treated the same way.

This sensitivity, this tendency to overreact to stress, is an important point to notice in regard not only to the XYY syndrome, but to almost any condition which predisposes a person to some kind of psychological weakness. But to XYY individuals, who are enigmatic in their personality development, such watchfulness applies especially, for they are extremely vulnerable to simple threats and stresses that most people would shrug off, or deal with, with relative ease.

In this regard, the contrast with Turner's syndrome is very sharp: girls with Turner's syndrome have an extraordinary stability in the face of adversity. It would almost seem that their syndrome not only inflicts upon them so many disadvantages in connection with their shortness, disfigurements and sterility, but also bestows upon them a protective advantage: they cope, and cope well, with adversity.

By contrast, there seem to be some people who are noteworthy because they have a vulnerability factor. Perhaps, at the present stage of knowledge, this is the most important lesson we can learn with regard to the behavior genetics of psychopathology. If there are particular traits and patterns of personality, or behavior, psychopathological or otherwise, that are specifically related to genetic patterns, then at the present time they must be either very rare and practically undiscovered. But a vulnerability factor, on a genetic basis? That is not so rare, and it seems the most sensible way to sum up the present status of knowledge.

This means that one does not anticipate that a person with a peculiar genetic or cytogenetic status will demonstrate a certain fixed stereotype of personality or pathology, but rather that he will show some kind of anomaly or deviation which will be an interactional product, a product of the interaction of the genetic vulnerability and the kind of stress that the environment has supplied.

But to return to the case of the XYY boy. When he was ten years old, his school counselor recorded some observations that are extraordinarily perceptive.

When the boy was first referred to the counselor as a six-year-old, newly admitted to school, the mother said that "he had violent temper fits and at times would wreck his toys and belongings." He was enuretic until the age of eight or nine. He was described as slow and a dreamer. His daydreams, according to his mother, were quite real to him.

These observations required four and a half typed lines, yet they say almost everything that is known at present about the XYY syndrome. The boy was subject to violent fits of temper at times; he was not a constantly bullying, aggressive person (to assume that the XYY individual is continuously aggressive is the first major error made by the news media in reporting this syndrome since 1966). He would wreck his toys and belongings, but only at times. Enuresis will probably be recorded more frequently as more cases of the XYY syndrome are uncovered. The slowness and daydreaming are also characteristics common to the syndrome.

There is a general tendency for XYY adults to be not only daydreamers but loners. One could possibly call them schizoid, but not schizophrenic; the safer word is "loners." They are not unable to relate as they sit and talk, and they can be very friendly and pleasant in a transient sort of way; but they do not encourage relationships or involvement in situations that have continuity and carry-through in their lives. They tend to plan their activities on an isolationist basis, so that one cannot quite predict what might develop tomorrow or next week.

When this boy was still six years old, his intelligence was tested and found to be in the dull-normal range (in the 80s). His thinking showed signs of perseveration; that is, after having been asked, and having answered a question, he was not able to make the shift to the next question, but instead tended to repeat the answer (or some part of it) to the antecedent question. Such behavior is noteworthy in a report on a patient of this type, because perseveration is supposed to be a sign of brain damage. His perception of his environment was described as unusual and, at times, bordering on the bizarre. The report indicated that the boy hallucinated, wisely refraining from speculation as to the causes, and characterized the boy as being uncertain of himself in dealing with others. At times, it observed, his hostility became quite marked. He was recommended for neurological and psychiatric examination, because he seemed, at the age of six, to be suffering from structural brain disease compounded by emotional problems.

At this early period, it was noted that the boy's father had had a psychiatric admission and evaluation first at the age of seventeen, with a diagnosis of possible schizophrenia; it was also noted that the mother tended to be remote. When she was interviewed in 1968, though it was obvious that she was genuinely concerned about her child's welfare, she spoke of it in the detached way one might expect a relative to talk about a child who was not related by blood, though living in the family.

During the early months of school, as a first-grader, the boy's academic work was very poor. He was known to behave peculiarly at times, as the report observed, "pulling a sweater over his head and putting his head down. He hears voices at times, seems confused and in a daze. His attention span is extremely short, and his social relationships are fair to weak. He has only one good friend, and he has been known at times, to hit children with no apparent reason."

This early school story can be understood when it is illumined by the later report, outlined above, of the difficulties he encountered upon entering junior high school, when once again his behavior very nearly became disrupted. It would seem clear, from his behavior at these two widely separated but extremely important times in his life, that to have to go from his home environment, where everything was familiar, to the school environment, where everything was strange, was for him a very special source of stress, almost a trauma, and his behavior deteriorated under that stress.

The subsequent history of this boy has been one of steady improvement, even with regard to his EEG. At the age of 10½ years, his EEG was abnormal, showing a typical seizure spike, though he has never been known to have a seizure. He was placed prophylactically on antiseizure medication. Gradually, the dosage has been lowered, and eventually the medication may be withdrawn entirely.

When his IQ was tested in 1963, at age 10½, it was still in the dull-normal range, as it had been when first tested at age six. By age 15, it was normal, and his nonverbal IQ was 111—one point above normal into the bright-normal range. Based on these several criteria, one sees the boy making progress.

At age 10½, he was referred by his school into a special research program for brain-damaged children, but he was not accepted because he seemed atypical, compared with other children in the program. At that time it was noted that he showed considerable twitching and choreiform movement, as well as other peculiar behavior. The interviewer observed: "He is a tall, thin, fair-haired boy who, when I introduced myself, offered me his left hand. His father and I commented on it at the same time, and the boy said nothing at that stage, but later, under questioning, he said that he gave me his left hand because his right one was occupied holding something. That was, in fact, untrue. He came toward the door at the office humming to himself and also muttering under his breath, and I heard him say, as he passed his mother, 'I think I'm going to kill you.' This was said in a very cheerful way and had no depth of aggression in it at all. He cheerfully entered the office and sat down, and throughout the interview he squirmed around in his seat with his eyes looking everywhere in the office except at me. He frequently giggled in a high-pitched way and hummed to himself. As the interview progressed, he often made comments to himself such as 'You can go on now;' 'That should be the end of that,' 'Well, I think it's okay,' all said in a half-tone under his breath, and brushed aside when I asked him to repeat what he had said."

Between that time and the date of his interview in 1968, the boy changed remarkably. Perhaps this change was owing in part to his having been enrolled in a special school for the so-called brain-damaged child, where some of the pressure of an ordinary schoolroom orientation toward achievement was taken off him. He is probably still liable to have regressions to his peculiar behavior, however. For example, in 1965 a report came from his teacher that "he appears to be distracted for various periods of time throughout the day talking and apparently listening to someone who is not there. He moves his lips, nods his head, raises his eyebrows, and chuckles or laughs. I have seen signs that make me believe he is masturbating in his cubicle in the classroom."

When he was seen in 1968, he was unable to give any information in the sex interview, because, with his nontalkative attitude, he was not really able to give any very deep information about anything. His mother, however, had not observed any signs of his having reached the stage of ejaculation; she had seen no semen stains on his underclothes or his bed sheets. His parents had not seen evidence of any romantic interests, no pictures, no involvements in such teenage activities as rock-and-roll, certainly no romantic approaches, and nothing to suggest an interest in a girlfriend.

Further study, of course, will reveal more of this boy's story. But when he was tested in 1968, his intellectual capacity seemed quite adequate, judging by the geometric drawing test, the IQ test, and other tests that were administered; he showed no deficit in auditory discrimination or direction sense; and his finishing of sentences was satisfactory, with no special indication of emotional problems. Apart from the fact that he was a rather peculiar, isolated loner, it was very difficult to believe that the history recorded prior to 1968 actually applied to this same boy, despite its obvious validity as part of his medical record.

Case 2: There is something very important, and perhaps pathognomonic of the behavior of the XYY individual, to be learned from the following story, told by a man with this syndrome, who had been detained in an institution because of a violation of the law.

As his occupational therapy and training while he was in the institution, he had taken up painting on canvas, and he became quite good at it. His story was that the other inmates knew that he hated to have anybody come up behind him and frighten him with a sudden noise, or poke him in the ribs. And so, with nothing much else to do in the institution, a lot of the inmates would torment him by doing just that. Since he really wanted to get out of the institution and go straight, it became necessary for him to exercise what was probably, for him, an almost superhuman act of self-control; to put his brushes down and lock himself away in his cell, because he had an almost undeniable urge to turn around and almost kill his tormentor.

An urge of this sort is uncannily similar to an epileptic seizure which is triggered by loud noises. This particular patient had an abnormal EEG, with a history of a few seizures, and was on seizure control with Dilantin (diphenyl-hydantoin) and Mysoline (primidone). The 15-year-old boy whose case is discussed above formerly had the seizure EEG pattern, but had never been known to have a seizure, and, at the present time, does not have an abnormal EEG.

The painter's story illustrates what may be the key to the behavior disorder in the XYY syndrome, namely, that there is an impulsivity (one might almost say, a paroxysmal impulsivity) and lack of regulation in the behavior. Very possibly, it is not only the regulation of aggressive and destructive behavior, perhaps including feeling, that is affected; the regulation of sexual behavior may be involved as well, and may turn out to be fairly peculiar in these people. Certainly, more evidence is needed, but so far the indications are that XYY individuals do not lead the ordinary, straightforward sex lives of males that one would expect to find, for example, in a random sample. Just how peculiar their sexual behavior may be, and how consistent the peculiarity from one person to another, are points that only additional cases can elucidate. Homosexuality, especially of the situationally-determined type, may prove to be atypically frequent in incidence.

Interactionism of Genetics and Environment: Norm of Reaction

In the case of the teenager discussed above, there is no point-for-point correlation between his extra Y chromosome and his behavior. However many points of similarity one might find among XYY individuals, they are not points of identity. Herein lies another illustration of how wise and necessary it is to use the modern genetic concept of the phyletic or genetic form of reaction. If one adds to this the concept of an environmental norm of variance, then what finally results is the product of interactionism. The genetic norm of reaction specifies an environment conforming to certain standards, within limits set by the phyletic history of the species, if genetic traits are to be able to express themselves according to the norm—and there are definite limits to how the environment may vary before it becomes so completely destructive that the genetic code is forbidden to express itself at all.

This kind of reasoning may be applied in the case of the XYY teenager, insofar as his behavior does seem to vary according to the kind of environment, with its stresses, in which his genotype exists.

In contrast to the nineteenth-century concept of genetics as part of a simple dichotomy (nature versus nurture, genetics versus environment, constitutional or innate versus acquired), the modern view is three-sided: on the one hand, genetics, the genotype; on the other hand, to coin a word, "environmentics"; and in the middle, the critical period. It is this interactionism, this meeting of the genotype with the environment-type at a critical period (often very limited— phyletically limited), that is so important and determinative of whatever phenomena follow. This model applies not only to morphological development, but to behavioral development in behavior genetics, as well.

Numerous environments must be taken notice of: the cellular environment, the intra-uterine environment; the perinatal environment; and the postnatal environment, which includes those special environments of the body, the senses and the social existence. As far as the social environment is concerned, it was formerly taken for granted in most animal learning experiments that all the animals were experimentally identical; but with greater knowledge, investigators became aware that, for example, the amount of handling of rats in an experimental colony during a critical early period of their lives will change the kind of response they subsequently give in various behavioral tests. In the prenatal environment, too, there are special factors to consider. For example, recent evidence shows that barbiturates may have a strong but as yet unknown effect, especially on a male fetus. When a female fetus is being masculinized in an experimental animal, the masculinizing effect of the hormone can be cancelled out by sufficient doses of barbiturates.[3] This is a fascinating and somewhat alarming concept, because of the drugs pregnant women take and our ignorance of how these drugs may differentially affect a male versus a female fetus.

"Family-tree Heredity" versus Sporadic Heredity

Traditionally, the popular definition of heredity is "family-tree heredity," which to many people means "tainted." Unfortunately, this unsophisticated view of heredity still persists even among educated people, a point well worth remembering in genetic counseling. The misconception can be cleared by differentiating "family-tree inheritance" of a dominant trait and sporadic heredity, which includes both unexpected mutational change and sporadic, both-parent transmission of a mendelian recessive.

A typical example of the latter type of sporadic heredity is the adrenogenital syndrome which, in girls, creates hermaphroditic external genitalia, and in boys has as its effect early virilization. Unless the girls are treated with cortisone, they also are virilized at an early age, as well. Unless they have studied biology, parents in whose offspring this condition appears are, because it is not in the family tree, often unable to understand that it is hereditary. It must be explained to them that the condition is the product of the meeting of two hidden carriers, producing an open carrier, by chance, in 25 percent of the pregnancies. This condition will occur only in the offpsring of an affected pair of hidden carriers. Thus, except in the case of experimental inbreeding, it does not show itself as traveling within a family tree over the generations, but it is, nonetheless, hereditary.

Sporadic heredity is differently exemplified in the case of a cytogenetic anomaly, of which several illustrations have been given above. For the purposes of genetic counseling, one explains that this type of hereditary disorder may appear only once in a nuclear family and in a family tree, in contrast to the mendelian recessive, which may appear several times in only one nuclear family in a family tree.

Nativism versus Environmentalism

Whatever the type of hereditary mechanism, the essential idea in the mind of either the layman or the professional, when he deals with heredity, is the idea of that which is somehow fixed and beyond his control. It goes variously by the name of constitutional, innate, physical, congenital and, of course, genetic. All these concepts are subject to severe limitation. The idea behind them all is that they point to something which is nativistic, as compared with environmentalistic. A rigid dichotomy between these two is untenable, as already pointed out. The real need is for a concept of interactionism. Nonetheless, theoretically there is a need to separate conceptually the nativistic from the environmental. The operational problem, however, in behavioral genetics is to find which behavioral traits to identify and trace in order to differentiate the native from the environmental component in their expression. Alternatively, before analysis has proceeded far enough to identify traits, one may resort instead to looking for global patterns.

Global Patterns or Syndromes

To identify a pattern of human behavior or development as nativistic in origin, one has traditionally needed certain supporting evidence to increase one's confidence in the inference of nativism. For example, usually one needed to know that the pattern is a long-term one; that it is persistent in spite of possible interference or interruption; and that it is a pattern evolving and developing over time. Such evidence should not be required dogmatically. There are many exceptions.

Three other types of supporting evidence have in the past given confidence to nativism in the explanation of a pattern of behavior. First is the presence of positive neurological signs, a good example of which is Huntington's chorea. Second is the presence of a measurable inborn error of metabolism, for which there are many examples from syndromes, recently identified, of mental deficiency associated with metabolic error (such as phenylketonuria). A third example of supporting evidence is that of a cytogenetic anomaly itself, in which the actual chromosomal error can be identified and visually displayed; an illustration which relates also to mental deficiency is Down's syndrome, with the redundancy of a number 21 chromosome.

Traits

Quite possibly we are only beginning to identify traits in human activity or behavior which, in the growing science or subscience of human behavior genetics, can be considered truly nativistic.

Color-blindness, for example, is well established as a genetic trait. In the past, it has been so much linked to physiological contexts that the fact of its determining a substantial portion of a color-blind person's behavior is easily overlooked. As proof, try talking to a color-blind person on matters of color discrimination, if he does not yet know of his color-blindness by testing, and if he does not know that you yourself are not color-blind by testing. Such a conversation provides opportunities for extraordinary disagreement, including angry attack and rage.

Taste acuity is another behavioral trait that is probably genetically determined—definitely so in some cases. Taste blindness for the bitter taste has been established in some instances of genetically induced hypothyroidism, and there are many other instances of a correlation of taste impairment with a disease syndrome.

Smell acuity might also be genetically determined to a greater extent than is realized at present. For example, some girls with the XO type of Turner's syndrome are deficient in smell acuity, and the mothers of these girls also have a degree of deficit.[6] A deficiency of the sense of smell has been found associated also with partial failure of pituitary gonadal stimulating hormone in boys (and sometimes girls) with delayed or imperfect puberty (Kallmann's syndrome). Smell acuity may also be related to genetics and behavior genetics insofar as there is a sex difference in smell acuity in favor of women; and in women themselves, the degree of acuity varies with the menstrual cycle.

Pain acuity is yet another of the behavioral traits that may be genetically determined. Petrie,[10] at Harvard, has shown that people may be classified according to their acuity for pain perception. She has delineated three types: the augmenters, the reducers, and the moderates. She has shown also that augmenters and reducers can be identified by psychophysical tests of several different modalities of sensory discrimination: for example, discrimination of differences in size or weight. Individuals are then found to correlate on these criteria with their discrimination of pain as either augmenters, reducers or moderates. Even more fascinating for the theory of behavior genetics is the suggestive finding that schizophrenic people may fall into the category of augmenters of sensation, including pain. They are people who need to escape from stimulation because the reverberation of a stimulus stays with them for too long. By contrast, people with so-called psychopathic personalities may tend to be reducers. They are people who need constant reinput of stimulation, since each stimulatory experience fades rapidly. It is obvious that an impressive theory of personality typology and behavior genetics could be constructed on the basis of this dichotomy.

Hearing acuity and hearing defects, it has long been known, may be associated with genetic determinants. As mentioned above, difficulty in auditory discrimination has been seen in individuals with Turner's syndrome. Whether one can hear properly has profound repercussions on all of one's behavior, especially in social interaction.

Locomotor activity is not a well-investigated trait among human beings, although some research has been done, for example, with regard to obese people. It is in animal running-wheel experiments by Curt Richter at Johns Hopkins, however, that locomotor activity has been shown clearly to be a genetically determined behavioral trait, and one that is sex differentiated.

Procedural Techniques: Family-tree Studies

The family-tree, or pedigree, method is the traditional one for establishing a hereditary origin for a trait, symptom or syndrome. When it works, it works well. But even for experts it has a disastrous built-in booby trap, that of "social contagion" or, one might say, social heredity. Manifestations of hysterial dissociation and suggestibility are classical examples. Everyone is familiar with family sayings that a child is dad's girl or mommy's boy, or that he takes after his uncle or some other member of the family. The search for resemblances begins at birth, when relatives proclaim that the baby takes after his father's side of the family, or his mother's. Everyone knows the story also of how a child has adopted some habit or mannerism of a family member. In an actual example, a mother has a phobia of poultry, having been terrorized as an infant by someone's rushing at her with a dead chicken. She avoids even the cooking of poultry and certainly the eating of any kind of bird. Her children are not like her except for one daughter, who incorporates this aspect of her mother's behavior into her own habit patterns and may even transmit it, as a habit, to someone in the succeeding generation.

The field of reading disability offers an excellent illustration of the danger of confusing heredity through the genetic code with heredity through the social code. There is one pedigree-type study by Hallgren[4] now widely cited, which claims to have proven a genetic basis for so-called developmental dyslexia. This study was not controlled for social transmission of attitudes toward school and learning to read. These social attitudes, or variables of personal interaction, are profoundly important in developmental dyslexia. They do not rule out the possiblility that a child who develops the condition may have a predisposition in the particular style of his cognitional functioning to become an underachiever, or one whose achievement is covert and self-sabotaged in its manifestation. However, the factors of social interactionism do make nonsense of any attempt to find a simple genetic mechanism for developmental dyslexia.

Sex Ratio Studies

In this method of genetic study, as in the pedigree method, the success of its application will depend on the trait under study. For example, in cases of the syndrome of testicular feminization (androgen insensitivity), the sex ratio will be disturbed in families that produce this condition. The number of normal girls is as expected, but the number of normal boys is too few. The explanation lies in the fact that children with the androgen-insensitivity syndrome have the morphologic appearance of girls and are considered to be girls, whereas actually they are genetically chromosomally males with the 46,XY chromosome constitution. Thus, even in the days before chromosome counting and karyotyping, it was possible to infer that these girls were genetic males, and not simply gonadal ones in whom there had been an error of embryonic differentiation of the anlagen of the ovaries: the gonads in these patients are not ovarian, but testicular in histological structure.

Such a neat demonstration is far less feasible in behavior genetics. For example, in 1940, Lang[7] (and several others since him) attempted to implicate a genetic mechanism for homosexuality by comparing the male-female ratio in the sibships of male homosexuals, with the ratio in the general population which, at birth, is 106 boys to 100 girls. He found some support for his hypothesis, as did his followers, in that the proportion of males was higher than expected. The different investigators obtained different figures, however, thus lessening support for confirmation of the hypothesis. The real pitfall, nonetheless, is not in the findings but in their use, for there is an alternative hypothesis which the investigators seem not to have entertained. One does not need to postulate a genetic tendency toward femininity in those brothers who constituted the excess of males in the families studied; one could postulate instead a tendency for an effeminate gender identity to differentiate more easily in boys whose families have a shortage of sisters and daughters. There are various subtle ways in which parents and siblings can put a premium on femininity when they are short a daughter or sister. The clues can be readily grasped by an infant or young child, who adjusts to them and is subsequently reinforced in his behavior by the approval and other rewards that may be bestowed upon him.

Evidence in support of this social interactional hypothesis, drawn from sex ratio data, was published by Slater in 1958.[12] He studied the sex ratios of the families not only of homosexuals, but also of male exhibitionists. In the exhibitionists' families, he found an excess of sisters, the ratio being 109 boys to 144 girls, instead of the expected 106 to 100. Surely the psychodynamic developmental mechanism here could be that a large audience of sisters in a family somehow induces the brother to be a show-off with his penis! If, subsequently, his psychosexual differentiation became anomalous, the anomaly might fairly easily stabilize as exhibitionism.

Ordinal Position Studies

The best known example of a genetic mechanism related to birth order is the occurrence of the chromosomal nondisjunction that produces mongolism or Down's syndrome. This nondisjunction, resulting in trisomy of chromosome

21, occurs more frequently in older mothers who have so-called change-of-life babies. I am not aware of any successful attempt to apply an ordinal-position hypothesis in behavior genetics as a means of attributing a genetic basis to a particular item or type of behavior.

Twin Studies

Twin studies have as venerable a history as pedigree studies in behavior genetics. I shall mention only a little recognized paradox, namely that *identical twins may be nonidentical.* It sounds a note of caution to the behavior genetics of twins.

The evidence for this paradox came from the work of cytogeneticists on monozygotic twins. In 1963, Bruins and coworkers[1] reported two sets of monozygotic twins that were discordant for trisomy 21—that is, for the supernumerary chromosome characteristic of Down's syndrome. They suggested that each twin of a pair had come from an original, single, fertilized egg, trisomic for chromosome G-21. At anaphase, when the zygote split and the twinning occurred, discordance for the extra chromosome also occurred. The resulting babies, with different numbers of chromosomes, qualify as being identical twins on the basis of the usual tests of blood grouping, dermatoglyphic patterns, and immunologic reactions, as tested by nonrejection of each other's skin grafts.

In 1966, Russell and coworkers[11] published a different kind of example of nonidentical identical twins. Both represented cases of gonadal dysgenesis and resembled Turner's syndrome. Twin one had an XO karyotype, that is, a chromosome count of 45,X, one of the X chromosomes being missing. Twin two had a karyotype which is an XO/XY mosaic; in other words, some of the cells are like those of twin one, whereas others have 46 chromosomes instead of 45, the extra chromosome being a Y instead of the X which would be expected in a girl with a female phenotype.

The children were verified for monozygosity. There was only one placenta present at birth. Palm prints and foot prints were as expected for monozygosity, as were the blood group antigens. There were many clinical similarities in physique and facial appearance, as normally found in monozygotic twins. The differences are, therefore, all the more remarkable.

Twin one had the gonadal streaks typical of Turner's syndrome, with internal female organs differentiated and external organs female, except for a slight enlargement of the clitoris. Twin two had, on the left side, a similar gonadal streak instead of an ovary or testis. On the right side, however, a gonad had differentiated and was in the inguinal canal. It proved to be an immature testis with seminiferous tubules, but no obvious Leydig cells. The uterus was not as well formed as in twin one, and the external organs were quite different; they were masculinized, with the result that the clitoris had the size of a small, improperly-formed penis. These sexual differences between the two children can be explained on the basis of the different karyotypes and their influence on embryonic differentiation.

With such remarkable differences in the sexual system, one would not be surprised to find quite different patterns of psychosexual differentiation in childhood, had the masculinized girl not been surgically corrected. There is still a possibility that differences in behavioral development may appear, insofar as the testicular structure in twin two may have exerted an organizing effect on the fetal brain, especially in the area of the hypothalamus, which would not have occurred in twin one.

The lesson to be learned from these children is that one should not automatically predict identical behavioral development in identical twins, because those whose behavior is different may, in fact, have differences in their genetic code. It will be rare in the study of, for example, schizopohrenic twins to be able to find differences in genetic code as dramatic as in this pair with the syndrome of gonadal dysgenesis. Here one complete chromosome made the difference. In the majority of cases, one would expect that only a small part of a chromosome might be involved. A small part, however, may be extremely influential in determining the behavior, or potential behavioral development, encoded in it.

Inbreeding

Animal Experiments. There is extensive literature on the selective inbreeding of animals for the production of special traits, including behavioral traits. The most common example is that of the temperament and behavior differences in dogs of purebred strain.

It is into the domain of science fiction that one projects the possibility of human behavioral-genetic inbreeding and the changes and improvements of the human race—perhaps its very viability even—that might thereby result. One can speculate, for example, on the consequence of breeding for a pure strain of sexual precocity and the abolition of childhood as we know it. People of this strain would be able to do their breeding in the early years of their lives and have all the years of adulthood unhampered by the obligations of childcare, except as grandparents.

Human Colonies. The nearest approach to pure-strain behavior genetics in human beings is not, of course, through experimental inbreeding, but through fortuitous inbreeding in isolated human colonies. Up to the present time, behavioral geneticists, as contrasted with medical geneticists, have not really taken advantage of isolated inbred colonies to any significant extent. Perhaps the reason is that they have not been able to establish, to their satisfaction, which traits should be enumerated or measured. One trait that has received some attention in inbred colonies is mental deficiency among the Amish of Pennsylvania and Ohio. The next step will be to view mental deficiency not only in terms of global patterns, but also as a matter of specific disability. Among the Amish of Pennsylvania, gross impairment of verbal intelligence, combined with a hearing deficit, has been demonstrated in some children, though constructional praxis and visual gnosis, as related to intelligent manipulations, were not impaired.[2]

Summary

Turner's (45,X) and Klinefelter's (47,XXY) syndromes are two cytogenetic syndromes, among others, that illustrate principles of behavioral cytogenetics. The testicular feminizing syndrome of androgen insensitivity in phenotypic females who are genetic males, is an example of a genetically based defect with profound sequelae on behavior.

Treatment of the genetic male fetus with antiandrogen and the genetic female fetus with androgen blocks the genotype from expressing itself and changes the phenotype of the external genitals to that of the opposite sex. By the use of hormones in experiments with fish larvae, it is possible to reverse the phenotype so completely as to produce XY females and XX males, both capable of breeding, and also to produce the new genotype of the YY male so as to compare its behavior with that of the normal XY male.

In human beings, the XYY syndrome in the male illustrates the importance of the principle of interactionism between genetics and environment. The principle of dichotomizing the inherited and the acquired is outmoded. Its replacement is a principle of trichotomy: heredity, critical period and environment, all three in interaction. The genetic code can express itself only with certain environmental limits, themselves phyletically set, beyond which the genetic norm of reaction is impaired, deformed or extinguished.

In genetic counseling, it is useful to distinguish "family-tree heredity" from sporadic heredity. In trying to separate nativism from environmentalism, particularly in behavioral genetics, one looks first at global patterns and then tries to analyze separate traits that are nativistic in the sense that, once established, they are relatively unsubject to environmental modification.

The major procedural techniques in behavioral genetics are family-tree studies, sex-ratio and ordinal-position studies, twin studies and inbreeding which in animals is experimentally designed and in human beings is the product of geographical or cultural isolation.

Acknowledgments

Mrs. Jean Booher assisted in the editing and final preparation of this manuscript. Dr. Shirley Borkowf kindly referred the teen-age XYY patient. Dr. D. Borgaonkar and Dr. P. Welch did the karyotyping of the XYY patients.

References

1. Bruins, J., Bolhius, J., von Bijlsma, J., and Nyenhuis, L.: Discordant monozygotic twins. Proceedings, XI International Congress of Genetics, The Hague, Netherlands, 1963.
2. Eldridge, R., Berlin, C. I., Money, J., and McKusick, V. A.: Cochlear deafness, myopia and intellectual impairment in an Amish family. *Arch. Otolaryng.* (Chicago) 88:49-54, 1968.
3. Gorski, R.: Sexual differentiation of the hypothalamus. In Mack, H. C. and Sherman, A. I. (eds.): *The Neuroendocrinology of Human Reproduction,* Springfield, IL, Charles C Thomas, 1971.
4. Hallgren, B.: Specific dyslexia ("congenital word-blindness")—A clinical and genetic study. *Acta Psychiat. Scand.* Supp. 65, 1950.
5. Hamilton, J. B., Walter, R. O., Daniel, R. M., and Mestler, G. E.: Competition for mating between ordinary and supermale Japanese Medaka fish. *Anim. Behav.* 17:168-176, 1969.
6. Henkin, R. I.: Abnormalities of taste and olfaction in patients with chromatin negative gonadal dysgenesis. *J. Clin. Endoc.* 27:1436-1440, 1967.
7. Lang, T.: Studies on the genetic determination of homosexuality. *J. Nerv. Men. Dis.* 92:55-64, 1940.
8. Neumann, F., and Elger, W.: Proof of the activity of androgenic agents on the differentiation of the external genitalia, the mammary gland and the hypothalamic-pituitary system in rats. *Amsterdam Excerpta Medica,* International Congress Series 101, Androgens in Normal and Pathological Conditions, pp. 169-185, 1965.
9. Neumann, F., and Elger, W.: Permanent changes in gonadal function and sexual behavior as a result of early feminization of male rats by treatment with an antiandrogenic steroid. *Endokrinologie* 50:209-225, 1966.
10. Petrie, A.: *Individuality in Pain and Suffering.* Chicago, University of Chicago Press, 1967.
11. Russell, A., Moschos, A., Butler, L. J., and Abraham, J. M.: Gonadal dysgenesis and its unilateral variant with testis in monozygous twins—related to discordance in sex chromosomal status. *J. Clin. Endocr.* 26:1282-1292, 1966.
12. Slater, E.: The sibs and children of homosexuals. In Smith, D. R. and Davidson, W. A. (eds.): Symposium on Nuclear Sex. New York, *Interscience,* 1958.
13. Witschi, E.: Hormones and embryonic induction. *Archives d'Anatomie Microscopique et de Morphologie Experimentale* 54:601-611, 1965.
14. Yamamoto, T.: Hormonic factors affecting gonadal differentiation in fish. *Gen. Comp. Endocr.* Supp. 1:311-345, 1962.
15. Young, W. C., Goy, R. W., and Phoenix, C. H.: Hormones and sexual behavior. In Money, J. (ed.): *Sex Research: New Developments.* New York, Holt, Rinehart and Winston, 1965.

Note

Originally published in *Seminars In Psychiatry,* 5:11-29, 1970, as an edited version of a tape-recorded lecture to first-year medical students. [Bibliog. #2.118]

Author's Comment:
XYY, The Law, and Forensic Moral Philosophy

A missing or an extra chromosome changes not only the body in a statistically predictable way, but also the mind, its brain, and brain-controlled behavior— thus casting serious doubts on the validity of the doctrine of free will and voluntary choice and control of behavior. The following editorial from *The*

Journal of Nervous and Mental Disease, 149:309-311, 1969 [Bibliog. #5.7], addresses this issue:

This year, 1969, marks the 10th anniversary of the now widespread technique of visualizing and counting chromosomes in man. Behavior cytogenetics has almost the same length of history, for it was early recognized that some abnormal karyotypes are associated with behavioral anomalies, specifically mental deficiency. In general, however, behavior specialists were slow to recognize the significance of the new technique of karyotyping human beings, perhaps because they were steeped in an anti-genetics tradition of social-environmental determinism.

The first report of an XYY karyotype was submitted by Sandberg *et al.* (2) in 1961. The XYY syndrome rested in quiet obscurity, however, until 1965, when Patricia Jacobs (1) and colleagues reported its excess incidence among very tall men held in an institution for dangerous criminals. The alleged link between masculine aggression and the extra Y chromosome became popular almost overnight, as the press carried headlines of rather spectacular murderers, suspected or proved to be XYY, in countries as far apart as Australia, France, and the United States. In the era of rioting, civil rights, and student unrest, violence was required to galvanize the public's attention to behavior cytogenetics. By contrast, the mental deficiency and many types of psychopathology, including some delinquency and crime, that were known for years to be associated with the XXY (Klinefelter's) syndrome had mobilized no one's attention to behavior cytogenetics.

The headlining of XYY reopens and dramatizes for the public the entire issue of personal guilt or blame; knowledge of right from wrong; will power, free will, and freedom of choice; and personal responsibility for one's own behavior.

My understanding of the civilization in which I participate is that we have been exposed to only two philosophies of human nature. One comes from the Old Testament, Plato, and St. Thomas Aquinas. It teaches the free will theory that man chooses his own actions. He is personally responsible for his own destiny. It is his personal duty and obligation to choose the narrow road of salvation and to reject the broad road of destruction. In the end, he will be forced to give an account of himself on the Day of Judgment. This is the judgmental philosophy of human nature on which the law is based.

The other philosophy of human nature is nonjudgmental and stems from Hippocrates, modern science, and Freudian psychiatry. It teaches a theory of determinism, including psychic determinism, namely, that man's motivation and behavior are, at least in part, determined by forces outside of his voluntary control. The theory of psychic determinism is, however, bedeviled by paradox: despite its label of determinism, it does not entirely relieve man of responsibility for his own behavior, for it half implies that man's duty is to make his unconscious motivations conscious. If need be, he should then revise, correct, and redirect them—presumably by will power, disguised officially under the name of insight.

The philosophy of our law courts, being primarily judgmental, commits its practitioners to finding and allocating blame. The exception, therefore, is traditionally imbedded in the famous M'Naghten rule which exempts a person from blame if he is incapable of knowing the difference between right and wrong—for this there is no valid test, only the opinion of ostensible experts who, under the conditions of the adversary system, do not readily agree.

Science, as compared with the law, is nonjudgmental. Medicine has an even longer history of nonjudgmentalism which has been recorded since Hippocrates. The physician betrays his trust if he blames a patient instead of treating him. For example, a physician does not scold a woman who becomes pregnant against medical advice; he supervises the pregnancy. Likewise, he treats a man who has venereal disease, even for the umpteenth time, or a man who mutilates himself, attempts suicide, or creates a factitious illness.

There really is no reconciliation of the judgmental philosophy of the law and the nonjudgmental philosophy of medicine as they now stand. That is why the XYY syndrome is proving to be forensically such an important test case. There is no doubt about the genetic defect. The question is: does this genetic defect lead directly to socially deviant and unacceptable behavior? There are those who argue that an XYY individual should not hide behind the excuse of his extra Y chromosome and must be accounted responsible for his actions.

Conversely, there are those who argue that, although the supernumerary Y chromosome does not cause crime, it exposes its possessor to an excessive risk of impaired personality differentiation and development. That is to say, the individual is, in some way or other as yet unspecifiable, more vulnerable to developing a behavior disorder, perhaps including impulsive aggression.

There almost certainly is a critical period early in life when vulnerability is at its maximum. If at that time in development the family and social environment are adverse, then the conjunction of vulnerability and adversity may produce a permanent damaging effect on all subsequent behavior.

In the XYY individual the permanent damaging effect may be in the form of a lowered threshold for temper tantrums, paroxysmal aggression, and unsolicited rage. (XYY men are *not* continuously aggressive.) The threshold may also be lowered for impulsively initiated sexual acts, some of which may be more or less exotic and unusual, depending perhaps partly on the response of the partner. Sudden and impulsive aggressive or sexual activity in the XYY male may be related to atypical brain function, since some such patients have an abnormal electroencephalogram, perhaps with actual epileptic seizures. The XYY syndrome syndrome thus relates the whole issue of moral and criminal responsibility to frankly abnormal brain functioning.

The XYY syndrome does not simply confront society with the question of whether the XYY individual is or is not responsible for his action if it is adjudged criminal. Rather it opens a much larger Pandora's box, namely the issue of what constitutes free will and moral responsibility of decision in all members of the human race, in all of their genetic and clinical variety.

It seems to me that man needs a new theory of human nature to present to the law, one that will take account of the fact that we are not all created equal, even before the eyes of the law. Some have more, some less, sense of moral judgment; some have more, and some less, resource for self-regulation of behavior. The differences sometimes, but not always, are a matter of heredity and chromosomes. Events before birth may have a lasting effect, as may events accompanying birth, to say nothing of what happens at critical periods of early development, both physically and socially. The brain, of course, is the focal organ of behavior, so that all behavior, good or bad, acceptable or not, eventually will be traceable to brain functioning.

Meantime, since there are very few occasions when science can predictably intervene to change behavior at its source in the brain, society needs to reexamine its policy of attributing equal responsibility to each individual for his own behavior. We need, in fact, nothing short of a complete redefinition of the Old Testament-based, legal philosophy of responsibility and punishment.

The legal system of the pre-Roman, pre-Anglo-Saxon Celts, it is said, was based on restitution, not retribution. To be adjudged guilty was to be required to make amends, not to be made to suffer simply for the sake of punishment. Here, perhaps, is a good principle on which to build penal reform.

In the absence of reform, one might envisage a reactionary nightmare of medievalism in which all XYY males would be adjudged as dangerous to society and exterminated. Even if the frequency of occurrence of XYY is as high as one in 500 births, as may be the case, the loss of manpower could easily be tolerated, economically speaking. What could not be tolerated would be the loss to society of its own moral conscience and its sense of human decency.

It is from the sense of human decency that man cries out for penal reform, away from the archaic and medieval penal philosophy that our society still lives by. Then to be found guilty will be equivalent to being found in need of rehabilitation or, in certain intractable disorders of behavior, in need of continuous surveillance with various degrees of restriction on personal judgment and choice of behavior.

In this new era of envisaged reform, today's question of whether the XYY male is or is not responsible for his behavior, including his crimes, will appear naive and oversimplified. The question will be: How much responsibility can he be *entrusted* with and what provisos and limitations are needed?

Then it will be possible, at long last, for the judgmentalism of the law and the nonjudgmentalism of science and medicine, represented by psychology and sociology, to join in the bond of a common morality and philosophy of responsibility, instead of being polarized and incompatible, as they are at present.

Will the extra Y chromosome of the XYY syndrome prove to be the catalyst of all this change?

References

1. Jacobs, P. A., Brunton, M., Melville, M. M., Brittain, R. P., and McClemont, W. F. Aggressive behavior, mental sub-normality and the XYY male. *Nature,* 208:1351-1352, 1965.
2. Sandberg, A. A., Koepf, G. F., Ishihara, T., and Hauschka, T. S. An XYY human male. *Lancet,* 2:488-489, 1961.

SEVEN

A Paradigm Shift from Heredity/Environment to Heredity/Critical-Period/Environment in Sexology

Psychoneuroendocrine Illustrations

Descartes gave the body to science, the mind to the church, and only the pineal gland to the unity of bodymind. Today, the disunity of body and mind persists in many bipolar guises: biological/psychological; organic/psychogenic; innate/ acquired; heredity/environment; and of special pertinence here, nature/nurture.

Nature is not the antithesis of nurture, however. The two may work in concert, and when they do so at a crucial developmental period, the old two-term paradigm is replaced by the new three-term one: nature/critical-period/nurture. The product of this concerted action, as has long been taken for granted in embryology, may in itself become established as the nature with which nurture yet again works in concert at a later crucial period in development. For example, the thalidomide baby learns to use a prosthetic limb.

The three-term paradigm of nature/critical-period/nurture applies also in behavioral science, as evidenced in the ethological concept of imprinting. In imprinting, a stimulus from the social environment (nurture) acts in concert with nature at a crucial period, and leaves a permanent effect, or imprint, on behavior.

From psycho/neuroendocrinology comes another example, namely, the syndrome of abuse dwarfism, in which abuse and neglect from the social environment (nurture) acting in concert with the pituitary-hypothalamic axis over a crucial period of development arrests the secretion of growth hormone and other pituitary hormones (Powell, Brasel, Raiti, & Blizzard, 1967). The outcome is an arrest of statural growth and eventually also of the onset of puberty. There is a concomitant arrest of intellectual growth and behavioral maturation, the brain correlates of which have not yet been ascertained. All three arrests—statural, intellectual and behavioral—may become permanently impaired, though some catchup growth takes place after the child is rescued from abuse and neglect (Money, 1977: Money, Annecillo, & Kelly, 1983).

Another example comes from experimental animal sexology, namely, the syndrome of induced hermaphroditism in sheep (Short and Clarke, undated). In this syndrome, the genetic sex and internal morphological sex (nature) is female, but the experimental injection of the hormone, testosterone, from the external environment (nurture) into the pregnant mother at a crucial period of gestation permanently masculinizes the external genitals and the brain's programing of subsequent courtship and mating behavior when the offspring reaches adulthood.

97

In human beings there are analogous syndromes, one of which is the spontaneously occurring adrenogenital syndrome of hermaphroditism (Simpson, 1980). In this syndrome, genetic programing (nature) to differentiate a 46,XX conceptus into a female is hormonally thwarted, as in the sheep, except that the masculinizing hormone is released into the internal environment (nurture) of the fetus, via the bloodstream, by its own malfunctioning adrenocortical glands at a crucial period of prenatal sexual differentiation of the external genitalia and the brain.

Whereas the hermaphroditic sheep is a prenatally-programed, hormonal robot, so to speak, the hermaphroditic human being is not. Postnatally, there is another crucial period during which nature acts in concert with nurture to determine the final sexual and erotic status. At this phase of development, nature is represented by the masculinized status of the external genitalia, the hormonal function of the adrenocortices, and also the sexual brain's readiness to continue masculine differentiation, if the baby is assigned and habilitated as a boy instead of a girl. Nurture is represented by input from the social environment as determined by the assigned sex and rearing, and by externally applied surgical and hormonal intervention for habilitation as either a boy or a girl.

The relative effects of nature and nurture can be observed in matched pairs of hermaphrodites, concordant for prenatal history, but discordant for postnatal history. That is to say, one of the pair grows up and is habilitated as a boy, and the other as a girl.

In three cases, 46,XX adrenogenital babies born with a penis (with penile urethra) and empty scrotum were habilitated anatomically, hormonally and by rearing as boys. Despite their chromosomal and original gonadal status as female, they grew up to be, except for sterility, indistinguishable from other men in their G-I/R (gender-identity/role), erotosexual practices included (Money and Daléry, 1976).

By contrast, babies with the same syndrome, some born with a penis and penile urethra, who were habilitated surgically, hormonally, and by rearing as girls, grew up differently (see Chapter 23). They were not like men, but women. However, erotosexually, some of them had a lesbian or bisexual status.

Thirty cases of the 46,XX adrenogenital syndrome in babies assigned, reared, and habilitated as girls were followed into adulthood (unpublished). In teenage, few of them made disclosures concerning romantic and erotosexual imagery, and they were atypical among their mates in being late to begin romantic and dating life. As they became older, more of them made personal erotosexual disclosures. Eleven of the 30 (37%) disclosed themselves to have had bisexual imagery and/or practice. Five (17%) in this group rated themselves as exclusively (n=2) or predominantly (N=3) lesbian. Only 12 (40%) of the 30 claimed to be exclusively heterosexual. The remaining 7 (23%) were noncommittal. These percentages were spectacularly dissimilar ($p < .001$) from those obtained from a clinical comparison or control group.

References

Money, J. The syndrome of abuse dwarfism (psychosocial dwarfism or reversible hyposomato-tropinism). Behavioral data and case report. *American Journal of Diseases of Children,* 131:508-513, 1977.

Money, J., Annecillo, C., and Kelly, J. F. Growth of intelligence: Failure and catchup associated respectively with abuse and rescue in the syndrome of abuse dwarfism. *Psychoneuroendocrinology,* 8:309-319, 1983.

Money, J., Annecillo, C., and Kelly, J. F. Abuse-dwarfism syndrome: After rescue, statural and intellectual catchup growth correlate. *Journal Clinical Child Psychology,* 12:279-283, 1983.

Money, J. and Daléry, J. Iatrogenic homosexuality: Gender identity in seven 46, XX chromosomal females with hyperadrenocortical hermaphroditism born with a penis, three reared as boys, four reared as girls. *Journal of Homosexuality,* 1:357-371, 1976.

Powell, G. F., Brasel, J. A., Raiti, S. and Blizzard, R. M. Emotional deprivation and growth retardation simulating idiopathic hypopituitarism. II. Endocrinologic evaluation of the syndrome. *New England Journal of Medicine,* 276:1279-1283, 1967.

Short, R. V., and Clarke, I. J. *Masculinization of the Female Sheep,* 16mm sound film, MRC Reproductive Biology Unit, 2 Forrest Road, Edinburgh Ehl 2QW, Scotland, U.K., undated.

Simpson, J. L. Disorders of sex chromosomes and sexual differentiation. In *Gynecologic Endrocrinology* (J. J. Gold and J. B. Josimovich, eds., 3rd edition). Hagerstown, Harper & Row, 1980.

Note

Written for the Symposium, "History, Heredity-Environment Interpretations, Ontogeny and Authenticity in Literature," Jerry Hirsch, Chairman, American Psychological Association, Ninetieth Annual Convention, Washington, D.C., 8/26/82. Expanded in the Newsletter of the Association of Sexologists, Vol. 2, No. 2, February/March, 1983. [Bibliog. #4.96]

EIGHT

Longitudinal Studies in Clinical Psychoendocrinology and Sexology: Methodology

Abstract

There are five universal exigencies of being human, against which a person's existence can be evaluated: pairbondage, troopbondage, abidance, ycleptance, and foredoomance. They constitute a template from which a standardized agenda or schedule of inquiry is generated, as needed, for a particular research investigation. The schedule of inquiry is painstakingly designed ahead of time so as to ensure coverage of all the variables relevant to a particular study. For economy of expense and effort, subjects conclude their own prior interview by summarizing it on tape, with the interviewer making a written record, verbatim, of what will become subheadings in the transcript. Inquiry progresses from an open-ended to a forced choice interrogatory. Topics in the public domain open the way to inquiry on personally sensitive issues. So also do parables drawn from actual cases and used as personalized narrative projective tests. A cumulative record, covering as many as 25 years, is indexed so that relevant material can be located, abstracted and classified for any particular study. A jury of two or more then uses the abstracted data to fill out a prepared data schedule, using its own standardized scoring or rating criteria. By contrast, an ordinary questionnaire uses standardized questions and each subject applies his or her own unstandardized scoring or rating criteria in answering them. In the final step the jury's ratings are tabulated on a master chart that consolidates the scores of a group of subjects and controls, ready for statistical analysis.

Introduction

Over the years, I've received from students and qualified professionals scores, if not hundreds of requests for the instruments or tools used to measure gender identity, sexual desire, aggressiveness, and other inferential constructs used in psychoendocrinology and sexology. In my lexicon, it is presumptuous and grandiose to use the terms, instruments and tools, as synonyms not for bench-science apparatus, but for clinical tests. Clinical psychoendocrinology and sexology are reliant for the most part on psychological tests. To call them instruments or tools gives a false sense of mensurational accuracy.

Three Categories of Test

There are three categories of test used in clinical psychoendocrinology and sexology. In category one is the test as a standardized sampling of a psychological function demonstrated in the here and now—for example, the intelligence test. It tests intelligence by requiring responses to questions and problems that necessitate the use of intelligence for their solution; and it presumes that the score is predictive of the level at which intelligence can be expected to function in general.

In category two is the test as a standardized scale of opinion, attitude, or self-evaluation—for example the personality inventory or questionnaire. Each item requires a forced-choice response of the either/or, multiple-choice, or numerical-rating type, thus limiting the range of information a respondent may provide. It is presumed that the items test not only verbalization but also the deeds or actions which that verbalization purports to represent.

In category three is the test as an interview with a standardized agenda or schedule of inquiry. It is also known as a structured interview, to differentiate it from a nondirective interview. The standardization in this type of test applies not to the fixed wording of both the questions and the forced-choice responses, as in a standardized scale, but to the agenda and to the scoring criteria used by the professionals who do the scoring.

Standardized-Agenda Interview

To avoid the stiltedness of fixed-word questions, each topic in an interview with a standardized agenda is deliberately introduced with open-ended inquiry. Open-endedness allows the respondent free rein to define the topic in terms of what it means to him/her personally. Subsequently, the inquiry becomes less open-ended, until eventually each particular topic may be closed with an interrogatory, employing forced-choice questions. Such questions are designed to get specific responses to specific details of chronology, prevalence, location, frequency, measurements, and so on.

An open-ended inquiry may be as straightforward as an announcement of the next topic on the standardized schedule of inquiry—for example, "Play. Tell me about your child's play." This straightforward approach is based on the premise that the topic is in the public domain and poses no threat of stigmatization, self-incrimination or breach of confidentiality.

In some instances, it is necessary to specify, not assume, that a topic is indeed in the public domain, even though it is also partly in the private domain. For example: "The bombing of abortion clinics has been in the news recently." If the respondent indicates familiarity with this news, it is then feasible to inquire as to his/her ideas about it. Thereafter, it becomes feasible to lead into more personal reference with respect to past history and future prospects regarding decisions about abortion.

If a topic is not in the public domain so far as a particular respondent knows, but is taboo-ridden and potentially stigmatizing and self-incriminating, then that topic may be opened up by utilizing what I have conceptualized as the parable technique. The parable is a story based on either a single or a composite case, selected because of the likelihood that it may have personal application to the respondent. For example, in counseling a teenaged or young adult woman with a history of treatment for the syndrome of congenital virilizing adrenal hyperplasia, I may quote from a case that illustrates my own research findings regarding the relative prevalence of bisexual fantasy and/or lesbian experience in the syndrome. The quote would draw attention to the fact that, as a teenager, the girl in that case was afflicted with extreme reticence and could not say anything about her own romantic, sexual, and erotic development until she had sufficient evidence that I could be entrusted with what she had to reveal. For the listener, the parable of this case serves as a narrative projective test, designed to elicit her own response, without imposing a forced-choice answer. At one extreme, she may respond with elective mutism, or with flippant evasiveness. At the other extreme, she may unlock and tell of the solitary torment she has been going through because of an unrequited and secret love affair with a female friend. Without the parable, she would not have been able to unlock, for she would have lacked evidence of my competence to be nonjudgmental in hearing her self-disclosure. She needed evidence that my ears would not explode when they heard her story!

The sportscaster technique with a detailed play-by-play account is the one to use when the informant is recounting a personal experience or encounter. Otherwise the account becomes too global and diffuse. Especially if the account involves an adversary relationship, the raw data become lost in inferential attribution of motivation and intent, in which there is a hidden agenda, namely, to cast the interviewer in the role of juror and to win a judgment against the adversary. Hearing the adversary's version helps to establish impartiality, all the more so if he/she also adopts the sportscaster technique of reporting.

Schedule of Inquiry

The scope of the agenda on a schedule of inquiry is governed by the scope of the hypotheses and concepts under scrutiny. It may be restricted, as for example, to information concerning the experience of erotic climax or orgasm. Such might be the case should a project be limited to the orgasmic effects of feminizing surgery, in a comparison of three syndromes, namely, 46,XX congenital virilizing adrenal hyperplasia; 46,XY hermaphroditism assigned and habilitated as female; and 46,XY male-to-female transexualism. Even so, it would be necessary to obtain ancillary information regarding sexual learning in childhood; erotic emancipation in adulthood; range of erotic practices; history of psychopathology that might affect the sex life; and history of love affairs and erotic pairbonding. Ideally, the sexual partner should supplement the patient's self-report. There should also be a supplemental health history, including the history of surgery, medications, and self-administered drugs.

A schedule of inquiry that has a restricted agenda is feasible when the research design is cross-sectional, which itself presupposes a sufficiently large sample population. By contrast, when the research design is longitudinal and developmental, the less restrictive the agenda on the schedule of inquiry, the greater the likelihood of recording and preserving information on variables that, only with the knowledge of hindsight, will prove essential to the formulation of hypotheses and explanations. There is, when a new field of inquiry is being developed, a need for a Lewis and Clark expedition, also known pejoratively by its detractors as a fishing expedition. To illustrate, when I first began research on the psychoendocrinology of hermaphroditism, I did not have a hypothesis concerning the function of juvenile sexual rehearsal play—nor even a name for it. However, there was a place under sex education in the schedule of inquiry for playing "doctor" and other sexual games, so that relevant information did get preserved.

The surest way to guarantee that information will be retrievable as given is to record it, verbatim. Videotaping preserves the image of the speaker along with the spoken word, but there is no system for transcribing the visual content in the same way as the auditory. With a schedule of inquiry, an interview can be recorded so that, with each change of topic, the words that indicate the new topic are simultaneously spoken and written verbatim on a sheet of paper, in capitals if spoken by the interviewer, and in lower case if by the respondent. These words then constitute subheadings. They are seen by the typist, and listened for. When they are heard, they are set in the transcript as subheadings. They facilitate the subsequent location and retrieval of information in the cumulative record, as well as the formation of a table of contents and an index.

There are some interviews, especially those with great emotional momentum, that need to be recorded from beginning to end. There are others that become too long-winded, digressive, and redundant. To record them in full would be uneconomic in both transcription cost and the time required of those who subsequently read them. In such instances, the interviewer keeps a list of topics covered, and concludes by enlisting the respondent to share the task of making a summary interview. The interviewer abridges for the summary those parts of the interview that were too wordy, and the respondent recapitulates those parts in which his/her own words are essential. The instances are rare in which a respondent is not able to say for the second time what he said the first. The proceedings of an hour can thus be reduced to fifteen or twenty minutes. With the microphone live, the summary interview may be extended to introduce additional topics for which the spontaneity of the first response is required.

Those who use a tape recorder as an electronic extension of their own memory use the same style of talking whether the microphone is on or off.

The respondent follows suit, and only rarely elects to have the microphone off. Listening to, or reading the transcripts of one's own interviews serves also as a valuable self-corrective.

Universals of the Agenda

In the case of hermaphroditism and other birth defects of the sex organs, a prospective, longitudinal study of development begins prenatally with the gestational history and continues with the clinical and social events of the birth history, and thereafter. As in astronomy, the investigator has no control over the timing of some events, nor of the variables that govern them and their consequences. He cannot design an experiment in which all variables are held constant except the one or two he is experimentally manipulating. In his research, he must cast a wide net, and catch as many variables as possible, so that he will not lose any that might subsequently prove important.

Confronted with this challenge, I have formulated the concept of five universal exigencies of being human (Money, 1957; 1984). They constitute a template against which to analyze the progress and trace the continuity of any biography in all of its components, clinical and nonclinical. They constitute also a template that, in its five categories, allows a place for all of the variables that may affect the development of an individual human life. Though it does not guarantee that all of the variables will be discovered, it does offer a guarantee against inadvertent omissions in the agenda of a schedule of inquiry.

The five universal exigencies of being human are, by name: pairbondage; troopbondage; abidance; ycleptance; and foredoomance.

Pairbondage pertains to parent-child and lover-lover bonding. Troopbondage pertains to becoming a member of a flock, herd, troop, or family. Abidance pertains to food, shelter, and clothing, and being sustained in an ecological niche. Ycleptance pertains to being named, nicknamed, classified, branded, labeled, or typecast. Foredoomance pertains to death as one's ultimate destiny, and to vulnerability to injury, defect or disease—either one's own, or someone else's.

The Psychohormonal History

It is self-evident that the five universal exigencies of being human involve not only the one person who might become a patient, but many others of the family and the troop as well. To illustrate: in the case of hermaphroditism and other birth defects of the sex organs, it is self-evident that professionals are initially involved as much with the parents as the neonate, and that they consult not with the newborn baby, but with the parents. Thus, the postnatal longitudinal biographical history of a person born with a birth defect of the sex organs (and of everyone else, as well) begins with reports from the person who did the delivery, and with reports from the parents of their experience of the delivery and what happened to them in the next few days or weeks.

The records from the prenatal and neonatal period are the beginning of what will become, in the long term, the consolidated, developmental history. The components of this consolidated history comprise the intramural clinical and laboratory history from each division of the hospital in which the individual has been seen; the surgical history; the history from extramural clinics and hospitals; the history from social service, penal, academic, and other institutions in which the person has been known; and the psychohormonal unit's history.

The psychohormonal history, like the rest of the clinical history, is cumulative over time and changes of personnel. The potentially adverse effects of personnel changes, which are inevitable in a longitudinal study, are minimized by having all interviews subdivided or shared among two or more interviewers. In this way, the patient and family establish a sense of belonging in the psychohormonal unit, and not just to a single person. They also have a chance to reveal themselves differently to different interviewers—male and female, black and white, old and young. Cohesiveness and unity among interviewers is achieved by means of a joint session of summing up, in which interviewers, patient, and family all participate. This joint session circumvents problems of secrecy and evasiveness.

The joint interview allows a child, as well as an older patient, to be an active collaborator in his/her case management, and not a victim of what may be experienced as nosocomial stress and abuse. It allows diagnostic and prognostic information to be given incrementally and in such a way that it does not traumatize, but has a therapeutic and preventive effect. It prevents the possibility of traumatic disclosure later in life when, under the freedom of information act, any patient has legal access to his/her own medical files. Even earlier in life, a young person can be traumatized by inadvertently overhearing personal clinical information, or by seeing his/her own clinical files. The young are also likely to read or to see on television documentaries of their own syndrome, or to study it in biology class.

There is a more traumatic and a less traumatic way of presenting even bad news. For example, it is traumatizing to tell a girl that she is a male with male chromosomes, but not traumatizing to explain that nature creates some XY girls and some XX boys among many other varieties of karyotype, and that she is an XY girl—and so on.

Professionals may avoid the entrapment of pejorative, stigmatizing, and traumatizing idiom, which is derived from the search for pathology, by writing all reports in the expectation that a copy will eventually be read by the patient. This criterion is automatically satisfied when the summary of an interview is made in the patient's presence with him/her collaborating.

Longitudinal Research Reports

The consolidated history, not the patient, is the data base for outcome research. Each specific outcome study begins with identifying those records that qualify for inclusion, according to the criteria established with respect to diagnosis, treatment history, present age, geographical availability, and such like. The pages of each record are sequenced chronologically and according to the classification of a standard Table of Contents (for example, Endocrine History, Surgical History, Hospitalization History, School History, Social Agency History, Psychological Testing, Psychohormonal Unit Interviews, and so on). The pages are then numbered so that the history can be indexed in the way that a book is indexed.

The index is a conceptual index, not a terminological one. The conceptual categories are decided upon in relationship to the purposes and hypotheses of each particular investigation. They are discussed, critiqued, and revised in detail, ahead of time. They derive from the basic theoretical issue or issues involved. For example, the conceptual categories in one investigation may be: gender-transposition; neonatal dissension regarding assigned sex; marital-sexual discord; and family psychopathology; whereas in another investigation they may be romantic dating, age of onset of puberty, academic progress, and history of sexual learning.

After the history is indexed, the next step is to tabulate on a personal data sheet the data relevant to each conceptual category, and then to reduce the content of the tabulation to a number. The simplest reduction is binary, that is a rating of present or absent with respect to a given characteristic. The next degree of complexity is a three-point rating scale, such as, strong/medium/weak, or severe/moderate/mild. A rating scale of more than three points is not excluded, but is typically avoided because the degree of precision it implies turns out to be spurious. If there is a problem of agreement betwen two independent raters, then another rater, or more than one, is coopted to form a jury. If the jury remains divided, then the rating is put into a special category, namely, undecided.

The aforesaid method of reducing data has an advantage over subjects' (patients') own ratings, for they have each their own subjective criterion standards. When the same two or three trained personnel do the ratings they bring the same criterion standards to each case. This is the objective type of scoring that is routine in, for example, the Wechsler Intelligence Scales.

This objective scoring method is eminently suited to longitudinal studies based on clinic histories. The developmental history of each individual is unique, despite the shared commonality of the same diagnosis, prognosis, and treatment. The clinical history of each individual differs, especially with respect to chronology, frequency, and duration of contacts. It cannot be otherwise when the subjects are human beings who cannot be experimentally controlled and regimented like experimental animals.

Each clinical history of each individual differs also with respect to the informant and the source of information from which a given rating is derived. For example, regarding parenting behavior manifested in juvenile play, the source may be direct observation of the child, the written report of a case worker, the taped and transcribed interview with a parent, or the retrospective recall (taped and transcribed) of the patient in later years. Either singly or in combination, these various sources can be accommodated to when the aforesaid method of rating is employed.

The final step in the consolidation of tabulated scores from each case into a master table which shows the number of subjects (or responses) in each category. These data can then be subjected to statistical evaluation. They lend themselves typically to simple statistical procedures, chiefly Chi-square, and T-test, in accordance with the standard methodology of science, though multivariate analysis is sometimes applicable.

References

Money, J. Five universal exigencies, indicatrons, and sexological theory. *Journal of Sex and Marital Therapy*, 10:229-238, 1984.
Money, J. *Psychologic Study of Man*. Springfield, IL, Charles C Thomas, 1957.

Note

Written for the International Symposium on Male Sexual Differentiation, organized by Claude J. Migeon, June 15-17, 1985, at the John Hopkins University and Hospital. Published also in *Journal of Developmental and Behavioral Pediatrics*, 7:31-34, 1986. [Bibliog. #2.300]

NINE

Five Universal Exigencies, Indicatrons and Sexological Theory

Abstract

In sexology as science, except for the special case of introspection, on which the defense of mind-body dualism rests, raw data are obtained, like the raw data of all the other sciences, through the special senses and exteroceptive observation.

In Table 1 are shown the verbs and nouns that are needed to relate the five special senses of the observer to the observed, as stimuli are transmitted to their destination from their source. Some of these terms sound somewhat unidiomatic, which is no accident. It is precisely because vernacular English was not designed for scientific usage that some needed terms have been lacking—to the detriment of theoretical mindbody unity.

Another missing term in sexology as science is a generic one for any type of unit of raw data. The gap can be filled with the new term, indicatron, in recognition of the fact that sexology's units of raw data all serve to indicate something. Since exactly the same applies to the raw data of any science, then sexology and the other sciences share the same premise. The sociopsychological and the biomedical sciences from which sexology conjointly derives are not separated as being of the mind and the body respectively. They are unified in indicatronics, the science of indicatrons, in which the split between body and mind is semantically irrelevant.

The indicatrons of sexology can be classified under five universal exigencies of being human: being pairbonded, troopbonded, abidant, yclept, and foredoomed.

Introspection and the Mind

Hermeneutically, if I say that I can have an orgasm better than you can, then I can defy you to prove otherwise. You can never inhabit my orgasm and know it at first hand. The same would apply, had I been born with a congenital absence of the sense of pain (as was one of my patients who underwent a testicular biopsy without anesthesia or analgesia). You can never inhabit my pain and know it at first hand. Less esoterically, had I been born color blind, only if you were color blind too could you dare to assume that your visual universe and mine were shared.

My premise is that it is a courtesy of empathy we extend to one another when we assume that our introspective universes of discourse are identical. The assumption is wrong, no doubt, many more times than we ever discover.

It is a courtesy, therefore, if I allow you to attribute to me, and vice versa, certain projections from your own introspective universe—projections about the way it feels to be joyful, sad, angry, humiliated, afraid, guilty, ashamed, creative, amused, limerent (love-smitten), erotically aroused, ecstatic, born-again; or to have an ego, a conscience, an unconscious, and, yes, indeed consciousness itself.

Introspective Projections

One knows today that it is Freud who, as recently as this century, bears chief responsibility for projecting into your soul (his term) and mine his formulations of its preconscious and unconscious, its id and superego, and its ego as the self of consciousness. He bears no responsibility for the soul itself, nor for the spirit, nor for the conscious mind or consciousness: they had all been projected into place since time unrecorded, along with various resident demons and spirits.

Most probably, some prehistoric ruler-priest, or conclave of ruler-priests, striving for understanding, created these metaphysical concepts, just as Freud created his more recent ones. They became imbedded in the very idiom of the vernacular language, so that there is no escape from them in everyday life. To question them is heresy!

Cartesian Dualism

Descartes, in the 17th century, was guilty of this heresy, but he adroitly protected himself by separating mind and body at the site of the pineal gland, keeping the body for science, and returning custody of the mind, and with it the soul, to the church. It is this Cartesian dualism that still haunts us today. Among sexologists, it manifests itself in the split between psychogenic and organic causation.

To digress, briefly, now into biography: I align myself among those greatly concerned with mindbody unity. It was imperative for me to do so when I began my career in psychohormonal research, because it is impossible to operate in two universes of discourse simultaneously. Hormones and behavior can be construed as interactive, but hormones interact with mental and spiritual forces no better than they do with the occult and astrological.

Motivational Teleology

Teleology appears in sexology in the guise of motivation theory borrowed from psychology and psychiatry. Hormone theory is ateleological. It replaces teleology with cybernetic feedback theory. Teleology and nonteleology do not mix. My solution has been to eschew motivation theory, and to use interactionism, or cybernetic feedback theory instead.

Motivational teleology in psychology and its subspecialty, sexological psychology, has its origins in self-observation or introspection which is a special case of the principle of solipsism. It is on this principle that the defense of mind-body dualism exists.

The solipsism of introspection directly affects only psychology as a science, and the other sciences only indirectly. Introspection provides raw data from a sample the size of which, by definition, is precisely and invariably never larger than one. If you are this one person, and if you are the psychologist as scientist, then as soon as you enlarge your sample to include others than yourself, then your raw data are not obtained introspectively by yourself. Instead, they are obtained like the raw data of all the other sciences, through your own special senses from sources beyond the self—that is to say, by extrospective observation.

The Lexicon of Exteroception

Exteroceptive raw data of sexology as a psychologist's science are seen and heard. To a lesser extent, some data are tacted (touched or felt), and to a still lesser extent smelled or tasted. To see, to hear, to tact, to smell, and to taste—whereas these are the five verbs, there are not in vernacular usage all five corresponding nouns (Table 1).

The logical symmetry of science requires, however, that the substantive unit of seeing should be a see; of hearing, a hear; of tacting, a tact; of smelling, a smell; and of tasting, a taste. These are the generic names of the units of raw

TABLE I

10 Nouns and 10 Verbs Needed for Scientific Precision in
Registering Raw Data (Indicatrons) from Source to Destination

AT THE DESTINATION		AT THE SOURCE	
Verb	Noun	Verb	Noun
to see	a see	to show	a show
to hear	a hear	to say	a say
to tact	a tact[1]	to touch	a touch
to smell	a smell	to odor[2]	an odor
to taste	a taste	to flavor	a flavor

[1]Tact, the noun, is an old synonym for a touch or a touching. It is an analogue of contact. Hence the feasibility of the verb, to tact. To tact something is to feel it, but feel has too many other meanings to be precise enough. A tact encompasses more than the recognition of a touch in its restricted sense, as in she tacted the touch of his finger on her arm. A tact is comprised of a range of qualities: pressure, temperature, resistance, consistency, moisture, motion, tickle, rub, scratch, prick, cut, etc.

[2]The creation of the verb, to odor, permits the giving off of an odor (to be smelly), to be distinguished from the recognition of it (to smell it). The Anglo-Saxon terms would be to stink and a stink, but they imply too strongly in current usage that the smell is offensive.

data at their destination, that is to say as you or I register or know them subjectively—with or without the aid of instrumentation.

Since there is no guarantee of equivalency between data as received at their destination and as transmitted at their source, the logic of science further requires names for the units of raw data at their source. It is idiomatic to see a sight, an image, a show, a display, and so on; and to hear a sound, a voice, a saying, a speech, a story, and so on. But none of these nouns exactly fits the bill, for each is too specific and fails to be all-inclusive enough. Nouns that would be sufficiently inclusive could be formed by adding to nouns the prefix en- (to make happen), as in to ensee, to enhear, to entact, to ensmell, and to entaste, meaning to send out a signal that for the recipient is, respectively, a see, a hear, a tact, a smell, and a taste. These words do not, however, sound idiomatic enough to be adopted in usage.

An alternative is to take nouns that are already currently accepted, namely, a show, a say, a touch, an odor, and a flavor, and to use them as verbs—to show, to say, to touch, to odor, and to flavor (Table I).

Indicatrons

Regardless of their source of origin, the units of the raw data of psychology, including the psychology of sex as science have no generic name. Behaviors, the plural term of recent vintage, and its derivatives like verbal behaviors, and sexual behaviors, do not rectify the deficit. In recognition of the fact that psychology's units of raw data all serve to *indicate* something or other to the psychologist as scientist, they can all be categorized as *indicatrons*. The principle under which they are subsumed can go by the name of *indicatronics*.

The criterion of an indicatron is that it can be, if visible or audible, recorded on video and audiotape, respectively, independently of the meaning attributed to it. So also can temperature. The indicatron is primary, the meaning secondary. Instrumentation to record touches, odors, and flavors independently of their meaning is presently either rudimentary or lacking. Nonetheless, the principle of the separation of the indicatron from its meaning still holds. Without adherence to this principle, sexology fails to be a science.

The same indicatron may have more than one meaning attributed to it. The meaning is thus not a primary datum but a secondary one. In fact, it is a first order interpretation derived from the indicatron. To illustrate; a videographic still shot of a gaping mouth and a face and neck muscularly tensed and strained may be interpreted to mean agony, rage, terror, ecstasy, breathless exhaustion, or sexual orgasm. The actual interpretation requires the added evidence of more indicatrons, either shown or heard.

For science, it is an error to use a first order interpretation as if it were a primary datum or indicatron. This error is endemic in psychology and the behavioral sciences, sexology included, to a far greater degree than in the other sciences.

As a principle, indicatronics is an analogue of ethics, insofar as it applies across all sciences. In all of the sciences, not only in psychology, the raw data, whether obtained with or without instrumentation, are indicatrons that serve to indicate something. Psychology, traditionally the science of mind, is thus not set apart from the other sciences. In sexology, for example, psychology is not set apart from endocrinology. Indicatronically, the two are compatible, and can be united as psychoendocrine sexology. So it is that the polarity between mind and body can be circumvented and rendered scientifically irrelevant and obsolete.

Obsolescence of Dualism

Obsolescence of mind-body dualism in science is not only long overdue but now, more than ever, inexorable. In the emerging era of sexual neuroscience, the possibility of definitively demonstrating causal relationships between sexual neurochemistry, and sexual behavior, and vice versa, becomes increasingly close to realization. Achievement of this realization is utterly dependent on having the same universe of discourse for a unified neurobehavioral science of sexology, which is precisely what the principle of indicatronics provides. Without this unification, sexual neuroscience will forever be tilting at chimerical windmills of the mind, like lack of sexual desire, or performance anxiety, for example, which are derivative interpretations from primary data, but not the primary data, or indicatrons, themselves.

A unified neurobehavioral sexology approaches causality on a two-way street. The hormone-behavior direction has long been known, and there are many examples, ranging from the effect of castration on erection and ejaculation to the effect of prenatal sex-hormonal sequelae on later sex-dimorphic behavior. The behavior-hormone direction is exemplified in anorexia nervosa, in which food abstinence induces amenorrhea. A more recently discovered, rather dramatic example is the syndrome variously known as psychosocial dwarfism, abuse dwarfism, or reversible hyposomatotropic dwarfism. In this syndrome, growth hormonal deficiency induces statural dwarfism, and gonadotropin deficiency induces pubertal failure. Both deficiencies correlate with child abuse, and are reversible upon rescue. Hormone levels become normal, and statural and pubertal catch-up growth begin, along with improvement in IQ and behavioral maturational deficiency.[1, 2]

Biomedical science has long prided itself on being scientific because it travels only the one-way street from organic determinants to behavior. Behavioral determinants that enter the organism through the special senses have been disenfranchised as nonorganic, which is to say as psychologic, social, spiritual, or occult. There is no justification for this disenfranchisement, as gender-identity/role (G-I/R), like native language, well exemplifies. Neither native language nor G-I/R is present on the day of birth, though both need at birth a healthy brain (a human brain) for their subsequent assimilation. Both then become imprinted into the brain. Thereafter, they cannot be eradicated except by a neurosurgeon's knife—or possibly by a stroke.

There should be nothing remarkable about the premise that exteroceptive light waves entering the organism through the eyes, sound waves through the ears, and similarly the other special senses, should share power with genes and internal chemistries in governing the organism and its functions and practices. Let it not be forgotten that there is a biology of learning and of remembering. Indeed, everything mental is also biological. Without a brain, there is no mentation. Only spooks, spirits, and the occult lay claim to exist sui generis, inaccessible to science.

Significatrons

Indicatrons are the building blocks of larger composites, *significatrons,* which have their own meaning or significance attributed to them. For those who find utility in neologism, and are not offended by their brevity, the subcategories of significatrons are *behavioron,*[3] *imageron,*[4] *verbaton, dictaton, graphicon,* and *praxicon.*

Frank Beach,[5] in 1969 analyzed the sequential components, or behaviorons, of mating and copulatory behavior in rats. Since then, animal sexologists have been able to adhere to the same system, greatly enhancing the accuracy of their science. They have adapted it to other species, but not yet to human beings.

An imageron[4] is a composite unit of images privately experienced, as in a dream, daydream, fiction, or fantasy. An imageron is made publicly known only insofar as it is transposed into indicatrons that are heard or seen, i.e., words, graphics, sculptures, dances, or enactments. Transposing an imageron into tactual, olfactory, or gustatory indicatrons is possible, but less prevalent. An imageron transposed into words becomes a verbaton or, if it is spoken, a dictaton. In graphics, it is a graphicon, and in acts or practices, a praxicon.

In sexology, some imagerons are the imagistic units of a paraphilia. They exist in fantasy prior to being transposed into the praxicons of a paraphilic ritual or enactment. They may be kept private and undisclosed. Or they may be revealed as narratives, paintings, photographs, or movies. Or they may be observed or participated in as an erotic drama that culminates usually in orgasm.

Systematrons

A *systematron* is one of a set of great organizing principles or concepts that permit order or system to be imposed on what otherwise is a chaotic multiplicity of indicatrons and significatrons. In the ancient adversary tradition of law and theology, the organizing principles that apply to human behavior are the polarities of right and wrong, truth and falsity, guilty and not guilty, righteous and unrighteous, spiritual and carnal, voluntary and involuntary, and approval and punishment. These polarities still permeate sexology, not only forensic sexology, but clinical and research sexology also.

In the development of biological sciences in the nineteenth century, there developed an increasing polarization of teleological vitalism and materialistic determinism. The same polarization spread into sexology and other biosocial sciences, with teleology represented as motivation, and materialism as behaviorism (later behavior modification and biofeedback).

In motivationism, various and selected motives, needs, drives or instincts, as they have been variously named, became the great organizing principles or systematrons. The most important ones, as it turned out, were named with words of Greek or Latin etymology, for they could be modified with suffixes that would not fit onto words of Anglo-Saxon, Nordic, or old French origin. Thus sexuality, hostility, instinctuality, intellectuality, passivity, impulsivity, compulsivity, creativity, aggressivity all may be endowed with motivational power, whereas think, dream, know, laugh, fight, fear, choose, and so on, may not.[6]

Motivationism, by addressing itself to the old polarity of voluntary and involuntary, gave new emphasis to involuntary motivation that may be irrational. In some instances, involuntary motivation was attributed to the unconscious, where it hides, unknown and forever unknowable if, in hiding, it is perfectly concealed.

Behaviorism addresses itself primarily to the old polarity of approval and punishment. It boasts that it has no great organizing principles but one, namely, the relentless determination or shaping of any and all behavioral responses as a consequence of reward (approval) or punishment.

Motivationism and behaviorism stand in relationship to one another as thesis and antithesis in need of synthesis. To add a note of personal biography, I now know, with the knowledge of hindsight, that my own formulation of synthesis began in 1945 with a paper later published as "Delusion, Belief and Fact."[7] Its sequel was an unpublished paper read at an international science congress in New Zealand in 1947, in which the teleology of universal drives was replaced by the pragmatics of universal exigencies of being human. As a graduate student, I later discovered in cultural anthropological theory another formulation of the concept of universals, namely the universal culture pattern.[8] Application of the universal exigencies of being human to societies as well as individuals was my next project, eventually expanded into a book.[6]

Synthesized and reduced to their smallest possible number, the universal exigencies of being human are five in number, namely, to be pairbonded, troopbonded, abidant, ycleped, and foredoomed.

Universal Exigencies of Being Human

Pairbondage

Pairbondage means being bonded together in pairs, as in the parent-child pairbond, or the pairbond of those who are lovers or breeding partners. In everyday usage, bondage implies servitude or enforced submission. Though pairbondage is defined so as not to exclude this restrictive connotation, it has a larger meaning that encompasses also mutual dependency and cooperation, and affectional attachment. Pairbondage has a twofold phyletic origin in mammals. One is mutual attachment between a nursing mother and her feeding baby, without which the young fail to survive. The other is mutual attraction between males and females, and their accommodation to one another in mating, without which a diecious species fails to reproduce itself.

Male-female pairbonding is species specific and individually variable with respect to its duration and the proximity of the pair. In human beings, the two extremes are represented by anonymous donor fertilization versus lifelong allegiance and copulatory fidelity.

Troopbondage

Troopbondage means bondedness together among individuals so that they become members of a family or troop that continues its long-term existence despite the loss or departure of any one member. Human troopbondage has its primate phyletic origin in the fact that members of the troop breed not in unison but asynchronously, with transgenerational overlap, and with age-related interdependency. In newborn mammals, the troopbonding of a baby begins with its pairbonding with its mother as the phyletically ordained minimum unit for its survival and health. After weaning, it is also phyletically ordained for herding and troop-bonding species that isolation and deprivation of the company of other members of the species or their surrogate replacements is incompatible with health and survival. Nonhuman primate species are, in the majority of instances, troopbonders like ourselves.

Abidance

Abidance means continuing to remain, be sustained, or survive in the same condition or circumstances of living or dwelling. It is a noun formed from the verb, to abide (from the Anglo-Saxon root, *bidan*, to bide). There are three forms of the past participle, abode, abided, and abidden.

In its present usage, abidance means to be sustained in one's ecological niche or dwelling place in inanimate nature in cooperation or competition with others of one's own species, amongst other species of fauna and flora. Abidance has its phyletic origin in the fact that human primates are mammalian omnivores ecologically dependent on air, water, earth, and fire, and on the products of these four, particularly in the form of nourishment, shelter, and clothing, for survival. Human troops or individuals with an impoverished ecological niche that fails to provide sufficient food, water, shelter, and clothing do not survive.

Ycleptance

Yclept is an Elizabethan word, one form of the past participle of to clepe, meaning to name, to call, or to style. Ycleped and cleped are two alternative past participles. Ycleptance means the condition or experience of being classified, branded, labeled, or typecast. It has its phyletic basis in likeness and unlikeness between individual and group attributes. Human beings have named and type-cast one another since before recorded time. The terms range from the hap-hazard informality of nicknames, that recognize personal idiosyncracies, to the highly organized formality of scientific classifications or medical diagnoses that prognosticate our futures. The categories of ycleptance are many and diverse: sex, age, family, clan, language, race, region, religion, politics, wealth, occupa-tion, health, physique, looks, temperament, and so on. We all live typecast under the imprimatur of our fellow human beings. We are either stigmatized or idolized by the brand names or labels under which we are yclept. They shape our destinies.

Foredoomance

Doom, in Anglo-Saxon and Middle English usage meant what is laid down, a judgment, or decree. In today's usage it also means destiny or fate, especially if the predicted outcome is adverse, as in being doomed to suffer harm, sickness or death. A foredoom is a doom ordained beforehand. Foredoomance is the col-lective noun that, as here defined, denotes the condition of being preordained to die, and to being vulnerable to injury, defect, and disease. Foredoomance has its phyletic origins in the principle of infirmity and the mortality of all life forms. Some individuals are at greater risk than others because of imperfections or errors in their genetic code. Some are at greater risk by reason of exposure to more dangerous places or things. All, however, are exposed to the risk, phy-letically ordained, that all life forms, from viruses and bacteria to insects and vertebrates, are subject to being displaced by, and preyed upon, by other life forms. Foredoomance applies to each one of us at first hand, in a primary way, and also in a derivative way insofar as it applies also to those we know. Their suffering grieves us; their dying is our bereavement.

The Five Exigencies in Sexological Practice

Because we are a diecious species, it is an absolute requirement of procreation that egg and sperm meet together and combine. Whereas that egg-sperm con-junction may be effected by an intermediary, as in a case of in vitro fertilization or donor insemination, normally conjunction of the male and female genitalia is necessary, no matter how transiently. Genital conjunction normally entails some degree of social intercourse between the two people, ranging in degree from rudimentary and brief, to complex and long-lasting.

One way or another, either peripherally or centrally, partially or globally, pairs and not singles are the subject matter of sexology and its application in sexual medicine. Historically, sex therapy developed as couple therapy. Even in individual sex therapy, the missing partner is represented in absentia, in most of the treatment. The focus of treatment is, in other words, on some facet of pairbondage that is inadequate, deficient, or impaired.

Whereas it is sexologically correct to define the unit of health care as the partnership, not as the lone individual, it is not correct to stereotype the relationship between the two people as the cause instead of, sometimes, the effect of a presenting sexuoerotic complaint. True, the universal exigency of pairbondage and its vicissitudes may often be the first of the universals to investigate in making an initial evaluation of a presenting complaint. People do use their sex organs to feud with, passively or actively, as well as to reconcile with. Nonetheless, there are other agendas in their lives also that have an impact on erotosexual health. Because these agendas belong not to the universal exigency of pairbondage, they may readily be haphazardly overlooked. For this reason, the other four universal exigencies take their place in any completely thorough evaluation.

If the presenting complaint is, for example, erotosexual inertia (so-called lack of sexual desire), focus on pairbondage may lead nowhere, if it is at the expense of troopbondage. For example, neglect of the history of troopbondage might allow a juvenile history of pathological family violence, erotic sadism, and mother-son incest to remain unspeakable and undisclosed.

With the same complaint in another case, there may be no headway made until a detailed inquiry on the universal exigency of abidance discloses that, in order to support his family, a man works two jobs. In addition, he is undernourished, and is regularly fatigued through lack of sleep. Sexuoerotic inertia is a derivative symptom.

In a third case with the same presenting complaint of erotosexual inertia, the missing piece of information may remain missing until inquiry is directed toward the universal exigency of ycleptance. Only then can the patient reveal his mortification in childhood at having been teased for getting his puberty as early as age five. In addition, his parents restricted him excessively, having been advised that he might become a sexual maniac and rapist. His early diagnosis had not only residual secondary effects, but also prompted a new diagnostic workup for the possibility of a hypothalamic/pituitary lesion.

The fifth universal exigency, foredoomancy, may also take its toll in relation to sexuoerotic inertia. Disownment or disavowal of premonitory symptoms, or even of an announced diagnosis of disease in oneself, is so common that it is wise not only to get a transcript of a patient's prior medical record, but also to inquire systematically about injuries, ailments, medications and street drugs that may not be on record. For the same reason, a physical examination is obligatory, with special attention in sexual medicine to genital adequacy, deficiency, or impairment. Not only a major pathology, but also any apparently trivial thing, such as an unsightly circumcision or protruding clitoris, may have a debilitating derivative effect on genitoerotic function.

The disease of others needs to be considered. Without specific inquiry, it took one particular patient a year to mention, and then only in passing, that his present round of complaints coincided with the addition to his household of his mother. She was a cantankerous person, frequently hospitalized, formerly with a diagnosis of schizophrenia, to which now was added cancer.

As exemplified in the foregoing, the five universal exigencies of being human serve as mnemonic and heuristic criteria against which to investigate, classify, and evaluate information about people and their lives in health and in failing health. They have great clinical utility in safeguarding against the inadvertent omission of crucial, and sometimes diagnostically decisive cues as to the etiology of presenting complaints.

These five universal exigencies of being human do not cause anything. They constitute a great phyletic template, so to speak, of principles within the confines of which our very existence takes place. It is within this template that the scientific search for causalities that shape us is conducted. These causalities are not polarized. They are neither nurture nor nature in provenience, but both together, integrated. They are not motivational and they are not behavioral, separately. They belong not to the body alone, nor to the mind alone, but to the bodymind. They apply to humankind in general, and to the biography of each individual life. They have their genesis in phylogeny. They are logical categories within which we all have our being. They inhabit us, so to speak, and we have no escape from them.

Coping Strategies

The human organism has three generic strategies for coping with the five universal exigencies: adhibition, inhibition, and explication. These strategies are under the governance of bodymind and should not be attributed to such inferential entities as unconscious motivation, voluntary choice, or will power.

Adhibition and inhibition derive etymologically from the same Latin root, *habere,* to have or to hold. The verb, adhibit, means to engage, take, let in, use, or apply. Inhibit means to restrain, hinder, check, or prohibit. Thus adhibition is characterized by actively becoming engaged in doing something, gaining mastery or control of a situation, accomplishment, and fulfillment. Inhibition is characterized by becoming actively disengaged, avoiding or circumventing a situation, yielding, and being thwarted or deprived

Explication derives from the Latin, *explicatus,* meaning unfolded. To explicate means to explain, interpret, or attribute meaning to an experience, situation, signal or stimulus. Thus, explication as a coping strategy is characterized by actively construing, inferring, conceptualizing, formulating, designating, evaluating, confabulating, and, in general, trying to make sense of what happens.

The aforesaid three coping strategies are generic insofar as they are inferential abstractions derived from particular coping tactics. Any particular coping strategy or tactic is classified as being primarily adhibitory, inhibitory, or explicatory, but each has the other two strategies represented as either secondary or tertiary, respectively. The ratio of the mix allows each particular strategy or tactic to have a three-way interpretation. Thus a major episode of depression, though primarily inhibitory and incapacitating from the viewpoint of the sufferer, is secondarily adhibitory, insofar as it has a manipulatory, tyrannical effect on others. It is tertiarily explicatory insofar as its genesis is misattributed by the sufferer, often to the extent of being delusional and self-persecutory. The coexistence of these three interpretations constitutes the basis on which psychodynamic hypotheses are constructed by scholars of psychodynamics.

The following is a listing of particular coping strategies or tactics which are presented descriptively in *The Psychologic Study of Man* (1957). They are classified according to the three generic categories of coping strategy.

Adhibitory Strategies or Tactics

Preservation
Orderliness, hoarding, and ritual
Constant exertion
Risk exploits
Protest exploits
Mating protests
Surrogate displacement
Impersonation
Addiction

Inhibitory Strategies or Tactics

Fixation and regression
Disownment
Phasic disownment
Phobia
Sleeping spells
Depression
Suicide
Mutilatory sacrifice of body parts
Organ and limb amnesias
Visceral amnesias
Autonomic dysfunctions
Gestural and vocal automatisms
Seizures and paroxysmal states

Explicatory Strategies or Tactics

Causal explanation
Mirth and the comic

Fantasy
Dream
Hallucination
Depersonalization

References

1. Money, J., Annecillo, C., Kelly, J. F.: Abuse-dwarfism syndrome: After rescue, statural and intellectual catchup growth correlate. *J. Clin. Child Psychol.* 12:279-283, 1983.

2. Money, J., Annecillo, C., Kelly, J. F.: Growth of Intelligence: failure and catchup associated respectively with abuse and rescue in the syndrome of abuse dwarfism. *Psychoneuroendocrinology* 8:309-319, 1983.

3. Money, J.: Paraphalia and abuse martyrdom: Exhibitionism as a paradigm for reciprocal couple counseling combined with antiandrogen. *J Sex Martial Ther.* 7:115-123, 1981.

4. Money, J.: The development of sexuality and eroticism in humankind. *Q Rev. Biology* 56:379-404, 1981.

5. Money, J., Ehrhardt, A. A.: *Man and woman, boy and girl: The differentiation and dimorphism of gender identity from conception to maturity.* Baltimore, Johns Hopkins Press, 1972.

6. Money, J.: *The psychologic study of man.* Springfield, IL, Charles C Thomas, 1957.

7. Money, J.: Delusion, belief and fact. *Psychiatry* 11:33-38, 1948.

8. Wissler, C.: *Man and culture.* New York, Crowell, 1938.

Note

Originally published in *Journal of Sex and Marital Therapy,* 10:229-238, 1984; and written for a Round Table Discussion on Mind-Body Interactions, XIII International Congress of the International Society of Psychoneuroendocrinology, Tubingen, 1982. The section of coping strategies, specifically written for this publication, is adapted and revised from *The Psychologic Study of Man* (1957). [Biblog. #2.283]

Author's Comment: Motivation versus Threshold

In the foreword to a long review of clinical findings on gender identity for the 1943 Nebraska Symposium on Motivation (Money, 1974), the concept of threshold is used to circumvent the pitfalls of both teleological and mechanistic thinking, as follows.

This is the Nebraska Symposium on Motivation. Therefore, I think it fair and appropriate for me to tell you at the outset that I don't subscribe to the doctrine of motivation! In general, and in the study and theory of sex in particular, drives, instincts, needs, or motivations are impossible concepts for me to handle empirically and operationally. For me, they belong in history's storage closet along with teleology, phlogiston, vital forces, and demonic possessions. Of course, I am able to converse with patients and other people whose idioms they are. In fact, I may even reciprocate their use in interviewing for a sexual history. But an idiom is not an organizing principle or concept of science. And it is as an organizing principle that I reject a sexual drive, an instinct, a need, or motivation.

That is not to say, however, that I would substitute a mechanistic stimulus-response principle whereby sexual man and woman become scientistic robots—not at all. As a first principle, I accept sexual behavior, like all of man's behavior, as a kinetic or dynamic system by definition. I do not need to put drive into it. Like the solar system, it goes; that is the scheme of things. My job and yours as scientists is to figure out the principles of the system's going. Here I can be a little facetious and say that we're figuring out its "go-itivity" or its "go-ationality,' if you can tolerate these bastard graftings of Latin suffixes. I am being more than a little facetious here because it is, in fact, true that without Latin and Greek suffixes most of motivation theory would have had no vehicle for its existence.

Some years ago I wrote a short paper on linguistic resources and psychodynamic theory. It is fascinating to see that we are victims of language when it comes to basic principles. For example, one always has to use some other psychic force or drive to explain dreams, because one can't have a word like "dreamivity" or "dreamuance" that explains something else. Anything that is known to us by Anglo-Saxon or Nordic root is something that has to be explained by something else which has a Latin or Greek root.

I've found it possible to make headway if I substitute for motivation the concept of *threshold*—threshold for the release or inhibition of behavior. Then I can clasisfy the types of behavior released or inhibited, the primary types being lexical versus gestural. In another way one might say imagistic versus signalistic or, in simplest English, voice talk versus body talk. The concept of threshold is really an extraordinarily useful one. It conveys a great advantage of continuity and unity to what would otherwise be disparate and divided. Thus I—and you too—may look for threshold differences in the release or the inhibition of sexual behavior. The threshold may apply to behavior attributable to genetic programing, or to prenatal hormonal programing, or to toxic programing, or to circulating hormonal programing at puberty, or after puberty to pheromonal programing—pheromones being stimulating odors, recently under investigation for the first time in primate sexuality.

You and I may also look for differences of threshold with regard to visual image programing of erotic arousal. There is an implication for sex differences here, in that men are much more girl watchers than women are boy watchers. Men have at puberty nature's own presentation of a pornography show to them in their wet dreams and their masturbation fantasies, in a way that women are not so programed for visual imagery. One could go on, one step further up the ladder, and say that thresholds can be studied with regard to activation or inhibition in social-history programing. The top of the ladder would represent traumatic or deteriorative change in the central nervous system—change in the threshold for release or inhibition of sexual behavior. In that respect the temporal lobe of the brain is particularly important. A lesion of the temporal lobe is very likely to change sexual behavior thresholds in some way or another. But the deteriorative process could also be a matter of disease in the genitalia themselves, and not simply of sexual pathways in the brain.

You see then that the concept of threshold does indeed have great value because of the great spectrum that it applies to. It helps to tie what would otherwise be a lot of loose ends together. It allows me to think developmentally or longitudinally also in terms of stages or experiences that are programed serially, or hierarchically or cybernetically.

No longer do I need to be enslaved to such worn-out platitudes of dichotomy as nature versus nurture, the biological versus the social, the innate versus the acquired, or the physiological versus the psychological. All these dichotomies capitalize on the very ancient, pre-Platonic, pre-Biblical dichotomy of the body versus the mind, or the physical versus the spiritual. This body-mind dichotomy is now so ingrained a principle of our vernacular or folk metaphysics that it is something very difficult for us to get rid of. Yet as scientists I believe we have to find our way around it. Otherwise it spells total disaster to the development of sexual science today, and tomorrow, and in the future.

Reference

Money, J. Prenatal hormones and postnatal socialization in gender identity differentiation. *Nebraska Symposium on Motivation,* 21:221-295, 1974. [Bibliog. #2.170]

TEN

New Phylism Theory and Autism: Pathognomonic Impairment of Troopbonding

Abstract

A phylism is a unit of existence, part of an individual's species heritage. It is neither nature nor nurture, but a phyletically dictated product of the interaction of both at a crucial developmental period which may be either prenatal, postnatal, or both. In the syndrome of autism, the phylism of troopbonding is specifically impaired, and other phylisms may be hypertrophic. The phylism of limerent (lover-lover) pairbonding is not impaired, and it may be the source of discordance with other members of the troop. Shyness is an attenuated manifestation of autism. The etiology of impaired troopbonding may be heritable, and almost certainly will prove to be neurochemical also, probably as an analogue of the Lesch-Nyhan syndrome. The lives of autistic children are subject to secondary shaping by the environment of living.

Phylism Defined

It is traditional to polarize nature and nurture; heredity and environment; organic and psychogenic; instinctual and learned; constitutional and acquired; and so on. The principles in each instance are global and diffuse. Therefore, their explanatory power is global and diffuse. What is needed is a breakdown of the global and diffuse into smaller and more pragmatic components. Hence the new concept, phylism.

The term, phylism, is derived from the Greek, phylon (Latin phylum), and is related to phyletic and phylogeny. A phylism is a unit or building block of our existence that belongs to us, as individuals, through our heritage as members of our species. Some phylisms have everyday names, like breathing, coughing, sneezing, hiccupping, drinking, swallowing, biting, chewing, pissing, shitting, fucking, laughing, crying, walking, grasping, holding, sweating, touching, hurting, tasting, smelling, hearing, seeing—the complete list has not been counted. Others have Latinate names, like thermoregulation, salt-regulation, osmolality, immunoregulation, and so on. Still others have not yet been given names, or have been named only recently, for example, pairbonding and troopbonding.

Most of the aforesaid terms fulfill the criterion of discreteness, that is, they name each phylism as separate and distinct, and with non-overlapping boundaries. There are other terms, however, that are too diffuse and that have too many meanings to have much scientific utility, for example, feeling, anxiety, fear, dependency, hostility, loving, repressing, resisting, and so on. Terms that are too diffuse, and that carry multiple shades of meaning, name phenomena which, by very reason of their name, cannot be pinned down and held constant enough for further scientific investigation.

Nature/Crucial-Period/Nurture

Both the nature and the nurture of a phylism are phyletically dictated or programed. Thus a phylism cannot be ascribed to either nature alone, or nurture alone. It is the product not of a two-term equation, but of a three-term one: nature/crucial-period/nurture. Nature and nurture interact during a crucial period of development to produce a phylism. The crucial period may be prenatal, in which case nurture takes place within the womb, and the environment is intrauterine. If the crucial period is postnatal, then the extrauterine environment expands to include the exteroceptive stimuli of the special senses, especially the eyes and the ears. Exteroceptive programing of the brain through the special senses is, as conventionally defined, learning.

Some learning is transient and trivial. Crucial-period learning, however, can be permanent and ineradicable, witness the example of native language. A native language inhabits the brain so permanently that it cannot be eradicated except by a neurosurgeon's knife—or perhaps by a trauma or stroke.

Phylisms: Prenatal/Postnatal

Some phylisms are already in existence and manifested before birth, though subsequently they will be responsive to various and different stimuli. For instance, the phylism of rhythmic heartbeat and circulation of the blood exists long before the baby is born, though subsequently the heart-rate is able to change to faster or slower in response to stimuli as divergent as drugs and dangerous threats.

The phylism of breathing, by contrast, although all set to go before birth, requires exposure to air while the baby is still life-supported through the umbilical cord, immediately after having been born, before it actually gets going. The phylism of sucking is performed in utero as thumb sucking, and has been observed prenatally by x-ray or sonogram. After birth, this phylism becomes activated in response to the nipple, and still later in life to a wider range of stimuli. The phylism of erection of the penis, like sucking, has also been observed by sonogram in utero, whereas the various diversity of stimuli that can induce an erection take effect progressively—soon after birth, later in infancy, in childhood, and in teenage.

Bonding

Infant-mother pairbonding in the newborn period has been named and studied only within the past quarter century.[1] It constitutes a phylism and is, developmentally, the first manifestation of bonding. It is essential to survival, and perhaps is also a precursor of lover-lover pairbonding later in development. Developmentally, it antedates another bonding phylism, namely troopbonding, which begins to manifest itself as attachment to members of the household other than the mother, and later as attachment to agemates.

Troopbonding and Autism

In the histories of autistic children, one may obtain evidence to the effect that, as newborns, they seemed to be aloof and self-isolating, instead of strongly mother-bonded. But it is in the impairment of troopbonding that autistic children are most extensively handicapped, so much so, that one may postulate failure to troopbond as pathognomonic of the syndrome of autism. Impairment of the phylism of troopbonding is the primary pathology in autism.

On the basis of the hypothesis that impairment of the troopbonding phylism may be highly specific, it follows that much in the symptomatology of autism that is otherwise puzzling becomes less so. For a child deficient in troopbonding, people become irrelevant and neglected, except as moving objects in space—comparable, by analogy, to colors in the sight of the colorblind, or to injurious harm in the apperception of the congenitally painblind (pain-agnostic).

Without troopbonding, linguistic communication with members of the troop also becomes irrelevant and neglected. Since the phylism for language is not itself impaired, however, private linguistic, numerical and related symbols may be used elaborately—even hypertrophically, in feats of mnemonic, intellectual, and calculational virtuosity, formerly known as the phenomenon of the idiot savant.

Such hypertrophy and virtuosity may be precocious, as in the extraordinary case of Nadia[2]. At the age of three and a half, this autistic girl repetitiously sketched carrousel horses and riders, modeled from pictures, with the graphic skill of an accomplished art-school senior.

Hypertrophic Phylisms

The drawings of Nadia, and analogous feats of other autistic children, suggest the hypothesis that the process responsible for impairment of the troopbonding phylism in autism may also be responsible for, or associated with either hypertrophy and/or precocious maturation of other phylisms. The phylism of repetition, for example, may fall into this category, and be responsible for monotonous repetition of mannerisms, vocalisms, and rituals.

The phylism for object-constancy may be similarly affected, and be responsible for obsessional orderliness of time and place. The phylism for rotational motion and giddiness, if affected, would be responsible for the spinning that is characteristic of some autistic children. The phylism for rocking motion is probably not specifically related to autism, but rather to isolation and neglect which triggers rocking in diverse contexts. Likewise headbanging which, paradoxically, hurts only initially, and then induces euphoria, perhaps by releasing analgesic and euphoriant endorphin from the brain's own opiate system.

Limerent Pairbonding

It is no more possible for an ordinary person to inhabit the experiential universe of an autistic person than to inhabit an egg inside its shell—and the same holds true in reverse. The autistic and nonautistic are forever mismatched, and so become potential adversaries in a no-win, no-lose, power struggle. Feuding may revolve around the phylism of limerent (lover-lover) pairbonding.[3]

The phylism for limerent pairbonding, unlike that for troopbonding, is not impaired in autism. Nonetheless, since socializing is usually a precursor to meeting and pairbonding with a lover and sexual partner, expression of the phylism for limerent pairbonding becomes impeded. In consequence, the matching of an autistic with a nonautistic partner has a high probability of being a mismatch—of being reciprocally discordant instead of concordant. The love affair is one-sided and unrequited.

The feuding and misunderstanding that may ensue are exemplified in the biography of a girl with a diagnostic history of both autism and 45,X Turner's syndrome, and with a history of treatment for both. By age sixteen, she was hormonally adolescent, puberty having been induced by treatment with estrogen, as is necessary in Turner's syndrome.

From the family's point of view, their adolescent daughter was jealous of her younger brother, aged thirteen, angry and spiteful toward him, and yet devoted to him. She was irrationally dictatorial about what color of socks he could or could not wear, about washing his socks for him, and about requiring him never to walk around the house with bare feet, always to wear long pants even for summer sports, and never to expose bare skin above his socks.

From the girl's point of view, her brother and her family were negative. She could not explain herself. She had fits of despaired rage and destructiveness. Only after months of frequent therapy was she able to give words to her own point of view: after showing his bare feet and bare legs, what would it be next? Eventually she was able to speak about a very explicit fantasy of having sex with her brother, which was stated in the past tense of delusion as history. The more mean she was to her brother, the more desperate she became at being unable to control herself, which led only to more anger and destructiveness. She wanted romance and marriage, like her sisters, but had no strategy except to wait for it to happen. Her conversations were characterized by residual autistic verbalisms, but by far the greater handicap was her ineptitude in social reciprocity. She was not only shy but oddly idiosyncratic as well.

Shyness and Autism

Shyness and social ineptitude, without a prior history of autism, may represent an attenuated manifestation of the same phylismic deficit of troopbonding that, in more intense degree, produces autism. To illustrate this hypothesis, I am able to draw on a comparison between a girl and her maternal grandmother's sister. Each of these two people had a history of having required extensive psychiatric help, including hospitalization. The child's diagnosis was autism of the most severe degree. The woman, had, at one time in young adulthood, been given a diagnosis of schizophrenia, from which she subsequently became wholly rehabilitated as both a profoundly shy person and an internationally esteemed genius among creative artists. She compared her own shyness with that of her grand-niece in the following anecdote. She was on one occasion visiting the child's parents, when company arrived. She gravitated away from the roomful of people into the empty hallway, still visible through the open door, but with a rapid avenue of escape available. There in the hallway, she found that the child also had gravitated away from the people, and was hidden from their view. She recognized that, quite independently, each of them had had the same reaction. It was one with which she had been familiar all her life—hovering in a doorway, or near a stairway, ready to slip away and be alone, should the presence of people become too jeopardizing. She recognized that, whatever the unknown entity that made the company of people, especially strangers, jeopardizing to her, her grandniece had a stronger, and more incapacitating degree of it than she did, herself.

Heredity and Neurochemistry

If this unknown entity is heritable, it is not X-chromosome linked, but it must be heritable in such a way as to be transmissible in variable degrees of penetrance, according to a principle familiar in genetics.[4] The variability may be in either severity, or age of onset of symptoms or both. Whether or not it should prove to be heritable, this unknown entity will undoubtedly prove to be biochemical, and more specifically neurochemical. There is a remote possibility of its being associated with the phenomena of autoimmunology.[5] It is all but certain that it will prove to be responsible for the governance, in the brain, of the phylism of troopbonding, and hence for the etiology of autism. Here lies the direction of future research.

Lesch-Nyhan Syndrome

The etiologic principles involved in autism have an analogue in the Lesch-Nyhan syndrome.[6] A phylism impaired in this syndrome is the phylism of biting and chewing. Affected children (the syndrome manifests itself only in males) bite and chew their own lips and fingers and destroy them. This self-mutilation represents a failure of discrimination similar to that which occurs when a mammalian mother, delivering her young, fails to discriminate between the baby and the placenta so that, beginning with biting and chewing the umbilical cord, she proceeds to cannibalize the baby. Its squealing does not stop her; nor does the Lesch-Nyhan boy's screaming from his own pain stop him.

The Lesch-Nyhan syndrome is genetically transmitted to males as a recessive trait carried on the X chromosome. Girls are protected by their second X chromosome. The defective gene is responsible for deficient production of the enzyme, hypoxanthineguanine phosphoribosyl transferase (HGPRT) which, in turn, is responsible for overproduction of purine, which in turn floods the body fluids with uric acid. The process by which the enzymatic deficiency affects brain neurochemistries that govern the phylism of self-mutilatory biting and chewing has not yet been worked out.

Secondary Shaping

As children with autism grow up, the full repertory of their atypical behavior will reflect not only the primary phylismic anomalies of the syndrome, but also the secondary shaping of them in the environment of living. Neglect in the back wards of an institution for the retarded will shape a very different product than will a disciplinary academy, and both will be different from a nonjudgmental recovery home that recognizes the basic phylismic anomalies as handicaps which, though they impose constraints, do not inevitably incapacitate, and in at least a few individuals permit the development of unique talent and creative achievement.

Conclusions

The determinants of phylisms as manifested in everyday life are neither entirely nature nor entirely nurture, but the product of the interaction of the two in varying proportion at a crucial period or periods of development. Phylismic theory is not teleologically causal and motivational, on the one hand, nor mechanistically causal, on the other. It is, however, dynamically causal, for it allows for multiple determinants to influence one another in dynamic interaction, including cybernetic or feedback interaction. It is a theory that makes the juxtaposition of biology and psychology anachronistic, and unifies the two in behavioral science and neuroscience research. Autism research is one of the beneficiaries.

References

1. Trause, M. A., Kendall, J., Klaus, M. Parental attachment behavior. pp. 789-799 in *Handbook of Sexology* (J. Money, H. Musaph, eds.). Excerpta Medica, Amsterdam, New York, 1977.

2. Selfe, L. Nadia. *A Case of Extraordinary Drawing Ability in an Autistic Child.* Academic Press, New York, 1977.

3. Tennov, D. *Love and Limerence: The Experience of Being in Love.* Stein and Day, New York, 1979.

4. Money, J., Hirsch, S. R. Chromosome anomalies, mental deficiency and schizophrenia: A study of triple X and triple X/Y chromosomes in five patients and their families. *Archives of General Psychiatry* 8:242-251, 1963.

5. Money, J., Bobrow, M. A., Clarke, F. C. Autism and autoimmune disease: A family study. *Journal of Autism and Childhood Schizophrenia* 1:146-160, 1971.

6. Gardner, L. I. *Endocrine and Genetic Diseases of Childhood and Adolescence.* 2nd ed. pp. 1056-1059, Saunders, Philadelphia, 1975.

Note

Originally rejected by the *Journal of Autism and Developmental Disorders* and published in *Medical Hypotheses,* 11:245–250, 1983. [Bibliog. #2.268]

PART II
Gender-Identity/Role
[G-I/R] Differentiation

ELEVEN

Hermaphroditism: Recommendations Concerning Assignment of Sex, Change of Sex, and Psychologic Management

Criteria of Sex

The homespun wisdom of medically unsophisticated people confronted with a newborn hermaphrodite usually guides them to assign the baby to the sex which it most resembles in external genital appearance. This procedure is, after all, only an extension of the age old practice of inferring, on the basis of a single glance, that the reproductive system in its entirety is either masculine or feminine. Before the advent of modern surgical and microscopic techniques, there was no way better than the homespun one of deciding the sex to assign to an hermaphrodite. After the advent of modern surgery and microscopy, it was assumed that gonadal structure, as revealed by microscopic examination of sections of gonadal tissue, was the ultimate criterion to use in assigning the sex of an hermaphrodite.

This microscopic criterion was the basis of Klebs' well known classification of hermaphrodites in 1876.[1] Klebs recognized the true hermaphrodites who possessed both ovarian and testicular tissue, male pseudohermaphrodites with only testicular, and female pseudohermaphrodites with only ovarian tissue. It was widely assumed that gonadal structure would determine sexual outlook and desires, even in those cases where gonadal structure and secondary sexual characteristics at puberty were paradoxically contradictory. Thus, it was taken for granted that the microscope would reveal the real sex of pseudohermaphrodites and decide the issue of their rearing. Only when the microscope revealed true hermaphroditism did the physician have an open choice in assigning the sex of rearing.

Klebs' archaic classification has survived despite the fact that it was made before anything was known of endocrine secretions and sex hormones; before any extensive psychologic research had been done on the determinants of the psychologic phenomena of sexual outlook and orientation; and before a reliable technique of chromosomal sex determination had been developed. Notwithstanding endocrine, psychologic and chromosomal discoveries, in the present day there are still many people, medical and lay, who unquestioningly accept the gonadal criterion, though the newly discovered technique of chromosomal sex determination from a skin biopsy[2, 3] has tempted some enthusiasts to adopt a chromosomal criterion instead.

Our studies of 65 ambiguously sexed people have demonstrated that it is extremely unwise to use a single criterion like gonadal structure or chromosomal pattern in assigning an hermaphrodite to one sex or the other. In view of what is currently known about the chromosomes of hermaphrodites and the contradictions which may exist between them and other signs of sex, the chromosomal criterion should be given a minor place and should never be used as the ultimate criterion. (Use of the chromosomal criterion alone would lead to absurdities in the case of, for example, patients formerly diagnosed as having ovarian agenesis. During the past year, it has been discovered that a large proportion of them are chromosomally male.[4] They have entirely feminine external genitals and internal accessory organs. It is inconceivable that any physician would recommend such a person to live as a male). Likewise with the gonads, the contradictions that may exist between them and other signs of sex are so great that the gonadal criterion should not be the exclusive one. The criteria to be more seriously considered and appraised for their relative importance are: external genital morphology, hormonal sex (with due recognition of the frequent difficulty of predicting hormonal sex before puberty and of the possibility of corrective hormonal intervention); and the gender role established and ingrained through years of living in a sex already assigned.[5, 6]

By the term, gender role, we mean all those things that a person says or does to disclose himself or herself as having the status of boy or man, girl or woman, respectively. It includes, but is not restricted to sexuality in the sense of eroticism. A gender role is not established at birth, but is built up cumulatively through experiences encountered and transacted—through casual and unplanned learning, through explicit instruction and inculcation, and through spontaneously putting two and two together to make sometimes four and sometimes, erroneously, five. (These statements do not represent adherence to a theory of environmental and social determinism, for experiences encountered do not dictate experiences transacted in a simple, point-for-point correlation. Transactions are frequently highly unpredictable, individualistic and eccentric, for reasons as yet not fully ascertained.) In brief, a gender role is established in much the same way as is a native language.

From our studies of the life adjustments of the patients in our series, we have found it definitely advantageous for a child to have been reared so that a gender role was clearly defined and consistently maintained from the beginning. When, in deference to the presumed importance of gonads, a change of assigned sex was imposed later than early infancy, the life adjustment was not significantly improved and was often made worse.

Varieties of Hermaphroditism

In this paper, it is not our intention to expound at length on the differential diagnosis of the various types of hermaphroditism[7, 8] but it will be pertinent to list, with comments, the seven categories which were found to be both exhaustive and mutually exclusive in making a survey of over 300 hermaphrodites reported in the English language literature between 1895 and 1951.[9]

Female Pseudohermaphrodites with Hyperadrenocorticism

The external genitals may appear almost normally female with slight to medium enlargement of the clitoris, or there may be a single urogenital orifice with enlargement of the clitoris; or, rarely, there may be a penile urethra and fused, empty scrotal sac. Physical growth and development is precocious and virilizing, but may be totally corrected with cortisone therapy.[10] Very early postnatal diagnosis is possible by means of urinary 17-ketosteroid assessment, without exploratory laparotomy. Plural incidence in a family is common, but is usually restricted to a single generation and a single marriage. Gonads and chromosomal pattern are female.

Female Pseudohermaphrodites with Phallus, Normal Ovaries, and Normal Mullerian Structures

There may be a single urogenital orifice with penis-like clitoris and a single urethral meatus in the urogenital sinus; or the clitoris may be so penis-like as to be supplied with a urethra serving as an auxilliary urinary outlet. Pubertal development is entirely feminine and reproduction is possible. Once the chromosomes have been established as female, this condition can be differentiated from the former on the basis of urinary 17-ketosteroid measurements, but it cannot be differentiated, on the basis of these two criteria alone, from true hermaphroditism which, so far as is known, is the only other variety of hermaphroditism in which female chromosomes may be present. A complete diagnosis, therefore, requires laparotomy and gonadal biopsy. The condition is extremely rare.

True Hermaphrodites

Ovarian and testicular tissue is present, either in one ovotestis, the other gonad being an ovary or a testis; in two ovotestes; or in one ovary and one testis. The nature of the chromosomes for all subvarieties has not been ascertained. In one case of true lateral hermaphroditism (left ovary, right descended testis, no gametogenesis) chromosomes were bilaterally female. Internal genital structures and external genitalia exhibit diverse degrees of ambiguity. Pubertal development may be masculine, feminine or ambiguous. Diagnosis requires exploratory laparotomy and biopsy of the gonads. No more than 60 cases have been reported in the European and American literature of the last century.

Male Pseudohermaphrodites with Well-Differentiated Mullerian Organs

The penis may be fully formed with penile urethra, or it may be hypospadiac. One or both testes may be cryptorchid. One testis may be atrophic. Mullerian structures often herniate into the groin or scrotum in the company of one testicle. Pubertal development is almost always masculine, sometimes rather eunuchoid, especially when cryptorchidism is bilateral and the penis hypospadiac. Diagnosis requires surgical exploration. Whether a female, as well as the usual male chromosomal pattern is compatible with this variety of hermaphroditism has yet to be ascertained.

Simulant Females with Feminizing Testes

External genital appearance completely simulates the normal female. The vagina is a blind pouch and, with very rare exceptions, the mullerian system is a cordlike vestige. The wolffian system is malformed or vestigial. The testes remain in an ovarian position or herniate into the groin. Pubertal feminizing is complete, except for menses, absence of which is the first sign of this concealed form of hermaphroditism in otherwise apparently normal women, unless the testes have previosly herniated. In some cases there is absence of pubic and axillary hair. Diagnosis requires biopsy of the testes which should not be removed since they produce estrogens and these patients always live like women. Familial incidence in several generations is common. The chromosomal pattern is male.

Cryptorchid Hypospadiac Males with Feminizing Testes

These cases resemble those in the former group except that the phallus is slightly or greatly larger than a clitoris, and that the blind vaginal pouch, usually present, opens into the sinus of a single urogenital orifice. The mullerian system is vestigial, and the wolffian system malformed or vestigial. Pubertal development is feminine, but not always strongly so. It is impossible to predict this feminization beforehand, except in cases of familial incidence. In infancy and childhood, therefore, these cases cannot be distinguished from those of the next group. Diagnosis requires testicular biopsy. Plural incidence within a family may occur. The chromosomal pattern is male.

Cryptorchid Hypospadiac Males

Historically, hypospadiacs have not been called hermaphrodites unless hypospadias is extreme, the scrotum bifid and the testes undescended. Careful scrutiny often reveals that such hypospadiacs have a blind vaginal pouch hidden beyond the single external urogenital orifice. There may also be a separate external orifice for a blind vaginal pouch. The phallus may be only slightly larger than a clitoris. A virilizing puberty cannot be predicted beforehand.

Diagnosis requires testicular biopsy. Plural incidence within a family may occur. The chromosomal pattern is male.

Sex Assignment: Neonatal Period

It should be the aim of the obstetrician and pediatrician to settle the sex of an hermaphroditic baby, once and for all, within the first few weeks of life, before establishment of a gender role gets far advanced. Some hermaphrodites are born with external genitals that look so completely masculine or feminine that ambisexuality is not suspected. The baby is unhesitatingly declared male or female and no question is raised perhaps for years. Early uncertainty is aroused only when the external genitals look ambiguous. It is our recommendation that, in assigning the sex in these ambiguous instances, consideration be given first to the appearance and morphology of the external genitals. If the external organs are so predominantly male, or so predominantly female that no amount of surgical reconstruction will convert them to serviceably and erotically sensitive organs of the other sex, then the sex assignment should be dictated by the external genitals alone. All further surgical and hormonal endeavor should be directed toward maintaining the person in that sex.

If the external genital anatomy of a neonate is thoroughly ambiguous and the possibilities of surgical reconstruction are equally promising in either direction, then gonadal and hormonal considerations may be more heavily weighted with regard to sex of assignment. On the basis of gonadal structure alone, however, it is frequently impossible to predict a virilizing or feminizing puberty. In the particular instance of hyperadrenocortical virilism in girls, it is possible to correct the hormonal incongruity by treatment with cortisone.

The chief objection to be raised against the recommendation of paying greatest attention to external genital anatomy in assigning the sex of a neonatal hermaphrodite is that the recommendation flagrantly disregards the issue of fertility. But this objection is more imaginary than real. No male pseudohermaphrodites or true hermaphrodites have been known to have become parents, and many have been proved sterile. Female pseudohermaphrodites, including hyperadrenocortical females regulated on cortisone, may become pregnant. When such female cases are diagnosed promptly at birth, it is precisely because of their obviously ambiguous genital appearance. Subsequent surgical feminization and hormonal regulation can be thoroughly successful, thereby preserving areas of erotic sensation, fortifying the feminine role and safeguarding the opportunity for eventual child bearing. The only exception to this generalization is the extremely rare case of a female pseudohermaphrodite with a fully developed penis and normal looking, though empty scrotum; but only an exceptional combination of circumstances would permit the diagnosis of female pseudohermaphroditism in such a baby in the neonatal period.

Postneonatal Period: Change of Sex

It is not in neonates, but in older infants and children that the most perplexing and difficult problems of sex assignment are encountered—problems of whether to change the sex already assigned. Even when fully aware of a baby's genital ambiguity, parents do assign it to one sex or the other before long. The language dictates that they refer to the child as he or she, and they cannot sit on the fence indefinitely before announcing the birth of a son or daughter. Using all the medical help available, parents make the best decision they can and thenceforth drift into the conviction that they have a son, or a daughter. They rear the child accordingly, despite the knowledge that they may have to make a change later, and the subtle processes by which a gender role is established have begun. The longer a change is postponed, the more difficult it becomes for parents to relinquish a son in favor of a daughter or vice versa. After a change, there is a time lag, maybe an extensive one, as parents readapt themselves, which is not without effect on the child. Neighbors and friends also find it difficult to accept the change, and even more difficult to forget it. Later in life the child is likely to be confronted with coarse jokes and reminders, unless the family had started life entirely afresh in a new community at the time of the change.

Difficult though it may be for parents and others to negotiate a child's change of sex, it is even more difficult for the child, once he or she has established a conviction of gender. It is not possible to state a fixed age at which gender awareness becomes established: as in other matters pertaining to development and maturation, it is not the same age for all infants. As a general guide, it may be said that the crucial age is somewhere around eighteen months. This claim is based on a study of 11 cases of change of sex; 4 of them were changed before nine months of age and subsequently assimilated their new gender role without identifiable signs of psychologic maladaptiveness. The other 7 were changed at or after fifteen months, the latest at sixteen years voluntarily, and the other 6 before school age. All of these 7 had assimilated their new gender role in varying degrees of pervasivenes, but all except one who was changed at two years and three months, subsequently evidenced at least one indisputable, chronic symptom of psychopathology. Severity of the symptom varied, though in no instance reached psychotic proportions. The incidence of psychologic maladaptiveness was conspicuously less frequent among cases with no history of change of sex.

Gender role is so well established in most children by the age of two and one-half years that it is then too late to make a change of sex with impunity. One must calculate the risk of ensuing psychologic disturbance. This risk may very occasionally seem worth taking, especially in cases of complete incongruity between assigned sex and external genital equipment, but psychiatric supervision and follow-up should never be omitted.

After the transition from infancy to childhood—which is another of those unfixed points in the developmental sequence, occurring some time between the ages of three and one-half years and four and one-half years—it is too late to impose a change of sex. In the exceptional instance of an hermaphroditic child who has privately construed that an error of sex assignment has been made, and who has secretly half-resolved on a change of sex, successful negotiation of a change may prove possible. But our experience has led us to believe that voluntary requests for change of sex in hermaphrodites belong to the teenage. Though such requests are rare, they deserve serious evaluation, for they are usually a culminating attempt to resolve years of well founded perplexity and doubt.

For neonatal and very young infant hermaphrodites, our recommendation is that sex be assigned primarily on the basis of the external genitals and how well they lend themselves to surgical reconstruction in conformity with assigned sex, due allowance being made for a program of hormonal intervention. For older hermaphroditic infants, children and adults, our recommendation is that first consideration be given to the degree that a gender role has been ineradicably established in the sex already assigned, and that changes of sex be scrupulously avoided, except in rare and carefully appraised instances.

The chief objection to be raised against this second recommendation, as against the first, is that it also flagrantly disregards the possibility of depriving the group of nonsterile hermaphrodites of fertility in adult life. The answer to this objection is that actual child bearing as distinguished from potential biological fertility is not determined by chromosomal, hormonal, and gonadal sex alone. It is also determined by the social encounters and cultural transactions of mating and marrying, which are inextricably bound up with gender role and erotic orientation. Gender role may be established so thoroughly and irreversibly, despite chromosomal, gonadal or hormonal contradictions, that it cannot be modified in accordance with a change of sex by edict. Thus a boy, changed to wear dresses once ovaries were discovered, may continue to think, act and dream as the boy he was brought up to be, eventually falling in love as a boy, only to be considered homosexual and maladjusted by society. Alternatively, after the change, the gender role may be partly modified, but only at the cost of psychologic disorder and symptomatology sufficiently disabling to prevent marriage. In either case, the plan to preserve fertile gonads carries the seeds of its own defeat by ensuring that fertility never culminates in reproduction.

Psychologic Management: Parents

When hermaphroditism is recognized at birth and there is doubt about the baby's sex, this doubt should be frankly revealed to the parents. It is preferable that they remain in as much doubt about the sex of their child as they were before delivery than that they have to contradict a public announcement of a son or daughter. When finally the decision is made, the parents will be firm in the conviction that they have a son, or else a daughter, and unequivocal definiteness is to the child's subsequent advantage.

SEXUAL DIFFERENTIATION IN THE HUMAN FETUS

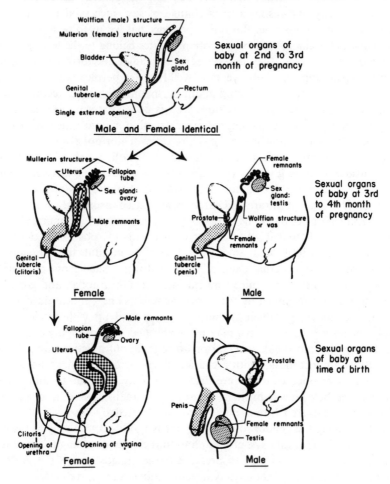

FIG. 1. Cross-section diagrams freely adapted from R. R. Greene and simplified for demonstrating to laymen the failure of complete sexual differentiation in hermaphroditism. (Drawn by Marie Vincent Kern.)

Ninety-nine times out of a hundred, the public construes an hermaphrodite as being half boy, half girl. The parents of an hermaphrodite should be disabused of this conception immediately. They should be given, instead, the concept that their child is a boy or a girl, one or the other, whose sex organs did not get completely differentiated or finished. A few simple embryological sketches[11, 12] showing the original hermaphroditism of all human embryos in

EXTERNAL GENITAL DIFFERENTIATION IN THE HUMAN FETUS

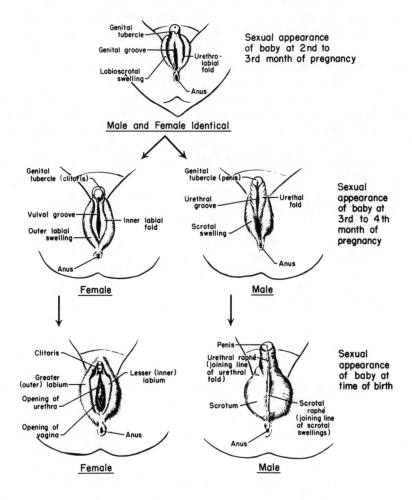

FIG. 2. Diagrams freely adapted from B. M. Pattern and simplified for demonstrating to laymen the failure of complete external genital differentiation in hermaphroditism. (Drawn by Marie Vincent Kern.)

the undifferentiated phase, and the late stage at which external genital similarity of males and females is still apparent, are of inestimable help in conveying this enlightening concept of genital unfinishedness (Figures 1 and 2). The average layman is totally ignorant of the fact that clitoris and penis, labia majora and scrotum, and labia minora and ventral skin of the penis are homologous structures.[13] In fact, many women are ignorant of the existence of the clitoris on their own bodies. It comes as a surprise, therefore, to the parents of, say, a female pseudohermaphrodite that the "male organ" is really a clitoris which did not shrink to normal size. Acquaintance with proper genital terminology is also of great practical importance in enabling parents to explain their child's deformity to grandparents and other close relatives without such emotion-laden and embarrassing expressions as "morphodite" and "not being right down there." More important still, a proper vocabulary equips parents to talk straightforwardly with the child and to answer questions as the need arises.

A special problem of vocabulary arises when talking truthfully with parents, should a decision have been reached to allow a contradiction between gonadal structure and sex of rearing in their child—which should, for example, ordinarily be the decision when, despite testes, the phallus is clitoral sized. Under such circumstances, it is preferable to refer always to abnormally formed gonads or sex glands, and not to testes. An abnormally formed gonad may look testicular under the microscope, and one may tell the parents that this is so, but to say it in this way is totally different in its emotional effect from bluntly saying that the gonad is a testis. Medical people know that they call a gonad a testis despite tubular atrophy, absence of sertoli cells, and interstitial cells which produce estrogens, but lay people do not know all this.

Most parents need to be told that their child is not destined to grow up with abnormal and perverse sexual desires, for they get hermaphroditism and homosexuality hopelessly confused.

Psychologic Management: Patients

The more manifest the signs of hermaphroditism, the more necessary are psychologic guidance and follow-up. As young as the age of two, hermaphroditic children begin to notice their difference from other boys or girls. Brought up as a girl, a child with a big phallus may, putting two and two together, tell herself that she is part boy. But not invariably. If she has seen only baby girls naked, she may conjecture that all girls develop a phallus as they grow up or, contrarily, if she has seen only older girls naked, she may conclude that her phallus will diminish as she gets older. Sooner or later, however, she comes to realize her oddity. It is preferable that such a child know from the time when she can first begin to comprehend it, that she has a clitoris like all other girls, but that it is too big, and will be made smaller surgically. With little boys, the simplest comprehensible explanation is that one day the surgeons will finish the penis so that the boy can stand up to urinate.

An hermaphroditic child needs only eyes and ears to know that the focus of medical attention is on his or her genitals, even if the hermaphroditism is concealed. Thus, far from burdening them with unnecessary worries, it is actually a lifting of the burdens of secret worries and doubts for the doctor to talk frankly with children. Truth is seldom as distressing as the mystery of the unknown. Older children, like their parents, can assimilate the concept of being genitally unfinished to replace ill-conceived theories of being part boy, part girl. As their comprehension permits, these older children also benefit from an explanation, with sketches, of failure of complete embryological differentiation. The amount of detailed explanation required is greatest for those hermaphrodites whose paradox is external and visible, and least for those with concealed hermaphroditism. If sterility is predictable, then it is preferable for a child to grow up with this knowledge rather than have it dramatically disclosed later in life.

One cannot, of course, say very much about the reproductive system without explaining the facts of reproduction. These items of information can be given quite intelligibly to young children, as they become ready to assimilate them, in terms of a baby nest or pouch, a baby tunnel or chute, an egg without a shell, and sperms that swim from the penis and up the baby tunnel in a race to see which one can win. Even more than most children, hermaphroditic youngsters whose genitals look ambisexual are at an advantage in having their curiosity about the difference between the sexes and the origin of babies satisfied by a responsible person: they are then not motivated to satisfy their curiosity in childhood sexual play and talk whereby they expose themselves to neighborhood ridicule and gossip. Given the facts about moral proprieties concerning the private things in life, along with the biological facts, our juvenile patients have proved thoroughly competent in conducting themselves appropriately. Like other children, they may or may not masturbate in private, and have not been medically forbidden to do so, but they have presented no neighborhood problems of sexual conduct.

The most complex problems of psychologic management arise in those hermaphroditic children who are exposed to equivocating indecision and doubt on the part of parents and physicians and whose sex is debated or ridiculed by their contemporaries, so that they do not establish their gender with unambiguous certainty. These ambiguously uncertain children include those subjected to change of sex after the early infancy period. The problems and time involved in handling these cases require the services of a specialist in psychiatric medicine.

Psychologic Management: Surgery

As a general psychologic rule, the earlier that signs of ambisexuality are corrected, the better, both from the parents' viewpoint and the child's. But operative decisions are always contingent on estimates of surgical safety and success. Concerning surgical safety, for example, it is risky for female pseudohermaphrodites whose hyperadrenocorticism is complicated by sodium loss to undergo surgery before salt retention has been firmly established. Concerning surgical success, except for clitoridectomy, greatest success with genital repair and reconstruction is usually obtained after the organs have grown and are of a good size to work with.

When surgical delay is indicated, children can accommodate to the impositions and embarrassments of a genital anomaly, but it is imperative that they be told about prospective medical and surgical plans. Without this information, they are likely to construe that they are freaks. With it, they can discuss and elaborate tactics for dealing with interim emergencies such as, in the case of hypospadiac boys, school urinary habits.

Not only should children be informed of prospective surgical plans, but also they should invariably be given a simple explanation of what to expect of an operation. A three year old girl about to be clitoridectomized, for example, should be well informed that the doctors will make her look like all other girls and women. Girls should also know, incidentally, that whereas boys have a penis, girls have a vagina—in juvenile vocabulary, a baby tunnel—as a double insurance against childish theories of surgical mutilation and maiming. It is also useful to inform children, as a matter of course, of preoperative and anesthetic routine and of what to expect postoperatively, for these apparently trivial details are the source of their most intense anticipatory terrors and misconceptions.

Clitoridectomy is the genital surgical procedure most likely to rouse psychologic debate among experts, particularly on the issue of loss of erotic sensation. We have sought information about erotic sensation from the dozen nonjuvenile hyperadrenocortical women we have studied. There has been no evidence of a deleterious effect of clitoridectomy. None of the women experienced in genital practices reported a loss of orgasm after clitoridectomy. All of the patients were unanimous in expressing intense satisfaction at having a feminine genital morphology after the operation. None of them had been antagonistic to the plan for clitoridectomy. Each had regarded herself as a woman and had established a feminine gender role. It would be most unwise to dictate clitoridectomy to a gonadal female who had established a masculine gender role and considered himself a boy or man. Formerly, complete clitoral extirpation was required in some hyperadrenocortrical females who had painful priapism of the amputated stump, but cortisone abolishes priapism so that amputation is nowadays sufficient. Though there is considerable evidence that an amputated clitoris is erotically sensitive, enough uncertainty remains to require conservatism in recommending clitoridectomy for hermaphrodites living as women in whom there is neither a blind vaginal pouch nor a vagina opening into a urogenital sinus.

When plastic reconstruction of the vagina is delayed until postadolescence, the patient should be made to feel free to request the operation whenever it suits her, and not only after she is engaged or married. It is unnecessarily embarrassing for a woman to have to explain and confess her vaginal shortcomings to a prospective husband.

Case Illustration

The following case report has been chosen to illustrate the type of case in which the pros and cons of a change of sex provoke considerable debate. The final decision in this instance was against a change of sex, chiefly on psychologic grounds which are spelled out and briefly documented in the report:

Introductory data: A diagnosis of hyperadrenocortical female pseudohermaphroditism was first made when the patient was three years and seven months old, at which time he was referred for psychologic appraisal. He had normal female internal reproductive structures, except that the vagina opened into the urethra near the bladder. He had already begun to virilize precociously in the typical hyperadrenocortical fashion. He had always lived as a boy. When he was born, the mother said, she was told that the sex of her baby was uncertain, but by the third day she was informed unequivocally that she had a son.

From the age of a year onward, the child had been hospitalized elsewhere, at approximately six-monthly intervals, for four successive stages of hypospadiac repair. The repair had not yet been completed and the child was still obliged to sit to urinate. The surgical consultant reported that further plastic surgery could be carried out to provide an adequately functioning penis, provided the mullerian system were removed, mucosa from the hidden vagina being used to fashion a penile urethra. The child could also be surgically feminized, with amputation of the phallus and construction of labia majora from the very rugose skin of what looked like an empty scrotum. Subsequent hormonal feminization could then have been induced with cortisone.

Family: The mother combined big-city flair and quick wits with the simple and artless folkways of a Scandinavian upbringing and meager education. She appeared to be a sincere, candid woman and mother, visibly harassed by the arduousness of synchronizing her son's hospitalization with all the other chores and duties of caring for her family. She gave the impression of not daring to give vent to her feelings and worries about her son lest, having let go, she find herself unable to resume mastery of herself again and carry on with her other responsibilities. Balancing the family budget was a constant responsibility, for her husband had been partially incapacitated for fifteen years by an inability to maintain postural equilibrium.

The family included five children: Bill, 19; David, 16; Bob, 7; Norman, the patient, 3½; Kate, the only girl, 1 year. There had been no other pregnancies.

The mother gave no sign of knowing that fresh doubts about the sex of her fourth child had arisen, and that the question of a change of sex had been asked. She had wondered initially when the child was a baby whether he were part girl. She had even wondered whether to give credence to her husband's conjecture that her intense longing for a daughter instead of a fourth son had caused the baby's genital ambiguity. Subsequently she had not for one moment conceived the child to be the daughter she had so much longed for. It appeared rather that she had made restitution for even a conjectured prenatal influence by accepting with redoubled certainty the maleness of the child and rearing him accordingly.

First impression of child: "As soon as he recognized my face as unfamiliar, he approached me, saying over and over again: 'Got to call my Mommy.' There was a look of stark terror about him, and a note of frantic urgency in his voice. He did not object to a genital examination, but kept perseverating, uneasily: 'The nurse cut my wee-wee.' I could not find much logical coherence between this and other reiterated sentences, and could not understand some of his baby-talk pronunciations. I was left wondering whether the child had some kind of cerebral defect, or whether he was simply in the midst of a hospital admission panic."

Intelligence test: The Revised Stanford-Binet Intelligence Scale was administered. Chronological Age three years and seven months; Mental Age two years and eleven months; IQ 81—dull normal level. The child was very friendly and cooperative. It was judged he did the best he was capable of on the test, but his general uneasiness at being in a hospital may well have had an adverse effect on his IQ score.

Interviews with child: The child was seen by each of the three investigators. Two of eight hours of conversation were recorded. He made an extremely cordial friendship with the man who saw him most frequently. With women he was slow to get friendly and at ease, which seemed to have some connection with his misconception that nurses, and not doctors, cut his penis as well as managing the postoperative procedures which hurt him.

With familiarity, the child's speech became easier to understand. It was rather more difficult than is usual with three and a half year olds to engage in logically coherent dialogue. Though his statements were not always linked coherently together and were sometimes childishly inconsistent, it was possible to trace a thread of continuity.

He came to the hospital, he said, because his mother brought him in the choo-choo train. And he also came to the hospital because: "The nurse cut on my wee-wee. The nurse hurt me. Cut on my wee-wee." Immediately he went on, reiterating: "I got to call my Mommy," so he tried to reach the telephone on the desk. "Got to call my Mommy. Take me in the choo-choo train. Home." By implication, he wanted to get out of the hospital before there was any more cutting on his wee-wee. Spontaneously he continued: "The nurse cut on Bobo's wee-wee" (Bob, his seven year old brother). It was not clear whether this was a statement of fact signifying that Bob's penis was small like his own, while the older brothers had large ones, or whether it was an expectation that Bob would be treated like himself. Kate, the sister, was mentioned next. She had no wee-wee. The nurse had cut it and taken it away. "Billy (the oldest brother) will bring Katie a new wee-wee," and other presents too. This new kind of organ was called a "koll wee-wee." It was the sort that Billy himself had. "Billy will bring me a koll wee-wee, too. Billy is nice to me."

Subsequently it was learned that the patient had spontaneously asked his oldest brother, Billy, away from home in the service, for "a new wee-wee," while talking on long distance with him. On the ward, the child was also spontaneous with impromptu talk about his wee-wee and its being cut, in conversation with the nursing and house staff. For all of his excessive penis-consciousness, he was not self-conscious in a prudish, embarrassed sense.

Like many infants, the child got muddled about the relationships of brother and sister. But he also got muddled about who were boys and who was girl in his family, which is unusual at three and a half. As for himself, by contrast, there was absolutely no question: he always answered definitively that he was a boy. In point of fact, to the many people who asked him his name, his reply was the single monosyllable: "Boy." He gave the name of his boy-dressed doll in the same way. Once when pressed for the doll's proper name, he tried to satisfy with: "Boy doll-girl," but there was never any such ambiguity about himself. Under similar pressure for his own proper name, he gave his age instead, saying one, two, three, with fingers held up, not quite sure of himself. Despite all this precision about being a boy at the cost of indecision about his name, he quickly agreed that his name was Norman when asked if it was.

In his general manner and bearing, the child was quite unlike little girls of his age and completely like other boys. The mother remarked on how boyish she found him—exactly as boyish as her three other sons had been. The house staff and nurses were unanimous that their impulsive feelings and responses to the child were as to other boys, not as to a girl nor an undecided misfit. Other children on the ward and in the playroom accepted him unhesitatingly as a boy. After his initial panicky reaction, he acted boisterously and full of boyish high spirits, without being seclusive, timid or inhibited. So far as could be judged, he was much relieved when informed that there would be no more surgery during his admission, but that when he got bigger his penis would not be taken away, but finished so that he could stand to urinate.

Psychological Appraisal

No one who had any sustained contact with this child could fail to observe that he was extraordinarily cognizant of his penis, even for an hypospadiac child, and alarmed by the history and prospects of its surgical alteration. In a typically childish way, he had grossly misconstrued his surgical experiences to signify that his penis was being mutilated and perhaps might suffer the fate he conceived had befallen his sister's genitals. His fantasied remedy for his plight was that his oldest brother would buy him a new and perfect penis. In an older person, this kind of reiterated illogical thinking would be identified as delusional and psychopathological, though it is regarded as benign in a child so young. It is not so completely benign, however, that one can afford to treat it casually and with indifference. The longer such misconceptions stay unrectified, they become increasingly ineradicable as a source around which more and more allied or derivative misconceptions cumulate. As this cumulative distortion of thinking and judgment progresses, there is reciprocal distortion of the balance between action and inhibition, between active meeting and mastering of life's challenges and control and discipline of actions and conduct, until a condition of frank psychopathological disorder is in evidence. At the age of three and a half, this child showed no signs of such disorder—only the signs that he was a good candidate in whom disorder might develop.

A very good way to promote development of psychopathological symptoms in this child would have been to subject him to a fifth genital operation to amputate the four-times-repaired hypospadiac phallus. So far as a change of sex for a child is concerned, one is, therefore, on the horns of a dilemma. On the one hand, to amputate the phallus without delay would magnify all the child's misconceptions and prove that they had been only too well founded, without in any way proving to him his femininity. On the other hand, delay of surgical feminization would leave strong genital evidence of maleness and impede assimilation and development of a new, feminine gender role and orientation.

The only conceivable way of making a change of sex and also of resolving this dilemma would be through an intensive program of psychiatric follow-up, both with the child and, to a lesser degree, with the members of his family, after the family had moved to an entirely new neighborhood. As a practical matter, this strategy was out of the question, for the family was impecunious and there was no other source of funds to meet all of the very costly exigencies.

For this child, the risk of change of sex ending in psychiatric disaster was judged too great to justify the change. The greater medical wisdom lay in planning for a sterile man to be physically and mentally healthy, and efficient as a human being, than for a probably fertile woman to be physically well but psychologically a misfit and a failure as a woman, a wife, or a mother. Accordingly, it was planned to prevent precocious epiphyseal fusion and too rapid advance of secondary sexual virilization by treatment with cortisone until the appearance of beginning feminization, and then to perform an ovariectomy and to discontinue cortisone. Completion of hypospadiac repair was postponed until the child was older and less psychologically menaced by this procedure.

Summary

There are seven variables which may operate independently of one another in hermaphroditism. They are: chromosomal sex; gonadal sex; hormonal sex; external genital morphology; accessory internal genital morphology; assigned sex and rearing; and gender role, including psychosexual orientation, which becomes built-up through experiences encountered and transacted. On the basis of chromosomal, gonadal and hormonal sex, seven varieties of hermaphroditism have been described, but these three criteria, singly or together, are never sufficient when practical decisions about assignment or change of sex have to be made. In the case of neonatal and very young infant hermaphrodites, we recommend that sex be assigned primarily, though not exclusively, on the basis of the external genitals and how well they lend themselves to surgical reconstruction in conformity with assigned sex, due allowance being made for a program of hormonal intervention, if indicated. For older hermaphroditic infants, children and adults, we recommend that first consideration be given to the degree that a gender role has been indelibly established in the sex already assigned, and that changes of sex be scrupulously avoided, except in rare and carefully appraised instances, in order to avoid hazardous psychiatric sequelae. Judged in conjunction with each of the seven clinically recognizable varieties of hermaphroditism, these recommendations make eminent practical sense. A case is reported to illustrate the methods of studying attitudes and diagnosing gender role and applying these concepts in practical decisions. The psychologic management of parents of hermaphrodites and of patients themselves, with special reference to genital surgery, derives in its specific details from a general policy of frank and straightforward discussion and explanation. A clear and explicit understanding of basic principles is a prerequisite to frank and straightforward discussion.

References

1. Klebs, E.: *Handbuch der pathologischen Anatomie.* August Hirschwald, Berlin, Germany, 1876; 1.Band, Zweite Albtheilung, 718.

2. Moore, K. L., Graham, M. A., and Barr, M. L.: The detection of chromosomal sex in hermaphrodites from a skin biopsy. *Surg. Gynec. and Obst.* 1953, 96:641.

3. Barr, M. L.: An interim note on the application of the skin biopsy test of chromosomal sex to hermaphrodites. *Surg. Gynec. and Obst.* 1954, 92:184.

4. Grumbach, M. M., Van Wyk, J. J., and Wilkins, L.: Gonadal dysgenesis, ovarian agenesis, male pseudohermaphroditism: Bearings on theories of human sex differentiation. Read at the 37th annual meeting of The Endocrine Society, June 2, 1955. *J. Clin. Endocr. and Metab.* In press. See also Vol. 14: 1270.

5. Money, J.: Hermaphroditism, gender and precocity in hyperadrenocorticism: Psychologic findings. *Bull. Johns Hopkins Hosp.* 1955, 96:253.

6. Hampson, J. G.: Hermaphroditic genital appearance, rearing and eroticism in hyperadrenocorticism. *Bull. Johns Hopkins Hosp.* 1955, 96:265.

7. Wilkins, L.: *The Diagnosis and Treatment of Endocrine Disorders in Childhood and Adolescence.* Charles C Thomas, Springfield, Illinois, 1950.

8. Wilkins, L. et al.: Hermaphroditism: Classification, diagnosis, selection of sex and treatment. *Pediatrics.* 16:287, 1955.

9. Money, J.: *Hermaphroditism: An Inquiry into the Nature of a Human Paradox.* Unpublished doctoral thesis, Harvard University Library, 1952; University Microfilms, Ann Arbor, MI, 1967.

10. Wilkins, L., Bongiovanni, A. M., Clayton, G. W., Grumbach, M. M., and Van Wyk, J. J.: The present status of the treatment of virilizing adrenal hyperplasia with cortisone: Experience of 3½ years. *Mod. Prob. Ped.* Vol. 1, 1954. (Supplement to *Annales Paediatrici,* Basle, Switzerland, and New York) p. 329.

11. Greene, R. R.: Embryology of sexual structure and hermaphroditism. *J. Clin. Endocr.* 4:335, 1944.

12. Patten, B. M.: *Human Embryology.* The Blakiston Co., Philadelphia, Pa., 1946.

13. Arey, L. B.: *Developmental Anatomy: A Textbook and Laboratory Manual of Embryology,* 5th edition. W. B. Saunders, Co., Philadelphia, Pa., 1946.

Note

Originally published in the *Bulletin of The Johns Hopkins Hospital*, 97:284-300, 1955, with J. G. Hampson and J. L. Hampson as coauthors. [Bibliog. #2.12]

Author's Comment: Update

This chapter and those that follow in Part II grew out of my 1952 doctoral dissertation (Money, Ann Arbor University Microfilms, 1967). They utilize the concept of gender role originally published in Money (1955, *Bull. John Hopkins Hosp.*, 97:253-264; see also Chapter 12, p. 153, footnote), and subsequently extended to include gender identity. In Chapter 19, the history of the usage of the term, gender, is traced from gender role to G-I/R, the acronym that unifies gender identity and role.

It has been the fate of the original and the immediate successors of this chapter that they have been misquoted by critics as exemplars of a simple-minded type of social-environmental determinism—a position that, right from the outset, I have explicitly disclaimed. In 1955, it required almost a decade of waiting for the appearance of new animal experiments showing a relationship between prenatal hormonalization of the brain and subsequent dimorphism of mating behavior. The earlier behavioral findings of Eugen Steinach in the 1920's, later confirmed by Vera Dantchakoff, namely that the experimental morphological masculinization of female guinea pigs in utero masculinized also their mating behavior, had become buried in the archives of science and were hardly known. Their reconfirmation in 1964 by William C. Young and his students initiated a vast amount of new activity, still continuing, that influenced all future concepts of hormones and behavior—as in the chapters of Part III, for example. Nonetheless, in the study of human hermaphroditism, there is still the evidence, as there was in 1955, of matched pairs, congruent for prenatal hormonal history and diagnosis, and discordant for sex of assignment and clinical habilitation (see Chapter 15). When they reach adulthood, such matched pairs are typically discordant also for G-I/R. One has the G-I/R of a man, the other of a woman, erotic and genitosexual aspects included. Such cases forbid the simple-minded acceptance of prenatal hormonal determinants of G-I/R. There is more about the complexity of G-I/R differentiation in boys and girls that remains still to be discovered. The same applies to monkeys. They also are influenced by the social conditions of rearing. Even the rat is proving not to be a hormonal robot, for the conditions of rearing influence these creatures also.

The term *chromosomal pattern* as used in this chapter refers to the sex chromatin. The method of actually counting and karyotyping the chromosomes was not discovered until 1956 (Tjio and Levan, *Hereditas*, 42:1-6) and was not ready for clinical application until 1959, four years after the publication of this article.

The father of the child in the Case Report was subsequently diagnosed as having multiple sclerosis, from which he became progressively incapacitated. The child became increasingly a victim of rejection and abuse. The information that he was born of an adulterous affair (as was his next older brother and younger sister) was revealed and subsequently used as a torment when he got into adolescent revolt at home. Surgical repair of his penis and urinary system was never totally satisfactory in its outcome. There were recurrent urinary infections. He married at age 25, and became emotionally and financially dependent on his wife as a multisymptomed, dependent invalid, unable to work and earn a living.

TWELVE

An Examination of Some Basic Sexual Concepts: The Evidence of Human Hermaphroditism

Introduction

Despite advancements of knowledge in embryology and endocrinology, most people have continued to make an absolute dichotomy between male and female—a dichotomy as seemingly axiomatic as the distinction of day from night, black from white. In psychology and psychiatry, this dichotomy is represented in the conception of predominant masculinity or femininity of the sexual instinct or drive.

A comprehensive theory of instinctive sexuality was first expounded to a medical audience by Freud at the beginning of the present century.[1] Developing and expanding earlier instinctive theories, Freud utilized, inter alia, the conception of innate bisexuality, namely, that instinctive masculinity and instinctive femininity are present in all members of the human species, but in differing proportions.

Freud construed his theory of innate and constitutional psychic bisexuality on the basis of embryological evidence as an hermaphroditic phase in human embryonic differentiation, and on the basis of anatomical evidence in congenital hermaphroditism itself. At a later date, he adduced the evidence of early experiments in endocrinology concerning hormonal reversal of sex in animals as a further support for his bisexual theory.

In an endeavor to ascertain if new and additional information relevant to psychologic theory of sexuality might be obtained from the study of hermaphroditism, the authors have, for the past four years, systematically been making psychologic studies of hermaphroditic patients. The work has been done in close cooperation with Dr. Lawson Wilkins who has been responsible for diagnostic, endocrine and other medical studies of the majority of the patients.

The sexual incongruities which occur in hermaphroditism involve diverse contradictions, singly or in combination, between six variables of sex.[2] These six variables are:

1. Assigned sex and sex of rearing;
2. External genital morphology;
3. Internal accessory reproductive structures;
4. Hormonal sex and secondary sexual characteristics;
5. Gonadal sex;
6. Chromosomal sex.

Patients showing various combinations and permutations of these six sexual variables may be appraised with respect to a seventh variable:

7. Gender role and orientation as male and female, established while growing up.*

Thus one is enabled to ascertain something of the relative importance of each of the six variables in relation to the seventh.

Patients in whom ambisexual contradictions exist include seven subgroups in the traditional diagnostic category of hermaphroditism,[2, 3] and a group traditionally diagnosed as ovarian agenesis but now more accurately named gonadal agenesis, or dysgenesis, since the chromosomal pattern is male[4, 5] (see Table I). We have studied 76 patients in all.

Chromosomal Sex

Barr's technique of chromosomal sex determination from skin biopsies has, since January 1954, revealed the chromosomal sex of some of our patients.[7, 8]† Though it is too early to make a final definitive statement, it appears reasonably likely that, among the eight varieties of ambisexual development, a female chromosomal pattern is always present in varieties 1 and 2, and a male chromosomal pattern in varieties 6, 7, and 8 (Table I). It happens that eight true hermaphrodites so far reported on have had a female, and four a male chromosomal pattern. The chromosomal sex of males in whom mullerian differentiation is relatively unarrested has yet to be elucidated. Gonadal agenesis (dysgenesis) may occur either in chromosomal males or chromosomal females who, in all other respects, are identically feminine.

In the interests of precision, only those patients from whom skin biopsies have been taken, and the chromosomal sex actually determined, are included in Table II. The 19 cases listed in this table are those in which there was a contradiction between chromosomal sex and the sex of assignment and rearing. In every instance, the person established a gender role and orientation consistent with assigned sex and rearing, and inconsistent with chromosomal sex. Thus, it is convincingly clear that the unity of gender role and orientation as male or female evidenced itself independently of chromosomal sex, but in close conformity with assigned sex and rearing.

---

*By the term, gender role, we mean all those things that a person says or does to disclose himself or herself as having the status of boy or man, girl or woman, respectively. It includes, but is not restricted to sexuality in the sense of eroticism. Gender role is appraised in relation to the following: general mannerisms, deportment and demeanor; play preferences and recreational interests; spontaneous topics of talk in unprompted conversation and casual comment; content of dreams, daydreams and fantasies; replies to oblique inquiries and projective tests; evidence of erotic practices and, finally, the person's own replies to direct inquiry.

†Chromosomal sex determinations were done by Dr. M. L. Barr and Dr. K. L. Moore at the University of Western Ontario.

TABLE I

Varieties of Somatic Ambisexual Development*

1. Congenitally hyperadrenocortical female 42
2. Female, with well differentiated phallus, normal ovaries and normal
   internal reproductive structures 2
3. True hermaphroditism 1
4. Male, with unarrested mullerian differentiation:
   (a) with normal penis and one or both testes cryptorchid 0
   (b) hypospadiac and cryptorchic 3
5. Gonadal agenesis (dysgenesis), with simulant female infantile body
   morphology and male chromosomes 11
6. Simulant female, with testes, blind vagina, mullerian vestiges and breasts 3
7. Cryptorchid male hypospadiac, with breasts at puberty:
   (a) with urogenital sinus 1
   (b) with blind vaginal pouch 0
8. Cryptorchid male hypospadiac:
   (a) with urogenital sinus 11
   (b) with blind vaginal pouch 2

                                                                        ─
                                                                        76

*For the purposes of this classification, the criterion of male and female is gonadal. The classification is based on the study of over 300 cases in the literature, in English, of the last half century.[6] Within each category, patients resemble one another closely enough to be strictly comparable as somatic units for the purpose of psychologic study.

Gonadal Sex

Among the 76 patients, there were 20 in whom a contradiction was found between gonadal sex and the sex of assignment and rearing (Table III). All but 3 of these 20 disclosed themselves in a gender role fully concordant with their rearing. Gonadal structure per se proved a most unreliable prognosticator of a person's gender role and orientation as man or woman, boy or girl. By contrast, assigned sex and rearing proved a most reliable one.

Hormonal Sex

To consider now the relationship between hormonal sex and gender role: hormonal sex must be distinguished from gonadal structure, for ovaries do not always make estrogens, nor testicles androgens. The ovaries of untreated hyperadrenocortical female pseudohermaphrodites are inert, and though their adrenal cortices produce an excess of estrogens as well as of androgens, androgenic activity dominates and the body is excessively virilized. The testes of male pseudohermaphrodites of the simulant female variety produce estrogens which feminize the body.

Table IV summarizes the data of the 27 patients who went through and

TABLE II

Chromosomes and Rearing Contradictory
19 Cases

CHROMOSOMES	Gonads	Endogenous Hormonal Sex	Internal Accessory Organs	External Genital Morphology	Assigned Sex and Rearing	Gender Role	Type of Ambisexual Development
♂	none	none	♀	♀	11 ♀	11 ♀	Gonadal agenesis (dysgenesis)
♂	♂	♀ 2 juv.	vestigial	♀	3 ♀	3 ♀	simulant female
♂	♂	1 ♂ 3 juv.	vestigial	⚥	4 ♀	4 ♀	cryptorchid male hypospadiac
♀	♀ left ♂ right	⚥	⚥	⚥	1 ♂	1 ♂	true hermaphroditism

TABLE III

Gonads and Rearing Contradictory
20 Cases

GONADS	Chromosomes	Endogenous Hormonal Sex	Internal Accessory Organs	External Genital Morphology	Assigned Sex and Rearing	Gender Role	Type of Ambisexual Development
♀	♀	♀	♀	⚥	2 ♂	2 ♂	female with phallus and ovogenesis
♀	♀	♂	♀	⚥	4 ♂	4 ♂	hyperadrenocortical female
♂	?	1 ♂ 2 juv.	♀	⚥	3 ♀	3 ♀	male with unarrested mullerian differentiation
♂	♂	1 ♀ 2 juv.	vestigial	♀	3 ♀	3 ♀	simulant female
♂	♂	4 ♂ 4 juv.	vestigial	⚥	8 ♀	5 ♀ / 1 ♀→♂ / 2 ⚥	cryptorchid male hypospadiac

TABLE IV

Hormonal Sex and Rearing Contradictory
27 Postpubertal Cases

ENDOGENOUS HORMONAL SEX	Chromosomes	Gonads	Internal Accessory Organs	External Genital Morphology	Assigned Sex and Rearing	Gender Role	Type of Ambisexual Development
♀	♀	♀	♀	♂	2 ♂	2 ♂	female with phallus and ovogenesis
♀	♂	♂	vestigial	⚥	1 ♂	1 ♂	cryptorchid male hypospadiac with breasts
⚥	♀	⚥	⚥	⚥	1 ♂	1 ♂	true hermaphroditism
♂	♀	♀	♀	⚥	18 ♀	17 ♀ / 1 ⚥	hyperadrenocortical female
♂	?	♂	⚥	⚥	1 ♀	1 ♀	male with unarrested mullerian differentiation
♂	♂	♂	vestigial	⚥	4 ♀	1 ♀ / 1 ♀ → ♂ / 2 ⚥	cryptorchid male hypospadiac

TABLE V

Internal Accessory Organs and Rearing Contradictory
18 Cases

INTERNAL ACCESSORY ORGANS	Chromosomes	Gonads	Endogenous Hormonal Sex	External Genital Morphology	Assigned Sex and Rearing	Gender Role	Type of Ambisexual Development
♀ > ♂	♀	♀	♀	⚥	2 ♂	2 ♂	female with phallus and ovogenesis
♀ > ♂	♀	♀	♂	⚥	4 ♂	4 ♂	hyperadrenocortical female
♂ > ♀ vestigial	♂	♂	1 ♀ / 2 juv.	♀	3 ♀	3 ♀	simulant female
♂ > ♀ vestigial	♂	♂	4 ♂ / 4 juv.	⚥	8 ♀	5 ♀ / 1 ♀ → ♂ / 2 ⚥	cryptorchid male hypospadiac
⚥	♀	⚥	♀	⚥	1 ♂	1 ♂	true hermaphroditism

TABLE VI

External Genital Appearance and Rearing Contradictory
23 Cases

PREDOMINANT EXT. GENITAL APPEARANCE	Chromosomes	Gonads	Endogenous Hormonal Sex	Internal Accessory Organs	Assigned Sex and Rearing	Gender Role	Type of Ambisexual Development
♂	♀	♀	♂	♀	15 ♀	15 ♀	hyperadrenocortical female
♂	?	♂	1 ♂ 1 juv.	⚥	2 ♀	2 ♀	male with unarrested mullerian differentiation
2 ♀ 3 ♂	2 ♂ 3 ♂	2 ♂ 3 ♂	2 Juv. 2 ♂ 1 Juv.	2 vestigial 3 vestigial	2 ♂ 3 ♀	2 ♂ 1 ♀→♂ 2 ♀	cryptorchid male hypospadiac
♀	♂	♂	♀	vestigial	1 ♂	1 ♂	cryptorchid male hypospadiac with breasts

TABLE VII

Male and Female Assigned Sex in
Patients with Same Diagnosis
55 Cases

Assigned Sex and Rearing	Gender Role	Type of Ambisexual Development
38 ♀ 4 ♂	37 ♀ 1 ⚥ 4 ♂	hyperadrenocortical female
8 ♀ 5 ♂	5♀, 1♀→♂ 2⚥, 5♂	cryptorchid male hypospadiac

beyond a puberty—or, in the case of hyperadrenocorticism, a precocious puberty-equivalent—in which hormonal influences produced a secondary sexual development contradictory of the sex in which they were living. Subsequently the contradiction was corrected with hormonal therapy and, where indicated, with plastic surgery. Psychologic data were gathered before treatment, when possible, otherwise retrospectively.

Of the 27 people whose hormonal functioning and secondary sexual body morphology contradicted their assigned sex and rearing, only 4 became ambivalent with respect to gender role as male or female. All four had been reared as girls. One, acting on his own initiative, began living as a man from the age of sixteen onward. The other three, while living as women, showed some degree of bisexual inclination. These four patients do not, in themselves, offer any convincing evidence of hormonal sex as a causal agent in the establishment of maleness or femaleness of gender role: the patient who lived as a man declined testosterone substitution treatment after surgical castration for malignancy, and the three who lived as women had been thoroughly feminized on estrogen substitution treatment. Moreover, the other 23 of the 27 patients established a gender role consistent with their assigned sex and rearing, despite the embarrassment and worry occasioned by hormonal contradictions. Like gonadal sex, hormonal sex per se proved a most unreliable prognosticator of a person's gender role and orientation as man or woman, boy or girl.

Internal Accessory Organs

Since the uterus is the organ of menstruation, and the prostate the major organ of seminal fluid secretion, it is necessary to compare maleness or femaleness of gender role with internal reproductive equipment. There were 17 cases in whom assigned sex and rearing were inconsistent with predominant male or female structures internally (Table V). Gender role agreed with rearing in 14 of these 17. The 3 remaining were the same three individuals as deviated in Tables III and IV.

In estimating the significance of the comparison in Table V, one must bear in mind that only rarely in hermaphroditism does either the uterus or the prostate reach full functional maturity, without medical intervention. Of the 17 cases, there were only 3 for whom this statement did not hold: though all three had a functional uterus, they had been reared as boys and had a thoroughly masculine gender role and outlook. So far as the evidence goes, there is no reason to suspect a correlation between internal accessory organs and maleness or femaleness of gender role.

External Genital Appearance

It goes without saying that the external genitals are the sign from which parents and others take their cue in assigning a sexual status to a neonate and in rearing him thereafter, and the sign, above all others, which gives a growing child assuredness of his or her gender. Nonetheless, it is possible for an hermaphrodite to establish a gender role fully concordant with assigned sex and rearing, despite a paradoxical appearance of the external genitals.

There were 23 among our 76 patients who, at the time they were studied, had lived for more than two-thirds of their lives with a contradiction between external genital morphology and assigned sex (Table VI). For one reason or another, they did not receive surgical correction of their genital deformity in infancy, but lived with a contradictory genital appearance for at least five and for as many as forty-seven years. In all but one instance, the person had succeeded in coming to terms with his, or her anomaly, and had a gender role and orientation wholly consistent with assigned sex and rearing.

It is not contended that these people encountered no difficulties in their lives. On the contrary, there was considerable evidence that visible genital anomalies occasioned much anguish and distress. Distress was greatest in those patients whose external genital morphology flagrantly contradicted, without hope of surgical correction, the sex in which they had grown up and established, indelibly, their gender role and orientation as boy or girl, man or woman. Distress was also quite marked in patients who had been left in perplexed confusion about the sex to which they belonged, in consequence either of parental or medical indecision, or of insinuations from age-mates that they were half boy, half girl. Uniformly, the patients were psychologically benefited by corrective plastic surgery, when it was possible, to rehabilitate them in the sex of assignment and rearing. Only one patient failed to take advantage of plastic surgery. Instructively enough, he was the person who, on his own initiative, changed his birth certificate and began living as a man from the age of sixteen onward. He was unable to summon up enough courage to have his genitals masculinized.

It is relevant to note in passing that psychotic symptoms in all of the patients were conspicuous by their absence. In remarkably few instances, evidence of neurotic symptomatology was apparent. In some, but by no means all patients, feelings of bashfulness, shame and oddity were to the fore, and they had great initial diffidence in talking about themselves.

Assigned Sex and Rearing

Chromosomal sex, gonadal sex, hormonal sex, internal accessory reproductive organs and external genital morphology—each of these five variables of sex has passed successively in review and has been compared first with assigned sex and rearing and, second, with the gender role and orientation as boy or girl, man or woman, which the person established while growing up. In only 4 cases among 76 was any inconsistency between rearing and gender role observed, despite the many inconsistencies between these two and the other five variables of sex.

Evidently there is a very close connection between, on the one hand, the sex to which an individual is assigned, and thenceforth reassigned in a myriad subtle ways in the course of being reared day by day, and, on the other hand, the establishment of gender role and orientation as male or female.

Gender Role and Orientation

In the light of hermaphroditic evidence, it is no longer possible to attribute psychologic maleness or femaleness to chromosomal, gonadal or hormonal origins, nor to morphological sex differences of either the internal accessory reproductive organs or the external genitalia. Conceivably, of course, instinctive masculinity or femininity may be attributed to some other innate bodily origin. For example, Krafft-Ebing[9] among others has suggested special brain centers. There is, however, no support for such a conjecture when, as may happen in hermaphroditism, among individuals of identical diagnosis, some have been reared as boys, some as girls (Table VII).

There are 55 cases represented in Table VII, including the only 4 in the whole series of 76 in whom ambivalence of gender role was found. The four had been reared as girls. Among the 51 remaining, 42 reared as girls had established a feminine gender role and orientation, while 9 reared as boys had established a masculine gender role and orientation.

From the sum total of hermaphroditic evidence, the conclusion that emerges is that sexual behavior and orientation as male or female does not have an innate, instinctive basis.

In place of a theory of instinctive masculinity or femininity which is innate, the evidence of hermaphroditism lends support to a conception that, psychologically, sexuality is undifferentiated at birth and that it becomes differentiated as masculine or feminine in the course of the various experiences of growing up.

Those who find the concept of instinct or drive congenial may choose to say that there is a sexual instinct or drive that is undifferentiated and genderless at birth. In that case, sexual drive is neither male nor female to begin with, and it can be assumed to have no other somatic anchorage than in the erotically sensitive areas of the body. So limited, sexual drive becomes a special example of a kinaesthetic or haptic drive—an urge to touch and be touched, an urge for bodily contact.

Those who find the concept of drive uncongenial may choose simply to say that in the human species there are erotically sensitive areas of the body, especially the genital organs, and that these areas are sometimes stimulated and used by oneself or another person. In the course of growing up, a person's sexual organ sensations become associated with a gender role and orientation as male or female which becomes established through innumerable experiences encountered and transacted.

Our studies of hermaphroditism have pointed very strongly to the significance of life experiences encountered and transacted in the establishment of gender role and orientation. This statement is not an endorsement of a simpleminded theory of social and environmental determinism. Experiences are transacted as well as encountered—conjunction of the two terms is imperative—and encounters do not automatically dictate predictable transactions. There is ample place for novelty and the unexpected in cerebral and cognitional processes in human beings.

Novelty and unexpectedness notwithstanding, cerebral and cognitional processes are not infinitely modifiable. The observation that gender role is established in the course of growing up should not lead one to the hasty conclusion that gender role is easily modifiable. Quite the contrary! The evidence from examples of change or reassignment of sex in hermaphroditism, not to be presented here in detail, indicates that gender role becomes not only established, but also indelibly imprinted. Though gender imprinting begins by the first birthday, the critical period is reached by about the age of eighteen months. By the age of two and one-half years, gender role is already well established.

One may liken the establishment of a gender role through encounters and transactions to the establishment of a native language. Once imprinted, a person's native language may fall into disuse and be supplanted by another, but is never entirely eradicated. So also a gender role may be changed or, resembling native bilingualism, may be ambiguous, but it may also become so indelibly engraved that not even flagrant contradictions of body functioning and morphology may displace it.

Case Illustration

The following illustrative case has been chosen because it shows convincingly how gender role and orientation may be fully concordant with the sex of assignment and rearing, despite extreme contradiction of the other five variables of sex.

Introductory data: The patient was twenty-four years old and married at the time of psychologic study. He had lived all his life as a male. Except for a small hypospadiac phallus and fused, empty labioscrotum, he was found to be anatomically and physiologically female when, at the age of eleven and one-half years, he entered a hospital because his breasts had begun to enlarge and his body had grown increasingly feminine in contour. His genital abnormality, of which there was no known familial incidence, had been known to exist since birth. The penis had not enlarged significantly with the onset of puberty. Its glans was completely hidden by wrinkles of foreskin. Although the urethral orifice was located at the base instead of the tip of the penile shaft, the boy was able to stand to urinate. Testicles could not be palpated. The scrotum was contracted and not in the least pendulous.

Exploratory laparotomy revealed a uterus, fallopian tubes, bilateral par-ovarian cysts, and two cystic gonads in the position of ovaries. The uterus did not connect with a normal vagina, but appeared to open into the upper urethra. No organs of the male reproductive system were discerned internally. The uterus, tubes and gonads were removed, especially as the parents thought their child should remain a boy. Only two sections of the gonads were examined micro-scopically. They revealed ovarian structure, with primordial follicles containing ova, a few intermediate forms of developing graffian follicles, and several large cyst-like structures lined with granulosa cells.

Postoperatively, male hormone therapy was instituted and continued regu-larly thereafter. When the patient was twenty-one, therapy was withheld for about nine months on a trial basis, with a result that he felt weak and easily fatigued. Two years later, in preparation for marriage, he underwent plastic surgery in order to transpose and straighten the penis. At this time he appeared quite masculine in stature, though the breasts had remained slightly enlarged. Facial hair required shaving every second or third day. The pubic hair was masculine in distribution and the voice deep. A small, soft prostate was palpable.

First impression: "At first sight and throughout the first meeting with this man, I kept thinking that nothing in his general appearance, manner or conver-sation betrayed a single hint of the information filed away in his medical record. He would pass anywhere as the advanced graduate student that he was. So much was he a young man, indeed, that I wondered briefly if it might be best to leave well enough alone and not risk stirring up doubts and forebodings. He quickly grasped the purpose of a psychological research study, however, and readily consented to cooperate."

Interviews: At all times the man talked fluently and spontaneously, un-perturbed by recording apparatus, with no signs of withholding information through embarrassment. He had been told that utmost discretion would be used in concealing his identity—which was an imperative expediency in view of his educational affiliations and associations—and that he would be able to censor the manuscript of the case report before its circulation or publication. Most of the interviews and tests were completed within a single week, with only one examiner, over a period of about fifteen hours. After that there were a few meetings, including two or three informal visits with the man and his wife during the ensuing two years, and a few written notes for another two years.

Family: Both the mother and the father were university graduates. Through their own efforts and achievements they had earned considerable social standing in the community in which they reared their family of three. The patient had two brothers, three years and fourteen years his junior. The family kept together as a quite closely knit unit. Judging from the patient's memories, comments and anecdotes, he was not idealizing when he said: "I think that my relationship with my family, although rocky in spots, has been very happy. I'm devoted to them all. . . ." He and his wife returned home for occasional visits.

Thumbnail self-sketch: "Well, I suppose I'm not an unattractive person for most people. I'm generally optimistic, I think. Probably a little on the lazy side when all is said and done. I probably don't work as hard as I ought to work. I have a pretty good head. It isn't the best head in the world, but it's better than average, and I'm really content with it even though I sometimes wish it were better. I think it's good enough and thank God for what I've got. I expect I'll in my own time do a decent job of living. I don't expect to be much better than average. I expect that I'm sort of average, average good, a little higher than average, in about everything. Average good, in the moral sense, average intelligent, average ambitious, and so on. And that my life will pretty much follow out what—this general route that's kind of set for me, by what I am. I'll do all right. I expect that I can have some pretty rugged things happen to me and it won't jar my general optimism too much. A lot of things I can think of I wouldn't like to have happen, but even so I imagine I'll get along all right no matter what happens because I manage to—for the reason that I am what I am and it has contributed to my average or slightly above average intelligence and so on and so forth, I am able to slough off a lot of stuff better than not. I don't think I'm too dangerously supersensitive or anything of that sort. I imagine I'll belong in the division of perfectly pleasant and not unuseful existence; I hope I'll be able to raise a batch of children that will be as happy as I think I'll be."

Day-to-day routines: At the time of the interviews, the man was well advanced toward obtaining a doctorate in one of the aesthetic disciplines. During the academic year he worked not only at his own studies, but also as a part-time instructor. Whether in the applied, historical or theoretical branches of his field, his accomplishment and achievement had been recognized as outstanding.

There were times, however, when he was not satisfied that he was concentrating on his work sufficiently. "I am ambivalent," he said, "about working harder and taking life easy. I don't expect to be much better than average; I have always been rather modest about my ambitions and expect it is founded on a certain amount of slothfulness. I probably don't work as hard as I ought to work."

The slothfulness, or taking life easy, as he called it, appeared in different guises. For example, he was as he said rather modest in his expressed ambitions for a career, contented to aim at a sure target rather than gamble for a great prize. Again, his account of the course of a typical day gave supportive evidence of a dilatory tendency, one very common in students, namely putting off assignments until the very last minute. The time thus gained was spent with his wife, or at some extracurricular study, or talking with and entertaining friends who might call. Fellow students were frequent callers, as the couple occupied an apartment near the college.

Easy-goingness was also apparent in the infrequency with which the man became agitated, irritated or angry. "I don't know that I've been really angry since I was a little boy," he declared. "Really right down at the guts angry I don't think I've been for a long, long time. I was considerably annoyed last year when one guy wouldn't give me $100 when I wanted it. But anger is kind of exhausting and I tend to avoid it if I possibly can."

It was not that the man was timid or self-effacing, nor a social isolate. While growing up he had always shared some interests with friends of his own age, especially his brother. "But I didn't make friends very easily," he said of grade school days. "And I wasn't a sportsman at all and I frequently got kind of kicked around because I didn't know how to hit a ball with a bat and that sort of thing. . . . But I never felt that life was giving me the blunt end of the stick." He avoided competitive team sports and gymnasium classes because of his genital condition, but joined various other school groups and clubs.

Before leaving high school, he had begun attending a summer colony workshop. There he made many lasting friendships, and there he later met his wife. His first trip abroad had been in childhood with his family, since which there had been others, including one with his wife.

Religious teaching and Sunday school attendance had not been part of the man's childhood experience. Not until college years did he give serious thought to religious, along with philosophical matters. After he met his wife who was devoutly Catholic, he found "Christianity started to make sense, perhaps because she had impressive, implicit faith, and good sense too. I overcame my family-derived horror of Catholicism," but he was far from dogmatic about his personal credo. With his wife he was a regular church attender.

Intelligence test: Wechsler-Bellevue Intelligence Scale results were as follows: verbal IQ 144; nonverbal IQ 133; full IQ 143. A high standard of accuracy was maintained on each subtest. The overall rating was at the level of very superior.

Somatic growth and appearance: After surgical arrestment of pubertal feminization, virilization was induced and maintained by substitution treatment with androgens.The young man had a straightforward understanding of these medical facts, as will become apparent in the following.

Sexuality: "As far back as I can recall, I was always aware of having a genital peculiarity. In our household we were always free and easy about nudity, so I knew I was different from my father and brother." But in the early years of childhood, "it just seemed that men were the superior sex and they had a better thing to pee with."

That the urinary implications of the anomaly were of major import initially was indicated by the first response to the request for earliest memories: "I remember myself squirting the hose. I think I squirted my father in the process. And it was lots of fun." This memory, dating from the age of two, had been reinforced from a photograph taken on the occasion; "and yet, when I look at it, it kind of brings me back, you know, that wonderful feeling of power you have when you're watering something! Well, it kind of brings back something of being a master in your own domain as you squirt this blasted hose around."

Also remembered were a couple of early childhood incidents when the boy and some playmates set up secret urine receptacles behind a garage and in the basement. There were "peeing contests" on a few occasions, including one in which the boys were amazed to find that a little girl was able to meet a challenge and "pee into a glass."

Sometimes experimentation became more frankly sexual, as when a small group of boys tried to stick assorted items into their orifices; but there were no mutual explorations. While still a young child, the boy learned not to expose himself, regardless of what the others did. His mother, who was less embarrassed by his anomaly than his father, had always talked to him, explaining that he was different from other boys and had special reason not to get into sex play.

"I took more care as I became more aware of the unconscious meannesses of children," he said, "and I got so that I could go to the toilet almost anywhere and manage it so that no one would see." Only once, in high school, did a boy who presumably had participated in infantile sex play make an oblique reference to his friend's genital anomaly. It was in connection with exemption from gymnasium classes. "I said: 'Oh that cleared up a long time ago,' and closed the subject as quickly as I could, but was really quite upset." One or two close contemporary friends were thought to have vague suspicions "that something is wrong." But apart from medical people, wife and family, "nobody else knows as far as I know; and I wouldn't like anybody else to know. I still have a fear that I would be made fun of, and that it would be talked about."

Sex was not a matter for harsh discipline or secrecy in the family. "I knew very early, about six or so, about the process of birth, about the kittens the cat had and where babies came from. It wasn't until I was in the ninth grade that boys told me about the sexual act. I didn't believe it though, and didn't quite dare ask my father. I finally did," but did not get a direct answer, and was eventually convinced from discussions with contemporaries and from comprehensive reading.

"Of course about then it began to dawn on me that I was singularly unequipped; and from then on it became a more acute worry, although it never bothered me very much. But I was aware of it. Other boys had talked about masturbation which I had never thought of up until that time. I had a hell of a time. I experimented for a year before I found out what was necessary, because the kids I knew used the term jerk off or pull off and I didn't know what physically you did. And I didn't realize you were supposed to have an erection to do this. Then I masturbated more or less continuously until I got married. But I never thought it was right; it seems wrong that you should use your head to get out of a trouble which is by the direct route of logic in nature unnatural."

At the age of eleven "to my great horror I discovered that I had breasts beginning to develop. This seemed quite a calamity. And it was from that time, after the exploratory operation, that I knew I would never have any children, and that was a kind of continual bother. Mother was quite sure that I would never marry;" and was very upset when, with the first serious love affair at nineteen "I said I was damn well going to get married, somehow. Even at sixteen I was thinking about it. Probably because I'd been told I couldn't ever get married anyway. And I had great moral difficulties because I was undecided as to whether I should marry this girl and whether I was going to give some girl a raw deal. Dad was more reticent about it, not knowing quite what to say; and my doctor didn't want to commit himself. But I went ahead anyway.

"In a sense my life has centered around this problem of getting married in that I have always wanted to get married. It's been one of the things that I was going to do, if it was humanly possible. That has been a controlling factor and a challenge all the way along, from some of my earliest memories. Patsy Jane, I can remember when we moved, I kissed her goodbye and took her pictures. I must have been about seven. And then I had a girl friend after that who continued to write to me." At high school there were the jealousies and rivalries over girl friends; the love notes; "the big fuss about who would dance with whom at dancing school"; the party games of post office; "and, if you were very lucky, the concession of a kiss." In the early college years there was the first serious affair "with Dorothy. And then the girl who is now my wife."

Of the findings at the exploratory operation "I still haven't gotten the whole works. I still don't know everything about it. But I've gathered that there'd been some kind of female apparatus in there by mistake and that it had been taken out. I also knew that they were looking for testes; and didn't find them. I guess they found a couple of ovaries or something too. That's about all I know about it."

Some weeks later the man did recall in a casual conversation that he had, at the age of eleven, been asked if he wanted to be a girl. The idea had no appeal. This knowledge, together with the evidence of enlarged breasts, apparently had more significance than that manifested in conscious awareness, witness the following passage of free association: "We ranged in size the same way as we ranged in age. And nobody could ever figure us out when we were on these trips together. They always thought we were some god-forsaken kind of damned pervert bunch. Nobody, obviously I was, I couldn't be the daughter or, or the son or, or Chloe wasn't Homer's daughter and he as', she couldn't be his wife very easily, and I wa', nobody could figure my relationship to; we even considered scratching the name of the institution off the side of the station wagon."

For the most part, however, the ambiguity of sexual status had been well thought out. Only once, in late childhood had there been "some experimenting with my brother, but we were pretty thoroughly frustrated and disgusted and gave that up as a bad job." It was during the college freshman year that the issue came really into focus. "I got to know vaguely of things about drinking; and some of the queer flabs around." One acquaintance "travelled with a weird group of avant-garde writers and knew an awful lot of the fairies around." A couple of homosexual guys in the dormitory committed suicide.

"One night a guy came up into my room and was lamenting about women— I hadn't heard from Dorothy for some time—and looked at me and said: 'Say, well, have you ever thought of trying anything else?' and gee, I about vomited on the spot, not knowing whether this was an offer or what. I began to think that maybe other people thought I was funny or something."

Sex was in mind frequently, "and I would think about all kinds of sex, what kinds there were, and then I would wonder if I was safe or not. Whether I would find myself liking it too much or something. Yet, if I ever started making any image of homosexuality, I could never get myself into it. It was always other people. Yet I could always think of myself as a possibility for the game. Physically I might have been the best bet in college for some joker. I presumed that some men might find me rather appealing because, well, I'm not a terribly hairy person, and my femininity, in other words, those things about me which are less masculine, less pronouncedly masculine.

"I was much concerned with my breasts at that time. Now I don't care about them, although I am careful how I dress. But at that time people did say things about them. That's something I hadn't thought of, but that might have had quite a lot to do with it. You see I had this tendency to be very conscious, or subconsciously aware of my breasts; and I suppose I always did make some kind of female association there.

"During all this time I was well into this affair with Dorothy; in which I knew consciously and rationally that I had every reason for feeling that I was perfectly okay because I knew perfectly well that I was attracted to women. I had been sneaking out against family opposition, and flying over to spend the weekend with her. And one of my undergraduate experiences was sleeping all night in the same bed with her. It was strictly a dry run, but it was great sport.

"The guys at school were all big talkers about women and I let it be known that I'd been a heller when I was in high school—which of course is very far from true—and was now going steady. There were some very vigorous parties, especially at the summer school resort, but I never had any affairs. I would like to have been around raising cain, but in addition to what vague moral feelings I had about it I knew damn well I couldn't. I was very lucky to have any instincts in that direction, I guess. I was taking testosterone; if I wasn't I don't think I would have given a hoot for anybody. I was also in a sense fortunate in falling in with a crowd that was all straight too. I don't think with my particular background I ever would have been very sympathetic to the fairy groups. It was too black and white like that, my family tradition, although there had never been anything very specific about it. I was lucky to be with a gang that were overtly sex happy and spending a lot of time running around finding it."

The resolution of sexual uncertainties was neatly illustrated in a dream, the only one which he could recall. It was dreamed nearly two years earlier, when he and two fellow instructors from the summer school had visited a man whom they thought homosexual. "I dreamed that I was in a church eating supper—stuffed cabbage leaves or something. Rae was with me and we were sitting with strangers at a table in front of the sanctuary. Homer and Chloe were at a table within the sanctuary. The altar was off in the transept. I looked up and in the first pew was this fairy wearing pearl earrings, lipstick and henna in his hair. He was with someone who looked like his mother and was grinning kind of silly. I laughed and went up and told Homer and Chloe to look at him. I came back and was concerned that Rae wasn't eating anything, so we went somewhere else and had supper together. It was a very happy dream. My big problems were resolved. Chloe and I figured it out. I wasn't a fairy because I was with Rae and was able to laugh at this other guy. And I was still able to talk to Chloe and Homer who were my friends, but who wonder about my marrying a Catholic girl and my feelings about Catholicism. And although Rae wasn't quite happy we went somewhere else and were very happy. I remember thinking kind of guiltily that she wasn't eating, because I was enjoying myself tremendously."

"Rae and I had a devil of a time trying to find out whether it was really all right for us to get married. We worried through that. We figured if we could get through that we could get through anything. So I think we can. Gee that was awful. Well, anyhow, we talked to my doctor and he said he thought it would be okay; and we talked to the Church and they said it was okay and so, with many a prayer, we took the giant step and got ourselves engaged and decided it was foolish to wait after you were engaged, and so we got married. At this point we feel, typically, that we're the luckiest people in the world."

Before being married he underwent a plastic repair of the genitalia so that the penis was more advantageously placed for coitus. "And Rae and I make out very well now, of course we're still just married, but it's a rough day when we don't get to bed at least once. And I consider that pretty normal for the first six months of married life. I've never felt that I was particularly abnormal in respect to the strength of libido, but that I seem to fit in the middle somewhere."

Since the age of twelve he had taken testosterone regularly except for one period of several months during which he felt a lack of energy and "probably a little bit of diminution of libido, but not enough to really worry about. I wasn't conscious of being completely apathetic." Ordinarily, there is plenty of erotic sensation localized in the penis. It erects very automatically. "In fact there was one time when I first started taking testosterone when I just needed to move and uff!—there she was, from the friction of my pants."

There is minimal fluid discharge at ejaculation, "but I have the sensation of ejaculation; I'm quite sure it's the same sensation. It may be greater or lesser intensity, I don't know. At any rate it's entirely satisfying. Of course we have had to experiment quite a bit, to find the best ways for Rae always to have an orgasm," since the erect penis is only about two inches long. "If she doesn't that makes me very unhappy."

A spontaneous gaiety in their marriage was clearly reflected in a passage of free association: "And we had good fun in bed the other day; gee it must have been two hours. We've felt good ever since." At this point he paused, checked himself, awakened from somnolence, laughed and said he had been thinking about examining his wife and of the day when she may get ambitious enough for fellatio in love making. "Rae's awfully nice. She's really awfully nice. I love her a great deal."

The blank-card story of the Thematic Apperception Test evoked a portrayal of family life around the meal table with the children whom they both took for granted they would rear. A family by adoption was, at that time, uppermost in mind, although the possibility of artificial insemination was not excluded. Some years later, the moral issues of artificial insemination having been thoroughly thrashed out, the wife became pregnant and gave birth to a child.

Psychological Appraisal

To all who knew him, it was perfectly obvious that this man had achieved conspicuous, all-round success in coping with life. Only those who knew his medical record knew of the odds against him. To the world at large he gave no signs of having had to surmount the tremendous obstacles imposed by the contradictions of his genital anomaly. He passed simply as an ordinary male college graduate—one of the more stable and well-adjusted.

The challenge to overcome genital defections was pervasive and of long standing: the man said so directly, as well as in unpremeditated sayings and test responses. In early childhood there had been peeing contests; at puberty a total lack of appeal in the idea of changing to live as a girl; in the teens a nagging uncertainty about genital mechanics but a determined resolution to get married; and finally plastic surgery of the genitalia and an erotically successful marriage.

For all its pre-eminence, sexuality did not blot out all else. Academically the man had always made superior achievement. Yet he disparaged himself as being slothful and lazy, and wondered if he might "fall down on the score of lack of penetrating enough intelligence." He spoke of daydream rivalries with a colleague "who is infinitely quicker in mind than I am, which irks me no end."

It seemed possible that the red-hot fire of this man's endeavor had burned in the service of psychosexual problems, and that it might not glow so intensely in the service of work and aesthetic creativeness. Allowing that one must speculate and not be sure in these matters, it also seemed that the kind of logical, systematic literalness requisite for solving psychosexual problems was incompatible with the flashy erraticness of creative insight, penetrating intelligence and a quick mind.

In discussing personal sexual matters, the man exhibited an astonishing degree of empirical detachment and logical reasoning. He had an accurate fund of information about himself which, presumably, had helped him to look at his own case with detachment. He had not been kept in the dark without answers to questions. He had not been obliged to jump to conclusions, putting two and two together for himself.

Judging from Rorschach and Thematic Apperception Test responses, he was the sort of person whose attention kept pretty well anchored to clear outlines in perceptual experience. He didn't venture too far with confabulation and make-believe. He described and analyzed instead. As most people would say, he was very realistic.

Fantasies and personal myths and symbol did not appear to occupy much of a place in the economy of his mental life. It would be brash to theorize about castration, Oedipus or other complexes, on the basis of evidence collected. Suffice it that the man said enough about his childhood relationship with his mother for the Oedipal attachment considered normal in boys to be attributed to him also, his somatic status notwithstanding. It was not an exaggerated or prolonged attachment. Eventually it gave way to a concern with girlfriend relationships and marriage, and with the anatomical problem of adequacy in intercourse.

Erotically, there is not a single doubt about the man's masculine orientation though, for those who seriously measure masculinity with a yardstick of pugnacity and aggressiveness, he will not get full marks. He rated himself as being a person slow to anger. His general behavior and demeanor confirmed his estimate.

This slowness to anger was a lack of aggressiveness in the narrow sense of belligerence. It did not include a lack of confidence and initiative making for tentativeness and hesitancy. It was an absence of attack but not of mastery. It was the substitution of strategy for disorganized fighting. At times it was also removal of oneself from provocateurs so that aggression was not aroused.

Though slow to anger, the man was not, then, inhibited and helpless. His control and restraint did not in this or any other context run to excesses; it was temperate and moderate. Thus vigilance was exercised lest the legitimate secret of his anomaly become public, but the secret was openly and frankly discussed under appropriate circumstances. The quality of vigilance and cautious moderation tempered most of his doings in life. His ambitions were modest, he said, and in fact they were, for he had talent and intelligence which would have justified even grandiose aspirations.

All in all, beyond every possible doubt, this person was psychologically a man. He was fortified with a diplomatic arrogance which adjusted to the human demands of the occasion, yet enabled him to choose and select his standards rather than run with the herd. He was meeting life most successfully without any suspicion of psychopathology. There was every reason to believe that he would continue to do so. His life is an eloquent and incisive testimony to the stamina of human personality.

Summary

Seventy-six hermaphroditic patients manifesting somatic ambisexual anomalies were studied psychologically and their gender role and orientation appraised. Gender role and orientation were compared with the sex of assignment and rearing, and with each of five other variables of sex, namely chromosomal sex, gonadal sex, hormonal sex, internal reproductive organs, and external genitalia. Gender role and orientation were found to be congruous with the sex of assignment and rearing in 72 of the 76 patients despite contradiction between this pair of variables and one or more of the other five. It was concluded that the sex of assignment and rearing was better than any other variable as a prognosticator of the gender role and orientation established by the patients in this group. The bearing of this finding on instinct theory in psychology and psychiatry was examined. A case report was given to illustrate how gender role and orientation may be fully concordant with the sex of assignment and rearing, despite extreme contradiction of the other five variables of sex.

References

1. Freud, S.: Three essays on sexuality. *The Standard Edition of the Complete Psychological Work of Sigmund Freud,* Vol. VII. Hogarth Press, London, England, 1953. See especially the first essay.

2. Money, J., Hampson, J. G., and Hampson, J. L.: Hermaphroditism: Recommendations concerning assignment of sex, change of sex, and psychologic management. *Bull. Johns Hopkins Hosp.* 1955, 97:284.

3. Wilkins, L., et al.: Hermaphroditism: Classification, diagnosis, selection of sex, and treatment. *Pediatrics.* In press.

4. Hampson, J. L., Hampson, J. G., and Money, J.: The syndrome of gonadal agenesis (ovarian agenesis) and male chromosomal pattern in girls and women: Psychologic studies. *Bull. Johns Hopkins Hosp.* 1955, 97:207.

5. Grumbach, M. M., Van Wyk, J. J., and Wilkins, L.: Gonadal dysgenesis, ovarian agenesis, male pseudohermaphroditism: Bearings on theories of human sex differentiation. Read at the 37th annual meeting of The Endocrine Society, June 2, 1955. *J. Clin. Endocr. and Metab.* In press.

6. Money, J.: *Hermaphroditism: An Inquiry into the Nature of a Human Paradox.* Unpublished doctoral thesis, Harvard University Library, 1952; University Microfilms, Ann Arbor, MI, 1967.

7. Moore, K. L., Graham, M. A., and Barr, M. L.: The detection of chromosomal sex in hermaphrodites from a skin biopsy. *Surg. Gynec. and Obst.* 1953, 96:641.

8. Barr, M. L.: An interim note on the application of the skin biopsy test of chromosomal sex to hermaphrodites. *Surg. Gynec. and Obst.* 1954, 92:184.

9. Krafft-Ebing, R. von: *Psychopathia Sexualis,* 7th edition. F. A. Davis Co., Philadelphia, Pa., 1930.

Note

Originally published in the *Bulletin of The Johns Hopkins Hospital,* 97:301-319, 1955, with J. G. Hampson and J. L. Hampson as coauthors. [Bibliog. #2.11]

Author's Comment: Seven Variables of Sex

In this chapter and in Chapter 11, the subdivision of sex into seven variables, each potentially independent of one another, grew out of my 1952 dissertation research. It was in a 1955 paper on hyperadrenocortical hermaphroditism (Money, *Bulletin of The Johns Hopkins Hospital,* 96:253-264) that the variables were first mentioned in print. The concept of sex as subdivisible was rapidly assimilated into the biomedical literature, as was the classification of its variables. By 1965, they were incorporated into the definition of sex as revised in the 24th edition of *Dorland's Illustrated Medical Dictionary* (Philadelphia, Saunders).

THIRTEEN

Sexual Incongruities and Psychopathology: The Evidence of Human Hermaphroditism

Introduction

Few people acquainted with Freudianism and its impact on the theories of psychology and psychiatry can fail to be aware that sexuality, in its broadest sense, has been given an important place in theories about the genesis of psychiatric disorders. It is appropriate, therefore, to examine the evidence of human hermaphroditism in relation to psychopathology.

During the past four years, the authors have studied and followed 94 hermaphroditic patients, juvenile and adult, in an attempt to ascertain, among other things, the status of their psychologic healthiness or nonhealthiness.

Before making an appraisal of psychologic healthiness in these 94 patients, it was necessary to separate them into subgroups the members of which were sufficiently similar, anatomically and physiologically, to permit valid psychologic comparison one with another. There are eight subgroups, representing eight varieties of hermaphroditism (Table I). A brief synopsis of the identifying signs of each variety has been published in an earlier paper (see Chapter 11).[1]

The sexual incongruities that one may find in hermaphroditism involve diverse contradictions, singly or in combination, between seven variables of sex (Table II).

In affirmation of evidence assembled in an earlier paper (see Chapter 12), it may be said that, in 95 per cent of our 94 cases, gender role and orientation corresponded unequivocally with the sex assignment and rearing, irrespective of incongruities between this pair of variables, on the one hand, and one or more of the other five variables of sex, on the other hand. In only 5 of our 94 patients, therefore, was there any question of psychologic nonhealthiness on grounds of a demonstrably ambiguous gender role and orientation.

Standards of Appraisal

To appraise psychologic healthiness and evaluate the severity of nonhealthiness is an extremely vexacious problem, to admit which requires no apology. There are no instruments to use, and no standardized routines of calibration to follow. We have collected extensive data on our patients using formal psychologic tests, casual interviews, recorded and transcribed systematic interviews, participant

TABLE I

Varieties of Somatic Ambisexual Development*

1. Congenital hyperadrenocorticism in otherwise normal female	48
2. Female, with well differentiated phallus, normal ovaries and normal internal reproductive structures	3
3. True hermaphroditism, i.e., with testicular and ovarian tissue both present	1
4. Male, with unarrested mullerian differentiation:	
(a) with normal penis and one or both testes cryptorchid	0
(b) hypospadiac and cryptorchid	3
5. Gonadal agenesis (dysgenesis), with simulant female infantile body morphology and male chromosomes	16
6. Simulant female, with testes, blind vagina, mullerian vestiges and breasts	7
7. Cryptorchid male hypospadiac, with breasts at puberty:	
(a) with urogenital sinus	1
(b) with blind vaginal pouch	0
8. Cryptorchid male hypospadiac:	
(a) with urogenital sinus	13
(b) with blind vaginal pouch	2
	——
	94

*For the purpose of this classification, the primary differentiation is by the criterion of gonadal sex. This practice reflects the traditional medical and surgical approach which prevailed until recently, whereby gonadal sex is the *real sex* and the classification of hermaphrodites threefold, namely, true hermaphrodites and male and female pseudohermaphrodites. Our findings do not justify the choice of this gonadal criterion as the *exclusive,* or even as the *primary* criterion, from the standpoint of psychologic and behavioral study, nor for purposes of wise clinical practice. Nonetheless, the gonadal criterion offers a convenient basis for medical classification and discussion. See bibliographic references 2 to 7, inclusive, for further, comprehensive information concerning the varieties of hermaphroditism.

observation of behavior, and interviews with relatives.* We have done follow-up studies on the great majority of patients once or twice a year, or more often, dependent on the feasibility of a return journey to the hospital. On the basis of all available data, we have exercised our clinical judgment, separately and as a group, and rated each patient on a graduated scale that has four salient points:

> — healthy
> — mildly nonhealthy
> — moderately nonhealthy
> — severely (morbidly) unhealthy

We have always been in agreement about the rating of each patient.

A rating of healthy, mentally or physically, is not synonymous with being perfect or ideal according to some preordained standard, not even the standard of the statistically typical or normal. It may, for example, be statistically typical or normal, but not healthy, for members of a population to have beriberi or

*Further details of the method of gathering information are given in Money and Hampson.[12]

TABLE II

Seven Variables of Sex

1. Chromosomal sex (8, 9).
2. Gonadal sex.
3. Hormonal sex.
4. Internal accessory reproductive structures (10).
5. External genital morphology.
6. Sex of assignment and rearing.
7. Gender role and orientation established while growing up.

endemic goiter. Nonetheless, healthiness and statistical typicalness become nearly more synonymous when a random sample of individuals is drawn from a large and heterogeneous population, for such a sample discloses the wide range of variability encompassed by the typical or normal.

In general medicine, a rating of healthy is consistent with a wide range of individual differences in height, weight, pulse rate, blood pressure, blood count, 17-ketosteroid excretion, threshold of resistance to microorganisms, and so forth. In psychologic medicine, also, a rating of *healthy* is consistent with a wide range of individual variation. To be rated healthy, it was not necessary for patients to be devoid of problems, conflicts, perplexities and anxieties, nor devoid of specialized modes of personality functioning. It was necessary only that they were encountering their various experiences and carrying out their various transactions in life without evidence of persistent mismanagement or incompetence of a degree that required other people consistently to make exceptional provisions for them or show special consideration toward them.

A rating of *nonhealthy* signifies that a person fails, in some way or other, to negotiate the encounters and transactions of life, unless other people grant special considerations or exceptional provisions of one sort or another. The kind of consideration or provision required varies according to the type of non-healthiness and its degree, whether mild, moderate or severe. Thus, congenital IQ impairment of severe degree may require permanent custodial supervision, whereas an equally severe disorder, such as compulsive immobility except when walking backwards, may require psychiatric hospitalization and psychotherapy. A rating of nonhealthy does not, per se, give any indication of the duration, onset, cause or prognosis of a disorder. Cognitional impairment, for example, is psychologic nonhealthiness whether associated with tertiary syphilis, with con-genital cerebral defect, with prolonged schizophrenic deterioration, with transient toxic delirium, or with chronic self-depreciation, anxiety and dread.

A patient with a rating of *mild nonhealthiness* is a person who, from a layman's point of view, would usually be credited as normal and well adjusted. On the basis of increased information obtained in psychologic investigation, however, it is found that the person negotiates life in a series of encounters and transactions that intermittently reach a crisis of stressfulness. During these periodic crises, some special considerations and exceptional provisions are needed in order that the person can again pick up the threads of living. The special considerations and provisions may come from family, friends, employer or a professional expert. A brief series of psychiatric consultations is, in certain instances, as expeditious a provision as any that can be made.

The people to whom a rating of *moderate nonhealthiness* is applied are usually recognized by laymen as slow, retarded, nervous, neurotic, maladjusted, emotionally disturbed, or beset by psychologic problems. Diagnostically, the psychiatric nomenclature applicable to such people is not restricted to the neuroses, but may include character disorders, personality trait disorders, delinquency or mental deficiency, among others. Moderately nonhealthy people are competent at negotiating some of the ordinary encounters and transactions of life, but their lack of healthiness is great enough to require that they be granted special considerations and provisions, of some sort or other, by many different people and in many different contexts of living, for an indefinite period of time. One special provison may be psychiatric treatment, more or less regularly, over a period of years, but without prolonged hospitalization or constant psychiatric supervision.

A rating of morbid or *severe nonhealthiness* is applied to people who are chronically, or for a long period, unable to negotiate any of the ordinary transactions and encounters of life without such special considerations and provisions as constant protection, constant supervision, indefinite custody or prolonged therapeutic treatment. Inexpert and lay opinion usually concedes that such people are not psychologically healthy, though the degree of nonhealthiness is commonly underestimated. Technically, the rating of severely nonhealthy applies to most psychoses. It may also apply to the most severe and disabling neuroses, to addictions, to chronically criminal and so-called psychopathic personality disorders, to extensive cerebral and cognitional impairments, gross mental deficiency, and so forth.

Distribution of Ratings

The distribution of psychologic healthiness and nonhealthiness ratings among the 94 patients, according to variety of hermaphroditism, is shown in Table III.

Severely Nonhealthy

The most noteworthy finding of this study of psychologic healthiness in hermaphrodites is the conspicuous absence of severe psychologic disorder. The rating of severely nonhealthy was appropriate for only one among our ninety-four patients. This patient, an hyperadrenocortical female pseudohermaphrodite mentally defective since birth, tested with an estimated IQ no higher than 40 by the time she was five years old. No other patients required a rating of severe psychologic nonhealthiness. None was psychotic and none required psychiatric

TABLE III

Psychologic Healthiness Ratings of 94 Patients

Variety of Hermaphroditism	Healthy	Mild	Nonhealthy Moderate	Severe	Total
1. Adrenal ♀	28	12	7	1	48
2. Nonadrenal ♀	3	—	—	—	3
3. True	1	—	—	—	1
4. ♂, mullerian differentiation	1	—	2	—	3
5. Gonadal agenesis	14	1	1	—	16
6. ♂, simulant ♀	7	—	—	—	7
7. ♂, hypospadiac, breasts	1	—	—	—	1
8. ♂, hypospadiac	8	3	4	—	15
Total	63	16	14	1	94

hospitalization, though one patient told that her older sister, an hyperadrenocortical female like herself, had been hospitalized ten years earlier with a diagnosis of dementia praecox, since which time she had been living at home on the farm, though only partially recovered.*

Moderately Nonhealthy

The fourteen patients rated moderately nonhealthy were, apart from their rating, a diverse and heterogeneous group. They ranged in age from three to thirty-seven years. Three were adults, six were in the teenage, and five below the teenage.

   With one exception, all of the patients knew from visible anatomical evidence that they were genitally deformed. The exception was a patient with gonadal agenesis and male chromosomes who looked like a girl and had been reared as a girl for all of her fourteen years. Four older female patients with hyperadrenocorticism, living as women, were severely virilized before treatment was begun. Two younger female hyperadrenocortical patients had been reared first as girls, then as boys, and a third had had several hypospadiac repairs, as a boy, from an early age. Two siblings, cryptorchid hypospadiac males with clitoral sized phallus, were living as boys, one having been changed from living as a girl at the age of five. There were two other cryptorchid hypospadiac males. One, with medium sized phallus who had been reared as a girl, changed on his own initiative to live as a man at the age of sixteen. The other, living as a boy, was a high grade mental defective. Finally, two cryptorchid hypospadiac males with well differentiated mullerian organs, both reared and living as girls, were also high grade mental defectives.

*The rareness of psychosis among hermaphrodites was corroborated in a survey of the literature (13). Among 248 postadolescent cases of hermaphroditism, there were 5 instances of psychosis: 2 senile dementia, 1 manic-depressive, 2 schizophrenia. There were also 3 cases of epilepsy, 3 of gross mental deficiency and 2 of suicide. Visible hermaphroditic anatomy was present and of apparent causal significance only in the two instances of suicide and one instance of schizophrenia, paranoid type.

Though they all received the same rating of moderately nonhealthy, these fourteen patients displayed widely diverse signs and symptoms of psychologic nonhealthiness. In three cases, the chief disability was an IQ (Wechsler) in the 60s, near the upper limit of the mental defective rating. The commonest disability, irrespective of IQ, was an excessive operation, in some form or other, of inhibitory and control functions of the personality. In half of the patients, this inhibitory excess showed up as a psychologic growth failure: relative to age and IQ, these patients evidenced in some degree a babyish lack of accomplishment and mastery.

Inhibitory excess also showed up, in all except two of the patients, as a chronic and sometimes excruciatingly pervasive syndrome of shyness, bashfulness, diffidence, reticence and inarticulateness. This syndrome was most in evidence whenever social transactions and conversation pertained in any way to eroticism, sexuality or romance.

The immobility of excessive inhibition, especially when tears or preliminary signs of weeping are added, may signify apprehension, anxiety, fear and dread. One patient, an older hyperadrenocortical woman, had a chronically recurrent syndrome of anxiety and dread, complete with concomitant physiologic signs of anxiety. Five of the younger patients manifested acute episodic bouts of anxiety intense enough to be called terror, especially in connection with hospitalization.

The immobility of excessive inhibition may signify not only anxiety and fear, but also sullen, stubborn antagonism. There were three patients in whom it was often difficult to distinguish antagonism from anxiety.

Two of the fourteen patients did not manifest a preponderance of the inhibitory function of personality. Each took the bull by the horns, so to speak, and met the challenge of the sexual dilemma head on. One changed from living as a girl to living as a man, and the other, despite severe adrenocortical virilization, entered compulsively into sexual relations with a series of boyfriends. Both these people negotiated their lives, however, only by resorting to stimulants and sedatives, including alcohol, in large doses. Each had assorted neurasthenic and psychosomatic complaints, and each was subject to intermittent depressive, moody spells.

Whether inhibitory control or assertive mastery predominated in personality functioning, in none of the patients was there an undue degree of bizarre perception and judgment, nor of cognitional idiosyncracy such as hallucination, confabulation or delusion.

Mildly Nonhealthy

The composition of the group of sixteen mildly nonhealthy patients does not differ in any clearly distinguishable way from that of the group of fourteen rated moderately nonhealthy. The sixteen ranged in age from four to fifty years. Eleven were adults, two were in the teenage and three below the teenage.

As in the less psychologically healthy group, there was only one patient (with a diagnosis of gonadal agenesis and male chromosomal pattern) who had no visible anatomical evidence of genital deformity. In the moderately non-healthy group, four patients underwent a reassignment of the sex of rearing, three of them after the age of four years; in the mildly nonhealthy group, three patients underwent a reassignment of the sex of rearing, all before the age of four years. Four of the group of sixteen were juveniles with hyperadrenocorti-cism (of whom two were also sex reassignment cases). Eight more with the same syndrome had reached adulthood as severely virilized women before cortisone therapy was available; one of these, married, had the chronically invalid person-ality expected in a person dying, as she was, with cancer. The remaining two patients in the group were cryptorchid hypospadiac males with female looking external genitals who had been reared, though with indecision, as girls.

By contrast with the moderately nonhealthy patients, none of the mildly nonhealthy had an IQ at the mentally defective level. The majority manifested in one form or another a mild excess, either chronically or intermittently, of inhibi-tion and control in personality function. In one patient, inhibitive collapse was a direct sequel of widespread metastatic cancer. In four patients, inhibition showed up chiefly as introverted shyness and cautious guardedness along with, maybe, an occasional outburst of righteous self-justification. In two other patients, in-hibition showed up chiefly as intermittent moody spells of despondency border-ing on depression. In yet two other instances, inhibition had a more specifically amnesic guise, and the patients had transient hysteric conversion symptoms. Another patient had a speech inhibition, namely stuttering and stammering. There were three patients, living as women, who had homosexual desires and inclinations. One of these, an introverted and shy person, had not been a partner in homosexual practices; the other two, whose erotic practices had been bisexual, were not introverted and shy in day-to-day routines and affairs.

In addition to the two bisexual patients, there were three other patients in whom the signs of mild nonhealthiness signified not inhibition but a makeshift, inexpedient effort of mastery. The three patients were living as girls. One had a compulsion to check locks and switches more than once before going to sleep at night. One did some compulsive stealing, notably of a watch from the home of friends. The third, an infant, had intermittent episodes of temper tantrum and screaming.

In the mildly, as in the moderately nonhealthy patients, disturbances of per-ception, imagery, thought or judgment were lacking. Only one patient was in-clined to be autistic in thought as well as introverted and inhibited in demeanor.

Healthy

The composition of the group of sixty-three patients with a rating of psycho-logically healthy differs from that of the nonhealthy groups on two major counts. The first count is this: the proportion of juveniles is greater among the healthy than the nonhealthy. A rating of healthy was given to nine adults, seventeen teenagers and thirty-seven preteenage children, of whom eighteen were below the age of five. Table IV shows the comparative distribution of patients according to age and to rating as either healthy or nonhealthy.

The preponderance of healthy juveniles (Table IV) is statistically significant at between the 2 percent and 1 percent level of confidence (chi-square: 6.19). This preponderance of juveniles may signify either that the investigators were more lenient in appraising children, or that nonhealthiness was more difficult to identify in children than adults, or that nonhealthiness was less prevalent among children than older people. The last of the three alternatives is considered almost certainly the correct one.

Greater prevalence of psychologic healthiness among the juvenile rather than the older hermaphrodites can be accounted for with the hypothesis that the juveniles had not experienced the impact of their hermaphroditic paradox in its full force, either because they had not lived long enough to do so, or because they had received corrective therapy from an early age, or because they had a form of hermaphroditism which did not declare itself as a visible ambisexuality.

There was no evidence that the psychologic growth and development of hermaphroditic babies during the first weeks and months of life was influenced by their hermaphroditic status, unless indirectly as a concomitant of parental doubts and dreads. The infants became most psychologically vulnerable when they grew old enough and experienced enough to know and recognize that they were genitally neither entirely boy nor entirely girl. Their vulnerability increased as they grew older, if their externally visible secondary sexual development was incongruous with the sex of assignment and rearing.

The relationship of psychologic vulnerability to age was particularly well exemplified in the hyperadrenocortical patients (Table V). Among the 20 preteenage patients rated as healthy, 13 were under the age of five years. They were being reared as girls. Each of the thirteen was unacquainted with her sexual ambiguity, owing either to her infancy or the early institution of corrective therapy, or both.

Hyperadrenocortical hermaphrodites for whom corrective therapy is instituted in infancy resemble another group of juvenile hermaphrodites who have no visible signs of their sexual anomaly. These others are simulant females who have a perfectly normal female body morphology, externally, which is contradicted by a male chromosomal pattern, by improperly differentiated mullerian organs, and by testes that paradoxically secrete estrogens after puberty. Very similar are the patients with male chromosomal pattern, immature normal mullerian organs, and gonadal agenesis. Patients in both categories are unhesitatingly declared girls at birth and grow up as psychologically healthy girls.

The preponderance of these female looking patients (with or without gonads) with a healthy rating is the second major count on which the group of 63 patients rated healthy differs from the nonhealthy groups. Only 2 of the female looking patients were rated nonhealthy whereas 21 (9 juvenile and 12 teenage or adult) were rated healthy. The prevalence of psychologic healthiness among

TABLE IV

Distribution of 94 Cases According to Age
and Psychologic Healthiness or Nonhealthiness

	Preteenage	Teenage and Adult
Healthy	37	26
Nonhealthy	9	22

TABLE V

Age and Psychologic Healthiness of 48 Hyperadrenocortical Patients

	Preteenage	Teenage	Adult
Healthy	20	6	2
Mildly nonhealthy	2	2	8
Mod. nonhealthy	2	3	2
Severely nonhealthy	1	—	—

these female looking hermaphrodites may be accounted for with the hypothesis that they were not confronted with sensory evidence of hermaphroditic incongruities to disturb healthy psychologic functioning. The fact that chromosomally they were male, or that the gonads were testicular in structure was irrelevant to their psychologic healthiness as girls.

Some patients whose external body morphology and appearance was ambiguous looking and incongruous also had been assigned to and reared in the sex which contradicted their chromosomal and gonadal sex. Thus, there were 4 hyperadrenocortical females reared as boys; 2 females without the adrenal syndrome reared as boys; 3 males with well differentiated mullerian structures reared as girls; and 8 cryptorchid hypospadiac males reared as girls. Of these 17 individuals, 8 were rated as psychologically healthy. It is not possible to correlate the nonhealthy ratings of the other 9 with their chromosomal or gonadal status. Their ratings reflect rather the disruptions of a reassignment of sex—4 cases—and, in two instances, congenital mental deficiency. In short, other things being equal, it proved quite possible for a patient to grow up psychologically healthy in the sex contradicted by chromosomes and gonads, and partially contradicted by genital appearance.

Reassignment of Sex

Hermaphrodites who are assigned to one sex at birth and subsequently reassigned to the other sex are a particularly instructive group with reference to psychologic healthiness and nonhealthiness. There were 14 patients whose sex was reassigned, the youngest at one month of age, the oldest, on his own initiative, at sixteen years of age.

TABLE VI

Psychologic Healthiness Ratings on 48 Teenage and Adult Patients

	Body Morphology and Appearance	
	Ambiguous	Unambiguous
Healthy	12	13
Mildly nonhealthy	12	2
Mod. nonhealthy	8	1

Ranged in order of age at the time of reassignment of sex, and rated for healthiness at least six months and at most twenty-one years later, these cases show clearly that the later in life a reassignment of sex, the greater the chance and the intensity of psychologic nonhealthiness.

Of 7 patients whose sex was reassigned between the ages of one and six months, 6 were rated healthy and 1 mildly nonhealthy.

Of 4 patients whose sex was reassigned between the ages of fifteen months and three years, 1 was rated healthy, 2 mildly nonhealthy and 1 moderately nonhealthy.

Of 3 patients whose sex was reassigned between the ages of four and sixteen years, all were rated moderately nonhealthy.

The symptoms of nonhealthiness in these patients were varied and diverse. The patients themselves did not connect their symptoms with their earlier change of sex, except for the thirty-seven year old man who himself had decided, at the age of sixteen, to cease living as a girl. Two other patients spoke about their change of sex, not from personal recall, but on the basis of subsequent hearsay. One, a boy of seventeen, had been changed at five years of age. The other, a girl of five, had been changed at five months of age, and subsequently reminded by other children that she had formerly been a boy; on account of her clitoral enlargement, she was also teased about turning back into a boy.

Neighborhood ridicule about being a freak and a half boy was prominent in the life of another girl, not subjected to a reassignment of sex, who was rated moderately nonhealthy. Other patients encountered more subtle insinuations about their authentic masculinity or femininity, and elaborated their own grave doubts and misgivings as well.

All in all, the ridicule, insinuation or misgivings of other people, as well as the about-face of a reassignment of sex, appear to have been very fruitful antecedents and concomitants of psychologic nonhealthiness in hermaphrodites, especially after the period of early infancy.

Visible Somatic Ambisexuality

Some hermaphrodites reach the teenage or adulthood living in the sex partially contradicted by their genital morphology or secondary sexual characteristics, or both. One might expect that life would present these patients with quandaries and problems over and above the usual and that, consequently, a high proportion of them would be rated nonhealthy.

There were 32 teenage and adult patients who looked ambiguous in body morphology and appearance, and 16 who did not. Their ratings for psychologic healthiness were distributed as follows (Table VI).

Some of the ambiguous looking patients would, without doubt, have warranted a rating of nonhealthy irrespective of their hermaphroditism. Nonetheless, it still appears from Table VI that ambiguity of genital and secondary sexual development facilitates psychologic nonhealthiness. This finding is not surprising. The surprise is that so many ambiguous looking patients were able to grow up and achieve a rating of psychologic healthiness or of nonhealthiness of only mild degree.

Hyperadrenocortical Patients Treated with Cortisone

So far in this presentation, it has become evident that hermaphrodites whose somatic ambisexuality does not publicize itself have a psychologic advantage over those for whom the reverse holds. Similarly, those patients whose incongruities and contradictions are corrected at an early age have an advantage over those whose treatment is delayed.

Hermaphroditic patients for whom corrective treatment, surgical or hormonal, is delayed until the late teens or older do not have their quandary automatically resolved in its entirety once surgical or hormonal corrections are effected. Psychologically, they are confronted with a program of readaptation to the demands and expectancies of life, and their readaptation may be prolonged and beset with difficulties. The syndrome of readaptation, as it may be called, was most clearly evident in patients whose corrective treatment did not get under way until they were well beyond the ordinary adolescent age. Owing to the recency of the discovery of cortisone for correcting hyperadrenocorticism in female pseudohermaphrodites, it happens that women with this severely virilizing syndrome had lived longer with conspicuous hermaphroditic incongruities uncorrected than any other of the patients in our study.

There were 8 hyperadrenocortical patients, ranging in age from twenty-three to forty-nine, who did not receive cortisone until adulthood. Some had had adrenal surgery earlier in life, and some genital reconstructive surgery, but all had remained hormonally virilized to an extreme degree. All had been reared as girls, were living as women, and had no intention whatsoever about changing to live as a man. They were profoundly embarrassed by what they considered the affliction of virilism. They considered feminizing treatment highly desirable and looked forward to the onset of menstruation and breast growth, as well as to a redistribution of hair growth along feminine lines.

For all of their desire to be rid of the stigmata of virilism and to undergo the physiological changes of a female puberty, these women had, nonetheless, found some sort of adaptation to life as virilized, abnormal looking individuals. Only one of them had married. One other had led an active sex life with boyfriends. Another was engaged and planned to marry at some unspecified time in the distant future. Love affairs and sexual relationships were excluded from the adaptation made to life by the remaining five patients.

Psychologic impedances associated with delayed attainment of a normal physiologic female puberty were twofold. The first impedance appeared to be associated very specifically with, indeed to be an effect of, realignments of body metabolism and functioning during the first week of cortisone therapy. The initial cortisone (or hydrocortisone) dosage for adults was 100 mg. a day for approximately a week until urinary 17-ketosteroids were sufficiently suppressed, and then 75 mg. every third day. During the first week, patients reported diverse subjective changes in feeling and perception, their reports coinciding with the onset of generalized edema and sodium retention.* One exceptionally articulate patient reported that she felt a vague and diffuse tiredness, weakness, depression and pessimistic gloom in which all of the tasks and problems of living seemed hopelessly magnified. Simultaneously, she felt a contradictory feeling of restlessness, as though sitting on the side of a volcano that might blow up. There was no accompanying thought content, but an urgent sense of responsibility to keep everything under control and to prevent an explosion. In addition to these two contradictory feeling states, the patient described an unpleasant somatic feeling of a bloated, over-full stomach and insatiable, ravenous hunger.

All of these disturbing feelings disappeared after the new electrolyte balance was established and the cortisone dosage was lowered. In the meantime, however, the patient's psychologic distress was magnified by what she construed as contempt and disdain from the nursing and house staff when she reported the first changes of feeling. Subsequently, she emphasized how adversely she had been affected by the belief that her doctors thought she was a fraudulent neurotic and complaining hypochondriac. She also emphasized how greatly she had been restabilized when the psychiatrist listened seriously to her descriptions of her feelings and reassured her that her experiences were not unique and would be transient. Like several other patients, this woman was well enough informed, from the popular press, about ACTH and cortisone psychoses to be panicky lest she were losing her mind as a result of receiving cortisone.

It is remarkable, though so far unexplained, that juvenile and teenage patients have not shown any signs of these peculiar reactions to the initial week of cortisone treatment.

The younger patients were also exempt from what proved to be the second impedance associated with delayed attainment of normal female puberty, name-

---

*The full clinical picture was discovered and investigated in three patients. It was not indubitably absent in any patients, but was probably overlooked in those treated earliest in the series. Edema and sodium retention appear to be lessened or absent when metacorten is used instead of cortisone or hydrocortisone, but feeling and mood changes are not necessarily eliminated.

ly, the negotiation of adolescence alone, completely without the group enter-prises and social encouragements of age mates. The more successfully the older women had come to terms with life as virilized individuals who could not expect to be attractive to men, the more difficult did they find the social and psycho-logic transition of adolescence after hormonal feminization and physiologic puberty began. Arrived anachronistically at a stage in life when their wildest romantic daydreams at last had a chance of coming true, these women found themselves awkward, inexpert and unself-assured at living the role of debutante, fiancée, lover, or perhaps, wife. So anachronistic an adolescence brought moody spells of depression and diverse bodily symptoms of severe anxiety in its train, four of these older women in particular having been so affected periodically.

Some of the older teenage girls also manifested similar signs of difficulty in coping with an anachronistic adolescence. By contrast, the preteenage girls, precocious in their virilism and also precocious in their feminizing response to cortisone, mixed socially with other adolescents somewhat older than themselves and negotiated the psychologic transition to adulthood with considerable facility, even if they had formerly been psychologically somewhat upset. Evidently, there are optimal growing periods for psychologic as well as somatic growth. Evident-ly, also, it is no easy matter to turn the clock back once an optimal period for psychologic growth and development has run its course.

Summary

Ninety-four hermaphroditic patients, representing eight varieties of hermaphro-ditism, have been under comprehensive psychologic and psychiatric study, and their psychologic healthiness has been appraised. On a four point rating scale, the 94 cases were distributed as follows: 63 healthy, 16 mildly nonhealthy, 14 moderately nonhealthy, 1 severely nonhealthy. The one severely nonhealthy patient was a congenital mental defective. Absence of psychosis, or rather lack of a high incidence of the so-called functional psychoses, is considered the most noteworthy finding of this study.

There was a marked tendency for mild and moderate nonhealthiness to show up as an excess of inhibitory and control functions of the personality. The symptoms included, among others, retardation of psychologic growth and personality development relative to IQ and life age; depressive moody spells; sullen and anxious bashfulness and shyness; and extreme but circumscribed diffidence and guardedness pertaining to sexual and romantic situations.

A rating of healthy was more common among infants and juveniles than among teenagers and adults, doubtless because the younger patients in our series had not experienced the impact of their hermaphroditic paradox with the same full force as the older patients had.

A rating of healthy was also more common among patients whose body morphology, irrespective of gonads and chromosomes, was unambiguous looking than among those whose sexual appearance was equivocal.

Patients whose sex of rearing was contradicted by chromosomal or gonadal sex were not necessarily destined to receive a nonhealthy rating. Reassignment of the sex of rearing after the early months of life was extremely conducive to subsequent psychologic nonhealthiness. Corrective surgical, hormonal or psychologic procedures were more beneficial if applied during infancy or childhood than later. Adaptation of a physiologic normalcy first induced during adulthood was seen to be a complex and difficult psychologic process, notably in adult hyperadrenocortical female pseudohermaphrodites newly feminized on cortisone therapy.

References

1. Money, J., Hampson, J. G. and Hampson, J. L.: Hermaphroditism: Recommendations concerning assignment of sex, change of sex and psychologic management. *Bull. Johns Hopkins Hosp.* 1955, 97:284.

2. Wilkins, L.: *The Diagnosis and Treatment of Endocrine Disorders in Childhood and Adolescence.* Charles C Thomas, Springfield, Illinois, 1950.

3. Wilkins, L., Grumbach, M. M., Van Wyk, J. J., Shepard, T. H. and Papadatos, C.: Hermaphroditism: Classification, diagnosis, selection of sex and treatment. *Pediatrics.* 1955, 16:287.

4. Wilkins, L., Bongiovanni, A. M., Clayton, G. W., Grumbach, M. M. and Van Wyk, J. J.: The present status of the treatment of virilizing adrenal hyperplasia with cortisone: Experience of 3½ years. *Mod. Prob. Ped.* (Supp. ad *Annales Paediatrici*). 1954, 1:329.

5. Grumbach, M. M., Van Wyk, J. J. and Wilkins, L.: Chromosomal sex in gonadal dysgenesis (ovarian agenesis): Relationship to male pseudohermaphrodism and theories of human sex differentiation. *J. Clin. Endocr. and Metab.* 1955:15:1161.

6. Hampson, J. L., Hampson, J. G. and Money, J.: The syndrome of gonadal agenesis (ovarian agenesis) and male chromosomal pattern in girls and women: Psychologic studies. *Bull. Johns Hopkins Hosp.* 1955, 97:207.

7. Morris, J. McL.: The syndrome of testicular feminization in male pseudohermaphrodites. *Am. J. Obst. and Gynec.,* 1953, 65:1192.

8. Moore, K. L., Graham, M. A. and Barr, M. L.: The detection of chromosomal sex in hermaphrodites from a skin biopsy. *Surg. Gynec. and Obst.* 1953, 96:641.

9. Barr, M. L.: An interim note on the application of the skin biopsy test of chromosomal sex to hermaphrodites. *Surg. Gynec. and Obst.* 1954, 92:184.

10. Jost, A.: Problems of fetal endocrinology: The gonadal and hypophyseal hormones. *Recent Progress in Hormone Research:* The Proceedings of the Laurentian Hormone Conference, Vol. VIII, p. 379. Ed. by G. Pincus, Academic Press Inc., New York, N.Y. 1953.

11. Money, J., Hampson, J. G. and Hampson, J. L.: An examination of some basic sexual concepts: The evidence of human hermaphroditism. *Bull. Johns Hopkins Hosp.* 1955, 97:301.

12. Money, J. and Hampson, J. G.: Idiopathic sexual precocity in the male. *Psychosomat. Med.* 1955, 17:1.

13. Money, J.: *Hermaphroditism: An Inquiry into the Nature of a Human Paradox.* Unpublished doctoral thesis, Harvard University Library, 1952; University Microfilms, Ann Arbor, MI, 1967.

Note

Originally published in the *Bulletin of The Johns Hopkins Hospital,* 98:43-57, 1956, with J. G. Hampson and J. L. Hampson as coauthors. [Bibliog. #2.15]

FOURTEEN

Imprinting and the Establishment of Gender Role

Introduction

Psychologic study of hermaphrodites sheds some interesting light on the venerable controversy of hereditary versus environmental determinants of sexuality in its psychologic sense.

Human hermaphrodites of whatever variety are persons born with some degree of sexual ambiguity, anatomically and physiologically. Since they are neither exclusively male nor exclusively female, hermaphrodites are likely to grow up with contradictions existing between the sex of assignment and rearing, on the one hand, and various physical sexual variables, singly or in combination, on the other. These physical sexual variables are five in number, namely, (1) chromosomal sex, (2) gonadal sex, (3) hormonal sex and pubertal feminization or virilization, (4) the internal accessory reproductive structures, and (5) external genital morphology.

In view of the various ambisexual contradictions that may be found in hermaphroditism, one may ask whether the gender role and orientation that a hermaphrodite establishes during the course of growing up is concordant with the sex of assignment and rearing, or whether it is predominantly concordant with one or another of the five physical sexual variables.

Psychologic Studies

During the past five years, we have investigated the sexual psychology of 105 hermaphroditic patients[1-5] of different diagnostic varieties and of all ages. The majority of them were, after their initial hospital appearance, followed from year to year. From observational notes, recorded interviews, and formal psychological tests, we obtained enough data from these patients to be able to appraise their gender role and orientation as masculine, as feminine, or as ambiguous. It was then possible to compare the gender role and orientation that each patient had established with the sex which had been assigned in infancy and in which the patient had subsequently been reared. It was also possible to compare the gender role and orientation with each of the five physical variables of sex, taken severally.

The resulting comparisons demonstrated that the sex of assignment and rearing is consistently and conspicuously a more reliable prognosticator of a hermaphrodite's gender role and orientation than is the chromosomal sex, the gonadal sex, the hormonal sex, the accessory internal reproductive morphology, or the ambiguous morphology of the external genitalia. There were only 5 among the 105 patients whose gender role and orientation was ambiguous and deviant from the sex of assignment and rearing. By contrast, for each of the five physical sexual variables, there were between 23 and 30 patients—not always the same persons*—whose sex of assignment and rearing was incongruous. In some patients this incongruity involved only one physical variable, but in most of the patients more than one physical variable was involved. Thus, some patients were predominantly female with respect to the physical variables of sex but, having been reared as boys, had the sexual psychology of a boy, or man—and vice versa for patients reared as girls.

The clinching piece of evidence concerning the psychologic importance of the sex of assignment and rearing is provided when, among persons of identical physical diagnosis, some are reared as boys, some as girls. It is indeed startling to see, for example, two children with female hyperadrenocorticism in the company of one another in a hospital playroom, one of them entirely feminine in behavior and conduct, the other entirely masculine, each according to upbringing. As a social observer, one gets no suspicion that the two children are chromosomally and gonadally female, for psychologically they are entirely different.

Further supportive evidence concerning the importance, psychologically, of the sex of assignment and rearing is provided by cases of reassignment of sex by edict. Among our cases there were 14 patients who underwent a reassignment of sex after the early neonatal weeks. Of these 14, there were 9 below the age of 2 years 3 months at the time of the change; with 3 exceptions, they appeared subsequently to have negotiated the change without even mild signs of psychologic nonhealthiness. By contrast, only one of the five children older than 2 years 3 months at the time of reassignment of sex could possibly be rated as psychologically healthy. One infers that once a person's gender role begins to get well established, an attempt at its reversal is an extreme psychologic hazard. Psychologic nonhealthiness was markedly less common in patients without a history of sex reassignment than in those with one.†

Practical Applications

The practical and clinical applications of our studies and findings have been spelled out in detail in two papers already published.[6,7] In briefest summary, our findings point to the extreme desirability of deciding, with as little diagnostic

---

*The individual patients represented in each of the five categories, one for each physical variable of sex, were not identical, owing to the inconsistencies of physical contradictions in hermaphroditism; but some patients required entering in more than one table.

†In actual fact, the incidence of psychologic nonhealthiness among our 105 patients was surprisingly rare; frank psychosis was entirely absent, except for one instance of schizophrenia of long duration.

delay as possible, on the sex of assignment and rearing when a hermaphroditic baby is born. Thereafter, uncompromising adherence to the decision is desirable. The chromosomal sex should not be the ultimate criterion, nor should the gonadal sex. By contrast, a great deal of emphasis should be placed on the morphology of the external genitals and the ease with which these organs can be surgically reconstructed to be consistent with the assigned sex. In cases of female hyperadrenocorticism, good surgical feminization is possible almost without exception, and these patients can, of course, also be hormonally regulated as females when treated with cortisone. Other surgical considerations being equal, the earlier surgical reconstruction of the genitals is done, the better. When operations must necessarily be delayed until later childhood or adolescence, it is sound psychologic medicine to take children into one's confidence and explain the whys and wherefores of what is planned on their behalf. Clitoral amputation in patients living as girls does not, so far as our evidence goes, destroy erotic sensitivity and responsiveness, provided the vagina is well developed. If clitoridectomy is performed in early infancy, the chances of undesirable psychologic sequelae are negligible.

Theoretical Considerations

Theoretically, our findings indicate that neither a purely hereditary nor a purely environmental doctrine of the origins of gender role and orientation—of psychologic sex—is adequate. On the one hand, it is evident that the unity of gender role and orientation is not determined in some automatic, innate, or instinctive fashion by physical, bodily agents, like chromosomes, gonadal structures, or hormones. On the other hand, it is also evident that the sex of assignment and rearing does not automatically and mechanisticaly determine the gender role and orientation: the small group of five patients whose sexual outlook diverged somewhat from that of the sex to which they had been assigned prevents so simple-minded a view of environmental determinism. Rather, it appears that a person's gender role and orientation become established, beginning at a very early age, as that person becomes acquainted with and deciphers a continuous multiplicity of signs that point in the direction of his being a boy, or her being a girl. These signs range all the way from nouns and pronouns differentiating gender to modes of behavior, hair cut, dress, and personal adornment that are differentiated according to sex. The most emphatic sign of all is, of course, the appearance of the genital organs. Presumably, it is the very ambiguity of the external genitals that makes hermaphrodites so adaptable to assignment in either sex, though it requires to be emphasized that the less ambiguous our patients could be made to appear as a result of well-timed plastic surgery and hormonal therapy, consistent with their rearing, the sturdier was their psychologic healthiness.

The salient variable in the establishment of a person's gender role and orientation is neither hereditary nor environmental, in any purist sense of those terms, but is his own decipherment and interpretation of a plurality of signs, some of which may be considered hereditary or constitutional, others environmental. His decipherment of social and environmental signs, whether under the impact of deliberate training and inculcation or through the more casual and haphazard lessons of experience, appears to be markedly more significant than has traditionally been allowed in medical and scientific theories.

Establishment of one's gender role and orientation appears to have much in common with establishment of one's native language. Bilingualism may be native. So also may a gender role and orientation be ambivalent. A native language eventually becomes ineradicable. So also does a gender role and orientation.

Ineradicability of psychologic functions established after birth is seldom given credence in most psychologic theory. There are many medical analogies, however. Bone development, for example, can be effectively influenced in rickets and cretinism only before maturity is reached. Thereafter, deformities of bone growth associated with these diseases become ineradicable.

There are some recent findings in animal psychology that give credence to the viewpoint that psychologic functions, such as gender role and orientation, may become so ineradicable as to appear innately instinctive. We refer to the investigations of Dr. Konrad Lorenz, in Austria, and with one of his examples we shall close.[8] Guided by his own exemplary reasoning, Lorenz experimented and discovered that wild mallard ducklings, immediately upon being hatched, could be induced to react to him as if he were their mother. In contrast with graylag goslings, which unquestioningly accept the first living thing they meet as mother, the mallard ducklings were panicky until they heard the quacking noise usually made by the mother mallard duck. Lorenz imitated the quacking of a mallard mother for half a day, almost continuously, waddling about in a squatting position, lest this height-width ratio produce a visual configuration that dispersed the ducklings in terror. After quacking and waddling with the newly hatched creatures for the first half-day of their lives, Lorenz became established for them as mother. The truly amazing sequel, however, is that the ducklings responded to Lorenz as if he were their mother from that day onward. They trailed behind him on his local excursions, and from the sky or the fields they came flying or running at the sound of the mallard notes he imitated.

Summary

Over a period of five years, we have made a comprehensive psychologic study of over 100 patients born with diverse varieties of hermaphroditism. With rare exceptions, it was found that the sexual psychology of these patients—their gender role and orientation—was consistent with their sex of assignment and rearing, even when the latter contradicted chromosomal sex, gonadal sex, hormonal sex, the predominant internal accessory reproductive structures, and the external genital morphology. Though the sex of rearing could transcend external genital morphology in psychologic importance, absence or correction of ambiguous genital appearance was psychologically beneficial. Reassignment of the sex of rearing after the early months of life was, without doubt, psychologically injurious.

References

1. Money, J.: Hermaphroditism, gender and precocity in hyperadrenocorticism: Psychologic findings, *Bull. Johns Hopkins Hosp.* 96:253-264, 1955.

2. Hampson, J. G.: Hermaphroditic genital appearance, rearing and eroticism in hyperadrenocorticism, *Bull. Johns Hopkins Hosp.* 96:265-273, 1955.

3. Hampson, J. L.; Hampson, J. G., and Money, J.: The syndrome of gonadal agenesis (ovarian agenesis) and male chromosomal pattern in girls and women: Psychologic studies, *Bull. Johns Hopkins Hosp.* 97:207-226, 1955.

4. Money, J.: Hampson, J. G., and Hampson, J. L.: An examination of some basic sexual concepts: The evidence of human hermaphroditism, *Bull. Johns Hopkins Hosp.* 97:301-319, 1955.

5. Money, J.; Hampson, J. G., and Hampson, J. L.: Sexual incongruities and psychopathology: The evidence of human hermaphroditism, *Bull. Johns Hopkins Hosp.* 98:43-57, 1956.

6. Money, J.; Hampson, J. G. and Hampson, J. L.: Hermaphroditism: Recommendations concerning assignment of sex, change of sex and psychologic management, *Bull. Johns Hopkins Hosp.* 97:284-300, 1955.

7. Hampson, J. G.; Money, J., and Hampson, J. L.: Teaching clinic: Hermaphroditism: Recommendations concerning case management. *J. Clin. Endocrinol.* 16:547-556, 1956.

8. Lorenz, K. Z.: *King Solomon's Ring: New Light on Animal Ways,* New York, The Thomas Y. Crowell Company, 1952.

Note

Originally published in *Archives of Neurology and Psychiatry,* 77:333-336, 1957, with J. G. Hampson and J. L. Hampson as coauthors; and written in recognition of having in 1956 received the Hofheimer Prize of the American Psychiatric Association for an "outstanding contribution to the advancement of psychiatry." [Bibliog. #2.17]

FIFTEEN

Matched Pairs of Hermaphrodites: Behavioral Biology of Sexual Differentiation from Chromosomes to Gender Identity

Serial Determinants

Gender identity in adulthood is the end product not of an either-or determinism of heredity versus environment, but of the genetic code in serial interaction with environment. From the time of conception, the genetic code unfolds itself in interaction, first with the intrauterine environment, then the perinatal environment, the family environment, and eventually the more extended social, biological, and inanimate ecological environment. Interactionism is a key principle, but an even more basic key is the principle of serial sequence of interaction.

Serial interactionism means that interaction between the genetic code and its environment, at a critical or sensitive developmental period in an individual's existence, from conception to death, may leave a permanent ineradicable residue upon which all else is subsequently built. This residue may be so indelible or insistent in its influence as to resemble the potency of the genetic code itself. Moreover, such indelibility or insistence may be residual to what has traditionally been referred to as learning—in which case learning should be referred to as imprinting, in recognition of the persistence and durability of its influence.

In a bygone era of medicine and behavioral biology, the differentiation of a person's sense of gender identity was confidently accepted as innately or instinctively determined. Among authorities of this bygone era, there was less confidence as to whether the innate determinism was genetic, gonadal (by reason of posesssing ovaries, testes or, rarely, ovotestes), or hormonal. But there was an agreement of sorts, among these erstwhile experts. They wrongly agreed, in hermaphroditic cases of doubt owing to incompleted anatomical differentiation of the external sex organs at birth, that the sex of the gonads somehow had paramount importance in dictating what the sex of assignment and rearing should be. Therefore, they tried to palpate two testes—if not descended, then in the groin. These palpated lumps might be defective and infertile. No matter. The expert, in his ignorance, might omnisciently decree that an infant, despite a deformed hypospadiac penis resembling a mildly enlarged clitoris, be assigned and reared as a male—though Nature's effort to make a complete male had obviously been thwarted.

Today, one knows better than to use a single, dogmatic criterion, like gonadal sex, on which to base the decision of sex assignment and rearing in cases of congenital ambiguity of the reproductive anatomy. When all the variables, from chromosomal sex to fertility, have been properly evaluated and prognosticated, the one that ultimately takes preeminence over all others is the criterion of erotic applicability in adulthood. It is useless to assign (or reassign) an hermaphrodite as a male, if all the medication, surgery, and psychotherapy in the world will fail to enable that individual to function in an adult erotic relationship as a male—and likewise in the case of female assignment.

Effect of Androgen Insensitivity on Differentiation

No matter what the genetically determined antecedents and components of gender-identity differentiation, the postconceptional and postnatal determinants can, in test cases, completely override them. The syndrome of androgen insensitivity (testicular feminization) in genetic males provides a graphic example of the extent to which the genetics of the sex chromosomes can be overridden in gender-identity formation. In this syndrome, suppression of the genetic program carried by the XY chromosome pair is itself a genetically transmitted trait. It has its effect at the cellular level by preventing cellular uptake of testosterone, the androgenic sex hormone of the male. The cells of the embryo and fetus are thus unable to utilize their quota of the testosterone released in normal amounts by the body's own testicles.

In consequence, the embryonic testes fail to inhibit, as they should, the primal tendency of the internal and external reproductive organs to differentiate as female. The failure is incomplete, so far as the internal organs are concerned, so that the uterus is poorly formed and incapable of menstruating at adolescence. By contrast, the failure of the testes to hormonally masculinize the external organs is total, with the result that the anlagen of these organs differentiate as 100 percent female. The baby is born with a female appearance so that, as for all babies with the same genital anatomy, she is announced and registered as a girl. It will not be until much later that a discrepancy will be recognized between the anatomical appearance, on the one hand, and the gonads and XY chromosome pattern, on the other.

Very occasionally, the syndrome will be recognized in infancy, because of the appearance of the testicles as lumps in the groin, as they try in vain to descend. Occasionally also, an infant might be diagnosed in the course of a family checkup, when an adolescent sister has been diagnosed after a gynecologic examination for failure to menstruate. This latter age is, in fact, the most usual one when a diagnosis is made. By this time, the girl has developed her own breasts and a normal female body contour, for her body has continued to be cellularly unresponsive to male sex hormone, now being released in normal adult amounts by the Leydig cells of her own testes. Her body cells have responded only to the normal amounts of estrogen, the feminizing hormone, normally released by the testicles of normal males.

The girl with the androgen-insensitivity syndrome spends her infancy and childhood exposed to the same family and social influences as her normal sisters, cousins, and friends. She is reacted to as a girl, and she responds as one. Her gender identity differentiates as that of a girl. She shares the play interests of other girls her age, and in teenage she develops the same romantic and dating interests. Despite the bitterness and deprivation of infertility, and of knowing about it ahead of time, she typically gets married and achieves her motherhood by adoption. She is indistinguishable from other mothers on her street. No one, except her closest family and her medical advisers, knows, or even suspects, the uniqueness of her status as a genetic and gonadal male, though she is an hormonal, morphologic, and psychologic female. Her case is a prime example of how little the genetic program of the XY chromosome pair can achieve, of and by itself alone, when its proper developmental environment—cellular through social—is changed as a consequence of a quite limited biochemical impairment, itself genetically determined.

Experimental Antiandrogenism

Though a genetic factor is responsible for initiating the train of events that produces human beings with the androgen-insensitivity syndrome, an analogous condition can be initiated in animals with no abnormal genetic trait. In this case, the hormonal environment of the fetus is changed at a sensitive period, critical for the differentiation of the external genitalia, by injecting the pregnant mother with a synthetic hormone that has an androgen-antagonistic effect. The sons are then born with the external genital anatomy of the normal female. Their testes remain undescended in the abdominal cavity where, if subject to no further antiandrogenic treatment, they will secrete masculinizing hormone at puberty. However, masculinization can be prevented by removal of the testes, and feminization can be induced by cyclic injections of estrogen and progesterone. Then the animals will go periodically into heat, as regular females do, and will respond sexually as females to the males that try to mount them. The males respond to them in the same way as they do to normal females.

The feminizing effect of antiandrogen on the sexual differentiation of the male was discovered by Neumann and his colleagues in West Berlin. Their experiment illustrates the principle, first demonstrated by Jost in Paris some 20-odd years ago, that Nature's first intention in sexual differentiation is to make a female. Jost had castrated fetal rabbits in utero and found that all, regardless of genetic sex, were born with the morphology of females. With no gonads and no gonadal hormones at the critical period of fetal life, differentiation of the external genitals is always female. Something must be added, namely male sex hormone, usually supplied by the fetal testicles, to initiate masculine differentiation of the primitive anlagen of the external sexual organs.

Neumann illustrates this principle humorously when he says that the story of Adam and Eve really should be retold. Eve would be created first, instead of

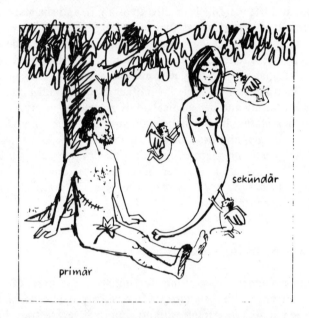

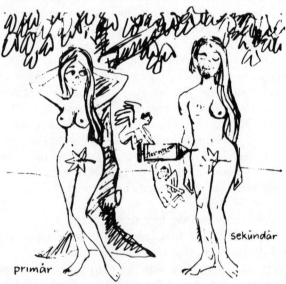

FIG. 1 Nature's first intention in sexual differentiation is to make a female. So perhaps the story of Adam and Eve might be retold, with Eve no longer being created from Adam's rib, but with Adam being made out of Eve by an injection of testosterone. [Courtesy of Friedmund Neumann.]

from Adam's rib. Then an archangel would appear with a big injection needle and, by injecting woman with testosterone, create man.

Male Hermaphroditism: Matched Pair

With this principle of masculine differentiation in mind, let me describe another kind of hermaphroditism in man—that of a genetic (XY) male who is defective in developing the clitoris small enough to qualify as feminine, or since it's a genetic male, one should say a penis large enough to qualify as masculine. Such an example was a baby assigned as a female and raised that way. The father considered it malpractice when his local gynecologist told him nearly 11 years later that he had a son instead of a daughter. Fortunately for the girl, she ended up at Johns Hopkins, where she was given surgical feminization in two stages— the first for external appearance at the age of 11, and the second at the age of 19 when her insufficient vagina was lengthened.

Hormone treatments can do a great deal when they are started early enough. In this case the girl was beginning pubertal masculinzation when we first saw her. But by surgical removal of the gonads and, therefore, of the male hormones, and with female-hormone replacement treatment, by age 19 she was a good-looking, feminine-acting girl. She was in love with a boyfriend who was number two in her experience. When she came to the hospital, number one was so anxious to be reinstated after being jilted that he took his vacation and visited her every day while she was recovering from her vaginoplasty. She still turned him down! Her psychosexual identity, as this anecdote indicates, had differentiated effectively as female.

This girl's example shows how complete can be a transformation, under an experiment of Nature of this type. It demonstrates that there is no preordained, mechanistic relationship between the genetic and genital structure, on the one hand, and the masculinity or femininity of behavior on the other. This lack of a direct determinism between genetics, anatomy, and sexual behavior is even more vividly demonstrated when the case of the girl is matched against one of the same genetic and somatic diagnosis, in which the assignment and rearing has been not as a girl, but as a boy. This boy was recognized as genetically ambiguous at birth and, after some uncertainty, assigned as a male. Masculine repair of the genitalia required multiple admissions throughout childhood, and was finally successful, though the corpus of the penis is rather small. The testes at puberty secreted androgen in sufficient amount to induce spontaneous adolescent virilization. Fortunately the body was not androgen-insensitive, nor even partially so, with resultant breast growth and impotence, as is sometimes the case. The prognosis regarding fertility is unsure, as is the possibility of transmission of the genital defect to male offspring, should there be any. From infancy onward, the boy's psychosexual differentiation as manifested in his behavior, and in what he says, has been masculine. In adolescence, his romantic interests and imagery

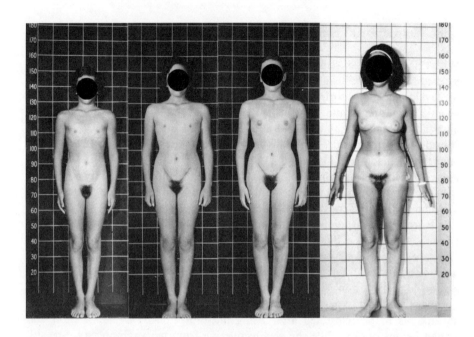

FIG. 2. This genetic (XY) male—shown at ages 11, 12, 13, and 19—was always raised as a female. At age 11 the mixup was discovered, and she got the first part of her surgical feminization; at 19 she received further feminization surgery. Her complete differentiation as a female shows how complete such a gender transformation can be.

emerged as masculine. There was nothing that marked him as particularly different from his high school age mates.

The boy and the girl of the preceding case are theoretically important because of the sameness on which their differences are built. Both are genetically male with the XY sex-chromosome pair, and both were exposed before birth to the same fetal-hormonal environment. In infancy and childhood they were somatically similar, but they were exposed to quite different behavioral experiences. They developed correspondingly different behavior in relation to gender role and the differentiation of a gender identity. This remarkable antithesis in psychosexual (and sexo-behavioral) differentiation is indicative of a general principle: namely, that gender-identity differentiation is phyletically programed in the human species to take place largely after birth, and also to be dependent to a large degree on stimulation from, and interaction with, the social environment.

Adrenogenital Female Hermaphroditism:
Four Matched Pairs

The foregoing principle can be found illustrated also in matched pairs of individuals who are genetic females with the XX sex-chromosome pair. Let me now present four matched pairs of cases of female hermaphroditism of the type known as the adrenogenital syndrome. In this syndrome, masculinizing of the genetic female fetus is initiated by a genetic anomaly that blocks the production of the hormone cortisone, in the adrenal cortex, and releases a masculinizing hormone instead. In a few rare instances masculinizing is so complete that the genital tubercle of the fetus develops not into a clitoris but a penis. The result is a genetic female born with a normal-appearing penis and empty scrotum. The tabs of skin that should form the labia minora of the female behave in the normal masculine developmental manner and wrap themselves around the protruding phallus to make a urinary tube in it. This genetic female will actually urinate through the penis. The outer swellings that should form the labia majora do the masculine maneuver of fusing in the midline to create an empty scrotum. Inside the body there are two ovaries and a uterus.

In the first matched pair, one baby was considered a boy a birth. Co-incidentally, symptoms of salt loss finally pointed the way to an accurate diagnosis, but too late to make a sex reassignment. The boy was allowed to stay living as a boy. Surgery was done in the masculinizing direction. The other baby, also because of acute salt loss, nearly died in the first few days after birth, and then was recognized diagnostically. After consultation with the parents (a very important thing, I might add, to get them to understand that doctors are not out of their heads when they tell them that their child with a penis is a girl), feminizing surgery was undertaken, and the baby was assigned and raised as a girl. Here again when two children have the same genetic sex, the same fetal hormonal history, and the same sexual anatomy at birth, it is possible to deflect one child to be raised and to develop a gender identity as a boy, and the other one as a girl.

In the second example, one child was again assigned as a boy and one as a girl. Each had masculinized external genitals, but not to the extent of a complete penis. We did not see them for treatment until they got to be around ten years old, by which time somebody had realized that something must be wrong. These were cases of imperfect, improper workup and diagnosis at the time of birth. When no treatment is given to genetic females with the adrenogenital syndrome, adrenal cortical androgen continues to be produced in excess and has its masculinizing effect—particularly noticeable by age ten as early virilizing sexual maturity. In the case of the child growing up as a boy, early virilizing was not too bad, but for the child growing up as a girl, it was a terrible mortification. The boy didn't like being sexually mature at so young an age, because no children like to be freaky and abnormal-looking, but at least he had the confirmation of being a boy. Nor did he like the final stigma of short stature, around five feet, as a consequence of early maturation.

Following diagnosis, both children and their careers continue unchanged, as boy and girl, respectively. The boy was able to maintain his body's masculinization, even without special treatment. Having had his penis repaired in childhood, he eventually got married. He did not keep his first marriage for too many years, but did not return to bachelorhood because of this, nor feel that he was unmasculine. He tried again in a second marriage. Here is further evidence of the extraordinary importance and power of postnatal events and conditions in directing the differentiation of psychosexual identity.

The girl's story is opposite, involving hormone treatment with cortisone in order to permit the ovaries to produce feminizing puberty. Despite the years of hormonal masculinization, behavior, outlook and ambitions were female in orientation. However, the girl's confidence as an erotic person, capable of an erotic life, and worthy of a boyfriend and a marriage was much delayed in maturing. (I've had to pilot quite a few of these girls through their anguish at feeling that they have a history of having been a freak, and that somehow this will be intuited by the boy who first has a sexual relation with them—that maybe he will find something wrong.) I have counseled this girl and her boyfriend, as they plan to get married, and she's finally triumphed. She's actually a very attractive young woman. The only telltale sign of her earlier medical history is a narrow configuration of the hips, because their fate was already settled by the time cortisone therapy was begun, owing to the years of the male-hormonal influence on the fusion of the bones.

The next two people, who again have the same adrenogenital diagnosis as the previous four, were recognized at birth. They were given the modern cortisone treatment (discovered in 1950) to regulate the adrenocortical glands and make them function normally. Physically they both grew at a normal rate in childhood, without early virilizing, so ugly for a girl. At puberty, the girl got her breast development from her own ovaries, which were allowed to come into estrogenic hormonal action instead of being suppressed by malfunctional adrenocortical glands. The boy, also maintained on cortisone to regulate somatic growth, got his masculinization by being given injections of testosterone. His ovaries, uterus and fallopian tubes had been surgically removed. He got testicles implanted as artificial prostheses. His penis had been repaired early in life. The girl, at a time soon after birth, had had a reconstruction of the vulva and vagina. Now both of these people have their romantic interests in teenage, appropriate respectively to their lives and roles as boy and girl.

There is a special, very fascinating point to mention here. This girl, like others of similar diagnostic and treatment history, has a certain special flavor to her behavior. Although completely acceptable as a female in our society today—not as a lesbian, not falling in love with other girls—she is a tomboy and puts marriage second in her life. Also, she is very bright and has her sights set

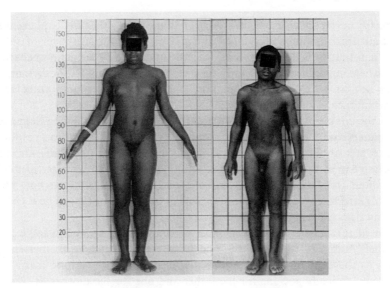

FIG. 3. Both these people are genetic females
with the adrenogenital syndrome. The one on
the left was identified at birth as a boy, the one
on the right as a girl. But in both cases the
assignment was uncertain, and the uncertainty
was conveyed to the growing children. Both, at
age 11, changed their sex identity.

on a high-level academic career. (These people, by the way, tend to have high
IQs.) Maybe she will get married one day, and maybe she will have a child, but
she's not strongly "turned on" by maternalism. Parenthood and a sex life are
something that she can, apparently without sacrifice, postpone.

The final example consists of two people whose position in life, by late
childhood, was that somebody must have been a knave or a fool who put them
in the wrong sex. As in the preceding six cases, each of them has the adrenogenital syndrome and is genetically a female. One, by age 11, thought he ought
to change from being assigned as a boy to live as a girl. The exact opposite
happened to the other one. In both cases, when the children were sent home
from the hospital at birth, the parents were left with the uncertain possibility of
a change of sex later, in view of the ambiguous appearance of the genitalia.
Consequently, the parents did not know exactly what kind of child they were
rearing—a boy or a girl. This type of uncertainty is as contagious as the
measles, and the children contracted it.

Now, if you're a girl who is not sure that you're supposed to be a girl
because of your funny-looking genitals, you have an alternative choice. It's a
simple law of binary logic that, if you feel everything is wrong the way you are,

maybe the correct way is the other way. I think therein lies the explanation of why both these children developed themselves in life as members of the sex other than that to which they were officially assigned. They finally reached the point where they felt that the only way they could belong to the human race was to be allowed to change. They both did, and now they both *do* belong to the human race.

In the course of their treatment I encountered two very telling documents. Both patients were electively mute on matters of sex; it was just too painful for them to talk about it. They were willing to be examined physically and to be cooperative in every way possible, but totally inhibited in the matter of talking. After about six sessions with the first of them, I found an illiterate note on my floor: "Dear Doctor, I do not wemt (want) to be a boy. I wemt to be a girl, just (like) my sisters. From Stanley."

I used this note as a parable, three or four years later, when talking with the other youngster who also suffered from elective mutism on matters pertaining to the dilemma of sex. From this second patient, among many other documents, I finally got one for the father and one for the mother. It was on a particular day when it was very important for the parents to get a message in person directly from the child, so they could be sure that their child was not being forced into a decision in the hospital. The situation was very tense and dramatic as this 11-year old, after a period of listening and doodling, finally wrote, with all the strength of his dyslexic and pre-primer level of achievement: "I gotta be a boy." Nobody had any doubts after that.

The lesson of my story of the four pairs of adrenogenital cases, each with the same genetics and each with the same prenatal history, is once again that— if we ever needed any convincing of it—one must always understand in matters of the biology of sexual behavior that a chain of interactive events leads from the genes to the final product. Only very rarely might one find a direct correlation on a cause-and-effect basis between genetics and any other single variable and behavior.

Note

Originally published in *Engineering and Science* (California Institute of Technology) Special issue: *Biological Bases of Human Behavior,* 33:34-39, 1970. Edited from the transcript of the Caltech "Conference on the Biological Bases of Human Behavior." [Bibliog. #2.120]

SIXTEEN

Determinants of Human Gender-Identity/Role

1. Principle of Differentiation and Development

Sexual behavior in man, like the sexual anatomy itself, is by reason of man's place in the phyletic scale, dimorphic. That is to say, its growth from its inception onward is simultaneously a process of differentation as well as of development. This fact tends to have been overlooked historically in psychiatry, which has spoken mainly of psychosexual development. Sexual theory has been impoverished thereby.

Reduced to its barest essentials, traditional sexual theory in psychiatry is built on two constructs: libido and identification. Libido, the instinctual sexual force, has not been conceived of as sexually dimorphic, per se, though possibly as bisexual. Manifest difference in behavior between the sexes has been regarded conceptually as secondary to libido and mainly as the developmental product of identification: to somewhat oversimplify, little girls identify with their mothers, little boys with their fathers. It is possible, though by no means justified, to account for identification exclusively in terms of stimulus-response and reward-reinforcement theory. Thus, there has grown up a strong current tradition of explaining differences in behavior between the sexes—or deviations therefrom—as socioenvironmental or cultural in origin.

A theory in which the totality of dimorphism in sexual behavior is attributed exclusively to postnatal social and cultural determinants, is, a priori, open to the charge of being too narrow and simple. Moreover, notwithstanding the cogent evidence of the power of postnatal events in shaping gender identity and gender role in human beings, one would be hard-pressed to defend an exclusively cultural theory against the newly accumulating evidence of animal sexology on the fetal influence of hormones on the governance of sexual behavior by way of the central nervous system.

2. Principle of Sequential Differentiation

The antecedents of sexual dimorphism of behavior in human development are typically sequential, beginning with the genetic dimorphism of the sex chromosomes, XY for the male and XX for the female. Then follows the differentiation of the gonads and their differentiated fetal hormonal functioning, differentiation of the internal reproductive anatomy, external genital morphology, sex assignment at birth, rearing as a boy or girl, differentiation of a gender role and identity, of hormonal puberty, and differential response to falling in love, courtship, mating and parenthood.

3. Critical-Period Principle

Differentiation of the embryonic gonads is normally governed by the sex chromosomes, but only if the genetic code written into the chromosomes is permitted to express itself normally (the genetic norm of reaction) without interference or disruption at a critical period from an environment liable to produce distortions. The most dramatic distortion of the genetic code of the sex chromosomes is one in which their role as sex determinants is completely reversed. Yamamoto (1962) was able to bring about such a complete reversal in the killifish, *Oryzias latipes*, by exposing larvae to sex hormone. Exposed to estrogen, the female sex hormone, an XY larva destined to have differentiated into a male, thereupon differentiated into a female. Amazingly enough, this XY female was able to breed with a normal XY male and produce young. Twenty-five percent of the second generation larvae were then chromosomally XX (female), fifty percent XY (male) and twenty-five percent YY, which, if left untreated, would differentiate as males, but if treated with estrogen, would become YY females. In the succeeding generation, it was then possible to breed YY females with YY males, the resultant progeny all being YY and differentiating as males, if left unexposed to experimental hormone treatment. Yamamoto was also able to produce XX males by treating XX eggs with male sex hormone. The strongly and competitively masculine mating behavior of YY males has been studied by Hamilton et al. (1969).

Yamamoto's experiment is not the first in which the germ cells have been reversed to produce ova instead of sperms, or vice versa, while still retaining their reproductive fertility. Many years ago, Witschi demonstrated that over-ripe toad eggs all developed as morphologic males. Not only the genetic males, but also the genetic females had the appearance of males. They produced sperms, but without the male sex chromosome present in them (Witschi, 1956, 1965). Witschi and his co-workers (Chang and Witschi, 1955, 1956; Mikamo and Witschi, 1963) also succeeded in producing a similar reversal of genetic sex in toads by implanting sex hormones into the developing larvae. In 1964, Turner and Asakawa made a first step toward achieving the same result in a mammal by transplanting the gonads of fetal mice into a host animal, so that the fetal testis turned the fetal ovary into an ovotestis in which spermatogenesis progressed to the point of secondary spermatocytes. Burns (1961) had in 1956 used estradiol in the fetal opossum to convert a would-be testis into an ovotestis producing ovocytes.

It has not yet been reported experimentally possible to reverse the sex differentiation completely from that of the genetic sex of the fertilized egg in mammals. Nonetheless the fish and amphibian experiments demonstrate how profound can be the reversal of everything pertaining to genetic sex: morphology, behavior and fertility. These experiments require that one keep an open mind with regard to possible partial reversals of the expression of the genetic sex in human beings, perhaps of direct relevance to sexual psychopathology, from causes as yet unknown.

The fish and amphibian experiments also point out a profoundly important principle in the theory of heredity versus environment (perhaps more appropriately designated as genetics versus environmentics). It is a principle that transcends the old dichotomy between nature and nurture by introducing the concept of the critical period. There is only a limited period during which a fertilized egg may be tampered with and forced to reverse the program for which it is genetically coded. After this limited, or critical period, the die is cast and the program cannot be changed or, having been changed, cannot revert.

The die is cast regarding the differentiation of the gonads in the human species at around the sixth week after conception. In the XY embryo, the core of the undifferentiated gonad proliferates to form into a testis, and the rind becomes vestigial; whereas in the XX embryo, the rind proliferates, while the core becomes vestigial, to form an ovary.

4. Principles of Differentiation: Vestigiation versus Homologues

The principle of commencing with the anlagen for both sexes, then allowing one to proliferate while the other vestigiates, is one which nature extends from the differentiation of the gonads to the differentation of the internal reproductive structures from the müllerian and wolffian ducts, both of which are initially laid down in parallel. Here another principle first becomes evident, namely this: for the differentiation of a male, something extra must occur—something must be added. In the total absence of gonads, whether by experimental castration of the fetus in utero, or by reason of a cytogenetic defect as in Turner's syndrome (typically 44 + X = 45 chromosomes), the fetus will develop as a female. There is no doubt about it that nature's first disposition is to make a female. Morphologically, for a female to be differentiated, it is not necessary to have fetal gonads able to release hormonal substances; whereas, for the differentiation of a male, it is absolutely necessary to have them and they must be testes. These fetal testes must release the so-called müllerian-inhibiting substance which causes the homolateral müllerian duct to regress, thus preventing the formation of the uterus and fallopian tube on that side. The fetal testes must also release an androgenic or male-hormonal substance which prevents regression of the wolffian ducts, thus ensuring the differentiation of the male internal sexual structures. When the müllerian-inhibiting substance fails, it is possible to have a male born with fully differentiated uterus and tubes. So far as is known, this rather extraordinary anomaly does not have any subsequent primary influence on sexual behavior. In the case of unilateral failure of the müllerian-inhibiting substance, only a half uterus and one tube is formed; subsequent external sexual development is liable to be hermaphroditic, with attendant risks of anomalously affecting sexual behavior.

Differentiation of the external sexual organs comes after that of the internal organs and proceeds on the basis of an entirely different principle—the principle of homologues. Here nature begins with the same anlagen and uses them for sexually different purposes: the genital tubercle becomes either the clitoris or the penis; the genital folds become either the hood of the clitoris and the labia minora or the foreskin and the wrap-around of the penis which forms the penile urethra; and the genital swellings become either the labia majora or the scrotal sac, joined by the same median raphe that fuses the penile urethra. It is between the second and third month of fetal life in the human species that external-organ differentiation takes place.

5. Masculine Differentiation: Additive Principle

The differentiating principle at this stage of embryonic development is once again: add something to obtain a male. The something added is androgen. In the absence of androgen, a fetus will differentiate externally as a female, regardless of chromosomal sex; and in the partial absence of androgen, differentiation will be as an unfinished male, that is with incomplete fusion of the penile and scrotal skin, the penis being diminished in size and the testes possibly being undescended. Conversely, in the presence of a sufficient quantity of androgen even an XX fetus will differentiate externally as a male.

Brain Differentiation

At around the same time as the external genitalia differentiate (6 weeks after conception), fetal androgens begin to exert an influence also on the developing central nervous system. In the lower, estrous species, androgen administered to the fetus at the appropriate critical developmental period counteracts its primary disposition to develop, subsequently, the cyclic estrous function of the female. The findings of different investigators using different techniques (reviewed by Harris, 1964; Money, 1965; Money and Ehrhardt, 1972) converge on the hypo-thalamus as the responsible area of the brain. Nuclei in the hypothalamus govern, by way of their neural releaser-hormones, the pituitary gland's activity. The pituitary, in turn, by cyclically or noncyclically releasing its gonad-stimu-lating hormones, the gonadotropins, regulates the production of sex hormones from the ovaries or testicles.

The overall principle emerging from the foregoing neurohormonal (or neurohumoral) research is once again the familiar one: add something, andro-gen, to obtain a male. Whether the differentiation regulated by androgen follows the homologous pattern of the external genitals, or the vestigiation pattern of the gonads and internal organs, remains to be ascertained. One piece of evidence in favor of the vestigiation hypothesis is that of Fisher (1956, 1966) who was able to elicit simultaneous female (maternal) and male (mating) behavior in a male rat by injecting minute amounts of testosterone directly into the preoptic area of the hypothalamus. The schema of female behavior is dormant, of course, or vestigial in the male, under ordinary circumstances.

Masculinized Female Monkeys

The masculinizing experiments that have so far been performed on primates, as contrasted with subprimates, have not shown a direct effect on hormonal cycling as manifested in the menstrual cycle. There is some evidence, however, to indicate a fetal effect on the central nervous system that will eventually influence sexual behavior. For example, investigators at the Regional Primate Research Center, Beaverton, Oregon (Young, et al., 1965; Phoenix, 1966) have produced genetic female rhesus monkeys so effectively virilized in utero by androgen injections of the mother that they were born with a normal male-appearing penis and empty scrotum instead of a clitoris and vaginal orifice. In the juvenile years, these animals gained behavior scores for initiating play, engaging in rough-and-tumble play, making threatening gestures, and adopting the position in sexual play, that were closer to the scores of normal control males than to normal control females. As they approached puberty and adolescence, these anatomically masculinized females tended to lose the masculine trend in their behavioral scores, but the complete story has not yet been ascertained, and the complete repertory of appropriate tests remains to be performed.

Masculinized Human Females

In human beings, there are two clinical syndromes that are the counterpart of fetal monkey androgenization. One is the syndrome of progestin-induced hermaphroditism in females. The other is the female andrenogenital syndrome of hermaphroditism, specifically those cases in which masculinization is restricted to fetal life, its continuance after birth being prevented by treatment with cortisone. It is superfluous to the needs of this chapter to digress into a full clinical description of these two syndromes and their differential etiology, prognosis and therapy; see instead Wilkins (1965) and Money (1980). It is sufficient for present purposes to note that, regardless of etiology, one has here examples of females subjected to masculinization in fetal life sufficient to enlarge the clitoris and partially fuse the labia, so as to create the appearance of hypospadias in the male. This anatomical abnormality is surgically corrected soon after birth, so that the appearance looks correctly female, in agreement with the rearing. Hormonal function, either spontaneously or by regulation, is female, and puberty is normal in onset. What then of behavior?

The evidence to date (Ehrhardt and Money, 1967; Ehrhardt et al., 1968) is that fetal androgenization in the above two syndromes does indeed influence the subsequent development of behavior, though only to a limited extent. It does not induce a complete reversal of gender role and gender identity in the sense that a girl feels she ought to be a boy or would like to change her sex. Nor does it automatically steer her in the direction of lesbianism. But it does tend to make her a tomboy, as judged by self-declaration and confirmed by parents and friends. Her tomboyism is defined, perhaps above all else, by vigorous, muscular energy expenditure and an intense interest in athletic sports and outdoor activities in competition with boys. It is not especially associated with aggression and fighting. It is accompanied by scorn for fussy and frilly feminine clothes and hair-dos in favor of utility styles. It is incompatible with a strong interest in maternalism as revealed in the rehearsals of childhood doll play or in future ambitions for the care of tiny babies. It does not exclude the anticipation of romance, marriage and pregnancy, but these are regarded in a somewhat perfunctory way as secondary to a career. Career ambitions are consistent with high academic achievement and with the high IQ, which tends to be a characteristic of girls with the adrenogenital syndrome.

Antiandrogenism: Rats

The experimental opposite of fetal androgenization of the female is nonandrogenization or antiandrogenization of the male. The former can be achieved by means of fetal castration, a technically difficult operation even in a species like the rat in which the young are delivered fetally immature. Neonatal castration of the male rat does indeed preserve cyclic functioning of the pituitary, as in the female (Harris, 1964). The use of antiandrogen is even more dramatic in its effect. When such a hormone is injected, with the proper timing, into the pregnant mother, then the fetal testes of the genetic males become dormant and fail to supply androgen to the anlagen of the external genitalia. In consequence, the animal, to be specific a rat (Neumann and Elger, 1965), is born with completely normal-appearing female genitals. By castrating the animal to eliminate all further influence of its own testes and giving replacement doses of female hormones at puberty, it is possible to obtain normal female mating behavior from these genetic males (Neumann and Elger, 1966). The stud males of the colony do not distinguish them from normal females. The sex-behavior reversal is complete.

Androgen Insensitivity: Human

In human beings, two clinical syndromes are close counterparts of experimental antiandrogenism in animals, namely Turner's syndrome and the testicular-feminizing or androgen-insensitivity syndrome (Wilkins, 1965; Money, 1980). In both instances, fetal androgenization of the external genitals fails so that the baby is born with normal-appearing female external genitals. In Turner's syndrome, there are neither ovaries nor testes as a result of the chromosomal error responsible for the syndrome, so that fetal androgenization is an impossibility. In the androgen-insensitivity syndrome, the testes are present and the chromosomal sex is 44 + XY = male. The testes produce male sex hormone in an amount normal for a male, and at puberty they produce also female sex hormone in an amount normal for a male. It is not the testes that are at fault in this condition, but all the cells of the body which manifest a genetic inability to respond to male sex hormone. The body therefore responds to the testes' output of female hormone; it develops a normal female appearance, including breasts at puberty. There is no uterus, however, since the testes produced their müllerian-inhibiting substance early in embryonic life, thus causing its vestigiation.

The behavior of girls and women with either Turner's syndrome (Money and Mittenthal, 1970) or the androgen-insensitivity syndrome (Money et al., 1968; Masica et al., 1969) is indisputably feminine. They are not tomboys. In childhood their interest is in traditionally feminine play and activities. They show strong maternalistic interests in doll play from an early age, generally like to take care of children as they grow through childhood, and rehearse fantasies of romance, marriage and motherhood as their primary ambition for the future. They are bitterly disappointed when their case is diagnosed and they learn the prognosis of sterility and motherhood by adoption. When eventually they do adopt children, they make good mothers. Their sex-lives in marriage are the same as for anatomically normal wives selected at random and subject to the same vicissitudes—except for the probabilty of needing long-term hormonal therapy and, in some cases of androgen insensitivity, surgical lengthening of the vagina for ease in sexual intercourse.

6. Core Gender Identity: Principle of Dissociation

Babies who will in future be diagnosed as having the androgen-insensitivity syndrome are almost never diagnosed at birth or in early childhood, for the obvious reason that they look normally female. The same is true for Turner's syndrome, except that various of the possible congenital defects of this syndrome may bring the child to earlier medical attention. It therefore happens that the differentiation of gender identity in these female-appearing people cannot be studied except under the reinforcement of a rearing that is female, like their appearance. The real test of the influence of sex of assignment and rearing on psychosexual differentiation is better studied in cases of sexual anomaly where the visible appearance is hermaphroditically ambiguous so that people of the same diagnosis can be found, differing only in that some have been assigned, reared, and surgically and hormonally treated as boys, the others as girls.

This condition, though rare, is met often enough to demonstrate the extraordinary power of postnatal events on the differentiation of gender role and identity. The typical finding is that gender role and identity differentiate in conformity with the sex of assignment and rearing. This conformity can withstand various partial contradictions which include: 1) even the extreme of contradictory hormonal puberty such that a person raised as a girl virilizes like a boy or, being raised as a boy begins to grow breasts and pass menstrual blood through the urethra; 2) tomboyism of energy expenditure in a person raised as a girl; 3) imperfect pubertal virilization with a nonerectile stub of a penis in a person raised as a boy; and 4) a masculine type of threshold, in a person living as a woman, for erotic arousal in response to visual and narrative material as contrasted with the more feminine dependence on tactile stimulation.

There are exceptions, nonetheless, when gender identity does not differentiate in conformity with sex assignment. Disparity between the two is most likely to arise when the assignment itself is ambivalent. The parents may be given no medical conviction about their infant's sexual diagnosis, or even may be told to half expect that a sex change might be necessary later. Parental ambivalence can be further reinforced if the genitalia are left surgically uncorrected during childhood so that they not only are a reproach to the child, when he or she looks at them, but also may be the source of teasing by siblings, cousins or friends. Under such circumstances the child, sensing and then knowing full well that something is wrong, does not tolerate the cognitive dissonance of his ambiguity. It is very rarely that an hermaphrodite settles for an ambiguous or hermaphroditic gender identity. A resolution of ambiguity is achieved instead by the simple expedient of repudiating the attributed status, so obviously wrong and unsatisfactory, in favor of its opposite, which at least has the virtue of not having yet been proved wrong and unsatisfactory.

The subjective process of reassignment, when it occurs, usually takes place early during an hermaphrodite's childhood; for the resolution of an ambiguous gender identity cannot feasibly be postponed. To achieve formal recognition of the change then becomes something of a cause célèbre and a real driving force in life.

The question of whether or not the influence of fetal hormones on sex differentiation of nuclei of the hypothalamus may have any bearing on an hermaphrodite's conviction of the need for sex reassignment cannot at present be answered. One can simply note (Money, 1969) that the decision seems to be arrived at more frequently by male than female hermaphrodites, and is more likely to require a female-to-male change of status than vice versa—which may have more to do with ambiguity of anatomy and of diagnosis of hermaphroditism than with assigned sexual status, per se.

The fact that some few hermaphrodites do not consolidate their gender identity from infancy onward, but reach a point of self-reassignment, contrasts strongly with those who do, and for whom a sex reassignment by edict would be a disaster. In the sex assignment of hermaphrodites, it is still relatively common for an on-the-spot decision to be made at the time of birth and then to have to be changed later, after completion of a full diagnostic work-up. As a result, a reannouncement of the baby's sex has to be made. Provided the parents are correctly guided through this dilemma, it need have no adverse effect, then, or subsequently, on the differentiation of the child's gender identity.

It is sometime between the ages of twelve and eighteen months, depending on a baby's facility in the understanding and use of language, that a sex reannouncement becomes more than an adjustment problem for the parents alone, and one for the child as well. By the time he has command of names, nouns and pronouns differentiating the sexes, a boy has a clear concept of himself as a boy, and a girl of herself as a girl. There is now no such simple thing as a sex reannouncement: it will be a sex reassignment involving the child as a person. Psychologically, it is very serious business, for the child already has a self-identity as boy or girl; the core gender identity, to use a term increasingly in vogue, is already on the way to being firmly established. This is an aspect of psychosexual differentiation not accounted for in the traditional Freudian scheme of the oral, anal and genital stages of psychosexual development.

The differentiation of a core gender identity probably follows the same principle as the differentiation of the gonads and the internal reproductive organs. In other words, two systems are present to begin with, only one of which becomes finally functional. In the case of gender identity, however, the nonfunctional schema does not become vestigial, in the true sense, but is dissociated—coded as not to be manifested by oneself, but to be expected from members of the other sex, and responded to reciprocally. Thus a boy grows up to know how to to all the boy things, because he knows also how to expect a girl to do all the girl things, to which he himself responds. The brain coding involved resembles that in bilingualism, especially that kind of bilingualism found in an immigrant child who knows how to listen to the old people's language, though he himself declines to speak it.

7. Principle of Identification and Complementation

The two gender schemas which become coded in one's brain, one as suitable for one's personal gender identity/role, and the other to use in predicting and responding to the gender-dimorphic, or gender-coded role of the other sex, are differentiated according to the principles of identification and complementation.

Identification, a long-familiar principle, refers to learning that takes place by direct copying or imitation of a model. Complementation, not so familiar, refers to learning the behavior of another, so that one's own behavior complements or reciprocates it in response. Identification and complementation both take place according to the ordinary contingencies of reinforcement and avoidance learning. Each may involve either overt instruction and indoctrination, or covert assimiliation from experience.

In the usual nuclear family, identification is primarily with the parent of the same sex, and complementation with the parent of the other sex. Other members of the household may, however, augment or substitute for the parents. A missing identification figure, say a parent, may also be represented in absentia by a complementation figure at the same time as he/she plays the role of complementing the missing one.

With advancing age, a child's identification and complementation models extend beyond the household to include playmates, older children, and heroes and heroines of folklore, sports and television.

Identification figures in absentia do not require responsive reaction from oneself except, maybe, in fantasy. When present in person, an identification figure is not simply a model to copy, but also a person whose behavior needs to be reciprocated or complemented, regardless of sex. This kind of complementarity is age-coded, as between parent and child, siblings of different age, and members of the same age/peer group. It may also be coded according to social, racial, or health status, and so on.

Sexually dimorphic roles which become incorporated into one's own gender identity/role are of two types. Sex roles, in the strict sense, pertain to eroticism and the function of the sex organs. Sex-coded roles are those that by custom and tradition are differentially assigned on the basis of genital status. They pertain to work, play, dress, cosmetics and manners, and are not specifically related to eroticism and the functioning of the sex organs.

Under special circumstances in a developing child, the complementary and the identification schemas may become transposed. Such a transposition occasionally occurs in an hermaphrodite child, with a resultant decision in favor of sex reassignment. Some anatomically normal chidren reach the same transexual decision, on the basis of an etiology chiefly unknown. Transvestism and the extreme manifestations of effeminate homosexuality in males and virilistic lesbianism in females represent other, less complete forms of transposition of gender identification and complementation (See Table I). Gender transposition may occur under circumstances of severe personality disorganization associated with adolescent psychosis. A behavioral sex change may emerge still later in life, in certain rare cases of temporal lobe epilepsy, or as a consequence of senile brain deterioration, and may be manifest in the form of personality changes, among others, toward transvestism or homosexuality.

8. Principle of Masculine Vulnerability

Except for hyposexual syndromes, it is widely acknowledged that the incidence of psychosexual disorders is higher in males than females. The variety of psychosexual disorders is also greater in males than females; some of the more bizarre and exotic anomalies have not been recorded in the female. It is quite likely that one has here a by-product of yet one more manifestation of the principle of sexual differentiation, namely that something must be added to differentiate a male. The something added that makes the difference between female and male in psychosexual erotic functioning might well, once again, be androgen. Its site of action, or absence thereof, would undoubtedly be the brain. Its mechanism of action would most likely pertain to threshold sensitivity for erotic arousal from a visual stimulus or, perhaps, its evocation in imagery from a narrative stimulus. After puberty, it is males who are girl watchers, not females who are boy watchers. Teenaged boys use nude pictures as masturbation stimuli, but girls do not. At puberty, the boy is self-presented with realistic erotic images in dreams accompanied by orgasm; the girl is not. The very sexual performance of

TABLE I

Transpositions of Gender-Role/Identity in 3 × 2 Classification of
Intensity and Duration (with permission, from Money, 1975).

	Total	Partial	Fractional
Chronic	Transexualism	Effeminate male and virilistic female homosexuality	Sex-coded work and legal status
Episodic	Transvestism	Bisexuality	Sex-coded play, grooming and manners

the boy is categorically different from that of the girl, in that his penis must be aroused to erection before he can begin; and it must ejaculate in orgasm if reproduction is to be effected. In the girl, by contrast, it is possible for conception to occur without either arousal or orgasm. It is possible for the male to be erotically aroused by touch alone, a fact to which many long-married husbands can attest. But it is typically the visual image that lends an element of excitement and, above all, incites the male to be the one who takes erotic initiative. This principle of male initiative is widespread in the animal kingdom, and in many primate species is dependent on visual stimulation, the closest competitor being smell.

If nature seems always to need to add something to make a male, then she seems also more likely to fail in her effort. The birth ratio, 106:100, in favor of males, allows for more rapid wastage of the male, and the conception ratio, estimated at as high as 140:100 shows even more dramatically how easy it is for a male to fail. There are no definite figures available, but the vulnerability of the male is again demonstrated at puberty, when, in the clinic, partial or complete failure of hormonal puberty is more common than in the female (excluding the postpubertal problems of ovulatory and menstrual irregularity). In the matter of psychosexual arousal, nature's difficulty in differentiating a male again manifests itself in the greater number of males than females who are "turned on" by a wrong stimulus, that is, one that has positive arousal value when it should be either neutral, negative or partial. All the anomalies in a textbook of sexual psychopathology can be interpreted in terms of being aroused by the wrong stimulus. Sometimes it is almost possible to glimpse how the wrong connections between behavioral components can be established by reason of their proximity of representation in the nervous system, as MacLean (1965) has pointed out with respect to oral-anal representations in the limbic system.

Vulnerability to errors of psychosexual functioning has no single source of origin. In some few cases genetics can definitely be implicated, as in the case of the XXY (Klinefelter's) syndrome or the XYY syndrome. Men with either of these cytogenetic anomalies are likely to have some or other peculiarity of sexual behavior. XXY men are also prone to be weak in libido, as well as sterile.

Whether events in intrauterine life may predispose human beings to psychosexual errors later in life is uncertain. In animal experiments it has been found that androgenization of the female fetus can be blocked by barbiturates (Gorski, 1971). One wonders what effect, if any, sleeping pills taken by a pregnant mother may have on an unborn fetus.

The bulk of today's evidence points unquestionably to events in early postnatal life and infancy as of prime importance in relation to eventual psychosexual normalcy. Harlow's (1965) work with rhesus monkeys raised on dummy mothers and in isolation from playmates is too well known to need retelling here. It points to the hitherto unsuspected importance of clinging and the sense of touch in primate development. It points also to the need to be able to play at the appropriate critical period—sexual play included—if normal reproductive behavior and parenthood are subsequently to be achieved. A report from the chimpanzee colony in New Mexico (Kollar et al., 1968) shows that, like the rhesus monkey, these primates also are very vulnerable to errors of psychosexual function when captured from their normal jungle troop and imprisoned in captivity. In fact, their sex-behavior problems are uncannily human.

As for human beings themselves, there is no highly systematic body of knowledge concerning the contingencies between rearing and subsequent sexual behavior, though there is a store of clinical knowledge and hypotheses, too vast to be reviewed here. It is perhaps a safe generalization to say that almost any major disruption of a child's developmental experience, regardless of its origin or type, is a potential source of disturbance in subsequent psychosexual development—the more so the younger the child. The vulnerability of the psychosexual system to disturbance may simply reflect the fact that its differentiation is actively in progress during early childhood. It may also be a reflection of the fact that, in many societies, our own included, psychosexual development is subject to an excess of taboos, such as the taboo on sexual play in childhood. If one judges from the evidence of the other primates, then childhood sexual play is a necessary and normal rehearsal, in preparation for adolescence and adulthood. Perhaps we would do well to reexamine our policies on childhood sexual play as a determinant of adult sexual behavior.

9. Principle of Love as an Imprint

After the advent of hormonal puberty, a new milestone in psychosexual development is reached, namely the capacity to experience falling in love. Children in kindergarten have play romances and children in the so-called latency period (not so very latent, either!) may play at copulation games, but they rarely fall in love, unless precocious falling in love may itself be a specific sign of psychosexual maldevelopment. The capacity to be aroused and possessed by the stimulus of the love object is not simultaneous with puberty. It does not occur, for instance, in children with precocious puberty of infantile onset until they become older—twelve is probably about the youngest. By contrast, in children, most notably boys, with long-delayed puberty, it is possible though not routine to observe the experience of falling in love sometime from middle to late teenage, even when complete hormonal infantilism still persists (Money and Alexander, 1967). One suspects, therefore, that whereas one neurohumoral mechanism (or biological clock) in the hypothalamus turns on puberty by way of activating the pituitary, another mechanism, site unknown, activates the capacity to fall in love.

Falling in love resembles imprinting, in that a releaser mechanism from within must encounter a stimulus from without before the event happens. Then that event has remarkable longevity, sometimes for a lifetime. The kind of stimulus that, whether it be acceptable or pathological, will be the effective one for a given individual will have been written into his psychosexual program, so to speak, in the years prior to puberty and dating back to infancy. Especially in the case of psychopathology, a boy or girl may be shocked and guilty to be 'turned on' by an abnormal stimulus, while at the same time secretly fascinated and obsessed with it because of the sexual feeling it releases. The effective erotic stimulus may not initially reveal itself in full, so that there is some element of discovery and expansion to erotic experience with the passage of time. By and large, however, human beings stay remarkably stable in their erotic dispositions. Thus, it is not possible to teach a man or even a teenager to be, say, a masochist or a peeping-Tom; and a few teenaged exposures to homosexuality do not create an appetite for more. The appetite has to be there in the first place. Earlier in childhood, the power of exposure and experience is probably far more impressive and lasting. However, a great deal more work needs to be done on the after-effects of childhood sexual experiences. There seem to be distinct personality types so far as falling in love is concerned, and they may correspond to the augmenters and diminishers of sensation as described by Petrie (1967). At one extreme are people of (psychopathic or) sociopathic personality disposition, the Don Juan and nymphomaniac types who are the experts at one night stands. These are perhaps diminisher-people whose experiences fade quickly and stand in need of constant repetition and novelty.

By contrast, at the other extreme are the augmenter-people who cannot let an experience go. It reverberates and enlarges in their memories, and haunts them. The love affairs of many schizoid and schizophrenic people have this quality. They may have an anguished love affair without ever declaring themselves to the partner; or even possibly conduct the whole love affair with an imaginary partner by way of a photograph.

The majority of mankind, of course, falls somewhere between these two extremes. Each tends to judge the other from within the solipsism of his own "egg shell" as being like himself. But the fact is that we are quite differently determined so far as sexual behavior goes.

10. Androgen-Libido Principle

When a teenager who has a syndrome of sexual infantilism nonetheless has a falling in love experience, it is not as intense and full-bodied as it will be once he is given effective hormone replacement therapy. The sex hormones do not in any way govern the cognitional content of eroticism—they do not cause homosexuality, for example—but they do affect the intensity and frequency of its expression, though without exercising total responsibility in this respect. Androgen is probably the libido hormone for both sexes (Money, 1961a; Herbert, 1967; Trimble and Herbert, 1968) though some women, notably those with androgen insensitivity, seem to be able to function adequately without it. Normal women tend to report a more receptive attitude of wanting to be possessed at around the time of ovulation, which is when the estrogenic phase of the menstrual cycle is in the ascendant. Estrogen tends to be an inhibitor of androgen. At the menstrual phase, when progesterone levels are higher, and androgen may be less inhibited, women are more likely to take an initiating role of inducing the male. The birth control pill may change this cycle, but in a way that seems to depend on the formulae of the different brands (Grant and Pryse-Davies, 1968). According to newly accumulating evidence from Hamburg and from Johns Hopkins (Money, 1968), antiandrogens may prove to be very beneficial in enabling certain sex criminals to gain a measure of control over their otherwise ungovernable sexual behavior. The effect is reversible when the medication is stopped, without adverse side effects. The same medication promises also to be helpful in the regulation of violent temper outbursts in some temporal lobe epileptics (D. Blumer, personal communication).

The hormonal changes of pregnancy have no routinely systematic effect on a woman's sex life. The mechanics of carrying a baby affect different women differently, as does the psychologic effect of the meaning of pregnancy and parenthood. Being a parent affects husband and wife equally and may have a profound effect, it goes without saying, on their opportunities for sexual behavior.

As with the hormonal changes of pregnancy, those of the menopause have no systematic effect on woman's sex life, except insofar as the vaginal mucosa may become atrophic and too dry, with an adverse effect on sexual intercourse. This effect can be reversed by the judicious prescription of estrogen (which also will serve as a protection against osteoporosis). The direct effect of the hormonal changes of the menopause on mood and temperament varies widely, as does the effect of the psychologic meaning of having reached the end of childbearing; consequently, both of these effects themselves bear no systematic relationship to postmenopausal sexual behavior. It is important for many couples to know that the menopause does not mark the end of woman's sexual desire and ability. Her sexual life may continue, and even be improved, far into old age.

The male's sex life also may continue far into old age, unmarked by any such dramatic hormonal event as the menopause of the female. The refractory interval between erections and between orgasms lengthens as age increases, but with great individual variation. Failing potency may be improved in older men whose own androgen levels have declined by the judicious prescripton of testosterone. Impotence not associated with a falling-off in androgen production is not improved by treatment with hormones, and the same holds true for frigidity in women.

Apart from the aging effect, deficit or impairment of sexual behavior and its frequency has many different etiologies, requiring considerable astuteness to establish a diagnosis. It is necessary to consider that the symptom of deficient or impaired sexual activity may be a sequel to: a genetic defect; an error of metabolism; an endocrine error; a mechanical, neurological or circulatory defect; a traumatic injury; an adverse psychologic reaction to illness (for example, after a heart attack); a primary psychiatric disorder (especially depression); a disturbance of personality and the interpersonal relationship of sex; or a lack of sufficient timing, variety or novelty of stimulation.

An excess of sexual activity is more often regarded boastfully as an asset rather than as a symptom. Yet it may be a symptom, especially when it represents a change from a former lesser level, together with a change in the type of behavior. The most likely diagnostic considerations then are: an endocrine error; a neurological error (particularly a trauma, tumor, or senile atrophy of the brain); a primary psychiatric disorder (especially mania or hypomania); or a disturbance of personality and the interpersonal relationship of sex.

11. Principle of Genitopelvic Sensation

It all but belabors the obvious to say that one of the determinants of sexual behavior is the integrity of the sexual organs with which coitus is performed. Yet the fact of the matter is that large amounts of sexual tissue can be removed without destroying the capacity for erotic response (Money, 1961b). Following amputation of the penis, whether by accident or because of malignancy, orgasm is retained. Sexual desire remains as before, sometimes creating a serious problem of morale in being unable to satisfy the partner.

A more complete loss of penile tissue is entailed in sex-reassignment surgery for male transexualism, for the corpora are extirpated and only the skin retained as a lining for the new vagina (Jones et al., 1968). Postoperatively and living as females, transexuals claim they experience erotic satisfaction in the female sexual role, and some report a climactic feeling of orgasm which, if different than they formerly experienced as males, satisfies them more because they are able to be in the female role.

Penile tissue is not lost but the corpora are, in many cases, functionally destroyed as a sequel to priapism. Erection is impossible. Here again orgasm and desire for intercourse are retained, while the morale may be seriously injured.

The morale problem is, by contrast, quite different in cases of paraplegia (Money, 1960) where the loss is not of genital tissue, but of all spinal cord connection with the brain. The genitalia are able to respond reflexly to local tactile stimulation, but the patient has no feeling and awareness of what has happened. A paraplegic male has no erection in response to erotic thoughts and imagery. The nearest he gets to an orgasm is by dreaming one, and even sexual dreams disappear as the years pass after the paraplegic injury occurred. The paraplegic knows that he has lost his sex life and would elect, if he could, to have it returned, but there is none of the quality of urgency and frustration found in men whose genitals can perform only a part of their sexual function without completing it. Signals from the genitals are obviously a principal component or determinant of sexual behavior.

In women as in men, ablation of genital tissue is compatible with the retention of erotic sensation and orgasm. The evidence comes from women who undergo radical resection of the vulva for epidermoid cancer, and from hermaphroditic females whose hypertrophied clitoris is resected or extirpated. According to the evidence of genital ablation, an orgasm is an orgasm regardless of the stimulation that triggers it—which is precisely the verdict of the Masters and Johnson (1966) research into the human sexual response. These authors effectively put to rest the ghost of the old controversy of the clitoral versus the vaginal orgasm as a determinant of mature sexual behavior in the female.

12. Principle of Dimorphic Signals

Over and beyond the specifics of genitopelvic sexual behavior, there is a vast amount of human behavior that is sexual in the sense that it is dimorphic in relation to gender: what men do one way, women do another. This kind of gender-related behavior ranges from fashions of dress to conventions of work and earning a living, from rules of etiquette and ceremony to labor-sharing in the home. Though these various stereotypes of what is masculine and what is feminine may ultimately derive from such fundamental sex differences as urinary posture, menstruation, childbearing, lactation, stature, weight, and muscular power, the conventions themselves are defined by custom and may be arbitrary and subject to sudden changes of fashion or slow changes in the cultural pattern. It does not matter that they change. It is the fact that they exist in any given time and place that counts, for we human beings are sensitively dependent on our cognition of the signals and cues emanating from others—they are determinants of our own sexual behavior, just as are plumage differences in birds. We differ from birds in being able to adapt and change the signals historically, but cannot obliterate them altogether. There is no more convincing evidence in support of this principle than the fact that the average man or woman tends to accept the impersonation put forth by a transvestite or a transexual—provided of course, that it is a perfect or near-perfect impersonation. It is then possible to accept the impersonation, even after the truth is known, as being more genuine than the sex of the sex organs. It is even possible for a psychosexually normal person to fall in love with a transexual impersonator. Resolution of the incongruity between impersonation and the sex organs is then achieved by responding to the impersonator as someone beset by misfortune who is deserving or needing medical or surgical help. There is no more cogent illustration of how compelling is the influence of the senses over that of judgment in determining sexual behavior!

13. Principle of Cultural Determinants

Cultural tradition determines not only the criteria of sexually dimorphic behavior, but also various criteria of sexual interaction. The variety of possibilities is extensive but not limitless, although the limits have not yet been catalogued. Variability can be classified as pertaining to the following characteristics of partnerships:

—age: same or disparate
—physique juvenile, adolescent or adult
—sex: same or opposite
—kinship: related or not related by blood, clan or race
—caste or class: same or different
—number: unity or plurality of partnerships
—time: sequential or contemporaneous partnerships, or one partnership only
—span: transient or constant partnerships
—privacy: public or concealed
—accessories: plain or modified by material artifacts, e.g., personal ornament, visual erotica, contraceptive device, etc.

To illustrate: the people of the lake region of northern Sumatra live in a cultural tradition that permits an age difference in a sexual partnership, ranging over the entire spectrum of physique, but only in homosexual and not heterosexual partnerships. In late childhood, it is not decent for children to stay sleeping in their parents' single-roomed house. A girl takes her sleeping mat to the home of a widow or old woman who accommodates about half a dozen girls who range in age from prepuberty to late adolescence. A boy joins a group of a dozen to fifteen males, his own age or older, who sleep in a boy's house specially constructed for them. There he learns from the adolescents and young men how to participate in paired homosexual play with them or older boys:* primarily mutual masturbation of penis held against penis, maybe anal coitus, but never fellatio. All members of the group may over a period of time become one member's partner, in rotation. Relationships are not necessarily unobserved, but they are always in pairs, not in larger groups. Partnerships among group members do not involve falling in love, but they are constant up to the point where a young man opts to leave the group by marrying. No man is permitted to remain a bachelor.

When he is ready to marry, a young man asks his close friends to join him in a prescribed etiquette of approaching the chosen girl's family and his own family, to see if they have the wealth to pay the bride price and put on a wedding festival.

The young man in search of a wife narrates the procedure of his courtship to his companions in the boys' house. Once married, he discloses details about

---

*Information about homosexuality among females is conjectural among males, as talk about sexual activities, except between husband and wife, is taboo between the sexes.

sexual intercourse. In this way information is transmitted down the generations, and a young adolescent is prepared to anticipate his graduation from the era of homosexual experience to heterosexual falling-in-love and marriage.

The homosexual era in adolescence, by sequestering the sexes, ensures that young women will be virgins until married. The sanctions against premarital sex are stringent, so that a girl who is discovered in transgression probably commits suicide. Once a marriage is effected, the parties discontinue homosexuality, though men away on working parties in the jungle may temporarily resume them.

By contrast with the allowable age disparities in homosexual partnerships, the heterosexual partnership is formed between people of like age in young adulthood, or else the girl may be younger, in her teens, than the man, in his twenties. The relationship between the pair may be as close as cousins, but there is no special kinship obligation in the choice of a partner. There is a preference for partnerships within the racial-linguistic group. Marriage is the first and only heterosexual partnership, except for remarriage after the early death of one of the spouses. A marriage cannot otherwise be broken. Being married is, of course, publicly announced. The coital relationship of marriage is, by convention private and unobserved, except that young children may awaken when the parents are copulating. They then must not disclose their observation, but ignore it. According to the formalities of the culture, they learn about sex not at home, but from their adolescent and young adult friends.

Changing Sexual Traditions in Our Society

The cultural traditions of a lakeside village in Sumatra have been able to survive intact for an unspecified number of generations, but now, under the impact of cultural contact through education and broadcasting, these traditions are yielding to change. Change is a hallmark of the cultural traditions of our own society in the present age of instantaneous broadcast communcation, nuclear-space technology and, in matters sexual, effective contraception and effective venereal disease control. Whereas to some, the change in sexual traditions is anathema, to others it is utopia, but to none is it very clear, what, exactly, is happening. In terms of the seven schematic categories above-listed, one may suggest the following. There has been no change of tradition with respect to a preference for pairing couples of similar age, with continuing toleration of a few exceptions of disparity within the adult years. There is still a rigid rule against juvenile sexual play, though the age of "sex education" is subject to radical downward revision, amidst sometimes acrimonious social controversy. There is no issue more heated than that of the rights of adolescents and young adults to have sexual and love affairs premaritally, with or without intention to marry and/or have children. The trend is toward greater freedom. Sanctions against homosexuality are being examined and eased, though ambivalently, in favor of consensual agreements between adults. Problems of kinship in mating continue to be singularly unimportant, so long as the incest taboo is respected. The issue of miscegenation is so explosive that it can scarcely be mentioned in public and political discussion, perhaps because it is a foregone conclusion that black-white intermarriage will become routine. Class and caste preferences and distinctions in sexual pairing remain otherwise about the same as ever.

The leading pressure point of change in our society's sexual traditions would seem to be toward a greater plurality of sexual relationships, for females as well as males, on a basis of mutual reciprocity. This change is registered in sequential more often than contemporaneous plurality of relationships, before or after marriage. Even contemporaneous relationships are constant, over a period of time, rather than transient. Availability of effective contraception is undoubtedly the material artifact that underlies this cultural change, though in the case of serial marriage and divorce, with children to be supported, the economic and legal emancipation of women is also a major factor. Despite the plurality of partnerships, the preference is still for episodic monogamy or fidelity, rather than running more than one affair contemporaneously. However, a new institution, its future still uncertain, is the "swinging scene" of partner exchanging and group sex, coexistent and compatible with contractual marriage and long-term loyalty and emotional allegiance to one partner.

Participation in any sexual relationship outside of marriage is still subject to at least a partial need for concealment, though increasing freedom is accorded to young adults to be frank and open about their nonmarital sexual liaisons and living together. Coitus itself is still subject to the rule of privacy, though some group participants are indifferent to being observed or to engaging in activities with more than one partner simultaneously.

Whether or not these changes in sexual tradition constitute a sexual revolution (or reformation), or are simply variations of basic primate behavior has become a subject for rhetoric and politics as well as for science and medicine. The reader must formulate his own conclusions.

14. Principle of Nativism versus Culturalism

The juxtaposition of nature versus nurture has long been a favorite topic of argument pertaining to the behavior of human beings. Fascination with the topic stems ultimately from the issue of free will versus determinism. Nature is cast in the deterministic role of imperatively governing an inevitable and inexorable destiny variously named as biological, hereditary, constitutional, instinctual, and innate or inborn. Nurture by contrast is cast in the probabalistic role of optionally governing a modifiable and reversible fate, variously named as social, environmental, acquired, learned and developmental.

Irrespective of terminology, the conceptual problem lurking in the nature-nurture dichotomy is that the two interact. They are not independent variables. Table II presents a new conceptualization of how to differentiate the inevitable from the optional in a 2 × 2 × 2 scheme which simultaneously differentiates the phylographic from the idiographic, and the nativistic from the culturistic. That which is phylographic is species shared, whereas the idiographic is personally unique. Both may be either nativistic or cultural in origin, and, either way, may exist as imperatives or options.

TABLE II

Nativism and Culturalism as Determinants of Gender-Identity/Role,
Classified Simultaneously with Phylographic versus Idiographic, and
Imperative versus Optional Determinants (with permission, from Money, 1975).

		Nativistic	Culturistic
Phylographic (species shared)	Imperative	Menstruation, gestation, lactation (women) vs. impregnation (men).	Social models for identification and complementation in gender-identity differentiation.
	Optional	Population size, fertility rate and sex ratio.	Population birth/death ratio. Diminishing age of puberty.
Idiographic (individu- ally unique)	Imperative	Chromosome anomalies, e.g., 45,X; 47,XXY; 47,XYY. Vestigial penis. Vestigial uterus. Vaginal atresia.	Sex announcement and rearing as male, female, or ambiguous.
	Optional	Getting pregnant. Breast feeding. Anorectic amenorrhea. Castration.	Gender-divergent work, law, cosmetics and grooming, child care.

The cells of Table II may be filled in for a variable other than that of gender-identity/role, the variable which is here appropriate.

The two-word term, "identity/role," is actually redundant, since identity and role are opposite sides of the same coin. The self perceives its own identity, whereas others can only infer it from its role manifestation, which is both verbal and nonverbal. People tend to dichotomize identity and role, instead of keeping them a unity.

References

Burns, R. K. (1961) Role of hormones in the differentiation of sex. In: (W. C. Young, ed.) *Sex and Internal Secretions*. (Williams and Wilkins, Baltimore.)

Chang, C. Y. and Witschi, E. (1955) Breeding of sex-reversed males of *Xenopus laevis Daudin. Proc. Soc. Exp. Biol. Med.* 89:150-152.

Chang, C. Y. and Witschi, E. (1956) Genic control and hormonal reversal of sex differentiation in Xenopus. *Proc. Soc. Expo. Biol. Med.* 93:140-144.

Ehrhardt, A. A., and Money, J. (1967) Progestin-induced hermaphroditism: IQ and psychosexual identity in a study of ten girls. *J. Sex. Res.* 3:83-100.

Ehrhardt, A. A., Epstein, R. and Money, J. (1968) Fetal androgens and female gender identity in the early-treated androgenital syndrome. *Johns Hopkins Med. J.* 122:160-167.

Fisher, A. E. (1956) Maternal and sexual behavior induced by intracranial chemical stimulation. *Science* 124:228-229.

Fisher, A. E. (1966) Chemical and electrical stimulation of the brain in the male rat. In: (R. A. Gorski and R. E. Whalen, Eds.) *The Brain and Gonadal Function.* Vol. III of *Brain and Behavior.* (University of California Press, Berkeley.)

Gorski, R. A. (1971) Sexual differentiation of the hypothalamus. In: (H. C. Mack and A. I. Sherman, eds.) *The Neuroendocrinology of Human Reproduction.* (Charles C Thomas, Springfield, Illinois.)

Grant, E. C. G. and Pryse-Davies, J. (1968) Effect of oral contraceptives on depressive mood changes and on endometrial monoamine oxidase and phosphatases. *Br. Med. J.* 3:777-780.

Hamilton, J. B., Walter, R. O., Daniel, R. M. and Mestler, G. E. (1969) Competition for mating between ordinary and supermale Japanese medaka fish. *Anim. Behav.* 17:168-176.

Harlow, H. F. and Harlow, M. K. (1965) The effect of rearing conditions on behavior. In: (J. Money, ed.) *Sex Research, New Developments.* (Holt, Rinehart and Winston, New York.)

Harris, G. W. (1964) Sex hormones, brain development and brain function. *Endocrinology* 75:627-648.

Herbert, J. (1967) The social modification of sexual and other behavior in the rhesus monkey. In: (D. Starck, R. Schneider and H. J. Kuh, eds.) *Progress in Primatology* pp. 222-246. (Gustav Fisher, Stuttgart.)

Jones, H. W., Schirmer, H. K. A. and Hoopes, J. E. (1968) A sex conversion operation for males with transsexualism. *Am. J. Obstet. Gynecol.* 100:101-109.

Kollar, E. J., Beckwith, W. C. and Edgerton, R. B. (1968) Sexual behavior of the ARL colony chimpanzees. *J. Nerv. Ment. Dis.* 147:444-459.

MacLean, P. D. (1965) New findings relevant to the evolution of psychosexual functions of the brain. In: (J. Money, ed.) *Sex Research, New Developments.* (Holt, Rinehart and Winston, New York.)

Masica, D. N., Money, J., Ehrhardt, A. A. and Lewis, V. G. (1969) IQ, fetal sex hormones and cognitive patterns: Studies in the testicular feminizing syndrome of androgen insensitivity. *Johns Hopkins Med. J.* 124:34-43.

Masters, W. H. and Johnson, V. E. (1966) *Human Sexual Response.* (Little, Brown, Boston.)

Mikamo, K. and Witschi, E. (1963) Functional sex-reversal in genetic females of *Xenopus laevis,* induced by implanted testes. *Genetics* 48:1411-1421.

Money, J. (1960) Phantom orgasm in the dreams of paraplegic men and women. *Arch. Gen. Psychiat.* 3:373-382.

Money, J. (1961a) Components of eroticism in man. I: The hormones in relation to sexual morphology and sexual desire. *J. Nerv. Ment. Dis.* 132:239-248.

Money, J. (1961b) Components of eroticism in man. II: The orgasm and genital somethesia. *J. Nerv. Ment. Dis.* 132:289-297.

Money;, J. (1965) Influence of hormones on sexual behavior. In: (A. C. Degraff, ed.) *Annu. Rev. Med.* Vol. 16, pp. 67-82. (Annual Reviews, Inc., Palo Alto.)

Money, J. (1968) Discussion: Clinical effects of agents affecting fertility. (Antiandrogen to control behavior.) In: (R. P. Michael, ed.) *Endocrinology and Human Behaviour.* (Oxford University Press, London.)

Money, J. (1969) Sex reassignment as related to hermaphroditism and transsexualism. In: (R. Green and J. Money, eds.) *Transsexualism and Sex Reassignment.* (Johns Hopkins Press, Baltimore.)

Money, J. (1975) Nativism versus culturalism in gender-identity differentiation. In: (E. Adelson, ed.) *Sexuality and Psychoanalysis.* (Brunner/Mazel, New York.)

Money, J. (1980) Hermaphroditism and pseudohermaphroditism. In: (J. J. Gold and J.B. Josimovich, eds.) *Gynecologic Endocrinology.* 3rd edn. (Harper and Row, New York).

Money, J. and Alexander, D. (1967) Eroticism and sexual function in developmental anorchia and hyporchia with pubertal failure. *J. Sex Res.* 3:31-47.

Money, J. and Ehrhardt, A. A. (1972) *Man and Woman, Boy and Girl: The Differentiation and Dimorphism of Gender Identity from Conception to Maturity.* (Johns Hopkins Press, Baltimore.)

Money, J., Ehrhardt, A. A. and Masica, D. M. (1968) Fetal feminization induced by androgen insensitivity in the testicular feminizing syndrome: Effect on marriage and maternalism. *Johns Hopkins Med. J.* 123:105-114.

Money, J. and Mittenthal, S. (1970) Lack of personality pathology in Turner's Syndrome: Relation to cytogenetics, hormones and physique. *Behav. Genet.* 1:43-56.

Neumann, F. and Elger, W. (1965) Proof of the activity of androgenic agents on the differentiation of the external genitalia, the mammary gland and the hypothalamic-pituitary system in rats. *Excerpta Medica, Int. Congr. Ser 101: Androgens in Normal and Pathological Conditions,* pp. 169-185.

Neumann, F. and Elger, W. (1966) Permanent changes in gonadal function and sexual behavior as a result of early feminization of male rats by treatment with an antiandrogenic steroid. *Endokrinologie,* 50:209-225.

Petrie, A. (1967) *Individuality in Pain and Suffering.* (University of Chicago Press, Chicago.)

Phoenix, C. (1966) *Psychosexual Organization in Nonhuman Primates.* Paper delivered at the Conference on Endocrine and Neural Control of Sex and Related Behavior. (Puerto Rico, Dorado Beach.)

Trimble, M. R. and Herbert J. (1968) The effect of testosterone or oestradiol upon the sexual and associated behavior of the adult female rhesus monkey. *J. Endocrinol.,* 42:171-185.

Turner, C. D. and Asakawa, H. (1964) Experimental reversal of germ cells in ovaries of fetal mice. *Science* 143:1344-1345.

Wilkins, L. (1965) *The Diagnosis and Treatment of Endocrine Disorders in Childhood and Adolescence,* Third ed. (Charles C Thomas, Springfield, Ill.)

Witschi, E. (1956) *Development of Vertebrates* (Saunders, Philadelphia.)

Witschi, E. (1965) Hormones and embryonic induction. *Arch. Anat. Microsc. Morphol. Exp.* 51:601-611.

Yamamoto, T. (1962) Hormonic factors affecting gonadal differentiation in fish. *Gen. Comp. Endocrinol,* 1, 311-345.

Young, W. C., Goy, R. W. and Phoenix, C. H. (1965) Hormones and sexual behavior. In: (J. Money, ed.) *Sex Research, New Developments* (Holt, Rinehart and Winston, New York.)

Note

Originally published privately for limited circulation to Johns Hopkins freshman medical students in *Readings V, Sexual Behavior, Introduction to Psychiatry and the Behavioral Sciences;* Baltimore, Department of Psychiatry and Behavioral Sciences, The Johns Hopkins University, 1969. The manuscript was actually written for a comprehensive textbook that failed to materialize. It appeared instead in *Progress in Group and Family Therapy* (C. J. Sager and H. S. Kaplan, eds.); New York, Brunner/Mazel, 1972. With minor revisions, it was republished in the *Handbook of Sexology* (J. Money and H. Musaph, eds.), Amsterdam/New York, Excerpta Medica, 1977. [Bibliog. #2.151]

SEVENTEEN

Phyletic and Idiosyncratic Determinants of Gender Identity

Sequential Determinants

If you have ever taken for granted that your own personal gender-identity was, after the fashion of a Platonic ideal, immanent in your genes at the moment of conception, needing only time for its inexorable unfolding, then you were wrong. Not only time was needed, but also an appropriately programed environment, because the program transmitted in the genes—the genetic code—does not express itself in a vacuum. The genetic code requires a permissive environment in which to express itself. Otherwise the code-carrying genes, and the chromosomes on which they cling, die and express nothing at all. The limits of permissiveness are phyletically prescribed and need to be empirically defined, species by species, for any given entity or variable. One such variable is gender identity of which the mirror image is gender role.

The environment in which the genes live and on which they are dependent for their survival is initially the cytoplasmic environment that surrounds the nucleus in which the genes themselves are located. In experiments on the frog, the genes in the nucleus of a cell have been shown to behave quite differently when they are located in a cell in the intestine as compared with when that same nucleus is implanted into an enucleated egg of the same species. The nucleus surrounded no longer by its intestinal cytoplasm, but by ovarian cytoplasm instead, can respond as the nucleus of an ovum and produce a tadpole, a replica of its one parent (Gurdon, 1968; Gurdon & Woodland, 1968).

Not only the cytoplasmic, but also the extracellular environment will influence the way in which the genetic code expresses itself. The critical or sensitive developmental period, especially in embryonic life, is of key importance in this respect. Thus, by changing the hormonal environment of the embryonic anlagen of the genital anatomy, one can experimentally dictate that a genetic male will differentiate the reproductive organs of a female.* In the mammal, the experimental formula is this: remove the testes before they become embryonically active. The converse of this experiment is the masculinization of the genetic female. Experimentally it is more difficult to masculinize the internal than the external organs. The latter is easy. All that is needed is to inject the pregnant mother with sufficient dosages of testosterone during the critical days of fetal external genital differentiation.

---

*Documentation for the statements made in this and succeeding paragraphs, together with a complete bibliography, will be found in J. Money and A. A. Ehrhardt. *Man and Woman, Boy and Girl: The Differentiation and Dimorphism of Gender Identity from Conception to Maturity.* Johns Hopkins University Press, 1972.

In fish and amphibians, the influence of the extracellular hormonal environment on the genetic code of the fertilized egg is even more spectacular. With the sex-appropriate hormone dissolved in the water of the larvae of the killifish, *Oryzias latipes* (Yamamoto 1962), genetic males will differentiate as phenotypic females, and genetic females as phenotypic males. Estrogen reverses the genetic males and androgen the females. In each of these reversals, the individuals will be able to breed as members of their phenotypic sex. A genotypic-XX-phenotypic-male, if bred with a normal XX female wil produce only XX females. A genotypic-XY-phenotypic-female, if bred with a normal XY male will produce 25% YY males. Thus, by experimental environmental manipulation, it is actually possible even to change the male genotype, from XY to YY, in the killifish.

In human beings the external genital phenotype is sometimes hormonally reversed not experimentally, but as a result of spontaneous changes of the hormonal environment of the fetus in utero—or, more rarely, as a result of iatrogenic hormonal changes coinciding with the critical period of external genital differentiation. In such a case, a genotypic female may, indeed, be born with a penis and empty scrotum and, conversely, a genotypic male with a vulva and abdominal testes. When such a baby is born, the appearance of the external genitalia—the external phenotypic sex—determines the sex of assignment and the sex of rearing, provided there are no associated tell-tale diagnostic signs that lead to a contrary decision. Thereafter, if the sex of rearing is unambiguous, psychosexual differentiation, that is to say the differentiation of gender identity, takes place concordantly with the phenotype of the external genitals and the sex of assignment, irrespective of genetic sex.

Figure 1 represents schematically the sequence of determinants or events that lead to the differentiation of gender identity in childhood and adulthood. The figure can be interpreted metaphorically as a relay race, each entity being the equivalent of a runner that carries the program for gender identity differentiation and passes it on to a successor. Each runner must translate the program into instructions comprehensible to his successor. In some instances there may be paired successors, as happens when fetal sex hormone passes on instructions partly to sex-organ morphology and partly to pathways in the central nervous system. One recipient of such a distribution may be time-delayed in carrying out its part of the program, as when the gonads delay the secretion of sex hormone postfetally until the age of pubertal onset.

With each change in the transmission of the program of gender-identity differentiation, there exists the possibility that an error may be introduced and subsequently transmitted. It is an empirical task to ascertain and catalogue potential errors and their consequences—a task which is by no means complete at the present stage of the history of sexual science. Errors before birth do not, it would appear, have an automatic, direct-line, causal effect on the differentiation of gender identity, but only by way of changing the risk or probability of what may happen in the later stages of differentiation. To illustrate, consider the case

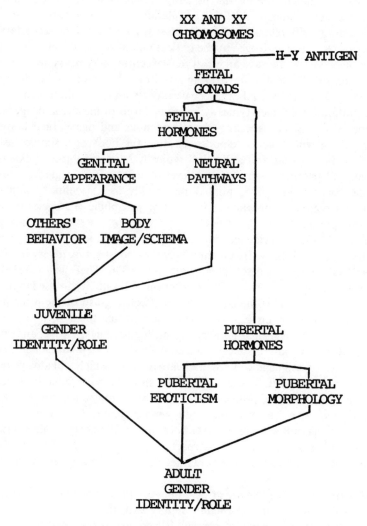

FIG. 1. Schematic representation of the sequential nature of the
determinants of gender-identity/role [G-I/R] differentiation.

of one of the cytogenetic anomalies, the inclusion of an extra X chromosome
into the XY chromosomal constitution of a genetic male (Klinefelter's, or the
47,XXY syndrome).*

The supernumerary X chromosome does not preordain any unique feature
of subsequent gender identity, but it does put the individual into a population at
risk for impairment of central nervous system functioning and psychological

*Parallel illustrations may be drawn from the 47,XYY and 45,X (Turner's) syndromes.

development. Included among the psychopathologies likely, though not pre-destined, to appear in members of this population at risk are errors or anomalies of gender-identity differentiation. This increased risk may well be secondary to a deficiency of testicular androgen at the critical phase of fetal development when the hormone is known to have an effect on the central nervous system. Alterna-tively, or additionally, fetal cells carrying an extra X chromosome, as do all cells of the body in XXY individuals, may be weakly responsive to androgen.

In adulthood XXY men typically have low levels of plasma androgens, and their pubertal virilization is weak. Given exogenous androgens, their bodies do not utilize them with a good response, as does the body of a simple castrate. One consequence is that an XXY adult typically has the subjective experience and behavioral manifestation of a low level of sexual drive, regardless of how the gender identity has differentiated postnatally as masculine, feminine or bisexual, and regardless of whether unusual or paraphilic tendencies in sexual behavior are present or not.

The bulk of today's evidence, particularly from the study of hermaphroditic biographies, points to the early postnatal years as constituting a very important developmental epoch in gender-identity differentiation. There is a parallel here with native language. According to the criterion of his ability to use language, a child by the age of five, at the latest, has an effective grasp of the principles of linguistics embedded in his native tongue. At that age there is, however, still enough flexibility for a second language to be acquired as if native, and spoken idiomatically and without an accent, which will seldom be possible later. None-theless, the second language will not eradicate the first, which will always remain subject to rapid reacquisition, even years later, should it have fallen into disuse.

By the age of five, a child's gender identity is imbedded firmly, like the native language. As a system in the brain, gender-identity programs a develop-ing boy's own masculinely appropriate behavior and imagery while simultane-ously programing the feminine counterpart as the complement of the boy's own reactions in relationship with the other sex. The reverse applies to the devel-oping girl.

The years before age five are critical ones for the establishment of concord-ance versus discordance of the gender identity with the sex of assignment and with the prenatal components of gender. It is probable also that these are the years in which are established the behavior and imagistic anlagen of what will later be manifest as paraphilias, that is to say the behavioral disorders or errors of sexual functioning. The factors and experiences that lead to such errors are not yet systematically understood—only sporadically and anecdotally in terms of individual biographies. Thus, it is not clear whether experiences in later child-hood and at the onset of puberty may leave an indelible mark.

It appears reasonably clear, however, that paraphilias do not become estab-lished in adolescence, but that they manifest themselves then on the basis of what was programed earlier in the biography. The function of the hormones of puberty is to lower the threshold of responsiveness to the erotic image and to increase the frequency of erotic expression. This principle applies irrespective of the erotic contents of both the image and the behavior, and irrespective of whether it is socially defined as normal or abnormal.

Prenatal Androgenization

My purpose at this point is not to elaborate further on the postnatal components of gender identity differentiation, normal or otherwise, but to give special attention to the prenatal hormonal effect, specifically the behavioral sequelae of prenatal androgenization of the genetic female. There is a certain parallelism here between the observations made by Goy and his associates on the rhesus monkey and those made by myself and co-workers on human beings. In both cases, genetic females became androgenized in utero, so that the external sexual organs took on a masculine appearance. The human beings were surgically feminized at birth or soon thereafter, when the diagnosis (adrenogenital syndrome or progestin-induced hermaphroditism) was correctly recognized, and were assigned and reared as girls, with appropriate hormonal regulation as needed. A few, however, were not correctly recognized and were assigned and reared as boys, with appropriate surgical and hormonal intervention, as needed. The monkey hermaphrodites were not surgically corrected and not given postnatal hormonal treatment.

Tersely stated, the androgenized genetic females, monkeys and humans, developed behaviorally as tomboys. The monkeys gained scores more like those of normal male than female controls for rough-and-tumble play, for the initiation of play, for threatening and chasing play, and for mounting play.

Among the human beings, those raised as girls thought of themselves as tomboys and were so considered by others more than were their matched controls. They evinced a strong interest in vigorous outdoor energy expenditure at the expense of doll play and the rehearsal of maternal caretaking. They were not aggressive—an important point with reference to current hypotheses attempting to correlate aggression with androgen level—but they were capable of self-assertion, fighting if need be, for a position in the dominance hierarchy of childhood. Usually they underplayed the role of dominance assertion, in deference to the boys they liked to play with and who might otherwise not have accepted them. (Those reared as boys did not need to make this concession.) In keeping with their tomboyish play interests and activities, they preferred utility clothing styles and hair styles to decorative frills and curls, but did not repudiate feminine dressing-up for special occasions. They had little use for jewelry, but had no objection to perfume. From childhood onward, they envisaged themselves as giving preference to a nondomestic career as compared with a career as housewife and mother. They did not exempt themselves from marriage but rather projected marriage to a distant horizon. Those already in teenage were late in developing a romantic interest in boys, though not because of a lesbian preference instead. As a group they tended to be high in IQ and academic achievement, quite possibly on the basis of an enhancing effect of excess prenatal steroidal hormones on ultimate postnatal intelligence (unconfirmed). A point requiring further observation is that they may prove to be more easily aroused erotically by the visual image than are most women. In childhood, prenatally androgenized girls, unlike their monkey counterparts, did not manifest either more or less sexual play than their matched controls, presumably responding to the typical taboos of our culture in this respect.

Prenatally androgenized genetic females who are assigned and reared as girls, with appropriate and timely surgical correction and hormonal regulation, if needed, differentiate a feminine gender identity. Nonetheless, it is a feminine identity with a difference, the difference being the flavor, so to speak, of tomboyism contributed by the prenatal androgenic effect. This effect, if one may interpolate from experiments on lower mammals, is mediated by way of androgen-sensitive pathways in the fetal hypothalamus and, probably, the nearby structures of the limbic system. The effect of androgen is probably not sexually dimorphic in the sense of either/or, but rather in the sense of changing thresholds. Thus, a woman with the adrenogenital syndrome, late in getting married and apprehensive as to her mothering ability should she get pregnant, does eventually succeed in the parental caretaking function—in a fashion not unlike that of the child's father, if he is adept at infant care.

Fortunately for the fetally androgenized female reared as a girl, there is no cultural stigma attached to tomboyism in a girl in our society. The reverse is true for the fetally deandrogenized male reared as a boy. There is not even an acceptable name for him, like tomboy, unless it be that he is sensitive and artistic. Usually he is stigmatized as a sissy.

The change of threshold for sexually dimorphic behavior induced by fetal androgenization works in favor of the genetic female assigned and reared as a boy because of morphologic masculinization to the extent of having a penis and empty scrotum. Such a boy has no difficulty at all in differentiating a masculine gender identity in conformity with society's stereotype of what a boy and a man should be.

There is a theoretical principle to be drawn from the foregoing, the principle of phyletic and idiosyncratic interaction. It is incorrect to conceive of gender identity as the effect produced by a genetic ideal, in the Platonic sense of an ideal as an immanent cause awaiting its time. It is equally incorrect to juxtapose the genetic versus the environmental, for they are interactive. Likewise it is incorrect to juxtapose the biological versus the social, the innate versus the learned, or the constitutional versus the acquired, for they also are, respectively, interactive. More correctly, one might juxtapose the phyletic versus the idiosyncratically biographic.

The phyletic represents that which is shared by other members of one's species, or by other members of the same sex. Phyletic is not synonymous with genetic, but includes that which is the product of interaction between the genetic code, and its developmental environment, on the assumption that the developmental environment has been similar from individual to individual, with respect to those facets of the genetic code that they carry in common.

The idiosyncratic represents that which is not shared by the majority of the members of one's species of the same sex but is individual. This individuality may reside in the genetic code, or in some more or less unique factor in its developmental environment. A good example of the latter, already mentioned, is that of genetic females morphologically masculinized by androgen present in the fetal environment during the critical developmental period. The appearance of androgen in atypical amounts for a genetically female fetus so alters the subsequent stages of the program for gender-identity differentiation that the baby may be born with a penis, reared as a boy, and differentiated with a masculine gender identity that, apart from sterility, allows him to be behaviorally and psychologically indistinguishable from other husbands and fathers.

Summary

Sexual science is now sufficiently advanced as to show that it is anachronistic to dichotomize heredity and environment, biological and social, or innate and acquired with respect to psychosexual phenomena, including the differentiation of gender identity. One gains extra theoretical freedom and flexibility by juxtaposing instead the phyletically determined versus the biographically idiosyncratic. Both may be the product of interaction between the genetic code and its developmental environment.

References

Gurdon, J. B.: Translated nuclei and cell differentiation. *Scientific American* 1968:219:24-35.
Gurdon, J. B. & Woodland, H. R.: Cytoplasmic control of nuclear activity in animal development. *Biological Reviews* 1968:43:233-267.
Yamamoto,T.: Hormonic factors affecting gonadal differentiation in fish. *General and Comparative Endocrinology 1962*, Supplement 1:311-345.

Note

Originally published in *Danish Medical Journal,* 19:259-264, 1972, the first of a two-part series written for the Kristen Auken Conference on Sexology in Copenhagen, May 1972, convened by Preben Hertoft. [Bibliog. #2.153]

EIGHTEEN

Identification and Complementation in the Differentiation of Gender Identity

Chromosomal and Gonadal Dimorphism

The untutored mind of modern man knows of gray, of the land of the midnight sun, and of intersexuality, yet it retains its atavistic logic of dichotomies and thinks of black and white, day and night, male and female. Only with difficulty does it accommodate itself to the logic of gradations.

Conceptual dichotomism in man's thinking undoubtedly has an ancient phyletic foundation, nowhere more anciently founded than with respect to sexual dimorphism which in its very origins is genetic, namely in the chromosomal dimorphism of sex. Yet even chromosomal dimorphism is not an absolute. Some individuals are born neither with the normally expected XX or XY sex-chromosomal complement, witness the syndromes characterized as 45,X; 47,XXX; 47,XXY, 47,XYY and diverse sex chromosomal mosaics.

The same absence of absolutism in sexual dimorphism may be observed also independently of chromosomal sex, in the fetal phases of sexual differentiation that follow the earliest beginnings when chromosomal sex is established. Thus, the gonads may differentiate not as ovaries or testes, but as various combinations of both, either separately, or as a histological mixture, ovotestes.

Fetal Androgenization and Hypoandrogenization

After gonadal sex has been developmentally established, lack of dimorphic absolutism may again manifest itself in fetal hormonal functioning. An excess of male sex hormone, whether produced by the fetus itself (most commonly from malfunction of the adrenal cortices) or of exogenous origin, will allow the external genitalia of the chromosomal female to masculinize. Thus the genetic female with two ovaries and internal female differentation may be born with a grossly enlarged clitoris and partial fusion of the labia. In the extreme case, the clitoris becomes a penis and the labia majora fuse to become an empty scrotum.

The counterpart of such masculinization of the genetic female occurs not as an influence of female sex hormone on the genetic male fetus, but as a failure of its male hormonal function. There are two types of failure. One is the failure of the embryonic testes to release their mullerian inhibiting substance, with the consequence that the uterus and fallopian tubes differentiate and persist in an individual otherwise differentiated as male. The second type of failure is that which occurs when the embryonic and fetal testes fail to release male sex hormone, or when the target cells prove incapable of utilizing the male sex hormone that is released (androgen insensitivity syndrome). In the extreme case, the genetic and gonadal male then differentiates the external genitalia of a female. In the less extreme case, the male organs are incompletely differentiated, with the penis small, its urinary canal unfused, and its urinary orifice in approximately the female position.

The hormonal exceptions to the rule of dimorphic absolutism that manifest themselves, as above, in ambiguity or hermaphroditism of the external genitalia influence also the differentiation of pathways in the brain. More accurately, one makes an inference to this effect on the basis of experimental animal studies and human clinical observations. In brief, it appears that the prenatally androgenized genetic female has no difficulty postnatally in differentiating gender-dimorphic behavior culturally ascribed to the male, provided the sex of assignment and rearing has been consistently as a boy, with concordant surgical and hormonal treatments. The same individual assigned as a girl, with appropriate surgical treatment and hormonal regulation, differentiates a female gender identity but with a tomboyish temperament. This tomboyism means, in brief, hypertrophy of interest in athletic energy expenditure, exploratory curiosity, and capacity for competitive rivalry and dominance assertion in boys' play groups, together with hypotrophy of interest in the childhood rehearsals of maternalism as manifested in dollplay.

The counterpart of tomboyism in the androgenized girl is a kind of behavior in the hypoandrogenized boy for which there is no term in English. It is not sissiness, for sissiness implies effeminacy and homosexuality, but rather a quietism against which much effort is needed in order to match the behavioral demands that boys put on one another. Such quietism facilitates feminine behavioral development and feminine gender identity differentiation in a hypoandrogenized genetic male assigned and reared as a girl, with appropriate surgical correction as needed. In cases of total androgen failure, no feminizing surgery is needed, nor is hormonal therapy at puberty, since the body responds only to its own testicular estrogens, being insensitive to androgen. Pubertal insensitivity to androgen creates an insoluble problem when the child has been reared as a boy, for no amount of hormonal treatment will produce a masculine body build, masculine secondary sexual characteristics, and masculine aging and maturity of appearance.

Pairs Concordant for Diagnosis, Discordant for Rearing

Androgenization of the genetic female, and hypoandrogenization of the genetic male demonstrate, in their respective ways, the lack of dimorphic absolutism with respect to those aspects of gender-dimorphic behavior subject to prenatal hormonal influence: babies of either genetic sex can be assigned and reared as boy or girl. Then, typically, they differentiate a gender identity concordant with the sex of assignment and rearing, albeit flavored or tinted, so to speak, by the particular prenatal hormonal brain influence. Despite their value for science, however, matched pairs of hermaphrodites concordant for the prenatal variables of sex, and discordant for assigned sex, rearing, and gender-identity differentiation, do not have quite the same dramatic impact, heuristically, as does another type of case.

This other type is that of a normally born boy who in early life underwent traumatic ablation of the entire penis as a result of an accident of circumcision by cautery. The total number of such cases has not been recorded. Some few are known to have been reared as boys, but are lost to follow-up. Within the last ten years, two cases are known in which the posttraumatic dilemma was resolved in a decision to reassign the baby as a girl, following appropriate first-stage feminizing surgery of the genitalia—with the second stage, namely construction of a vaginal cavity, to follow in adolescence after a feminizing puberty has been induced by estrogen replacement therapy. The oldest of these two children is now in middle childhood. Her gender specific behavior as a girl is quite remarkably evident by reason of its contrast with that of her identical twin brother. Her appearance and behavior as a girl elicit sex-appropriate behavior toward her from other people. At school her medical history is not known or suspected. The mother is explicitly aware of reinforcing and encouraging feminine behavior in the girl, and masculine behavior in the boy. The father simply takes for granted that one behaves as a girl, the other as a boy, and he responds accordingly. The end of the story, scientifically, will be written with the development of romance and falling in love in adolescence. One predicts then that the girl will continue the feminine gender identity already differentiated, basing the prediction on adult cases of male hermaphroditism with feminine sex assignment, rearing, and gender identity differentiation.

Hermaphroditic Sex Reassignment

Cases of sex reassignment, like the foregoing, occur also in some cases of hermaphroditism when the initial decision later proves to have been unwise. Usually it is not feasible to decide on a sex reassignment after an infant has begun to grasp sex differences imbedded in linguistic and other conventions and to apply them to the self. Thus, between eighteen months and two years of age is usually the limit for an imposed reassignment, unless it is later evident that differentiation of the gender identity has been equivocal. The age of eighteen months, however, is sufficiently advanced for it to become quite evident to parents and other adults that they do, indeed, have different programs and expectancies in their own behavior toward a boy as compared with a girl. Moreover, these programs and expectancies exist independently of the child's own sex-specific appearance and behavior, and can be changed if the child's sex is reassigned. There is no doubt, nonetheless, that a parent's behavior is reinforced by the sex-appropriate appearance and behavior of the child. Thus, the change of clothing style and haircut is of major importance in facilitating the change in parental behavior when their child's sex is reannounced—to say nothing of the appropriate surgical change of the genitalia. Visible changes also influence other people's responses to the child and as the child's behavior reciprocates a feedback effect is established.

Complementation and Identification Models

Sex reassignment demands that father and mother both reorient themselves and their behavior toward the child. Thus, the father whose erstwhile son comes from the hospital reassigned as a daughter no longer can act as a male identification model for a son, but must become a male complementation model for a daughter. Simultaneously, the mother changes from a complementation to an identification model. The principle is nicely illustrated in an anecdote given by the father of a son-become-daughter. Back from the hospital, the little girl showed an enthusiasm for copying her four-year-old brother's rough-house dancing, to be a big shot, like him. The father's impulse was to hold his daughter close to him in partner-to-partner dancing. Rebellious at first, she soon recognized her favored position, whereupon her brother wanted to share it. The father's reaction was negative. He taught his son to dance with his mother, instead, all four being together each evening for the children's play time with their parents.

Ideally, there will exist reciprocal concordance between parents regarding their respective roles as identification and complementation models, so that each reinforces the role of the other in interaction with the child. Discordance between the parents in this connection introduces ambiguity and conflict into the child's gender-identity differentiation. The roles of complementation and identification may both then become impaired in the child, and to a greater or lesser degree transposed or translocated, part of one being affixed to the other, and vice versa. Ideally, both parents—and other people too—agree on both roles, so that a child can establish each with clearly demarcated boundaries.

Clarity of the boundaries is more important than the content of the two roles themselves. In fact, there is no absolute dichotomy of male and female identification roles and their complements. The invariates or imperatives may be condensed to four: males impregnate, and females menstruate, gestate and lactate. Other criteria of sexual dimorphism of behavior are either derivatives of these irreducible four, or are optional according to time and place—as is obvious in studies of historical and cultural anthropology. In today's world, there is plenty of scope for reciprocal change with respect to the optional content and definition of male and female roles, in keeping with the new feminism of the Women's Liberation Movement. Ideally, for each child, both parents will agree on the change, even though reciprocal change is not predictably easy to achieve.

Ideally, also, the child's own family will not be socially isolated in its definition of the two roles, since such social isolation easily stigmatizes a child among his age mates, and may force him to choose between parents and peers.

Gender Schemata in the Brain

Differentiation in the postnatal phase of gender identity by means of identification and complementation (manifestations of both types of behavior being reinforced by both parents) requires, by implication, that the two patterns of gender-dimorphic behavior be encoded in the brain. In normal development, the one gender schema is encoded as positive, so to speak, which means identification, which means "this is how I do it." By contrast, the other, negatively coded, means complementation, which means "this is how it will be done by the other sex, and I shall respond in a complementary way."

Here again, to continue the thematic principle of this paper, there is no dichotomous absolutism. Part or all of the dimorphic gender schemata may become reciprocally translocated or transposed. Phenomenologically, the result is what is commonly considered to be a gender identity disorder, either minor or severe. As well as being either partial or complete, transposition may be also either chronic or episodic in its manifestations.

Transpositions in Gender Schemata

A partial chronic form of transposition is exemplified in the ordinary type of homosexuality in which there is a degree of discordance or dissociation between cognition of one's morphologic sex, on the one hand, and cognition of one's same-sex erotic partnership on the other, but not between morphologic sex and vocational, business, or recreational partnerships.

A partial episodic form of transposition is exemplified in genuine bisexuality, in which dissociation between cognition of morphologic sex and of erotic partnership alternates with episodes in which there is no dissociation. In other words, the partner is sometimes of the same sex, and sometimes of the other sex.

A complete chronic form of transposition is exemplified in transexualism, in which there is a more or less complete dissociation between cognition of one's morphologic sex and cognition of one's gender identity plus its expression as gender role. The transexual person has an intense conviction, or idée fixe, that the only way to resolve the paradox is by way of hormonal and surgical change of sexual morphology.

A complete episodic form of transposition is exemplified in transvestism, in which dissociation between cognition of morphologic sex and gender-identity/role alternates with episodes in which there is no dissociation. The dissociative episode has some kinship with a fugue state and is intimately associated with putting on the clothing of the opposite sex. A homosexual erotic partnership, that is, one with a person of the same morphologic sex, is optional while the transvestite is cross dressed. Also, the clothing may have a fetishistic stimulus value, heightening the possibility of erotic and coital performance in a heterosexual partnership.

The above four examples are ideal types, so to speak, with various gradations and subtypes found in actual clinical manifestation. One special subtype is that in which transposition between the two gender schemas is, in addition to being partial, unstable—subject to chaotic shifts and fragmentation. The resultant dissociation between cognition of morphologic sex and of gender-identity/role is unstable and disorderly, sometimes present, sometimes gone. It is likely to manifest itself primarily in the solipsistic privacy of thought and imagery, as in fantasy, dream or hallucination. Its public expression is likely to occur only in elliptical signs and symbols of either body language or verbal language. In its classic form, this type of dissociation is schizophrenic.

Brain Dysfunction

It is exceptionally rare to be able to trace a transposition of the gender schemata from its manifestation in behavior to its manifestation in demonstrable brain dysfunction. However, there are recorded cases in clinical neurosurgery which show that behavioral symptoms of such a transposition, in one case transvestism, may occur in connection with a brain lesion and the onset of temporal lobe epilepsy. Additionally, following successful temporal lobectomy for relief of seizures, the psychosexual symptom may disappear. One may then infer that the epileptogenic lesion opened a gating mechanism that permitted negatively coded behavior to escape, and that surgery, being successful, allowed the gate to close again. The escape of sexually dimorphic behavior that once was negatively coded is also symptomatic in some cases of brain deterioration in senility. The principle of escape is an example of the well known Jacksonian Law of Release which has hitherto been applied to the functioning of other brain systems, but not to sexual dimorphism as a brain system.

Clearly, the brain holds the secrets of the etiology of gender identity differentation and its transposition disorders—secrets that pertain to fetal hormones, childhood developmental learning, and the impairment of maturity. When the brain will yield up all of these secrets—who knows what the story will be?

Summary

There is no absolute dichotomy of male and female, even with respect to chromosomal and gonadal sex. Hyperandrogenism in utero masculinizes the genetic and gonadal female. Hypoandrogenism demasculinizes the genetic and gonadal male. Hyperandrogenized females differentiate a gender identity concordant with assigned sex and rearing, though as boys or girls they share those behavioral traits which in girls constitute tomboyism. Hypoandrogenized males also differentiate a gender identity concordant with assignment and rearing; and they lack tomboyish traits. Cases of sex reassignment in childhood hermaphroditism demonstrate that the same-sexed parent is an identification model, and the other parent a complementation model. Ideally they both agree on the boundaries of what constitutes sexual dimorphism of behavior. The irreducible imperatives of such dimorphism are that women menstruate, gestate and lactate, and that men impregnate. Complementation and identification are the basis of two gender schemata in the brain, which may possibly become reciprocally transposed, either partly or wholly, and either chronically or episodically. Transposition may be either stable and organized, or shifting and chaotic. Different types and degrees of transposition are manifested clinically as homosexuality, bisexuality, transexualism, transvestism and the schizophrenic type of gender-identity ambiguity. In very rare instances the behavioral manifestations of transposition can be correlated with demonstrable brain dysfunction.

Acknowledgment

Supported by USPHS Grants 5K03-HD18635 and 2R01-HD00325.

Notes

Originally published in *Danish Medical Journal,* 19:265-268, 1972, the second of a two-part series. [Bibliog. #2.152]
    The twins mentioned in this chapter have been lost to follow-up as a sequel to the invasion of their privacy by an unscrupulous television team from the BBC.

NINETEEN

Gender: History, Theory and Usage of the Term in Sexology and Its Relationship to Nature/Nurture

Abstract

A person's sexual status is conventionally defined on the criterion of the external sex organs, and this criterion is presumed to be concordant with the other criteria of sex. When the sex organs are deformed, as in hermaphroditism, or mutilated, their sex role is to some extent affected, whereas all the other manifestations of the person's masculinity or femininity may be intact. Gender, not sex, is the umbrella term which refers to the totality of masculinity/femininity, genital sex included. Gender role and gender identity are two sides of the same coin, gender-identity/role (G-I/R). G-I/R may differentiate to be discordant with one or more of the basic sex variables which are now listed in the definition of sex in Dorland's Medical Dictionary. G-I/R is the product not of either nature or nurture acting alone, but of both in interaction at crucial periods of developmental differentiation. The new paradigm is nature/crucial-period/nurture, not nature/nurture. Social scientists and sexologists are among those who, for the most part, have not made the paradigm shift.

Sex, Sex Organs, and Gender

It is not surprising that the recently idiomatic English term, *gender role* (first used in Money, 1955[1]), has proved difficult to translate into other languages. So also have the terms, *gender identity* and *gender-identity/role*. In 1955, it had proved similarly difficult for me to translate the term, *gender,* from language science to sexual science and have its new usage accepted. At first it sounded funny and idiomatically unfamiliar. Very rapidly, however, it became assimilated into both scientific and literary usage as a necessary supplement to the term, *sex.*

I first became aware of the terminological overload imposed on the word, *sex,* in my early studies of individuals born with a birth defect of the sex organs. Take, for example, the case of a child growing up as a boy with a miniscule penis, too small to urinate from while standing. He is in a position similar to that of a boy or man whose penis has been accidentally ablated. He may grow up to be masculine in all respects except that he cannot urinate or perform sexually as a male with his penis. Terminologically, one cannot say that his sex role is masculine because, insofar as his sex role with his sex organ is lacking or incomplete,

237

it is not. The way out of this terminological impasse is to say that his gender role is masculine in all of its extragenital manifestations, whereas in its specifically sexual, or genital and erotic manifestations, it is imperfect. The gender role (a definition is appended) is all-encompassing, like a big umbrella that houses all its heterogeneous components, of which the genital-sexual role is only one. Other components, according to traditional conceptions, are legal, educational, vocational, recreational, sartorial and cosmetic roles, and so on, that are male/female coded or stereotyped.

Male-Female Polarity: Hermaphroditism

Univariate, not multivariate determination of sex as either male or female has the status of an eternal verity. "Man and woman created He them," declares the book of Genesis, having first declared that "God created man in His own image." Taken literally, that implies that God is a manwoman God.

This ambiguity has its counterpart in pre-Biblical creation myths of an original unisex that divided into male and female. Plato tells how the two halves ever since have sought reunion. It is not so much the reunion, however, that has permeated the scientific thinking of humankind (not mankind or wom(b)ankind, but humankind!) as the absolute polarity of the division between male and female.

The phenomena of manwomanism, that is, hermaphroditism, belie the univariateness of the polarity of male and female, insofar as there exists in the hermaphroditic individual an incongruent combination of both male and female variables. Lord Coke, the great British jurist of the 16th century, attempted to deal with this incongruency by decreeing that a hermaphrodite may, by the common law of England, "be either male or female, and it shall succeed [i.e., inherit] according to the kind of sex which doth prevail."[2] Despite its common-sense wisdom, this decree did not specify the criterion by which to judge "the sex that doth prevail." Medicine and science of the time had no fixed criterion of sex. The association of testes with the male, and ovaries with the female had an ancient history; but there was no technique of surgical exploration for internal gonads, and no surgical anesthesia. Pregnancy was abstrusely attributed to the semen (the seed) of the male, in combination with the female's menstrual blood. Spermatozoa were unknown until 1677 when Antoni van Leeuwenhoek, addressing the Royal Society of London, reported having seen them under the newly invented microscope. The existence of the human egg was first authenticated by Carl Ernst von Baer in 1827.

By 1867, Klebs in Germany decreed the diagnostic criterion of sex in hermaphroditism, namely the histology of the gonads, that has remained in use for more than a century.[3] True hermaphrodites were decreed as those with ovary and testis or ovotestes. Those with two testes, or two ovaries were decreed to be not true hermaphrodites at all, but pseudohermaphrodites, that is, primarily males or females with secondary hermaphroditic ambiguity. Thus, except for rare cases of true hermaphroditism, the criterion of the difference between male and female was reaffirmed as univariate and absolute. Clinically, the spinoff from this dogma is that urologists claim male pseudohermaphrodites for enforced masculinizing surgery, and gynecologists, female pseudohermaphrodites for feminizing surgery. In addition, psychiatrists, or at least some of them, claim homosexuals for enforced change of orientation and behavior.

Multivariate Discordance

The Klebs nomenclature, variously qualified but still in use, is totally without prognostic value. It makes no provision for the fact that testes do not automatically predicate pubertal masculinization, and, vice versa, that ovaries do not automatically predicate pubertal feminization. Each syndrome of hermaphroditism, regardless of gonadal status, has its own developmental prognosis with respect to the variables of being male or female, masculine or feminine. The different variables may be discordant with one another, instead of concordant as they are usually expected to be in nonhermaphroditic people.

In my earliest studies of hermaphroditism,[2] I came to the realization that there is no absolute dichotomy of male and female. A person's sex must be specified not on the basis of a single criterion, but of multiple criteria. For example, it is possible to have the genetic sex of a male (chromosome counting became a routine laboratory procedure only in 1959), the gonadal sex of a male; the internal morphologic sex of a male; the external genital morphologic sex of a female; the hormonal pubertal sex of a female; the assigned sex of a female; and the gender-role and identity of a female. This is what typically happens in the androgen-insensitivity syndrome—and there are many other syndromes, each with its own story.

The only irreducible difference between male and female, in higher primates, is that males impregnate, whereas females menstruate, gestate and lactate—in other words, they have the babies. In some fish, even this reproductive difference is reducible, for they are able to change sex and breed as both male and female in one lifetime.

I first published a tabulation of the multivariate determinants of sex in 1955.[4] Very rapidly, they became idiomatic, and the conception of sex as multivariate and multivariately determined became assimilated into general medical and scientific thinking. By 1965, in the twenty-fourth edition, *Dorland's Illustrated Medical Dictionary* changed its definition of sex, listing and defining the multiple variables.

Eventually, I devised a diagram showing not only the variables of sex, but also the chronological sequence in which they exert their influence. This diagram, updated to include H-Y antigen, appears in Chapter 17, p. 225 (originally, Figure 3-1 in Money[5]).

In writing about ordinary people born without a hermaphroditic or other sexual birth defect, it is feasible to assume that sex is a univariate characteristic, simply because all of the multiple variables are concordant with one another. When, however, one or more of the variables is discordant with the others, there arises the issue of which variables to use, and which to disregard in defining the sex of the person.

Gender-Identity/Role [G-I/R]

In the theater, an actor plays a role. A good actor may even continue to play the role extramurally, while the production lasts. A gender role is not so ephemeral. It belongs to the person who inhabits it and lives in it every day, indefinitely. Thus a gender role is experienced not as a social script, dictated like the script of a play. Rather, it is experienced at first hand as one's own gender identity, and it is manifested to others in what one says and does.

Ideally, it should have been possible to have the unity of the private experience and the public manifestation of one's gender role guaranteed within the single term, *gender role*. In the 1950s, the social and behavioral sciences were not geared toward such a principle of unity, and so the two terms, *gender role,* and *gender identity* became part of the common usage.[6]

Inevitably, the existence of the two terms led to their false reification as independent entities. To reunify them, I have now adopted the practice of using the acronym G-I/R as a single term for *gender-identity/role*.

G-I/R: Dimensions

Hypothetically, G-I/R may be subdivided into dimensions which either are or are not irreducibly male or female. In mammals, though not in sex-changing fish, breeding roles are *irreducibly* male or female. In human beings, there are three categories of *reducible* roles: 1) sex-derivative, as in urinary posture, or hormone-governed muscular build; 2) sex-adjunctive, as in the extension of women's breast-feeding to overall food preparation, or men's territorial roaming to truck-driving; and 3) sex-arbitrary, as in cosmetic, sartorial, and grooming styles.

Most people experience and manifest their G-I/R as cohesive and unitary in dimension, whether as stereotypically masculine or feminine, or as an androgynous mixture of the two stereotypes. Others may have a greater or lesser degree of dualism, the extreme being the dualism of two names, two wardrobes, two personalities, and two occupations, one male and one female, respectively.[7]

In its genital-erotic dimension, a G-I/R may be heterosexual, bisexual, or homosexual in variable degree. Whatever its status in this dimension, the G-I/R may or may not incorporate some degree or type of paraphilic, hypophilic, or hyperphilic phenomenon. To illustrate: a man may have heterosexual G-I/R, but be inert or apathetic with respect to penovaginal coitus, his turn-on being klismaphilic, that is being given an enema by his woman partner, without the imagery of which he would remain impotent and anorgasmically hypophilic.

A Paradigm Shift Needed

A person's G-I/R is the product of neither nature nor nurture, heredity nor environment, acting alone, as is spelled out in Money and Ehrhardt.[8] To replace such simple polarization, what is needed is a theoretical earthquake that will bring into being a paradigm shift away from the two-term nature/nurture formulation, to the three-term, nature/crucial-period/nurture formulation. Nature and nurture interact during a crucial period of development. What they effectuate is serially added to by subsequent interactions, until the final product is permanently in place.

This three-term formulation has long been accepted in embryology. For nearly half a century, it has been also accepted as the basis of imprinting theory in animal ethology. But the paradigm shift that it represents still has not been generally accepted in the social and behavioral sciences—psychology included— though not through lack of a convincing model. This is the model of native language in human beings.

Native language inhabits a brain that must be human, and must have had a healthy and normal prenatal life. Only in postnatal life, however, does language actually get into the brain—extraceptively, of course, and typically from sound waves that enter the brain through the ears at a crucial period of development. Once language gets implanted into the brain, it stays there, as permanently ineradicable as if it had been programed there prenatally by genes, hormones, or other brain neurochemistries. Despite its postnatal origins in learning, native language can be eradicated only by a neurosurgeon's knife or, perhaps, by stroke or trauma.

This example of native language shows that permanence in the brain is not synonymous with innateness. That which becomes permanent may also be post-natal, and acquired by social learning. Thus, the much-vexed issue of whether G-I/R in human beings is innate or acquired, biological or learned, prenatal or postnatal, does not either quarrel or correlate with the issue of whether G-I/R is immutable or changeable.

G-I/R: Prenatal and Postnatal

In experimental studies of subprimates, it has been amply documented that reciprocal mating behavior of male and female is preprogramed, robot-like, into the fetal or neonatal brain by steroidal sex hormone.[8,9] Then at the first breeding season, the behavior of male and female emerges, robot-like, as is remarkably demonstrated in a film by R. V. Short and I. J. Clarke on prenatally masculinized ewes that mate as rams.[10,11] In primates, and in particular human primates, there is no such robot-like program. Except for the irreducibles (see above) of procreation, the influence of sex steroidal hormone prenatally is to set differential thresholds for behavior that is sex-shared, but threshold dimorphic. That is to say, in adulthood, either sex can manifest exactly the same behavior, but the threshold for its release is male/female divergent. Parenting behavior in rhesus monkeys is an example. It is the same in males and females; but in the father it is released only after prolonged cajoling and entreaty by the infant, whereas in the mother, the response is released momentarily.

The list of sex-shared/threshold-dimorphic behavior[5] includes:

General kinesis—activity and the expenditure of energy, especially in outdoor, athletic, and team-sport activities

Competitive rivalry and assertiveness for higher rank in the dominance hierarchy of childhood

Roaming and territory or boundary mapping or marking

Defense against intruders and predators

Guarding and defense of the young

Nesting or homemaking

Parental care of the young, including doll play

Sexual mounting and thrusting versus spreading and containing

Erotic dependence on visual stimulus versus tactual stimulus and arousal

In postnatal life the continued differentiation of G-I/R is, like native language, contingent upon input through the special senses into the brain. Smell, taste, skin senses, eyes and ears participate with different degrees of prominence at different crucial periods, progressively, in development. Ultimately, it is the eyes and ears that carry the major responsibility for continuing the differentiation of G-I/R as shaped by other people, in accordance with the traditions they transmit.

Identification and Complementation

Identification is one of the principles according to which G-I/R differentiation takes place in postnatal life. The term, *identification,* has long been in use to signify learning by copying, imitating, or modeling. In psychoanalytic theory, particular emphasis is given to the parent of the same sex as the model. In the differentiation of G-I/R, the model is not restricted to the parent. In childhood, age mates and leaders of the peer group may supersede members of the household as identification models. Popular heroes of sports and entertainment also serve the same function.

Complementation, or reciprocation, is the other principle according to which G-I/R differentiation takes place in postnatal life. This concept had its origin in hermaphroditic studies,[12,13] and in particular in the case of a child with a birth defect of the genitalia whose sex was reannounced from son to daughter at age 16 months. In the next couple of years, complementarity of this child's behavior as a girl in relation to that of her father and brother (and of theirs to hers) was clearly equal in importance to her identification with her mother as a model for behavior as a girl. Like identification, complementation takes place among friends within the peer group, and not only within the family.

The schemas of identification and complementation become locked into the brain where they function as templates in the governance of sex-dimorphic behavior. Identification is for the self and others identified as of one's own morphologic sex (or successful impersonators thereof); and complementation, vice versa. The more overlap or interchangeability between the two, the greater the degree of androgyny. The more rigid and extreme the male/female stereotyping of behavior, the less the overlap and interchangeability.

There may be some change in the degree of overlap and interchangeability during the course of a person's lifetime, but for the most part a person's identification/complementation quotient remains remarkably fixed in his/her G-I/R.

Transpositions

Fixity of G-I/R applies even in cases of male/female transposition, of which transexualism with hormonal and surgical sex reassignment, is an extreme example.

Gynemimesis, known in street language as being a "drag queen," applies to a person who lives full time as a lady with a penis and, if taking female hormone, breasts. Andromimesis is the converse.

Transvestism (the syndrome of transvestophilia, and not the act of crossdressing) is episodic male/female transposition of G-I/R. Each episode represents a very convincing male or female G-I/R with, respectively, its own name, personality, wardrobe, and occupation.

In homosexualism, there are varying degrees of transposition. If manifested in gesture and mannerism it is referred to as effeminacy in males, and as mannishness or lesbianism in females. In many instances there is no such manifestation, in which case the person is homosexual only in the sense of having a person of the same genital morphology as an erotic partner or lover.

In bisexualism, the erotic partner or lover may be of either sex. The bisexual ratio may symmetrically be 50:50 or, as is more likely, asymmetrical.

Male/female transpositions of G-I/R exclusive of procreative sex, genital sex, eroticism, and limerence (being love-smitten) apply to legal status, work, schooling, play, customs, and manners. These are the transpositions that generate the sometimes intense and partisan passions of sexual politics.

Sexual Politics

Partisanship in sexual politics polarizes on the body/mind split, for the body is readily ceded to nature and biology, and the mind to nurture and social science.

Except for the growing influence of neuroscience, theories of mind and motivation hold sway in today's sociology, social and clinical psychology, psychiatry, and psychoanalysis. The proponents of these disciplines have assimilated the concept of gender into their teleological theory of mind and motivation by isolating it from sex and the body. Sex they classify as biological or constitutional, and gender as acquired or learned.

This same polarization has also been espoused by some biologists and sociobiologists, intent on preserving their own definition of biological determinism in the genesis of sex differences in society. Sexual politics, it transpires, is in many instances their hidden agenda. They misuse biology to justify the dominance of the male, and to attack the contrary arguments of militant feminists. The latter, by contrast misuse biology by explaining it away. They substitute instead a mystique of social stereotyping and historical determinism that, by fiat, has a nonbiological existence. Each side quotes research material to bolster its own doctrines, and excludes that which does not. My own research has been assaulted from each side, since its theoretical position is biosocial, integrating nature and nurture, not polarizing them.

Neither side is yet intellectually ready to put into practice the unity of biological and social determinism in the brain, which is where the unification takes place. Social learning and memory are, let it never be forgotten, just as much biology in the brain as are genes, hormones, and neutrotransmitters. All share in both long-term and short-term programing of the brain and mind. That is the basic principle of the unity of bodymind.

Definitions

andromimesis: the condition in which a girl or woman manifests the features or qualities of a male in body language, bodily appearance, dress and behavior. There is no fixed vernacular synonym except, maybe, being a bull dyke, that is, a female homosexual who lives the role of a man, who may request breast removal but not genital surgery, and who may or may not request hormones to masculinize the voice, beard and body hair. *See also* gynemimesis.

gender: one's personal, social and legal status as male or female, or androgynous, on the basis of somatic and behavioral criteria more inclusive than the genital criterion alone.

gender identity: the sameness, unity, and persistence of one's individuality as male, female, or ambivalent, in greater or lesser degree, especially as it is experienced in self-awareness and behavior.

gender-identity/role (G-I/R): gender identity is the private experience of gender role, and gender role is public manifestation of gender identity. Both together are G-I/R.

gender role: everything that a person says and does to indicate to others or to the self the degree that one is either male or female, or androgynous; it includes but is not restricted to sexual arousal and response.

gynemimesis: the condition in which a boy or man manifests the features or qualities of a female in body language, bodily appearance, dress and behavior. The vernacular synonym is being a drag queen, or a lady with a penis, that is, a male homosexual who, living the role of a woman, retains his male genitalia, even though he may take hormones to grow breasts. *See also* andromimesis.

sex: [as defined in the 26th (1981) edition of *Dorland's Illustrated Medical Dictionary*] (L. *sexus*) 1. the fundamental distinction, found in most species of animals and plants, based on the type of gametes produced by the individual or the category into which the individual fits on the basis of that criterion; ova, or macrogametes, are produced by the female, and spermatozoa, or microgametes, are produced by the male, the union of these distinctive germ cells being the natural prerequisite for the production of a new individual in sexual reproduction. 2. to determine the sex of an organism. *chromosomal s.,* sex as determined by the presence of the XX (female) or the XY (male) genotype in somatic cells and without regard to phenotypic manifestation; called also *genetic s. endocrinologic s.,* the phenotypic manifestations of sex determined by endocrine influences, such as breast development, etc. *genetic s.,* chromosomal s. *gonadal s.,* the sex as determined on the basis of the gonadal tissue present, whether ovarian or testicular. *morphological s.,* sex determined on the basis of the morphology of the external genitals. *nuclear s.,* the sex as determined on the basis of the presence or absence of sex chromatin in somatic cells, its presence normally indicating the XX (female) genotype, and its absence the XY (male) genotype. *psychological s.,* the self-image of the gender role of an individual. *social s.,* the complex of attitudes, expectations, etc., that a society attaches to the male and female roles.

References

1. Money, J.: Hermaphroditism, gender and precocity in hyperadrenocorticism: Psychologic findings. *Bull Johns Hopkins Hosp* 96:253-264, 1955.
2. Money, J.: *Hermaphroditism: An inquiry into the nature of a human paradox.* Doctoral Dissertation, Harvard University Library, 1952. University Microfilms Library Services, Xerox Corporation, Ann Arbor, MI 48106, 1967.

3. Klebs, E: *Handbuch der pathologischen Anatomie.* Berlin, August Hirschwald, 1876; 1.Band, Zweite Abtheilung, 718.

4. Money, J., Hampson, J. G., Hampson, J. L.: An examination of some basic sexual concepts: The evidence of human hermaphroditism. *Bull Johns Hopkins Hosp* 97:301-319, 1955.

5. Money, J.: *Love and love sickness: The science of sex, gender difference, and pair-bonding.* Baltimore, Johns Hopkins University Press, 1980.

6. Money, J.: Gender role, gender identity, core gender identity: Usage and definition of terms. *J Amer Acad Psychonal* 1:397-403, 1973.

7. Money, J.: Two names, two wardrobes, two personalities. *J Homosexuality* 1:65-70, 1974.

8. Money, J., Ehrhardt, A. A.: *Man and woman, boy and girl: The differentiation and dimorphism of gender identity from conception to maturity.* Baltimore, Johns Hopkins Press, 1972.

9. McEwen, B. S.: Neural gonadal steroid actions. *Science* 211:1303-1311, 1981.

10. Clarke, I. J.: The sexual behaviour of prenatally androgenized ewes observed in the field. *J Reproduction Fertility* 49:311-315, 1977.

11. Short, R. V., Clarke, I. J.: *Masculinization of the female sheep* (film). Distributed by, MRC Reproductive Biology Unit, 2 Forrest Road, Edinburgh EH1 2QW, Scotland, U.K.

12. Money, J.: Differentiation of gender identity and gender role. *Psychiat Ann* 1:33-43, 1971.

13. Money, J.: Identification and complementation in the differentiation of gender identity. *Danish Med Bull* 19:265-268, 1972.

Note

Originally published in *Journal of Sex and Marital Therapy,* 11:71-79, 1985. [Bibliog. #2.291]

PART III
Homosexual/Bisexual/Heterosexual Gender Status

TWENTY

Gender-Transposition Theory
and Homosexual Genesis

Abstract

The genesis of homosexuality, and therefore of heterosexuality also, has traditionally been argued as either wholly biological or wholly social-environmental. The theory of gender transposition integrates findings regarding both prenatal hormonal programing of the sexual brain, and postnatal social programing.

Definition

Gender transposition is a generic term that characterizes diverse degrees of male/ female crossover, especially in erotic and sexual practice and/or imagery of the type conventionally classified as either masculine or feminine according to the criterion of procreation in two-sexed species. It includes the simple and sometimes time-limited phenomenon of having a partner of the same genital morphology as the self, with or without being pairbonded. It includes also the more extensive transpositions exemplified in the syndromes of transexualism and transvestism.

Role Inconstancy

In attributing cognitive order and system to their existence in a social environment of selectively withheld sexual learning, some children are more, and some less, versatile than others at dramatic play-acting and theatrical make-believe in gender-inconsistent roles and strategies.[1] Those who are more versatile constitute a population at risk for gender inconstancy and possible gender transposition, if they are born of parents whose reciprocal compatibilities and incompatibilities, in their careers as mother and father, and in their sex lives as husband and wife, remain perpetually unreconcilable. In this formulation, the key concept is that of versatility. If one defines gender transposition as pathology, then the concept is not versatility, but vulnerability to gender inconstancy and transposition.

The development of gender inconstancy and transposition can be observed, and has been documented in children as young as three to four years of age. It is either more exaggerated and frequent in boys than in girls, or else it generates more alarm in those adults who take action toward changing it. In our society today, sissy boys are severely stigmatized. Tomboyish girls are not.

In boys, gender transposition expresses itself in playing with girls' toys and associating with girls instead of boys, in wearing clothing and accessories of feminine style as often as possible, and in expressly wanting to be a girl. In the early stages of gender transposition, a child is able to walk, talk, and gesture like either a boy or a girl.

Less is known about gender transposition in girls than boys, in part because clinical referrals are less common. In general, gender transposition is less conspicuously expressed in girls than boys. It is more a matter of repudiating the historical stereotype of the idealized little girl than of impersonating a macho boy, though there are exceptions. In extreme cases, the girl with a gender transposition has a macho alliance with the father, and with the mother a contemptuous, dominating, and abusive relationship.

Father-Son Allegiance

Contrary to established beliefs, the fathers of sissy boys are typically blandly indifferent to the signs of their son's nonconformity to the standard of masculinity in boyhood development. They write it off as something the boy will grow out of.

For years, I did not know what to make of this indifference. I had no hypothesis until a few years ago when a psychiatrist consulted me about his own son, aged five, the younger of two children, both boys. He and his wife excluded the boy from a family appointment, ostensibly to spare him from stigmatizing himself as abnormal. They distanced themselves from one another, spatially and verbally. Their matrimonial relationship was that of wedded adversaries practicing insidiously clever strategies of mutual sabotage. For example, even though he was a professed agnostic, the husband criticized his wife for being religiously too laissez faire. She reacted by becoming a conservative fundamentalist. Family religious observances became a source of unending dispute.

The rift thus created was additionally widened in disputation regarding acoustic sensitivity. For her, loud music was noxious, so he was obliged to pursue his interest in live rock performances without her. In fantasy, he anticipated that his younger son would become his companion in music. The older son, by contrast, already at age eight coerced his reluctant father to share his all-boy interest in fishing and the outdoors.

Professionally trained to be self-analytic, this father was also self-revealing. After soliciting my prognosis of his son's cross-dressing and girlish inclinations, and hearing that it was not necessary to be pessimistic at age five, he asked why he was feeling so angry with me—and angry because of what I had said. My reply was to the effect that perhaps he didn't wholly want his son to stop cross-dressing, and did not want to be robbed of the one member of the family whom he might consider his special escort.

Subsequently I dictated a note "to put on record a new hypothesis or formula regarding the role of the father in the genesis of feminism in a son's G-I/R (gender-identity/role). This is the formula: the father covertly courts his son's allegiance, in place of what he finds missing in his wife, and casts him in the role of a wife substitute, if not for the present, then for the future." The son, for his part, may solicit his father's allegiance as a formula for keeping him in the household, and for preventing a parental separation. If the father had already gone, or even if he had died, the son's gender transposition may serve to solicit his miraculous return.

Within a family, the allocation or reallocation of roles is not necessarily covert. It is more or less inherent in the idea of naming or nicknaming a baby after an ancestor, parent or other relative, also in the wisdom of the kin regarding whom a particular child takes after. Parents have favorite children— mommy's boy, daddy's girl—just as children may favor one parent over the other, or one relative over another.

The young son who becomes self-allocated to the role of daughter, and thereby becomes a bonding agent who keeps the family intact, is likely to keep the role of bonding agent in perpetuity. The evidence of one longitudinal, outcome study[2,3] is such that a son reaches adulthood with not a transexual or transvestite gender status, but a nonparaphilic homosexual one.

Parental Compatibility/Incompatibility

There is now new preliminary evidence, unpublished, that the transpositional course of events may be changed if the child can be relieved of the self-imposed responsibility of keeping his parents together. In one case, that of a three year old, the gravity of the boy's responsibility for keeping the parents together could be measured against the intensity of the father's response when confronted with the possibility of losing a custody battle, in the event of divorce. That was absolutely out of the question, he said, so far as he was concerned, and he hinted darkly at homicide rather than permit it to happen.

The son's change away from girl-imitative behavior ensued with unexpected rapidity in the immediate aftermath of the family's first visit—a marathon five hours of individual evaluations and joint discussions. The change in the boy was concomitant with a change in the parents, as they achieved more focus on their compatibility, and less on their incompatibility.

They were strongly compatible in their professional and domestic lives, and equally incompatible in their sexual and erotic lives. In four years of follow-up, their sexual and erotic incompatibility has remained stubbornly intractable to change. Nonetheless, there was only one brief occasion when it threatened to bring an end to their compatibilities. It was then that a resurgence of effeminacy threatened in the boy. It was transient. It did not, as had been the case in the original diagostic toy-play sessions, generate dramas of desperation in which members of a toy family became victims of catastrophe, abusive violence and murder.

This boy's play enactments did not include any dramas of explicit erotic or sexual content. Nor was there a history of overtly initiated erotic or sexual conduct other than age-typical masturbation in private, which the parents did not condemn. If the boy experienced erotosexual imagery in dreams and fantasies, their content remained private and undisclosed. Explicit erotosexual fantasies with the father as partner have been retrospectively dated to boyhood by some young adult homosexual men, however.[4]

In a young child's development, gender transposition is a rudimentary and inchoate response to diffusely mixed covert and overt signals that seem to indicate that, by being a girl with a penis or a boy with a vulva, a child will somehow be more satisfactory to each parent. Thus, the two parents can be retained in or restored to an intact family unit and their continued allegiance to one another mutually ensured. This formulation sounds outrageous and absurd only if it is elevated to the status of being a sufficient, instead of only a necessary condition in the genesis of developmental gender transposition.

Prenatal Hormonalization: Adam/Eve Principle

In gender transposition, the phylogenetic basis of the transposition and its attachment to sex and eroticism is epitomized in the Adam/Eve principle, namely, nature's rudimentary principle of sexual differentiation, which is to differentiate a female and to have to add something to differentiate a male. In gender transposition, the successive phases of differentiation, beginning prenatally and continuing postnatally, do not proceed concordantly in the usual orderly fashion. Discordance may begin prenatally under hormonal influence so that, at birth, a baby is at risk postnatally for a transposed gender status, provided convergent social influences and experiences increase the risk.

Historically, gender transposition of the complete type was explained as hereditary. However, the hereditary attribution has proved too simple and is now anachronistic. The contemporary explanation is hormonal. Like its hereditary predecessor, the hormonal explanation applies to development that takes place before birth. This development is governed not by the genetic code directly, but by sex hormones that program the sexual differentiation of the brain.[5]

According to the Adam/Eve principle, simply stated, if the fetal brain is not hormonalized, it will develop from its early, sexually bipotential stage to be, like Eve, feminine. To be like Adam, it must be hormonalized. The hormone is testosterone or one of its derivative metabolites.

Masculinization/Defeminization

Brain hormonalization is not inevitably an all-or-none affair. It may be a matter of degree. It is possible to be masculinized without being also completely defeminized or, conversely, to be feminized without also remaining completely demasculinized.[6-10] Thus, it is possible for a boy to be born with a brain that is both masculinized and feminized (that is, not defeminized) to some degree—and correspondingly for a girl. At birth, and immediately after (see below), the masculine/defeminine ratio in boys, and the feminine/demasculine ratio in girls is potentially widely variable.

The source of variability could be spontaneous. It might be secondary to stress that changes the pregnant mother's own hormone levels, which can affect the fetus. It might also be induced within the intrauterine environment or through the placenta by substances breathed, swallowed or otherwise absorbed by the mother. For example, it is known that barbiturates may have a demasculinizing effect on a fetus; and that in the last half century literally millions of pregnant women have taken sleeping pills and other medications containing barbiturates.[11]

In most instances of gender transposition, regardless of degree, it is impossible to reconstruct the prenatal sex-hormonal history in retrospect. Ethically, it is not possible to conduct experiments on pregnant women in order to find out everything that needs to be known about the causes and the timing of prenatal masculinization and defeminization of the sexual brain in boys, and of its prenatal feminization and demasculinization in girls. Therefore, it is necessary to garner whatever evidence one can from spontaneously occurring clinical syndromes or so-called experiments of nature.

Clinical Syndromes

The relevant syndromes are those in which the prenatal sex-hormonal history is known to have been atypical because the baby is born with a sex-hormonally generated hermaphroditic (or intersexual) ambiguity of the reproductive organs. There are also syndromes in which the postnatal hormonal history is atypical, for example in adolescent gynecomastia, but in which the prenatal hormonal history has not yet been spelled out, though it too may be presumed to have been atypical.

In order to make an inference regarding the prenatal influence of sex hormones on the sexual differentiation of the brain, it is necessary to follow a patient clinically into teenage and young adulthood when masculine and feminine sexuoerotic behavior and imagery may be expected to be fully expressed.[12-16]

The evidence from clinical studies supports the hypothesis that there is in human prenatal development a sex-hormonal effect on sexual brain differentiation, but that it does not have a hormonal-robot effect of the type described for sheep and other subprimate animals. Rather, the effect is one of laying down a threshold so that behavior that is generally defined as masculine or feminine, respectively, is expressed either rapidly or unhindered, or only after surmounting a barrier. The only irreducible sex difference is that men impregnate, and women menstruate, gestate and lactate. Other behavior that is commonly regarded as sex different, including aggression, is actually sex shared. It is the threshold for its elicitation and expression that distinguishes most men from most women.

Postnatal Gender Differentiation: Identification/Complementation

Whereas sex hormones are responsible, prenatally, for programing individual variation in the sex-divergent thresholds of sex-shared behavior, postnatally the sex-hormonal influence goes into a period of dormancy. In girls, sex-hormonal dormancy begins at birth. In boys, by contrast, there is a great surge of testosterone beginning at about two weeks of age. It becomes spent by age three months and remains so until the onset of puberty.[17] The effect of this testosterone surge remains to be ascertained. It could be the grand finale of sexual brain differentiation, according to David Abramovich in Aberdeen (personal communication).

When the sex hormones flow again at puberty, they activate male/female erotosexual programs or schemas already differentiated in the brain. Contrary to popular assumption, they do not cause behavior to be masculine instead of feminine, or vice versa.[18-20] That is why, among other things, it is not possible to change heterosexuality into homosexuality, or the other way around, by giving injections of sex hormones.

During the period between birth and puberty, when male/female erotosexual programing of the brain is no longer affected by sex hormones, the special senses take over. The eyes, the ears and the skin senses, more than the senses of smell and taste, are the brain's gateways to information about the gender status and erotosexual programing of the people among whom the child grows up. Gender related information, like information about native language, is assimilated through usage and experience, and not simply as a product of training and indoctrination.

Listening and being heard are together imperative for the brain to be successful in allowing a native language to take up residence within it. Likewise, copying and practicing gender-divergent behavior together are imperative to the establishment of one's gender status within the brain. Gender copying is conventionally referred to as identification with persons assigned the same gender status as oneself. The converse, gender practicing, only recently has been referred to as complementation or reciprocation.[21] That which is assimilated and learned by way of identification is put into practice with persons not assigned the same gender as oneself. To illustrate, the little girl learns to dance by identifying with her mother or sister and copying them, but she dances with her father or brother, complementing them. The same two principles apply across the entire spectrum of gender divergent status, sexuoerotic rehearsal play included. Age mates have exceptional authority in transmitting gender dimorphic standards and stereotypes.

Sexuoerotic Rehearsal Play

Rehearsal of the positions of presenting and mounting is widespread in the age-mate play of early childhood primates. It has been most intensively investigated in rhesus monkeys (Goldfoot et al.,[22] and personal communication). Monkeys deprived of play grow up unable to copulate and breed. Restricting play to as little as a half-hour a day allows one out of three young ones to achieve the correct copulatory position, but a year or more too late. They grow up able to copulate, but their breeding rate is subnormal.

Monkeys allowed unrestricted play time, but only in all male or all female groups, engage in presenting and mounting play with one another when they become adolescent. Although normally reared partners of the opposite sex find them sexually attractive, they cower and are scared. A male does not mount a female, even though he inspects and touches her genitalia with curiosity. A female resists the approach of a male partner, who succeeds in copulating only if he is exceptionally gentle and skilled at not making her more scared. When back with their same-sexed friends with whom they played as juveniles, males continue to mount males, and females to mount females with a frequency unrecorded in males and females that grew up and engaged in sexual rehearsal play together as juveniles (David Goldfoot, personal communication, January 7, 1984).

Among human beings, the hallowed social policy of prohibiting, preventing and punishing erotosexual rehearsal play in late infancy and the juvenile years may interfere with the genital component of identification and complementation to a degree as yet barely suspected. Social failure to endorse healthy masculinity and femininity in erotosexual rehearsal play may very well permit this aspect of develoment to become permanently and irrevocably stunted—misrepresented or transposed in the brain.

Brain Schemas

Identification and complementation each have their representation or schema implanted in the brain. One is the schema of one's own gender status. The other is the schema of the other gender status to which one must complement one's own. On the basis of actuarial statistics, one expects that the identification schema will differentiate to be concordant with the morphology of the genitalia of the self, whereas the complementation schema will be concordant with the morphology of the genitalia of the other sex. It is when this expectation is not realized that one has a gender transposition. The degree of transposition is variable, from total or obligative to trivial or adventitious. A total, but episodic transposition is evident in cases of two names, two wardrobes, and two personalities—one male, and one female, each alternating with the other and having a different lifestyle and personality.

TABLE I

Gender Transpositions

	Total	Partial*	Adventitious
Chronic	Transexualism	Gynemimesis andromimesis, male androphilia, female gynophilia	Androgeny of gender-coded education, work legal status
Episodic	Transvestism	Androgynophilia (bisexualism)	Androgeny of gender-coded play, body-language, grooming, ornament

*Gynemimesis and andromimesis mean impersonating a female and a male, respectively, on a full-time basis.[24] Male androphilia means erotosexual attraction between men, and female gynophilia between women. Androgynophilia means erotosexual attraction, to some degree, to men and women.

Table I shows a 2 × 3 classification of gender transposition on the criteria of duration and degree of pervasiveness. By itself alone, a transposition is neither an asset nor a debit. It becomes one or the other on the basis of the value judgments, both informal and official, of other people.

References

1. Green, R., Money, J.: Stage-acting, role-taking, and effeminate impersonation during boyhood. *Arch Gen Psych* 15:535-538, 1966.
2. Money, J., Russo, A. J.: Homosexual outcome of discordant gender-identity/role in childhood: Longitudinal follow-up. *J Pediat Psychol* 4:29-31, 1979.
3. Money, J., Russo, A. J.: Homosexual vs. transvestite or transexual gender-identity/role: Outcome study in boys. *Int J Fam Psychiat* 2:139-145, 1981.
4. Silverstein, C.: *Man to Man: Gay Couples in America.* New York: Morrow, 1981.
5. Money, J.: The development of sexuality and eroticism in humankind. *Q Rev Biol* 56:379-404, 1981.
6. Baum, M. J.: Differentiation of coital behavior in mammals: A comparative analysis. *Neurosci Biobehav Rev* 3:265-284, 1979.
7. Baum, M. J., Gallagher, C. A., Martin, J. T., Damassa, D. A.: Effects of testosterone, dihydrotestosterone, or estradiol administered neonatally on sexual behavior of female ferrets. *Endocrinology* 111:773-780, 1982.
8. Nordeen, E. J., Yahr, P.: Hemispheric asymmetries in the behavioral and hormonal effects of sexually differentiating mammalian brain. *Science* 218:391-393, 1982.
9. Ward, I. L.: Prenatal stress feminizes and demasculinizes the behavior of males. *Science* 175:82-84, 1972.
10. Ward, I. L., Weisz, J.: Maternal stress alters plasma testosterone in fetal males. *Science* 207:328-329, 1980.
11. Reinsich, J. M., Sanders, S. A.: Early barbiturate exposure: The brain, sexually dimorphic behavior and learning. *Neurosci Biobehav Rev* 6:311-319, 1982.
12. Lewis, V. G., Money, J.: Gender-identity/role: G-I/R Part A: XY (androgen-insensitivity) syndrome and XX (Rokitansky) syndrome of vaginal atresia compared. In L. Dennerstein, G. Burrows (eds.), *Handbook of Psychomatic Obstetrics and Gynecology.* Amsterdam-New York-Oxford, Elsevier Biomedical, 1983.

13. Money, J. Daléry, J.: Iatrogenic homosexuality: Gender identity in seven 46,XX chromosomal females with hyperadrenocortical hermaphroditism born with a penis, three reared as boys, four reared as girls. *J Homosex* 1:357-371, 1976.

14. Money, J., Lewis, V. G.: Homosexual/heterosexual status in boys at puberty: Idiopathic adolescent gynecomastia and congenital virilizing adrenocorticism compared. *Psychoneuroendocrin* 7:339-346, 1982.

15. Money, J., Mathews, D.: Prenatal exposure to virilizing progestins: An adult follow-up study of twelve women. *Arch Sex Beh* 11:73-83, 1982.

16. Money, J., Schwartz, M., Lewis, V. G.: Adult erotosexual status and fetal hormonal masculinization and demasculinization: 46,XX congenital virilizing adrenal hyperplasia (CVAH) and 46,XY androgen-insensitivity syndrome (AIS) compared. *Psychoneuroendocrinology,* 1984.

17. Migeon, C. J., Forest, M. G.: Androgens in biological fluids. In B. Rothfeld (ed.), *Nuclear Medicine in Vitro,* 2nd ed. Philadelphia, Lippincott, 1983.

18. Parks, G. A., Korth-Schultz, S., Penny, R., Hilding, R. F., Dumars, K. W., Frasier, S. D., New, M. I.: Variation in pituitary-gonadal function in adolescent male homosexuals and heterosexuals. *J Clin Endocrin Metab* 39:796-801, 1974.

19. Sanders, R. M., Langevin, R., Bain, J.: Hormones and human sexuality. *Neuroendocrinol Letters* 5:129, 1983.

20. Sanders, R. M., Bain, J., Langevin, R.: Peripheral sex hormones, homosexuality, and gender identity. In R. Langevin (ed.), *Erotic Preference, Gender Identity, and Aggression in Men.* Hillsdale, NJ, Erlbaum, 1984.

21. Money, J.: Identification and complementation in the differentiation of gender identity. *Dan Med J* 19:256-268, 1972.

22. Goldfoot, D. A., Goy, R. W., Neff, D. A., Wallen, K., McBrair, M. C.: Social influences upon the display of sexually dimorphic behavior in rhesus monkeys: Isosexual rearing. *Arch Sex Beh* 13:395-412, 1984.

23. Money, J.: Two names, two wardrobes, and two personalities. J Homosex 1;65-70, 1974.

24. Money, J., Lamacz, M.: Gynemimesis and gynemimetophilia: Individual and cross-cultural manifestations of a gender coping strategy hitherto unnamed. *Compr Psychiat* 25:392-403, 1984.

Note

Originally published in *Journal of Sex and Marital Therapy,* 10:75-82, 1984. [Bibliog. #2.285]

TWENTY-ONE

Homosexual Outcome of Discordant Gender-Identity/Role in Childhood: Longitudinal Follow-up

Abstract

Nine of 11 boys with prepubertal discordance of gender-identity/role have been maintained in follow-up until young adulthood. All are known to be homosexual or predominantly so. None is known to be either a transvestite or transexual, though one formerly began the real-life test for transexualism and quit after 6 weeks. All nine have completed some postsecondary education, and all are well-achieved or better, occupationally. Secondary psychopathology in adulthood has not been obviously manifest. There was a consensus in adulthood that the nonjudgmentalism of those responsible for their follow-up over the years had had a strongly positive therapeutic effect on the boys' personal development.

Introduction, Sample, and Method

Prospective, longitudinal studies of childhood sexuality are rare. Few people are able to commit themselves to a longitudinal study and remain budgeted long enough to complete it. In addition, the sexual taboo of our society is particularly antithetical to the recognition of sexuality in childhood, let alone the study of it. Until recently, if a problem of gender identity showed up in a boy's development, the usual medical tradition was to prophesy that he would grow out of it at puberty. This tradition is completely contradicted by evidence of retrospective studies of the developmental antecedents of homosexuality, bisexuality, transvestism, and transexualism, all of which typically have a history dating back to prepuberty.

The purpose of this paper is to report the findings of the outcome in adulthood of discordant gender-identity/role differentiaton relative to the criterion of gross morphologic sex in five boyhood cases, with specific reference to occupational status, psychosexual status, and mental health status.

The follow-up period is from 15 to 22 years. The size of the sample, five, is small in absolute terms, but large in terms of the availability of such long-term follow-up.

In the middle 1950s, and as an extension of psychologic studies in hermaphroditism, a request went out from the psychohormonal research unit of The Johns Hopkins University and Hospital for referral of prepubertal boys with discordant gender-identity/role. In the period from 1955 to 1962, 12 referrals were made by pediatricians and/or school social workers.

The criteria for referral were: exceptional interest in dressing in girls' clothing; avoiding play activities typical of boys and preferring those of girls; walking and talking more like girls than boys; and stating overtly the wish to be a girl. The presence of overt homosexual erotic behavior was not specified as a requirement for referral and, indeed, was not a presenting symptom for any of these boys.

The patients referred did not represent a random or probability sampling from the general population of boys manifesting discordant gender-identity/role. The exact biasing factors are not known. There was no selective bias in favor of psychopathology or delinquency as usually defined, for the primary concern was gender-identity/role. There was also no consistent bias with respect to IQ, socioeconomic status, physique, or somatic status.

Of the 12 patients, 11 qualified for inclusion in the present follow-up study on the criterion of being now older than 23, the oldest being 29; 2 of the 11 were earlier lost to follow-up and remained lost. Of the nine remaining candidates for follow-up, two were reluctant to be seen in current psychosexual follow-up but are not lost; and the two remaining are presently untraced, though not written off as permanently lost, as they were seen for teen-aged follow-up within the past 7 years. The remaining five gave the data tabulated in this report.

Initially the patients were all followed annually, with intervening visits on a self-demand, no-charge basis until puberty was established. Subsequent visits were on self-demand until 1977, when the present follow-up was instituted. A longitudinal file has been kept on each patient. The files included: test data; transcribed, taped interviews based on a systematic schedule of inquiry; and notes of physical examinations and measurements from the pediatric endocrine clinic. In addition the files also included interviews with parents and/or other guardians, as appropriate.

Patients were called in for follow-up interviews, which were based on a systematic schedule of inquiry. The Cornell Medical Index, among other tests, was also administered to each patient as a source of inquiry regarding his general health.

The schedule of inquiry was drawn up specifically for this follow-up study. It consisted of 27 typed pages with space for the interviewer to record the responses. In the case of extended answers, a tape recorder was used and answers were transcribed. The topics of inquiry fell into categories dealing with education, indoor and outdoor recreational activities, hobbies, dress, make-up, jewelry and perfume, teasing, dreams, enuresis, sleep, self-image, parental relationships, employment and career, living arrangements, religion, nonromantic friendships and acquaintances, romantic friendships, aggressive/passive behavior, sexual activity, and any other special behavior. The follow-up evaluation required an average of 6 hours.

Occupational Status

The educational and occupational information in Table I shows that none of the nine individuals for whom the information is available was a vocational failure. Except for two who were completing a college education when last contacted, all were, at a minimum, economically self-supporting at the middle-class level or higher. Among the seven who were already employed, six were professionally trained and were working at a level consistent with their training and intelligence. The seventh had irregular work in his chosen theatrical career, and took a second job in order to augment his salary in the meantime.

TABLE I

Age, Education, and Occupation of Five Men with a History of
Discordant Gender-Identity/Role in Childhood*

Patient no.	Age in years at follow-up	Education completed	Occupation
564988	29	B.A.	Small business entrepreneur
076559	23	College 3 semesters	Paramedical
141178	29	H.S.	Professional theater
868999	24	B.A.	Pedagogy and small business entrepreneur
6900501	24	A few college credits	Waiter; non-professional theater

*Among the six persons not seen in current follow-up and not included in Table I, educational data are known about four persons. Of the four, one had attended college for a year when last interviewed; one received a bachelor's degree as an art student; one is a fine arts director; and one is a graduate in American literature.

In view of the association between stage-acting and childhood effeminacy reported by Green and Money (1966) for the same group of individuals in childhood, it is noteworthy that two of them have pursued their interests professionally, one of them to a high degree of recognition.

Psychosexual Status

Inspection of Table II shows that the stated request to be a girl during childhood did not persist into a stated request to be a woman in adulthood. The current absence of a request to be a woman is paralleled by an absence of seeing the self as a woman during current dreams. Since the dreams of childhood as formerly reported did not include seeing the self as a girl, it is possible that the dream content in childhood may be utilized as a prognosticator of the status of gender-identity/role in adulthood. This childhood dream content correlates in four cases

TABLE II

Gender Orientation: Reported Statements, Dreams, and Thoughts of Five Men
With a History of Discordant Gender-Identity/Role in Childhood

Patient no.	Stated request to be a girl during childhood	Stated request to be a woman, currently	Self seen as a woman in dreams, currently	Self seen as a girl in dreams in childhood	Thought of being transexual
564988	Yes	No	No	No	Never
076559	Yes	No	No	No	Never
141178	Yes	No	No	No	Never
868999	Yes	No	No	No	Never
6900501	Yes	No	No	No	Yes (see text)

with consistent absence of the possibility of the self as transexual. In the fifth
case the boy did, between the ages of 17 and 19, contemplate the possibility of
sex reassignment as a solution to what he perceived as his life's dilemma. He
went so far at the age of 19 as to embark on the real-life test of cross-dressing
and presenting himself socially as a woman. After 6 weeks he gave up, having
learned from the real-life test that sex reassignment was not for him.

TABLE III

Preferences in Clothing, Make-up, and Jewelry of Five Men with a History
of Discordant Gender-Identity/Role in Childhood

Patient no.	As a child dressed up as a female	Currently dresses up as a female	Wore make-up in childhood	Wore make-up at time of follow-up	Wore jewelry in childhood	Wore jewelry occasionally at time of follow-up
564988	Yes	Costume parties only	No	Costume parties only	Yes	No
076559	Yes	No	Yes	No	Yes	No
141178	Yes	No	Yes	No	Yes	No
868999	Yes	No	No	No	Yes	No
6900501	Yes	No	Yes	Minimal	Yes	No

By contrast with the cross-dressing interest as juveniles (see Table III), the
current interest is zero in four cases and in the fifth case is restricted to costume
parties.

With respect to the use of make-up and the wearing of jewelry, the change
from childhood to adulthood follows in the same direction as the change in
cross-dressing. That is to say, in daily life, none of the five men exhibits himself as being feminine by reason of what he wears. The only signs, if any, that
an observer might construe as being feminine would be subtle ones of body

TABLE IV

Romantic and Erotic Status of Five Men with a History
of Discordant Gender-Identity/Role in Childhood*

Patient no.	Had coitus with a female	Erotic status	Romantic involvement with females	Romantic involvement with males
564988	No	Homosexual	Yes	Yes
076559	No	Homosexual	No	Yes
141178	Yes	Predominantly homosexual	No	Yes
868999	Yes	Predominantly homosexual	No	Yes
6900501	No	Homosexual	No	Yes

*Among the six persons not seen in current follow-up and not included in Table IV, four are known to be homosexual in erotic status, and two are lost to follow-up.

movements. In four of the five, such signs were minimal at most, and in the fifth a little more obvious to those educated in what to look for.

With respect to current romantic and erotic status, Table IV shows that all five men considered themselves homosexual or predominantly so, as confirmed in their actual erotic behavior. Two have had the experience of copulating with females, but in a more perfunctory way than in their corresponding experience with males. One of these two appears to be in a phase of transition to a less perfunctory continued relationship with a girlfriend. One man who had not had sexual intercourse with a female described what he called a dating relationship with a girlfriend during his high-school years, subsequently totally discontinued. All five of the men have had romantic involvements or love affairs with males and two of them are in long-term living arrangements with their lovers. The other three men are living independently away from their parents. In all five cases, contact with the parents was maintained in the usual adult way when sons live away from their parents.

Mental Health

As stated in the section on Procedure, self-demand counseling was offered to all of the individuals in this study from childhood onward. All of the five seen personally for current follow-up expressed their approval of this arrangement, and particularly of the nonjudgmental attitudes they encountered in their visits. They volunteered that they had strongly benefited from their counseling sessions and believed that they were better able to accept themselves as healthy individuals because of them. None of the five men was evaluated as being in need of more frequent psychotherapy and none showed psychopathological symptoms requiring it.

Etiology

The starting date of the ideal longitudinal study of the outcome of psychosexual differentiation would be the day of conception; and the ideal prenatal methodology would be one in which the prenatal fetal hormonal history could be measured with greater precision than is today possible. Fetal sex hormones are known to influence brain pathways which in turn will subsequently mediate behavior that is to some degree sexually dimorphic: the relevant animal-experimental and human-clinical evidence is reviewed in Money and Ehrhardt (1972). This fetal-hormonal influence does not preordain masculine versus feminine behavior, but simply creates a threshold that will either help or hinder the manifestation of the one or the other, respectively. An excess of fetal androgenization of a genetic and gonadal female, for example, may induce a high degree of anatomical masculinization of the genitals. In extreme cases, there is instead of a clitoris a penis. In less extreme cases, the phallus looks like either a hypospadiac penis or a maximally hypertrophied clitoris. In some cases the baby is assigned, reared, and rehabilitated hormonally and surgically as a boy, especially when the phallus looks like a normal penis. Psychosexual differentiation then proceeds as masculine so that, in adulthood, the individual shows no signs of having a 46,XX chromosomal complement, nor of having been born with two ovaries (Money & Daléry, 1976). Conversely, when the postnatal medical biography is aimed at feminization, then the psychosexual differentiation, while not masculine, has a tomboyish underpinning, and it is easy for the girl to grow up to become bisexual or, in some instances, exclusively homosexual in young adulthood (Money & Schwartz, 1977).

In the present series of cases, there was no way of retrospectively retrieving information about the prenatal hormonal status of the individuals concerned. It is, therefore, purely speculative as to whether or not they were born with a prenatal hormonal disposition favoring the differentiation of a homosexual gender-identity/role. Nonetheless, such a possibility cannot be rejected. If one allows this possibility, one must equally allow also that the possibility does not automatically dictate the outcome. As in the case of native language, the outcome of psychosexual differentiation is, in nature's economy of things, heavily dependent on postnatal input from the social environment. The two principles involved are identification with people of one's own assigned sex, and complementation to those of the other sex. The most important models of identification and complementation are typically the parents.

In the present group of cases, there was no consistency of evidence as to whether the child encountered an exogenous difficulty in identification and complementation as compared with one that emanated from within the child himself. In some cases, the relationship between the parents was blatantly pathological, in others not. When the parents were caught in a pathological relationship, the nature of the pathology was not consistent among families. In some instances the mother was the power broker, in some the father, and in some neither dominated the other. The variability of family relationships was not noticeably different from that found in families who bring their children to the clinic with other diagnoses; and the same kind of variability could have been found in nonclinic families sampled at random. In brief, we did not recognize any consistent postnatal developmental formula to account for the fact that it was in psychosexual differentation and not in some other aspect of behavioral development, that the child encountered developmental difficulty. Different pathways led to the same destination.

In popular superstition, there is a commonly held dogma that boys are recruited to homosexuality by older homosexual boys or men. In the present sample, this was definitely not the case, for all the boys manifested the signs of gender-identity/role discordance which led to their hospital referral in the absence of known homosexual play. In all 11 cases, there was only one known instance of homosexual involvement in childhood. It happened at age 10 when the boy concerned woke up from sleep to discover his 16-year-old baby sitter having interfemoral intercourse with him. One of the reasons why the parents asked their pediatrician for a psychological referral following this incident was that they had some apprehension that their son, an adopted child, might have unwittingly invited the incident because of what they construed as signs of effeminacy. An interview with the teenager showed this not to have been the case. The younger boy is the one in the present series who, more than the others, grew up to achieve a fair degree of explicit bisexuality, partly with the help of continued therapy, self-initiated from age 16 onward.

There is another popular superstition that links the onset of homosexuality with the onset of hormonal puberty and, specifically, with a hormonal imbalance. The boys of the present series negate this superstition, for they all showed the developmental signs of what would later manifest itself as homosexuality well before puberty. The timing of the onset of puberty was within normal limits in all cases, and the degree of adolescent virilization of the body was evaluated as normal in the physical examination done by a clinical endocrinologist. The techniques of hormonal measurement were still relatively crude in those days, and were not expected to add significantly to the evidence of hormonal virilization as recorded in the physical examination. Hence there are no hormonal levels to report.

Diagnosis

In the present era of equal rights for both sexes and of the destereotyping of occupational, recreational, and legal sex roles, one may be called upon to justify the legitimacy of labeling a boy's behavior as girlish and then classifying it as pathological. In the present group of cases, it was not simply girlish or androgynous behavior that brought the boys to medical attention. Rather it was the pervasive discordance between the sex of the genitalia and the sex of the mind, so pervasive that each boy had developed a conviction that he should change into a girl, and that he should be able to do so by somehow or other losing his penis, for example, by praying to God to perform the miracle of having it wither and drop off. Other evidence of identification with girls and of adopting their socially coded roles, including their dress, was secondary to this rejection of the male anatomy. The manifestation of such discordance between genital anatomy and gender-identity/role eventually provoked concern in the parents, even in those cases in which either one or both of the parents were in covert collusion with the child. The concern at home was matched by concern at school, and was exceeded by peer abuse. Other children persecuted the boy as a sissy and excluded him from their companionship, usually quite cruelly.

At the time they were first seen, these boys were unable to widen their repertory of behavior to encompass that which in our society is stereotypically coded as male as well as that which is coded as female. They had no option of moving back and forth between both sets of stereotypes, which is the true mark of sexual liberation and of behavioral androgyny. They were trapped in one of the two stereotypes, the one in which they were victimized as freakish, and in which they suffered too much at the hands of a disapproving society.

There is no traditionally accepted diagnostic term for boys with a discordant gender-identity/role, the terminology utilized in this paper. It is incorrect to use the terms juvenile homosexual, transexual, or transvestite (see below, Prognosis).

Prognosis

When the men of the present study were first seen in childhood, the strategy of longitudinal follow-up had already been decided upon. In those days, as now, funding for projects on sexuality in childhood was impossible to come by, the taboo on sexuality in our society being what it is. Economic necessity thus joined with a basic policy decision to be as helpful as possible, with minimal intrusion into the lives of the boys and their families. They were offered follow-up on a self-demand basis without charge, on the understanding that an appointment would be sent out from time to time for the purpose of a check-up and progress report. One boy, with his mother's collusion, soon insisted on never coming to the hospital again, though his parents did not. Only two families became permanently lost to follow-up.

Apart from the two early drop-outs, enough is known of the remaining nine men to permit the statement that they did not develop as transexuals in adulthood. Since transvestites usually are rather theatrical about cross-dressing and not particularly secretive except with people who might punish or chastise them, it is probably correct to say that none of the nine is a transvestite, the evidence being quite definite in seven cases. The evidence is quite conclusive that in eight cases, including the one bisexual case, the boys grew up to be practicing homosexuals. The ninth might well be a case of erotic apathy and inertia, the details remaining undisclosed, except that he is not overtly heterosexual, and has exclusively gay friends.

There is no way of knowing to what degree, if any, the prognosis may have been altered by the minimal form of treatment given. Nonetheless, the follow-up does show that a syndrome that included cross-dressing in boyhood and appeared likely to be a precursor of transexualism, and possibly of transvestism, did not in fact turn out to be either. Presently there is no known way of establishing a differential prognosis regarding transexualism, transvestism, and homosexuality (or bisexuality) on the basis of discordance of gender-identity/role in childhood. If one judges by the retrospective biographies of adulthood, then the childhood precursor of all three outcomes in adulthood could be indistinguishable from one another.

As adults, none of the men is known to have complained about inadequacy of genital functioning—no impotence, premature ejaculation, anorgasmia, or other erotic disability. To use a newly emerging terminology, they had no difficulty with the second, the acceptive phase of functioning with a sexual partner. This is the phase in which the couple accept one another bodily, the sex organs included. It is preceded by the proceptive phase, the phase of courtship and solicitation, of attracting and being attractive. This is the phase of establishing a pairbond, otherwise known as falling in love. It is the phase in which the phenomenon of homosexuality essentially resides, for homosexuality is not, in fact, a sexual phenomenon at all, but a love phenomenon—an inability to fall in love with a person of the other sex, and an ability to fall in love with a person of the same sex as one's own. In consequence, the acceptive phase, when it follows the proceptive, does not lead on to the conceptive phase. Nonetheless, the conceptive phase of parenthood is not impaired. The men of the present sample all had a positive attitude toward children, and not a negative one, on the criterion of being able to be parental toward young children. They were able to develop a special avuncular relationship with their nieces and nephews, if they had them.

Treatment

In the present era of the ethics of informed consent and the rights of patients in medicine, some critics have questioned the morality of considering the problems of discordant gender-identity/role in childhood as symptoms requiring treatment. Thus, it is not possible to find out what might happen to psychosexual differentiation should a group of boys with discordance of gender-identity/role be transferred from the home of origin to, say, a children's recovery center or to foster homes for a period of time, as happens in the case of child-abuse dwarfism (Money, 1977), with ensuing catch-up growth, both statural and mental. At the present time it is also doubtful that one will be able to compare the effects of different forms of attempted intervention while the child stays living with the parents.

What can be said on the basis of the present findings is that the minimal form of treatment offered did no obvious harm. On the contrary, the verdict of those men interviewed in person during adolescence or young adulthood was, without exception, that they had benefited from having someone, especially in the juvenile years, whom they could expect to be totally nonjudgmental and willing to help in time of need, when they disclosed intimate and confidential information that brought scorn, disapproval, and stigmatization from many other authorities. It is quite possible that they were assisted to maintain self-esteem and self-respect, and to become successful human beings, unencumbered by secondary psychopathology, because of the early experience of nonjudgmentalism. They certainly do not fit the common and faulty stereotype of homosexuality as a form of sickness, degeneracy, or abomination.

Addendum

Three of the five adults here reported were among those previously reported as children (Green & Money, 1960, 1961).

References

Green, R., & Money, J. Incongruous gender role: Nongenital manifestation in prepubertal boys. *Journal of Nervous and Mental Disease,* 1960, 130, 160-168.

Green, R., & Money, J. Effeminancy in prepubertal boys: Summary of eleven cases and recommendations for case management. *Pediatrics,* 1961, 27, 286-291.

Green, R., & Money, J. Stage-acting, role-taking, and effeminate impersonation during boyhood. *Archives of General Psychiatry,* 1966, 15, 535-538.

Money, J. The syndrome of abuse dwarfism (psychosocial dwarfism or reversible hyposomatotropism): Behavioral data and case report. *American Journal of Diseases of Children,* 1977, 131, 508-513.

Money, J., & Daléry, J. Iatrogenic homosexuality: Gender identity in seven 46,XX chromosomal females with hyperadrenocortical hermaphroditism born with a penis, three reared as boys, four reared as girls. *Journal of Homosexuality,* 1976, 1, 357-371.

Money, J., & Ehrhardt, A. A. *Man and Woman, Boy and Girl: The Differentiation and Dimorphism of Gender Identity from Conception to Maturity.* Baltimore: Johns Hopkins University Press, 1972.

Money, J., & Schwartz, M. Dating, romantic and nonromantic friendships, and sexuality in 17 early-treated adrenogenital females, aged 16-25. In P. A. Lee, L. P. Plotnick, A. A. Kowarski, & C. J. Migeon (Eds.), *Congenital Adrenal Hyperplasia.* Baltimore: University Park Press, 1977.

Note

Originally published in *Journal of Pediatric Psychology,* Vol. 4, No. 1, 1979, pp. 29-41, with A. J. Russo as coauthor. [Bibliog. #2.239]

TWENTY-TWO

Iatrogenic Homosexuality: Gender Identity in Seven 46,XX Chromosomal Females with Hyperadrenocortical Hermaphroditism Born with a Penis, Three Reared as Boys, Four Reared as Girls

Abstract

This paper describes seven chromosomal and gonadal females with the adreno-genital syndrome who were born with a penis as a result of extreme fetal androgenization. Four of them were reared as girls and differentiated a female gender identity with tomboyism. The other three were reared as boys, differentiated a male gender identity, and performed sexually as men with women partners. Even though these men are by no means homosexual in the everyday meaning of the term, the sexual relation is homosexual on the criteria of chromosomal and gonadal sex. The prenatal hormonal environment as well as the social experience of the rearing have thus demonstrated a formula for creating the perfect female homosexual.

Introduction, Sample, and Method

This paper is one in a series of studies from the psychohormonal research unit of the Johns Hopkins University and Hospital on the effects of excessive fetal androgenization on subsequent behavior and gender identity in 46,XX chromosomal females with the adrenogenital syndrome. The adrenogenital syndrome is the result of a genetically recessive inborn error of metabolism due to an enzymatic defect in the biosynthesis of cortisol. By way of consequences, there is an excessive secretion of fetal adrenal androgen which in turn causes varied degrees of fetal masculinization of external and internal genital structures in the genetic female. The excessive amount of adrenal androgen secretion is not limited to the fetal stages; it goes on in the postnatal period, unless cortisone replacement therapy is given. When the treatment is started soon after birth and well regulated, the physical handicaps are minimized.

In the most extreme degree of masculinization, when excessive androgen is produced before the 12th week of fetal life, the urethra extends along the shaft of the hypertrophied clitoral organ, opening at the tip of the glans, so as to form a clitoral penis indistinguishable from a normal penis. The labioscrotal folds are completely fused to the extent that they look like an empty scrotum. In this anatomic type, the patient can at birth easily be mistaken for a male with bilateral cryptorchidism. This type is often referred to as Prader's type V (Prader, 1954).

Different subtypes of this syndrome occur where masculinization is the only manifestation, or associated with a tendency to salt loss, or with hypertension. A direct relation between the greater degree of masculinization of the genitalia and the salt-losing tendency has been reported (Qazi & Thompson, 1972; Verkauf & Jones, 1970). The salt-losing subtype may add life-threatening manifestations sporadically in times of illness or injury, and requires additional treatment for salt loss.

Cortisone replacement therapy, clitoridectomy, and vaginal exteriorization are required when the patient is to live as a female. Cortisone and testosterone replacement therapy and removal of the internal sex organs and of the gonads are required when the patient is to live as a male.

The purpose of the present paper is to show that complete embryonic differentiation of a penis in a genetic female does not preclude assignment, rearing, and habilitation as a girl with a feminine gender identity—albeit tomboyish—but, conversely, is consistent with assignment, rearing, and habilitation as a boy with a masculine gender identity. The secondary purpose is to comment on the etiology and theory of homosexuality.

The criteria for being included in this sample were threefold: (a) the diagnosis was adrenogenital syndrome; (b) the chromosomal sex was female; and (c) the patients presented at birth the extreme degree of masculinization of the external genitalia with penile urethra and fusion of the labioscrotal folds (see Figures 1, 2, and 3).

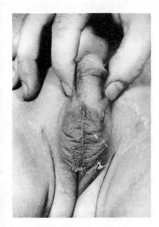

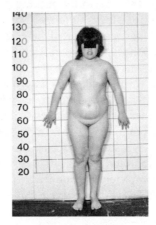

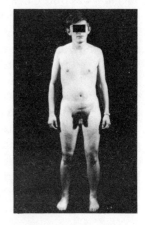

FIG. 1. Aspects of genitalia at birth.

FIG. 2. Girl at the age of 10.

FIG. 3. Boy at the age of 19.

Ten patients met these criteria. One born in 1955 died in an acute adrenal crisis in 1958; two others born in 1973 and 1974 are too young to be reported here. The seven remaining patients are described herein (see Table I). Six of them were referred to the psychohormonal research unit from the pediatric endocrine clinic of the Johns Hopkins Hospital. The seventh patient was seen by one of us in the Children's Hospital in Boston, courtesy of Dr. John Crigler.

The subjects were divided into two groups according to their sex of rearing. Group 1 includes three patients declared males without ambiguity at birth and raised from birth onward as males. The syndrome of adrenal hyperplasia was recognized before the genetic status; and surgical correction—namely, hysterectomy and ovariectomy—was done still later. Additionally, E. U. had prosthetic testes implanted in his scrotum when he was 13. Because in two cases the adrenogenital syndrome was not recognized neonatally, and cortisone replacement therapy not started until later, both subjects developed virile precocious puberty. As a consequence, the excessive acceleration of the bone growth created a discrepancy between physique age and chronological age in childhood. The premature fusion of the epiphyses explained the definitive short stature in adulthood (see Table I). In the ensuing part of this paper, patients of this group will be referred to, according to their sex of rearing, as boys.

Group 2 includes four patients raised as females. Three of them were declared males at birth and reannounced as females. Because of the death of an older sibling with ambiguous genitalia, a suspicion of female hermaphroditism was raised for the fourth subject at birth, and no sex was declared. She was announced a girl at the age of 6 days. For all four patients the syndrome of adrenal hyperplasia, as well as the genetic status, was recognized early in life. The first stage of surgical correction of the genitalia—penectomy and division of the scrotal fusion—was done without delay; the second stage—exteriorization of the vagina—was done later (see Table I). In the ensuing part of this paper, patients of this group will be referred to, according to their sex of rearing, as girls.

In summary, the seven patients reported here had a concordant prenatal history, but the postnatal history was completely discordant for patients of Group 1 and those of Group 2.

The basic procedure for the present study was to compile material from the patients' files. This was completed by a contemporary interview with the patient and such members of his or her family as were available. Additionally, extended telephone interviews were given to the three men and one girl, all of whom lived too distant for a contemporary visit to the Johns Hopkins Hospital. A standard data schedule of topics was followed, but the interviews themselves were flexible. Interviews were recorded completely or summarized on tape. The information relevant for the present paper was abstracted from the transcripts and then tabulated.

TABLE I

Descriptive Data of Sample (N = 7)

Patient:	E.U.	O.A.	O.I.	A.O.	U.T.	O.O.	I.I.
Date of birth	4/10/57	5/17/51	1/31/49	4/29/71	11/7/64	10/21/63	8/3/63
Sex announced as	Male at birth	Male at birth	Male at birth	Female at 6 days	Male at birth, female at 19 days	Male at birth, female at 8 weeks	Male at birth, female at 1 yr.
Age at first psychological report	13 yrs.	19 yrs. 6 mos.	6 yrs. 4 mos.	6 days	19 mos.	8 weeks	1 yr.
Age at last follow-up	18 yrs. 2 mos.	24 yrs. 3 mos.	26 yrs. 6 mos.	4 yrs. 1 mo.	10 yrs. 5 mos.	11 yrs. 7 mos.	12 yrs. 1 mo.
Age at surgery	13 yrs.	3 yrs. 6 mos.	7 yrs. 5 mos.	16 days/ 2 yrs. 6 mos.	1 mo./20 mos.	10 weeks/ 2 yrs. 9 mos.	1 yr./3 yrs.
Age at beginning of cortisone therapy	3 yrs. 6 mos.	11 days	4 yrs. 7 mos.	6 days	19 days	21 days	2 mos.
Age at determination of genetic status	12 yrs. 2 mos.	1 mo.	7 yrs. 5 mos.	6 days	19 days	8 weeks	10 mos.
Penile size in cm (age)	5 × 2 (13 yrs.)	6 × 2.5 (19 yrs. 6 mos.)	6.5 × 2.5 (5 yrs. 6 mos.)	2.5 × 3 (3 days)	3 × 1.5 (19 days)	3.5 × 1.4 (8 weeks)	2 × 1.2 (11 mos.)
Prosthetic testes	Yes	No	No	No	No	No	No
Salt-losing syndrome	No	Yes	Not proved	Yes	Yes	Yes	Yes
Family history of ambiguous genitalia	No	Yes[a]	No	Yes[b]	No	Yes[c]	No
Age at beginning of puberty	2 yrs. 6 mos.	11 yrs. 6 mos.	3 yrs. 6 mos.	Prepubertal	10 yrs.	11 yrs.	11 yrs.
Height in cm (age)	152 (18 yrs. 2 mos.)	160 (24 yrs. 3 mos.)	152 (26 yrs. 6 mos.)	96.2 (3 yrs. 9 mos.)	135.8 (10 yrs. 7 mos.)	133.8 (11 yrs. 7 mos.)	140 (12 yrs. 1 mo.)
Weight in kg (age)	58 (16 yrs.)	62 (24 yrs. 3 mos.)	78 (26 yrs. 6 mos.)	13.5 (3 yrs. 9 mos.)	38.2 (10 yrs. 5 mos.)	40.1 (11 yrs. 7 mos.)	91 (12 yrs. 1 mo.)

[a] Sibling with abnormal penis died at 3 weeks. [b] Sibling with ambiguous genitalia died at 1 week. [c] Two siblings with ambiguous genitalia died at 11 and 30 days.

Rehearsal of Sex-Coded Roles in Play Habits and Domestic Activities

For little girls, rehearsal of parental and domestic roles in play habits and child caretaking is a socially accepted and recommended stereotype, at least in our society. A little girl traditionally rehearses her future motherhood by playing the mother with her dolls, and her future as housewife by helping her mother with the domestic activities. On the other side of the spectrum, a similar and even stronger stereotype forbids the little boy to play with dolls and to show any interest in domestic work and infant caretaking.

The four girls did not follow exactly the stereotypic pattern. They played with dolls only rarely. They preferred traditional boys' toys such as cars, trucks, guns, and blocks. They liked to ride bikes or motorbikes. I.I.'s favorite hobby was to build models of cars. In the game of house, A.O. and U.T. rehearsed the role of mother. O.O. preferred the role of the father: She said she was going to work on her motorbike; and when she came back, her friend who played the role of the mother was supposed to have the supper ready for her. She also played the role of the doctor: She had a physician's kit and gave shots to her dolls who were supposed to be sick. When she was 5 years old, her mother observed her pretending she was pregnant: "She put a whole bunch of clothes underneath her dress and said, 'I am pregnant; I will soon have my baby.'"

The three boys followed more closely the socially stereotyped male pattern. None of them was interested in doll play. So far as a retrospective study can tell, their boyish play habits were unremarkable. When old enough, at age 12, E.U. liked to ride his motorbike with a friend in the desert near his home, to build models of funny cars, and to hunt and fish with his father. As a teenager he raised steers for financial gain as part of a school farm project. O.I. liked to ride his bike and to play Tarzan and cowboys. All three were interested in playing ball games with other boys.

The seven patients had in common their lack of interest in infant caretaking. When asked by their mothers to help with the housework, the three boys did so reluctantly. They preferred to play outside with their friends. When he was 13 years old, E.U. said, "I have to empty the trash, sweep the carpet, wash the truck and the car. I don't specially appreciate it." Every once in a while, O.A. and O.I. helped their mothers with the cooking. When he was 8, O.I. explained to us in a very proud way that he knew better than his father how to cook and that he had to teach him: "I can cook nearly about everything. My daddy can't even cook soup."

Two of the girls, U.T. and O.O., complained a lot about working in the house, but they did it for the reward of being allowed to play outdoor games. A.O. did not engage in any domestic work. I.I. cleaned her room and made her bed, but she did not help her mother with the housework, and did not cook.

Romantic Interests in Boyfriends/Girlfriends

As reported by his mother, E.U. had his first date when he was around 12. The couple used to dance together at school dances, and to hold hands. At one time, he wanted to kiss the girl, but she held back. At the age of 13, when queried about what it means to have a girl friend, he replied, "Well, it means that you like each other; you just don't care about anybody else. . . . Friendship, that's just when you see them every so often, but you never call them or anything. Whenever you're a little bit more than friendship, you like her a little bit more, and you call her, and this kind of stuff. And you spend money on her, and your wallet gets a little lighter than it usually is." At the time of the last psychological report, he had had four different girlfriends. He dated the last one for more than 1 year and was expecting to marry her.

Before he married his wife, O.A. had four or five different girlfriends, the first one when he was around 13 years old, with whom he engaged in kissing and petting.

O.I. reported having his first girlfriend when he was about 8. He engaged in petting and kissing with her when he was 9. More than 17 years later, he was able to recall her and to describe her physically. He claimed having had 19 different girlfriends before he met his future wife.

The four girls were too young to make appropriate statements on their romantic interest in boyfriends. One can infer from older patients with the diagnosis of adrenal hyperplasia but with a lesser degree of genital masculinization at birth that they will be "late bloomers" with respect to romantic interest in boys, and that the threshold barrier to erotic awakening will be rather high.

When she was 10 years old, U.T. doubted that she would go out with a boyfriend, if she were old enough, and if her parents gave permission, adding: "I have more important things I would like to do, like playing basketball." When she was 10 years old, O.O. declared that she knew that some of her friends went to boys' houses and they talked about which boy they liked best, but she was not interested in doing that. I.I. did not have any boyfriend, and her only interest in boys was to compete with them and to comment on how good or bad they were in the ball games.

Physical Energy, Tomboyism, and Cosmetic Interests

In early childhood, the three boys showed intense athletic interests, including outdoor preference, participation in rough sports, and competitiveness with other boys. These activities were not associated with fighting and aggression, which were conspicuous by their absence. Athleticism was commensurate with physique age rather than with chronological age. In early adulthood, O.A. was the only one who still engaged in regular sports. The two others, by reason of their short stature in adulthood, secondary to premature bone maturation prior to effective cortisone regulation, were somewhat restricted in their interests in competitive sports and outdoor activities.

The four girls followed the behavioral pattern of other girls with the adreno-genital syndrome, often referred to as tomboyism (Ehrhardt, Epstein, & Money, 1968). Their tomboyism included a profile of high energy expenditure in rough outdoor play. They showed a preference for boys over girls in peer contact, and they liked competitiveness with boys. U.T. explained, when she was 9 years old: "I'd better be good [at sports], because I substitute for a boy in the football game. I was not afraid of the ball, and he was. I was the only girl. . . . Two other girls are better than me in soccer, but I am the best at baseball." The mother of O.O. commented: "O. has a lot of initiative and determination." Later she added: "She is more out to have a lot of fun. I think she is a tomboy." This tomboyism was considered by the parents of the girls as a socially acceptable pattern. None of them tried to discourage it, and there was no excess of parental pressure toward more stereotypic femininity. The girls enjoyed being tomboyish in play, and were not rejected by their peers. This tomboyism did not include hyperactiv-ity nor aggressiveness. It was not accompanied by an overt desire to be a boy.

In keeping with their energetic outdoor recreation, the girls preferred to wear utilitarian and functional clothes, like slacks, overalls, and shirts rather than decorative dresses. They wore dresses on special occasions such as for going to church or coming to the hospital. The same trend carried over to accessories such as jewelry and hairstyling.

The clothing habits of the boys were unremarkable for a boy.

Reaction to Physical Handicaps

The four girls and one of the boys presented a severe salt-losing tendency. Consequently, the diagnosis of hyperadrenocortical hermaphroditism was recog-nized, and replacement therapy was initiated early in life. Under well-regulated hormonal therapy, the prognosis for physical development is variable, but within the normal range.

The girls can anticipate fertility. The three men knew of their inability to induce a pregnancy. One man and his wife decided to have children and, at the time of the last psychological report, had started a pregnancy by donor in-semination.

In childhood, two of the men did not benefit from early cortisone therapy, as the diagnosis of adrenal hyperplasia was not recognized until they developed precocious signs of male puberty. When the parents noticed the first signs of precocious development, they did not expect abnormal sexual behavior. Mrs. I. explained her attitude toward the precocious appearance of pubic hair: "When he got about 3½ years old, I noticed one day when I was bathing him, it seemed like he had a little straggly black hair and I kept trying to wash it off; and it would not come off. . . . His father is just a bear of hair; he has got it all over his body, on his back, shoulders, and everything. Well, I thought maybe the child might have inherited all that hair. I just thought maybe he was going to be like his father. I did not know nothing much about boys."

Because a faulty plan of case management was decided upon by an insufficiently informed physician, E.U. developed breasts when he was around 11 years old, in anticipation of menarche. This mortified him, and he tried to hide it from his friends and family. At the age of 13, he commented: "It started 2 years ago. . . . It was embarrassing. I kept quiet. You are just always scared that somebody will find out about it and they may start kidding you. I thought I would just have to live life like that. . . . One month ago, my mother told me about plastic surgery, that it could be removed. . . . I was overjoyed. I really could not wait until I could get here." His local doctor had told him he was a female, and should change to live as a girl, but he wanted no part of it. Mrs. U. had no doubt about her son's masculinity. When E. was 13, she said: "He has a sister, and they are just completely different. He does not think like a girl. He does not have the same interests, and right now the thing that I think made me very sure of it is that he has a girlfriend; and that to me was a relief—when he did—because that was just the clincher, that he was not a girl. So I just think he is a boy."

The three boys were told that their sex glands had to be removed because they could not get down in the scrotum. This explanation made the monthly testosterone injection more acceptable. The lack of testes, as well as their inability to induce a pregnancy, did not create any evident behavioral problem. O.I. and O.A. knew the possibility of having artificial testes implanted, but were not interested in it. E.U. was satisfied with his artificial testes.

Though their adult height was only 5 feet (152 cm), E.U. and O.I. did not overtly complain about it. O.I. commented on it by saying: "I am short, I am fat, but I have no complex."

Sexual Practices and Fantasies

According to what the mothers were able to disclose, and according to direct inquiry, none of the seven patients reported socially unacceptable childhood investigative sexual curiosity and play. There was no extreme shyness about appearing naked either in front of members of the family or during a physical examination.

The four girls were too young at the time of the last psychological report to give relevant information on this topic.

The three patients reared as boys, being adult at the time of the last psychological report, provided detailed information pertaining to their sex lives (Table II). All three began their sex lives before marriage, and found sexual intercourse pleasurable. Neither of the two married men reported extramarital sex. None of the three had difficulty in getting and maintaining an erection. E.U. appeared a little dissatisfied with his sex life and complained, at a time when receiving insufficient androgen, about his penis not getting hard enough to go deep enough. The other two, as well as their wives, were perfectly satisfied with their sexual function. All three reported orgasm by masturbating and by vaginal intercourse. They all ejaculate a small amount of a watery liquid, presumably of prostatic origin. They could not have a repeat orgasm over a short period of time in the manner typical of a woman. O.I. claimed, besides having pleasurable vaginal intercourse two to three times a week, that he masturbated two to three times a day. None of them reported any erotic behavior or fantasies toward men.

TABLE II

Sexual Function of the Three Males

	E.U.	O.A.	O.I.
Age at first masturbation	No information	13 yrs.	9 yrs.
Age at first vaginal intercourse	16 years	19 yrs.	20 yrs.
Premarital sex including vaginal intercourse	Yes	Yes	Yes
Frequency of intercourse	Once a week	3 times a week	2-3 times a week
Erotic stimuli	Visual	Touch	Visual
Erotic zones	No information	Genitalia	Genitalia
Attitude toward oral sex	No information	No experience	Pleased with it
Self-rating of satisfaction with sex life	Slightly dissatisfied	Very pleased	Very pleased

Social Mixing with Peers and Siblings

All seven patients were able to mix with and be accepted without difficulty by their age-mates either at school or in the neighborhood or in their family. The four girls were more engaged in social mixing related to competitive rough play and sports than in a long-term relationship with one single friend.

School Achievement and Career

The three boys finished their schooling around the age of 18. None of them went to college. E.U. obtained average grades in high school. From the age of 18, he worked with his father who owned a farm-supply business. Because of bad grades, O.A. dropped out of eighth grade at school when he was 17, worked as a cook for 4 years, and is presently working in construction with his father. O.I. dropped out of school around the age of 17 and is presently employed in a factory doing manual work.

At the time of the last report, A.O. was too young to go to school. U.T. obtained good results in the fifth grade and expected to be either a nurse or a veterinarian. O.O. was in the sixth grade. She was doing very well academically, and she expected to be either a doctor or an artist. I.I. had average academic achievement in the sixth grade. Her career expectancy was to be a car racer.

Discussion

Seven seem too few cases on which to report a basic psychological finding. But seven patients who are chromosomal and gonadal females with complete masculinization of the external genitalia are a large sample. Weldon, Blizzard, and Migeon (1966) reported an endocrine study of five adrenogenital patients with penile urethra and reviewed the relevant literature. O.I., U.T., O.O., and I.I. of this present paper were included in their report also. O.I.'s medical history has been reported by Jones and Scott (1971). Reference to the cases of O.I. and O.O. may be found also in Money (1970) and in Money and Ehrhardt (1972).

The three patients living as men are instructive for the theory of homosexuality, even though they are not by any means homosexual in the everyday meaning of the term. When each is with a partner sexually, it is a man with a penis who is copulating with a woman with a vulva. The man has a masculinized body form, and a masculine personality, so that other men recognize him as one of themselves, and other women respond to him unhesitatingly as a man. Hormonally he functions as a male, and did so also in the formative period of fetal life. Nonetheless, the gonadal sex at birth and the chromosomal sex (46,XX) are both female.

Thus, a formula for creating the perfect female homosexual—homosexual on the criteria of chromosomal and gonadal sex—is to take a chromosomal and gonadal female fetus and to flood the system with a masculinizing hormone during the critical period when the external genitals and sexual pathways in the brain are being differentiated. Then assign the baby as a boy at birth and rear him unambiguously as a boy, making sure that hormonal puberty, at the appropriate age, is masculinizing.

If this formula is interrupted at birth, as is the case of the four girls above, so that the baby is assigned and reared as a girl, surgically corrected as a girl, and hormonally regulated so as to have a feminizing puberty, then there is an increased, though not invariable, chance that she will have bisexual erotic imagery and/or experience. This statement is made on the basis of still unpublished data on a series of cases of the female adrenogenital syndrome in which the clitoral organ at birth was enlarged so as to resemble a penis, but one without a covered urethral tube. This bisexual girl, like nonbisexual girls with the same syndrome, has a childhood history of tomboyism and an adolescent history of being late to reach the romantic age of dating and boyfriends. She is capable of becoming pregnant and delivering a normal baby.

On the basis of the foregoing considerations, it is hypothetically reasonable to propose a prenatal hormonally induced component, in the central nervous system, of a bisexual or homosexual gender-identity/role in anatomically nonhermaphroditic individuals. This component does not automatically assert itself, however, but is dependent for its expression on one or more additional components from the postnatal phase of gender-identity/role differentiation. This postnatal component is almost certainly social. There is clear-cut evidence that it is not hormonal, even at the age of puberty, some dissenting reports notwithstanding.

It is technically a challenge to obtain data pertaining to a prenatal hormonal component of a bisexual or homosexual differentiation of gender-identity/role. One possible lead is to be found in a report by Doerner, Rohde, Stahl, Krell, and Masius (1975) who found that when homosexual males were tested with a dose of estrogen, the female hormone, their pituitary glands released luteinizing hormone in a manner that was more similar to control females than to control males.

The present report raises a pragmatic question as to whether, in the future, chromosomal females born with a penis should be assigned and reared as boys or girls. The issue is one of competing values, namely, preserving fertility, as a female, versus a smoother path through adolescence to adult psychosexual maturity and function as a male. The medical profession is divided. We are inclined to favor the masculine alternative as being the one beset with fewer difficulties, overall.

References

Doerner, G., Rohde, W., Stahl, F., Krell, L., & Masius, W.-G. A neuroendocrine predisposition for homosexuality in men. *Archives of Sexual Behavior,* 1975, 4, 1-8.

Ehrhardt, A. A., Epstein, R., & Money, J. Fetal androgens and female gender identity in the early-treated adrenogenital syndrome. *Johns Hopkins Medical Journal,* 1968, 122, 160-167.

Jones, H. W., Jr., & Scott, W. W. *Genital Anomalies and Related Endocrine Disorders* (2nd ed.). Baltimore: Williams & Wilkins, 1971.

Money, J. Matched pairs of hermaphrodites: Behavioral biology of sexual differentiation from chromosomes to gender identity. *Engineering and Science* (California Institute of Technology), 1970, 33, 34-39.

Money, J., & Ehrhardt, A. A. *Man and Woman, Boy and Girl: The Differentiation and Dimorphism of Gender Identity from Conception to Maturity.* Baltimore: Johns Hopkins University Press, 1972.

Prader, A. Der Genital befund beim Pseudohermaphroditismus feminimus des kongenitalen androgenitalen Syndroms. *Helvetica Paediatrica Acta,* 1954, 9, 231-248.

Qazi, Q. H., & Thompson, M. W. Genital changes in congenital virilizing adrenal hyperplasia. *Journal of Pediatrics,* 1972, 80, 653-654.

Verkauf, B. S., & Jones, H. W. Masculinization of the female genitalia in congenital adrenal hyperpalsia: Relationship to the salt losing variety of the disease. *Southern Medical Journal,* 1970, 63, 634-638.

Weldon, V. V., Blizzard, R. M., & Migeon, C. J. Newborn girls misdiagnosed as bilaterally cryptorchid males. *New England Journal of Medicine,* 1966, 274, 829-833.

Note

Originally published in *Journal of Homosexuality,* 1:357-371, 1976, with J. Daléry as coauthor. [Bibliog. #2.198]

TWENTY-THREE

Adult Erotosexual Status and Fetal Hormonal Masculinization and Demasculinization: 46,XX Congenital Virilizing Adrenal Hyperplasia and 46,XY Androgen-Insensitivity Syndrome Compared

Abstract

Among 30 young women with a history of the treated adrenogenital syndrome (CVAH), 11 (37%) rated themselves as bisexual or homosexual. Among a control group consisting of 15 women with the 46,XY androgen-insensitivity syndrome (AIS) plus 12 with the Rokitansky syndrome (MRKS), the corresponding figure was 2 (7%), both bisexual. Chi-square was significant beyond the 0.01 level. In Kinsey's 1953 sample 15% of women experienced homoerotic arousal imagery by age 20, and 10% had had homoerotic partner contact. The most likely hypothesis to explain the CVAH findings is that of a prenatal and/or neonatal masculinizing effect on sexual dimorphism of the brain in interaction with other developmental variables.

Introduction

In the human species, naturally occurring clinical syndromes must be relied upon to generate data that, in other species, can be more systematically generated in contrived experiments. For this reason, the congenital syndromes of intersexuality (hermaphroditism) are a prime source of information regarding the possible effects of fetal hormonal status on erotosexual status in young adulthood.

This paper has as its purpose the comparison of two syndromes in order to ascertain the likelihood of a prenatal hormonal effect on subsequent erotosexual status. One is the syndrome of congenital virilizing adrenal hyperplasia (CVAH) in the 46,XX fetus. The other is the complete androgen-insensitivity syndrome (AIS) in the 46,XY fetus.

On many of the variables of sex, the two syndromes are the antithesis of each other (Table 1). For present purposes, the most important of the antithetical variables is fetal hormonal sex, which in the CVAH fetus is masculinizing and in the AIS fetus is feminizing. (For details of the etiology, diagnosis, prognosis and treatment of both syndromes, see Gardner, 1975; Gold & Josimovich, 1980.)

280

Nature of the Syndromes

In the CVAH syndrome, fetal androgenization originates in a genetically recessive defect that interrupts the natural synthesis of cortisol, the hormone normally secreted by the adrenal cortices. In its place, an androgenic precursor hormone, androstenedione, is secreted instead. Androstenedione is metabolized into testosterone in the liver and elsewhere, some of which in turn is metabolized into dihydrotestosterone in target cells. Testosterone and dihydrotestosterone are the active hormones of masculinization. In the 46,XX CVAH fetus, the most extreme degree of masculinization of the external genitals results in a fully formed penis and empty scrotum (see Migeon, 1979, for details of the etiology, diagnosis and treatment of CVAH). In the less extreme degree, which is more common, there is clitoromegaly that resembles penile hypospadias, with a bifid labioscrotum and urogenital sinus. If the diagnosis is not established neonatally, the baby may be assigned and reared as a boy (Money & Daléry, 1976). In the absence of hormonal intervention, virilizing development, simulating normal hormonal puberty, will be early in onset and rapidly progressive. If the birth-defective genitalia, and in some instances an associated symptom of salt loss, do lead to a neonatal diagnosis, then the prevalent decision is to assign and rear the child as a girl. Corrective genital surgery is performed early in life. Long-term endocrine therapy with cortisol arrests any further virilizing from the adrenocortical error, normalizes growth, and allows puberty to be morphologically feminizing.

In the androgen-insensitivity syndrome (AIS), fetal deandrogenization originates in a genetic error which prevents either the binding or utilization of androgen within the nucleus of cells. The error is transmitted in the maternal pedigree, most likely as an X-linked recessive. Cellular insensitivity to androgen permits the 46,XY fetus not to masculinize. The external genitalia differentiate as those of Eve instead of Adam. The vagina is a shallow dimple or blind pouch, and there is no cervix or uterus, as the embryonic müllerian structures vestigiate under the influence of müllerian inhibiting hormone. At the time of puberty, the body morphology develops as feminine in response to testicular estrogen and rejection of androgen. Vaginal lengthening can be accomplished by dilation, failing which surgery may be resorted to.

The 46,XY androgen-insensitivity syndrome has a 46,XX counterpart in the Mayer-Rokitansky-Küster Syndrome (MRKS; Griffin *et al.*, 1976), which is characterized by congenital atresia of the vagina and vestigial müllerian structures (Table I). For the most part, MRKS occurs sporadically, without associated embryological anomalies, and without a known genetic anomaly. The relevance of this syndrome to the present report is that affected individuals cannot be distinguished behaviorally and erotosexually from those with AIS (Lewis & Money, 1983). Thus a pooled sample representing both syndromes may be used to augment the smaller size of a control group composed of AIS alone.

TABLE I

Variables of Sex in Three Syndromes

	CVAH*	AIS*	MRKS*
H-Y antigen	no	yes	no
Chromosomal sex	46,XX	46,XY	46,XX
Gonadal sex	ovarian	testicular	ovarian
Internal sex	müllerian	wolffian	müllerian
External genitalia	masculinized	feminized	feminized
Fetal hormonal sex	masculinizing	feminizing	feminizing
Pubertal hormonal			
sex (untreated)	masculinizing	feminizing	feminizing
Pubertal physique			
untreated	masculinized	feminized	feminized
treated	feminized	feminized	feminized
Gonadotropin secretion			
untreated	noncyclic	noncyclic	cyclic
treated	cyclic	noncyclic	cyclic
Menarche			
untreated	no	no	no
treated	yes	no	no

*CVAH, Congenital virlizing adrenal hyperplasia; AIS, androgen-insensitivity syndrome; MRKS, Mayer-Rokitansky-Küster syndrome.

Sample and Method

The group of 30 CVAH patients qualified for inclusion in the present study because they met the criteria of being over 17 years of age, of having been followed in the Johns Hopkins Psychohormonal Research Unit, and of having received postnatal cortisol therapy (available since 1950) beginning early enough to ensure that the virilization which had begun prenatally was prevented from escalating in childhood. Ten other patients who met these same criteria proved to have been lost to follow-up, and one other was excluded because of an additional diagnostic complication of petit mal epilepsy.

All 30 of the CVAH patients were born with clitoromegaly without urethral closure to form a penile meatus, and without complete labioscrotal fusion. Surgical reduction of the clitoris was performed neonatally or up to the third year in 21 cases, between ages four and six years in eight cases, and at age 9 in one mild case. The age of diagnosis and onset of hormonal therapy were neonatal (birth to two months) in 18 cases; between two and nine months in five cases; between one and two years in five cases; and one case each at age five and nine years (the mild case), respectively.

The control-comparison group consisted of 15 AIS patients augmented with 12 MRKS patients. These 27 patients met the criteria of being sixteen years of age (one patient) or older, of having been followed in the Psycho-hormonal Research Unit, of having amenorrhea, of having a history of some degree of vaginal atresia, and of having no associated congenital malformation except of the müllerian organs. Only one AIS patient who qualified for inclusion in the study elected not to participate, saying it was against her beliefs, and none was lost to follow-up. Three MRKS patients were lost to follow-up, and 12 were not.

Eleven of the 15 AIS women had undergone elective gonadectomy as a prophylaxis against possible future malignancy; they were maintained on cyclical estrogen replacement therapy. Twelve AIS and 11 MRKS women had had surgical vaginoplasty in their middle-to-late teenage years to lengthen the vagina. The others used the more recently revived nonsurgical method of dilation.

There are no epidemiological statistics on the frequency and prevalence of CVAH, AIS, and MRKS in the general population, and no data on factors that might have selectively influenced the number of affected patients seen at Johns Hopkins. Once registered as patients, however, their referral to the Psycho-hormonal Research Unit was on the basis of their diagnosis only. Thus there was no artifact of sampling that might bias the findings on gender-identity and erotosexual status. Therefore, such differences as do appear between the CVAH findings and those of the AIS/MRKS controls may be expected to be syndrome-related and not artifacts (see Schwartz, 1977, for additional information regarding the composition of the sample in all three clinical syndromes).

For each patient followed in this study the consolidated, longitudinal endo-crine/psychoendocrine history was updated with the transcript of a taped interview based on a schedule of inquiry especially designed to provide data on, *inter alia,* adolescent and young-adult erotosexual imagery and experience. The interview was conducted according to the principle of open-endedness first, with forced-choice subsequently. It was done either in person or, by appointment, *via* long-distance telephone. The history then was conceptually indexed and the data abstracted and tabulated into a master chart for statistical comparisons. In case of uncertainty regarding the numerical coding of data (on a two- or three-point scale) a consensus of a jury of two or more was required. This method relied on the pooled experience of trained investigators in applying rating criteria to data that, by reason of their clinical content and the patient's ethical right to know about her syndrome and to talk about it, could not be censored, and could not be presumed to be experimentally blind. Formal reliabiity testing would have required two juries, which was not possible. Jury policy was that, in case of doubt, a rating would disfavor rather than favor a proposition for which confirmation was being sought.

Results

Table II is constructed on the basis of each patient's personal self-evaluation of her erotosexual status on the spectrum of heterosexual/bisexual/homosexual. The basis of self-evaluation is two-fold: erotosexual arousal imagery in spontaneous fantasy, dream, or apperception; and erotic experience alone or with a participating partner. Patients who had experience also had imagery, whereas in a few cases imagery had not yet been expressed in practice.

TABLE II

46,XX Adrenogenital Syndrome (CVAH) Female Rearing:
Present Self-Rating on Erotosexual Status (Imagery ± Activity)

Rating	CVAH (n = 30)	Controls (n = 27)*
Noncommittal	7(23%)	0(0%)
Heterosexual only	12(40%)	25(93%)
Bisexual	6(20%)	2(7%)
Homosexual only or predominantly	5(17%)	0(0%)

chi square = 18.5; $p < 0.001$†

*Androgen-insensitivity syndrome (n = 15) + Rokitansky syndrome (n = 12).
†Omitting the noncommittal line so that n (CVAH) = 23, and n (Control) = 27 and combining bisexual and homosexual ratings then chi-square = 10.5; $p < 0.01$.

Table III confirms the findings of Table II, differing only in that the ratings were made by the investigators on the basis of information of a patient's actual history of erotosexual imagery and practice. The difference between the two tables is that the five CVAH patients who rated themselves as totally or predominantly homosexual were rated by the investigators as bisexual to some degree, on the basis of their actual histories of experience and imagery.

TABLE III

46,XX Adrenogenital Syndrome (CVAH) Female Rearing:
History on Erotosexual Status (Imagery ± Activity)

Status	CVAH (n = 30)	Controls (n = 27)*
Noncommittal	7(23%)	0(0%)
Heterosexual only	12(40%)	25(93%)
Bisexual	11(37%)	2(7%)

chi square = 17.7; $p < 0.001$†

*Androgen-insensitivity syndrome (n = 15) + Rokitansky syndrome (n = 12).
†Omitting the noncommittal line so that n (CVAH) = 23, and n (Control) = 27, then chi-square = 10.5; $p < 0.01$.

All 12 of the CVAH patients who were rated as only heterosexual and one of those rated as bisexual (Tables II and III) had experienced actual sexual intercourse. The corresponding incidence of sexual intercourse in the control group was 18 of the 25 rated as heterosexual and one of the two rated as bisexual.

Among the CVAH patients, five of the 11 homosexual/bisexual subgroup had experienced nongenital, romantic eroticism with a same-sexed partner, and four of these five had also experienced genital eroticism with a same-sexed partner. The corresponding incidence in the control group was one of two; the diagnosis of each of these two was AIS. They were predominantly heterosexual and only trivially involved in bisexualism.

The chi-square values of the comparisons in both Tables II and III are significant beyond the 0.01 level, thus leaving no doubt that the CVAH and the control group are, indeed, erotosexually different.

In both groups, the incidence of homosexual status with or without a bisexual component may be compared (Table IV) with the sample of Kinsey *et al.* (1953). In the Kinsey sample, the incidence of homoerotic arousal imagery in females by age 20 was 15%. In the present study, the corresponding percentages are CVAH, 37% and control group, 7%. In the Kinsey sample, the incidence of homoerotic partner contact in females by age 20 was 10%, whereas the patient study figures are CVAH, 17% and control group, 4%.

TABLE IV

Comparison of Homoerotic Incidence
in CVAH, AIS/MRKS, and Kinsey's Sample

	CVAH $n = 30$	CVAH $n = 23^*$	AIS/MRKS $n = 27$	Kinsey's sample
Homoerotic arousal imagery by age 20	37%	48%	7%	15%
Homoerotic partner contact by age 20	17%	22%	4%	10%

*Omitting seven noncommittal subjects.

In the control group, there was no homoerotic pairbonding with or without bodily contact. By contrast, in the corresponding five (17%) CVAH patients, there was homoerotic romantic pairbonding in the same-sexed relationship of the four who had homoerotic body contact and in the one who did not. This CVAH percentage increases from 17 to 22% if it is calculated with $n = 23$ (Table IV), omitting the seven CVAH patients who were erotosexually noncommittal and too inhibited to talk freely (Tables II and III). Correspondingly, the percentage of CVAH homoerotic imagery increases from 37 to 48%.

Discussion: Theoretical Formulations

The foregoing findings, provided they can be independently confirmed, indicate that individuals with the syndrome of 46,XX congenital virilizing adrenal hyperplasia (CVAH, also known as the adrenogenital syndrome) who are reared and habilitated as girls and women may differentiate an erotosexual status that is heterosexual, bisexual, or homosexual. The likelihood of a homosexual status, with or without a bisexual component, is increased relative to its frequency both in a normative control sample (Kinsey *et al.*, 1953) and in a clinical control sample which is a composite of two syndromes, the 46,XY androden-insensitivity syndrome (AIS) and the 46,XX Mayer-Rokitansky-Küster syndrome (MRKS).

One particular relevancy of AIS is that it occurs in a 46,XY fetus and represents a complete degree of fetal deandrogenization. The low incidence of a homosexual status in AIS women supports the hypothesis that the sex chromosomes *per se* do not directly contribute to the subsequent differentiation of a homosexual status, whereas fetal hormonal deandrogenization and morphological demasculinization may, indeed, do so. In addition to a history of prenatal deandrogenization, AIS women have a lifetime history of hormonal deandrogenization, which includes spontaneous feminization of the body morphology at puberty. Because of the normally female appearance of the vulva, they have a history of having been assigned and reared as girls from birth onward, and of having grown up as girls with a gender-identity/role (G-I/R) that is feminine in all of its components, not only the erotosexual one (Lewis & Money, 1983). The feminizing erotosexual sequelae of fetal deandrogenization in the AIS individual support the parallel hypothesis that fetal androgenization in the 46,XX CVAH individual has masculinizing erotosexual sequelae, in addition to the masculinization of body morphology that is subject to surgical and hormonal correction.

In experimental animal hermaphroditism, it has been well-established in some species that prenatal hormonalization programs sexual dimorphism in brain differentiation, which in turn programs the sexual behavioral dimorphism of mating behavior in adult life. The sheep, for example, is a veritable hormonal robot, as is dramatically shown in a film (undated) by Short and Clarke (Clarke, 1977). In their experiments, a daughter fetus was exposed to testosterone in intrauterine life. The timing and dosage were calculated so as to have an effect only on the brain, not on the genitalia. Thus, though such an animal appeared to be a ewe and secreted ovarian hormones, at the first mating season its mating behavior replicated that of a ram. It competed with other rams, and they did not respond to it as a ewe.

In human beings, and probably in primate species in general, there is no such prenatal hormonal "robotization". However, the present CVAH findings support the hypothesis of a masculinizing prenatal hormonal threshold effect (Money, 1981), which will interact variably with other subsequent factors that contribute to erotosexual differentiation on the heterosexual/bisexual/homosexual continuum.

This hypothesis is well illustrated in the 46,XX CVAH cases, in which the baby is born with a fully formed penis and empty scrotum, with a uterus and two ovaries internally. The hormone that masculinizes the external genitalia also has a prenatal influence on sexual dimorphism of the brain. If the baby is assigned as a boy (Money & Daléry, 1976) and the diagnosis is not suspected, the continuing elevated level of prenatal androgen of adrenocortical origin continues in postnatal life. Quantitatively, it mimics the surge of androgen from the testes, measurable in the blood-stream of male but not female babies, during the first three months of life (Migeon & Forest, 1983). The relationship of this surge to sexual brain dimorphism, though not known, is suspected by David Abramovich (personal communication) on the basis of his fetal and neonatal brain/ hormone studies to be masculinizing (Baum, 1979; Baum *et al.*, 1982; Nordeen & Yahr, 1982; Ward, 1977). Thus, the 46,XX CVAH baby with a penis who is assigned and reared as a boy is equipped for boyhood with masculinized brain thresholds. Even if later endocrine intervention in prepuberty temporarily permits ovarian hormonal function and morphologic feminization of the body (as happened in one case in the Money & Daléry, 1976, study), the masculine differentiation of overall gender-identity/role and its specific erotosexual component does not change to become feminized. The combination of prenatal and neonatal masculinization, external male genitalia, endocrine pubertal management as a virilized male, and childhood rearing and socialization as a boy completely outweigh the 46,XX chromosomal status and the ovarian gonadal status. The sexual life of such a person in adulthood is that of a man, complicated only by infertility.

In the babyhood of the present CVAH cohort there were 10 cases in which the diagnosis was established and cortisol treatment began within the first week of life. In two other cases,the corresponding date was two months of age, and in the remaining eight cases, it was six months or older. The degree to which deandrogenization was effectively maintained in the period immediately following the onset of treatment was variable. Thus it is likely that some of even the earliest-treated babies had a fluctuating androgen level, periodically elevated, in the earliest months or years of life, as the later-treated babies consistently did. It must be allowed, therefore, that the elevated homosexual/bisexual prevalence in the CVAH group later in life may be associated not only with prenatal but also with postnatal elevations of androgen reaching the brain.

The longer the adrenocortical androgen level remains high in CVAH, either initially or in periods of sufficiently monitored treatment, the greater the chance that the body will become virilized. Bodily virilization may itself negatively influence the feminine status of gender-identity/role and erotosexualism. In the pre-1950 era, prior to the discovery of cortisol therapy, CVAH women became extremely virilized in physique. In 23 such cases studied in the Psychohormonal Research Unit at Johns Hopkins, 30% had a history of homoerotic imagery in dreams and fantasies, and another 18% had homoerotic experiences in addition to imagery (Ehrhardt *et al.*, 1968).

Bodily virilization includes virilization of the genitalia, specifically pubic hair, and enlargement of the phallic clitoris, if it remains intact. This organ may reach its adult size prematurely, be more frequently erected, and more sensuous. If it has been surgically reduced or removed, the vulval area may react to an increased level of circulating androgen by becoming more erotically sensitive, with the capability of orgasm still present. Whether the criterion be erotic feeling or visual appearance, the external genitalia may exert a negative influence on the development of a feminine status of either erotosexualism in particular or of gender-identity/role in general. The longer the genitalia retain an abnormal morphology, the greater the likelihood of this negative effect. Even after corrective surgery, the genital morphology may be less than ideally feminine, so that the more aware a girl becomes of her genital difference, the greater the likelihood of a negative effect. There is so much diversity among CVAH individuals in their histories of genital morphology and genital surgery, and their effects, that it is not possible to generalize further on the basis of the available data.

It is known that, among primates, sexual rehearsal play with age-mates is prerequisite to subsequent sexual ability with breeding partners. Rhesus monkeys deprived of rehearsal play in infancy are unable to copulate and breed in adulthood (Goldfoot, quoted in Money, 1980). A child with a history of birth defect of the sex organs may well have a history of childhood sexual rehearsal play different from age-similar siblings or playmates. The sexual taboo that prohibits and punishes all children's sexual rehearsal play makes ascertainment of information about it sporadic and incomplete. Therefore, the possible effect of either the exercise or deprivation of early sexual rehearsal play on the erotosexual development of 46,XX CVAH children as heterosexual/bisexual/homosexual remains unascertained. By contrast, on the basis of available evidence, it is known that 46,XY CVAH boys who, like 46,XX CVAH girls, are excessively androgenized *in utero,* have virtually a 100% likelihood of growing up to have a heterosexual status, not a bisexual or homosexual one (Money & Alexander, 1969; Money & Lewis, 1982), regardless of variations in childhood social developmental experiences (sexual rehearsal play presumably included).

In childhood development, the first experience of a pairbonded love affair in which the mutual attraction is expressed as explicitly erotic and sexual may occur as early as age eight (Money, 1980, p. 148). More typically, it occurs postpubertally. In the CVAH cases of the present study, it was typical that in childhood the girls were energetic tomboys who fraternized with boys in their sports and vigorous outdoor activities, neglecting the more stereotypic play of girls. In their teenage years, at the age when boys become romantically interested in girls, the CVAH girls became misfits among their erstwhile male playmates (Schwartz, 1977). They did not develop a romantic interest in a boyfriend. This was the age when they became extremely diffident in their approach to matters of sexual learning and erotic development—more so than adolescent patients with other diagnoses. These were apparently unspeakable issues, shameful and embarrassing in a diffuse and inarticulate way and to be evaded at all costs, even if the talk pertained to the possible need of vaginal dilation or minor surgery to ensure vaginal adequacy. It was the persistence of this kind of evasion that explains why, in Tables II and III, there are seven cases listed as noncommittal. In the other 23 cases, advanced age brought increased sophistication and the ability to talk about apprehensions and anxieties regarding copulatory adequacy and pregnancy, or the moral self-condemnation of being erotically attracted to either sex, or the mortification of love unrequited by another woman. There were not any whose erotosexual status led them to define themselves as transvestites, andromimetics (Money, 1980), or transexuals demanding a sex reassignment.

The most likely hypothesis to explain the erotosexual diffidence of CVAH girls in their early teenage years is that they were inchoately aware that something about them was different from other girls of their age. Perhaps it was that they were late in maturing to the romantic age of dating and love affairs, just as they tended to be late in getting their first menses (though not breast development). In some of the girls this awareness may have extended to include an intimation that they would be romantically more interested in a girlfriend than a boyfriend, despite their moral self-disapproval of homosexual relationships. Their moral conflict may have further delayed their erotosexual development. If this hypothesis is correct, then it might be explained on the basis of the hypothesis of a developmentally delayed-action effect of prenatal and/or neonatal masculinization of sexually dimorphic brain thresholds.

The concept of sexually dimorpohic brain thresholds is dramatically illustrated in the mating behavior of parthenogenic whiptail lizards *(Cnemidophorus uniparens)* studied by Crews (1982). This is an egg-laying species that breeds without the union of male and female. There is no sperm-carrying sex in the species. The parthenogenic eggs do not need sperm to make them fertile. Nonetheless, when a parthenogenic whiptail is gravid with eggs, it goes through an as-if mating ritual with another parthenogenic, but nongravid, whiptail. The latter simulates the behavior exhibited by males in closely related two-sexed species and mounts its partner. At a different phase of the reproductive cycle, each parthenogenic lizard may reverse its as-if mating role.

Cnemidophorus uniparens and other parthenogenic species (Moritz, 1983) demonstrate that the two mating programs, stereotypically ascribed to the male and female respectively, are present in the brain of each individual lizard. By turns, each program is able to manifest itself in action, depending externally on the stimulus of the mate and internally on the hormonal phase of the reproductive cycle. The hypothesis that can be borrowed from these lizards and applied to human development is that, as a species, human beings have a basic ambisexualism of the brain and its imagery. However, the hormonal history prenatally, in interaction with the gender history postnatally, usually resolves the ambisexualism into unisexualism. In the case of the CVAH girl, the masculinizing prenatal hormonal history puts a constraint on the resolution of the brain's original ambisexualism into unisexualism. The ambisexual potential persists and facilitates the developmental differentiation of a bisexual gender status that manifests itself in bisexual erotic imagery and/or practice in adulthood.

The bisexual and homosexual phenomena in the CVAH group are defined by the criteria of their chromosomal sex (46,XX), gonadal sex (ovarian), and the sex in which they were hormonally and genitally habilitated and reared (female). If these same criteria are applied to the AIS group, then those who were rated heterosexual on the criterion of external genitalia and rearing (female), would be homosexual on the criteria of chromosomal sex (46,XY) and gonadal sex (testicular). An analogous paradox applies in 46,XX CVAH cases born with two ovaries and a penis and habilitated and reared as males. When they pairbond with a 46,XX woman, the two partners are female on the criteria of chromosomal and gonadal sex, but not on the criteria of external genitalia and rearing.

The cases presented in this report raise a profound and fundamental question as to the very definition of the concepts of heterosexuality, bisexuality and homosexuality. The most expeditious answer is that heterosexual/bisexual/homosexual status should be defined in terms of the genital morphology of oneself and the partner with whom one falls in love and becomes erotically pairbonded. Genital contact *per se* can be too casual, transient, or perfunctory to provide a satisfactory definition.

References

Baum, M. J. (1979) Differentiation of coital behavior in mammals: a comparative analysis. *Neurosci. Biobehav. Rev.* 3, 265-284.

Baum, M. J., Gallagher, C. A., Martin, J. T. & Damassa, D. A. (1982) Effects of testosterone, dihydrotestosterone, or estradiol administered neonatally on sexual behavior of female ferrets. *Endocrinology* 111, 773-780.

Clarke, I. J. (1977) The sexual behavior of prenatally androgenized ewes observed in the field. *J. Reprod. Fert.* 49, 311-315.

Crews, D. (1982) On the origin of sexual behavior. *Psychoneuroendocrinology* 7, 259-270.

Ehrhardt, A. A., Evers, K. & Money, J. (1968) Influence of androgen and some aspects of sexually dimorphic behavior in women with the late-treated adrenogenital syndrome. *Johns Hopkins Med. J.* 123, 115-122.

Gardner, L. I. (ed.) (1975) *Endocrine and Genetic Disorders of Childhood and Adolescence*, 2nd edn. W. B. Saunders, Philadelphia.

Gold, J. J. & Josimovich, J. B. (eds.) (1980) *Gynecologic Endocrinology*, 3rd edn. Harper & Row. Hagerstown.

Griffin, J. E., Edwards, C., Madden, J. D., Harrod, M. J. and Wilson, J. D. (1976) Congenital absence of the vagina: The Mayer-Rokitansky-Küster-Hauser syndrome. *Ann. int. Med.* 85, 224-236.

Kinsey, A. C., Pomeroy, W. B., Martin, C. E. & Gebhard, P. H. (1953) *Sexual Behavior in the Human Female*. W. B. Saunders, Philadelphia.

Lewis, V. G. & Money, J. (1983) Gender-identity/role: G-I/R Part A: XY (androgen-insensitivity) syndrome and XX (Rokitansky) syndrome of vaginal atresia compared. In *Handbook of Psychosomatic Obstetrics and Gynaecology*, L. Dennerstein and G. Burrows (eds.), pp. 51-60. Elsevier Biomedical Press, Amsterdam.

Migeon, C. J. (1979) Diagnosis and treatment of adrenogenital disorders. In *Endocrinology*, Vol. 2, L. J. DeGroot, G. F. Cahill, Jr., L. Martini, D. H. Nelson, W. D. Odell, J. T. Potts, Jr., E. Steinberger and A. I. Winegrad (eds.) pp. 1203-1224. Grune & Stratton, New York.

Migeon, C. J. & Forest, M. G. (1980) Androgens in biological fluids. In *Nuclear Medicine in Vitro*, 2nd ed., B. Rothfeld (ed.), pp. 145-170. J. B. Lippincott, Philadelphia.

Money, J. (1980) *Love and Love Sickness: The Science of Sex, Gender Difference, and Pairbonding*. Johns Hopkins University Press, Baltimore.

Money, J. (1981) The development of sexuality and eroticism in humankind. *Quart. Rev. Biol.* 56, 379-404.

Money, J. & Alexander, D. (1969) Psychosexual development and absence of homosexuality in males with precocious puberty: review of 19 cases. *J. Nerv. Ment. Dis.* 148, 111-123.

Money, J. & Daléry, J. (1976) Iatrogenic homosexuality: Gender identity in seven 46,XX chromosomal females with hyperadrenocortical hermaphroditism born with a penis, three reared as boys, four reared as girls. *J. Homosexuality* 1, 357-371.

Money, J. and Lewis, V. (1982) Homosexual/heterosexual status in boys at puberty: Idiopathic adolescent gynecomastia and congenital virilizing adrenocorticism compared. *Psychoneuroendocrinology* 7, 339-346.

Moritz, C. (1983) Parthenogenesis in the endemic Australian lizard *Heteronotia binoei* (Gekkonidae). *Science* 220, 735-737.

Nordeen, E. J. & Yahr, P. (1982) Hemispheric asymmetries in the behavioral and hormonal effects of sexually differentiating mammalian brain. *Science* 218, 391-393.

Schwartz, M. F. (1977) Athletics, friendships, dating, romance, and sexuality in adrenogenital females, aged 17-27, compared with females with androgen-insensitivity and Rokitansky syndromes. Doctoral Dissertation, Johns Hopkins University School of Hygiene and Public Health, Baltimore.

Short, R. V. & Clarke, I. J. (undated) *Film: Masculinization of the Female Sheep.* Distributed by MRC Reproductive Biology Unit, 2 Forrest Road, Edinburgh EH1 2QW, Scotland, U.K.

Ward, I. L. (1977) Exogenous androgen activates female behavior in noncopulating, prenatally stressed male rats. *J. Comp. Physiol. Psychol.* 91, 465-471.

Note

Originally published in *Psychoneuroendocrinology,* 9:405-414, 1984, with M. Schwartz and V. G. Lewis as coauthors. [Bibliog. #2.290]

Author's Comment: Bisexuality and Homosexuality

The following editorial viewpoint supplements the discussion section of this chapter. It appeared in the *British Journal of Sexual Medicine,* 10(94):14, 1983. [Bibliog. #4.95]

After conception and before the sex organs develop, everyone is bisexual because everyone has the embryonic beginnings of both types of sex organ. By the time of birth, however, differentation of the genitals has usually occurred. This differentiation is taken to indicate the sex of the baby, but, scientifically, there is still no way of ascertaining how sexuality is governed in the brain. It is highly probable, however, that sex-related pathways in the brain are programed to make it either easy or difficult to conform to one or the other of the strict gender stereotypes.

A new discovery in prenatal rat sexology, using brain implants of steroidal sex hormone, has revealed that experimental defeminization of mating behavior is governed predominantly in the left hypothalamus of the brain, whereas experimental demasculinization is governed in the right hypothalamus.[1] Thus, if someone is prenatally programed so that conformity to either the male or female stereotype is difficult, then learning experiences may lead them to develop either a role of transexual gender-identity or one of obligative homosexual gender-identity. It is likely, however, that he/she would develop some degree of bisexualism.

If one travels the manifest path of bisexuality, then, by the age of sexual maturity, one will almost certainly label oneself as homosexual. The explanation of this error is historical. Homosexuality has been considered a sin on a par with heresy and treason. Sinners are still labeled for their vices and not their virtues. Thus bisexuals are still singled out, not for their heterosexual but for their homosexual actions. In the 19th century, homosexuality became relabeled as not a sin but a sickness. Physicians dedicate themselves to sickness, and so they label their patients in terms not of their health but their pathology. Medicine still perpetuates the anachronism of labeling bisexuals by the homosexual, not the heterosexual, component of their behavior.

Times are changing, however, and homosexuality is gradually being seen as a social option. The bisexual is a person endowed with both a homosexual and a heterosexual option. Each option deserves equal social approval, for the bisexual did not choose his duality, nor can he or she choose to eradicate it.

The changes taking place have not yet affected, as greatly as they should, the lay and professional conception of bisexuality. Indeed, professionals need to address themselves to the task of beginning a reformulation of bisexual theory on the basis of evidence from the clinic, from research investigations, and from history and the arts.

Science must begin to develop a coherent body of knowledge about bisexuality, for current developments in biomedical engineering, especialy genetic engineering, make it quite likely that one day people will be able to spend part of their lives as men and part as women. Nature has already solved this problem for, in certain species of fish, breeding males can change into breeding females, and vice versa. One day reverse embryogenesis may permit the mammalian reproductive system likewise to regress and redifferentiate.

Reference

1. Nordeen E. J., Yahr, P. Hemispheric asymmetries in the behavioral and hormonal effects of sexually differentiating mammalian brain. *Science* 218:391, 1982.

TWENTY-FOUR

Homosexual/Heterosexual Status in Boys at Puberty: Idiopathic Adolescent Gynecomastia and Congenital Virilizing Adrenocorticism Compared

Abstract

In a nonbiased sample of 10 boys with idiopathic adolescent gynecomastia [IAG] matched with eight boys with treated congenital virilizing adrenocorticism [CVA], there were three cases of homosexual gender status, all three in the IAG group; and no cases of transexualism, transvestism or gynemimesis. Signs of gender incongruity in the three cases preceded the onset of puberty and appearance of breast growth. If, in these cases, gynecomastia and homosexual status are etiologically connected, then the connection probably originates prenatally, when sexual brain differentiation is hormonally influenced.

Introduction

This paper adheres to the clinical research method, long practiced in the Johns Hopkins Psychohormonal Research Unit, of matching two different syndromes on the criterion that each is admirably suited to be the reciprocal of the other as a control, comparison or contrast group. In the present instance, the two syndromes are idiopathic adolescent gynecomastia [IAG] and congenital virilizing adrenocorticism [CVA] (Williams, 1974; Gardner, 1975; Gold & Josimovich, 1980). Both syndromes occur in males.

IAG boys are presumed, though not proved, to have a normal prenatal and juvenile hormonal history which becomes atypical at puberty, when large breasts develop. CVA boys have an abnormal prenatal hormonal history, being flooded with a great androgenic excess from their own dysfunctional adrenocortical glands. Postnatal suppression of the excess can be effected, as in the patients of this study, by cortisol treatment. Normal virilization then ensues at puberty.

The purpose of this paper is to compare two groups, IAG and CVA respectively, on the criterion of behavioral conformity to the male stereotype and the criterion of heterosexual/homosexual status, in order to ascertain if there are behavior differences between the two groups, and if so, whether they might be attributable to a difference in the history of their hormonal status at puberty.

Nature of the syndromes

Idiopathic adolescent gynecomastia. Enlargement of the breasts in adolescent boys is in some instances associated with other pathology, as in the 47,XXY (Klinefelter's) syndrome and in the Reifenstein syndrome of partial androgen insensitivity with ambiguity of the external genitalia as a birth defect. More commonly, however, adolescent gynecomastia is idiopathic. The breast enlargement involves the nipples, areolae and underlying glandular tissue. It is not fat padding. The amount of enlargement may be trivial, self-limiting and transient; or, as in the cases included in this study, it may resemble, in magnitude and permanence, adolescent breast growth in girls.

Apart from breast growth, pubertal masculinization in boys with adolescent gynecomastia is within normal male limits, as are blood and urinary androgen and estrogen levels (Lee, 1975). Androgen (testosterone) is a precursor hormone of estrogen in males as well as in females. The sex difference lies in the ratio of the two hormones. In adolescent gynecomastia, it is possible that breast tissue is unduly sensitive to estrogen (or conversely unduly resistant to the competing effect of androgen) and so takes up more estrogen than normal. This is the hypothesis of target-organ sensitivity. Whether or not this hypothesis may apply to other target organs, especially the brain, is not known.

Congenital virilizing adrenocorticism. This syndrome is transmitted as a recessive genetic trait, and may occur in siblings of either sex. Only boys are included in the present sample. The genetic error expresses itself as an enzymatic defect in the synthesis of cortisol in the adrenocortical glands from early fetal life onward. Instead of cortisol, the glands release a precursor hormone which is androgenic in both chemical structure and endocrine function. Whereas in girls this androgen masculinizes the morpohology of the external genitalia in fetal life, in boys there is no corresponding overt external genital effect. Whether or not it may have a covert effect on sexual centers and pathways in the brain is not known, though animal experiments indicate such a possibility. Before corrective treatment with cortisol was establshed in 1950 (Wilkins, 1965; Lee *et al.,* 1977), the hormonal error, persisting postnatally, induced pubertal virilization prematurely, even as early as age two or three, and rapidly accelerated growth in stature. All of the boys in the present study were correctively regulated with cortisol from early infancy onward and became pubertal at the expected age.

Patients and Methods

In both syndromes, the size of the population at risk is unknown; so also is the proportion of that population that is referred to The Johns Hopkins Hospital. Though some private referrals may have been to other clinics, the Pediatric Endocrine Clinic was the destination of most referrals. Patients in that clinic were eligible for automatic psychohormonal referral and follow-up. In order to avoid too much age disparity, the sample for the present study was subject to the criterion that the year of birth was between 1958 and 1966. For those who qualified within this age range, there was no known systematic sampling bias, and no exclusions except for two cases in the IAG group for whom a psycho-hormonal appointment could not be arranged.

TABLE I

Data Descriptive of the Sample

Variable	IAG (n = 10)	CVA (n = 8)
Age first seen (yr-months)		
Mean	15-9	9-9
Range	14-0 to 18-8	3-6 to 15-10
Age last follow-up (yr-months)		
Mean	16-11	19-0
Range	15-1 to 20-11	15-10 to 22-0
Puberty onset, age (yr-months)		
Mean	13-8	10-11
Range	12-0 to 15-6	9-2 to 12-0
Puberty Stage V, age (yr-months)		
Mean	16-10	16-5
Range	15-5 to 18-9	15-3 to 18-0
Puberty complete, height		
Mean (cm)	177	166
Range (cm)	171 to 184	148 to 177
Puberty complete, weight		
Mean (kg)	71	62
Range (kg)	54 to 94	54 to 75
Puberty complete, HQ		
Mean	101	94
Range	97 to 107	84 to 102
Puberty complete, WQ		
Mean	104	90
Range	81 to 137	99 to 147
Reduction mammoplasty		
Recommended	10	0
Surgery done	7	0
Schooling by age 16		
Grade school only	0	0
High School drop-out	0	0
High School student	10	8
Employment, last seen		
Unemployed	1	0
Student, full-time	8	5
Wage earner	1	3

IAG = Idiopathic adolescent gynecomastia.
CVA = Congenital virilizing adrenocorticism.
HQ = Height quotient (actual height/expected height for age).
WQ = Weight quotient (actual weight/expected weight for height).

Phenomenological characteristics of the sample are listed in Table I. The two groups appear to be adequately matched. The CVA patients were typically seen at an earlier age than the IAG patients, because CVA symptoms are manifested first in infancy, whereas IAG symptoms are not recognized until puberty. CVA patients are more likely than IAG patients to prolong clinic contacts into adult life, because they require continued endocrine regulation.

The tendency for treated CVA patients to have an earlier age of pubertal onset than their IAG counterparts is consistent with the clinical fact that, without endocrine intervention, CVA boys begin pubertal virilization early in infancy. It is possible that the prenatal excessive androgenization of the treated CVA syndrome accelerates the onset of puberty. It is also possible that pubertal virilization will begin early in CVA boys if their endocrine regulation on cortisol should go out of balance for an extended period—not a likely possibility in the present sample. Despite the difference between the CVA and IAG groups in age of pubertal onset, the age of attaining Tanner's Stage V of puberty did not differ appreciably.

The earliest onset of puberty in some CVA cases was responsible for earlier epiphyseal fusion and shorter adult height relative to the IAG cases. Only three CVA patients had an adult height equal to or greater than the shortest IAG heights, and the latter were not exceptionally tall, but average.

The CVA youths were stocky and muscular, and not obesely overweight. By contrast, the IAG youths ranged form bean-pole thin through average to muscular-hefty or obesely overweight. Thus, there was no consistent relationship of gynecomastia to body build.

The two entries in Table I that express these height and weight statistics most succinctly are those for height quotient (HQ) and weight quotient (WQ). Both are calculated by dividing the measurement obtained × 100 by the measurement expected—the height expected for age, and the weight expected for height. When both obtained and expected measurements are the same the quotient is 100. The quotients in Table I show that the IAG group tended to be taller and heavier than the CVA group.

Table I also presents information on schooling and employment and indicates that the groups were matched on these variables, despite the aforesaid differences.

As expected, none of the CVA patients needed to be recommended for surgery, whereas reduction mammoplasty was an option for all of the IAG patients. Three of them did not take up the option and tolerated breast enlargement as the lesser of two evils.

For each patient there was a consolidated longitudinal endocrine and psychoendocrine history covering, at a minimum, the period from early puberty to advanced adolescence. The psychoendocrine history contained transcripts of a longitudinal series of taped interviews given by the patient and at least one other person, typically a parent, with whom he lived. In a flexible and unstilted way, the interviews covered a Schedule of Inquiry designed to cover topics and obtain information requisite to this study.

The consolidated histories were indexed for the information contained in Tables I and II. The necessary information was abstracted onto a personal data sheet and numerically reduced either quantitatively (for example, age or height requirements) or qualitatively on a rating scale (for example, five stages of puberty; behavioral evidence positive or negative; or behavior rated as high, average or low). The responsibility for rating was imposed on the investigators, not on the patient, so as to ensure uniformity of the criterion standards.

Finally, data from the individual sheets were consolidated into a master chart and tabulated.

Male Stereotypic Lifestyle: Conformity/Nonconformity

In Table II the findings are presented as ratings and ratios, in nine categories. The two samples are too small for comparative statistical calculations which, in any case, would mask the fact that three youths in the gynecomastia group accounted for the majority of the differences between the two groups. These were the three youths with a history, dating from prepubertal childhood, of having manifested evidence of incongruity between sex as defined by the anatomy of their genitalia, on the one hand, and by the manifestations of their gender-identity/role, on the other. The three were not otherwise recognizable as a subgroup, as for example with respect to the variables of Table I.

By contrast, the three did emerge as a subgroup according to the criteria of Table II. All three were either unsatisfied with or ambivalent about their male status. Two of them were homosexual and one was bisexual in amative orientation. This orientation had persisted until the age when most recently contacted, namely ages 17, 17½ and 21 yrs. respectively. All three had a history of cross-dressing at times, and their mannerisms and body-language had, since childhood, allowed other people to regard them as effeminate or homosexual. Only one of the three had a history of ever having participated in stereotypic male sports (in his case baseball, track and swimming). None of the three had a positive rating with respect to marriage and parenthood. All three were the victims of peergroup teasing regarding not only gynecomastia, but also the mannerisms by which they were stigmatized as homosexual. All three had a history of behavioral pathology—respectively, suicidal despair, germ phobia and school disruptiveness requiring special placement.

Table II indicates that these three youths were not alone in having a negative rating on marriage, parenthood or teasing. In both groups there were others with similar ratings, the majority of them being also in the gynecomastia group (see page 298).

Only with respect to history of teasing did the virilizing adrenocortical (CVA) group approximate the gynecomastia group. The CVA boys were teased because of being relatively short in stature, but it was benign teasing. The gynecomastia boys were more traumatically teased, and in six cases viciously so. 'He would come up and say: "Are you half boy and half girl?" And then he'd

TABLE II

Conformity and Nonconformity to Male Stereotypic Lifestyle
in Idiopathic Adolescent Gynecomastia (IAG, *n* = 10)
and Congenital Virilizing Adrenocorticism (CVA; *n* = 8) in Teenage Boys

Category	IAG	CVA
Male sexual status		
Satisfied	17(70%)	8(100%)
Unsatisfied or ambivalent	3(30%)	0(0%)
Orientation: imagery, dating, coitus		
Heterosexual	7(70%)	8(100%)
Bisexual	1(10%)	0(0%)
Homosexual	2(20%)	0(0%)
Cross-dressing history		
Negative	7(70%)	8(100%)
Postive	3(30%)	0(0%)
Male stereotypic sports history		
Participant	7(70%)	8(100%)
Nonparticipant	3(30%)	0(0%)
Attitude to marriage		
Positive	3(30%)	6(75%)
Negative or non-committal	7(70%)	2(25%)
Married		
Yes	0(0%)	1(12%)*
No	10(100%)	7(88%)
Attitude to parenthood		
Positive or taking chances	5(50%)	7(88%)
Negative or non-committal	5(50%)	1(12%)
History of teasing		
Negative	2(20%)	3(38%)
Positive	8(80%)	5(62%)
History of social isolation		
Withdrew from peers	5(50%)	0(0%)
Always a loner	2(20%)	1(12%)
Social participant	3(30%)	7(88%)
History of behavioral pathology		
Negative	6(60%)	6(75%)
Positive	4(40%)	2(25%)

*Only this patient was a father.

touch me, and I'd hit him,' one boy reported. Another boy said, 'The girls were
even turning against me . . . when I went into the hospital and got them
removed, I came home and some girl came up and said, "I heard you got your
titties cut off. . . . " It used to bother me a lot; but what they think is their
thoughts, and their thoughts can't harm me, I told myself.'

There were no boys in the adrenocortical group who were stigmatized as
homosexual. All eight of the group recognized themselves as heterosexual only.
Two of them were not positively oriented toward marriage and parenthood.
Otherwise, the ratings of the group as a whole were unimodal and in favor of
conformity to society's current stereotype of masculinity.

By contrast, the gynecomastia group was bimodal—three non-conformists and seven conformists, with respect to the masculine stereotype. Among the seven stereotypic conformists, four were discrepant in being not positively committed to marriage, and two of these four also were indefinite about becoming a parent, probably as a function of youthful age and/or subcultural traditions.

Behavioral Pathology

In the history of behavioral pathology (Table II), there was a trend toward dual polarity insofar as, in the two affected adrenocortical cases, pathology was of the exteroceptive type (rage attacks in one case and stealing, drugs and running away in the other). In two of the gynecomastia cases, one homosexually stigmatized, pathology was similarly exteroceptive. In the other two, both homosexually stigmatized, it was interoceptive (suicidal despondency and germ phobia, respectively).

Gynecomastia Self-construed

The shame and embarrassment of gynecomastia may be manifest in social withdrawal, especially from participation in activities requiring exposure of the naked or thinly-clothed chest. In Table II, the entry under History of Social Isolation shows that 50% of the gynecomastia youths did undergo a period of social withdrawal, whereas none of the CVA group did.

An adolescent youth with gynecomastia typically construes the development of his breasts as discordant with his ideal self-image (Schonfeld, 1961). He may think of them as knots, lumps or cancer; as a sign of a need to lose weight by diet or body-building exercise; or as a feminizing sign. Alternatively, he may say he attributed no specific significance to them.

The three who had been stigmatized by agemates as homosexual construed their gynecomastia differently from one another. One claimed not to have been worried except by a phobia of 'being put to sleep', on which account he forwent surgery. The other two had a reduction mammoplasty. One of these two was able to construe himself as being like his father who had asymmetrical gynecomastia. The other discounted his mother's early statement that all boys get knots in their breasts, and then discounted his own thought of turning into a girl with 'I thought probably the top is a girl's and the bottom is a boy's.' The two other boys who considered that their chests were changing like that of a girl did not fear that they were changing into a girl. 'I just ruled that out of my head,' one boy recalled. 'I said this is crazy.'

In the eight adrenocortical cases, there were no developmental phenomena that might have been self-construed as feminizing.

Discussion

In neither the foregoing data, nor in the IAG and CVA literature, is there evidence of gender incongruity or transposition of the type that would justify a diagnosis of either the syndrome of transexualism or transvestism [the syndrome of transvestophilia, which is not the same as the act of cross-dressing] (Money, 1969). Nor is there evidence of another transposition syndrome, gynemimesis, which in street language is known as being a drag queen—a lady with a penis and, in many instances, breasts grown as a sequel to exogenous estrogen, taken either with or without prescription.

There are many cases of transexualism, transvestophilia and gynemimesis in the files of the Johns Hopkins Psychohormonal Research Unit, but none with an additional diagnosis of idiopathic adolescent gynecomastia. The nearest approach to such a double diagnosis occurred approximately 20 years ago in a case of adolescent gynecomastia excluded from the present sample on the criterion of age. In this case, the boy with breasts had formulated for himself two alternatives: either he would become a woman or, failing that, a priest, each of which would presumably have eliminated his living as a male with a male lover. Homosexuality was morally and religiously reprehensible to him. Ultimately, however, that is the lifestyle to which he has reconciled himself.

It could, of course, be statistically fortuitous that three youths with a homosexual status turned up in an unbiased sample of 10 cases of adolescent gynecomastia and none in a control group of eight cases of male congenital adrenocorticism. The scholarly estimate of homosexuality of the type found in these three youths in the general population ranges from 3 to 5% (Kinsey, 1948; Livingood, 1972; Gebhard & Johnson, 1979). Therefore, the probability of finding three in a group of 10 is $p < 0.02$ to $p < 0.003$. Even if the figure of homosexuality in the general population were as high as 10%, three among 10 is marginally significant at the $p < 0.07$ level, which is striking, given the small size of the sample.

If the association between homosexual status and gynecomastia is not fortuitous, the alternative is that one might cause the other, or that both share a common determining factor in their developmental histories. For homosexuality to cause gynecomastia, the only known explanation is in terms of exogenous estrogen—available in some cosmetic creams; or by using someone else's prescribed oral contraceptive pills or estrogen pills; or by having a legitimate prescription. Usage may be overt or secretive, the latter in the manner of Munchausen's syndrome, as exemplified by a 12-year-old estrogen-ingesting transexual patient followed by Stoller (1968).

In idiopathic adolescent gynecomastia, if breast growth itself caused a homosexual status to develop, then there should be no prepubertal evidence of gender incongruity. In the three cases in this study, that condition was not met, and the same applied to the older patient, above-mentioned, not included in the present sample. Thus, there is no support for a hypothesis that a hormonal or other agent, active at the time of puberty, was responsible for both gynecomastia and homosexual status. Of course, the very fact of the coexistence of gynecomastia and heterosexual status in 70% of cases in the present sample also militates against such a hypothesis.

Thus, by a process of elimination, the connection between gynecomastia and homosexual vs. heterosexual status must begin before puberty. Hypothetically, it could begin as early as prenatal life or immediately thereafter, when, from animal studies, it is known that the sexually differentiating brain is sex-hormone sensitive. At this early stage, whether or not the precursor of the factor eventually responsible for gynecomastia would also be a precursor of the factor responsible for the postnatal differentation of a homosexual status might be dependent on either the timing or the intensity of influence, or both. Whatever the prenatal factor, it would be in the nature of a necessary but not a sufficient cause. It would set a threshold, disposition, susceptibility or vulnerability that, in turn, would influence the further differentiation of homo/heterosexual status in postnatal life. The postnatal phase might be inconsequential in some lower mammals, whose patterns of mating behavior may be set, robot-like, by prenatal hormonal programing exclusively. In higher primates, by contrast, postnatal erotosexual rehearsal play is, in infancy and early childhood, apparently, an additional prerequisite of male/female mating behavior, and also of male/female love-smittenness, known as limerence* (Tennov, 1979). Deprivation or negation of this play has divergent effects, depending on the vulnerability of the individual at risk.

The absence of homosexual status in the congenital virilizing adrenocortical syndrome in males applies not only to the present small sample, but also to an extended sample of more than 30 cases in which only one man† had a history of homosexual attraction. This low prevalence of homosexual status in the CVA syndrome may be attributed, hypothetically, to an excess of androgen and its presumed brain-masculinization effect in fetal life.

If this hypothesis is correct, then it would appear that the prenatal effect of excessive androgenization in congenital adrenocorticism in boys is to differentiate not only masculinized but ultramasculinized dimorphism of the sexual brain. Then it may be hypothesized that the erotosexual differentiation of postnatal life is resistant to influences that, had the brain been less masculinized, might permit a degree of either bisexuality or homosexuality to emerge.

---

*Pairbonded attachment of an erotic and sexual type in human beings lacked a one-word term in the English language until Tennov (1979), deliberately avoiding etymological antecedents, coined the new term, *limerence,* a noun from which a verb, adjective and adverb can be derived. Limerence is synonymous with being love-smitten, being in love, having fallen in love or having a love affair. Limerence may be requited or unrequited.

†There may well be more to learn from this man's case about hormonal history and homosexuality, for he had an atypical form of the CVA syndrome which passed unnoticed and untreated until, at age 35, he volunteered to participate in a family study. He had two male cousins, who were brothers, with the same variant of the syndrome. Both were heterosexual and fertile, one without ever having been treated with cortisol. There were no affected females in the pedigree.

Acknowledgment

Supported by USPHS grants HD00325 and HD07111.

References

Gardner, L. I. (ed.) (1975) *Endocrine and Genetic Disease of Childhood and Adolescence.* Second Edition W. B. Saunders, Philadelphia.

Gebhard, P. H. & Johnson, A. B. (eds.) (1979) *The Kinsey Data: Marginal Tabulations of the 1938-1963 Interviews Conducted by the Institute for Sex Research.* W. B. Saunders, Philadelphia.

Gold, J. J. & Josimovich, J. B. (Eds.) (1980) *Gynecologic Endocrinology.* Third Edition. Harper and Row, New York.

Kinsey, A. C., Pomeroy, W. B. & Martin, C. E. (1948) *Sexual Behavior in the Human Male.* W. B. Saunders, Philadelphia.

Lee, P. A. (1975) The relationship of concentrations of serum hormones to pubertal gynecomastia. *J. Pediat.* 86, 212-215.

Lee, P. A., Plotnick, L. P., Kowarski, A. A. & Migeon, C. J. (eds.) (1977) *Congenital Adrenal Hyperplasia.* University Park Press, Baltimore.

Livingood, J. M. (Ed.) (1972) *National Institute of Mental Health Task Force on Homosexuality: Final Report and Background Papers,* DHEW Publication No. (HSM) 72-9116. U. S. Government Printing Office, Washington.

Money, J. (1969) Sex reassignment as related to hermaphroditism and transsexualism. In *Transsexualism and Sex Reassignment,* R. Green and J. Money, (eds.). Johns Hopkins Press, Baltimore.

Schonfeld, W. A. (1961) Gynecomastia in adolescence: personality effects. *Arch. Gen. Psychiat* 5, 46-54.

Stoller, R. J. (1968) *Sex and Gender.* Science House, New York.

Tennov, D. (1979) *Love and Limerence: The Experience of being in Love.* Stein and Day, New York.

Wilkins, L. (1965) *The Diagnosis and Treatment of Endocrine Disorders in Childhood and Adolescence.* Third Edition. Charles C Thomas, Springfield, Illinois.

Williams, R. H. (ed.) (1974) *Textbook of Endocrinology.* W. B. Saunders, Philadelphia.

Note

Originally published in *Psychoneuroendocrinology,* 7:339-346, 1982, with V. G. Lewis as co-author. [Bibliog. #2.262]

TWENTY-FIVE

Gender Identity and Gender Transposition: Longitudinal Outcome Study of 32 Male Hermaphrodites Assigned as Girls

Abstract

The longitudinal case histories of 32 female-assigned male hermaphrodites aged 18 or older were indexed and abstracted for evidence of variables related to gender transposition, i.e., bisexualism, lesbianism, or sex reassignment to live as male. The prevalence of transposition was biased because of the referral of cases selected for reassignment. Childhood stigmatization, either subtle or blatant, because of the birth defect of the sex organs correlated with gender transposition ($p < .001$) and was related to the age of feminizing surgery ($p < .05$), which often coincided with the age of gonadectomy. Variables not significantly correlated with gender transposition were: neonatal ambivalence regarding the sex of announcement; feminizing or masculinizing puberty; presence or absence of müllerian organs; and gross family pathology. Physicians encountered no moral problem with sex reassignment as the chromosomal and gonadal sex were male.

Introduction

This paper is one of a series dating from Money, 1952 and 1955, on the sexology of the syndromes of hermaphroditism. Their purpose has been to differentiate the variables and determinants of what is variously known as psychosexual development, gender identity, gender role, and G-I/R (gender-identity/role) in both its sexuoerotic and extragenital aspects. A defining characteristic of their design has been to compare individuals concordant for diagnosis but discordant for the sex in which they are assigned and registered, and in which they grow up. This design applies to the present two-part study of G-I/R and gender transposition in male hermaphroditism, of which this is the first part. It is a long-term outcome study of male hermaphrodites assigned and registered as girls, some of whom in adulthood are heterosexual as women, some bisexual or lesbian, and some heterosexual as men after sex reassignment. Its purpose is, by applying a series of eight strategies, to identify variables that do and do not contribute to the development of varying degrees of female-to-male gender transposition as defined below (see Strategy 1).

The sample is a heuristic one. It includes all 32 cases of female-assigned male hermaphrodites aged eighteen or older for whom a longitudinal, consolidated clinical and sexological history was on file.

The method of obtaining sexological data, of indexing and abstracting the consolidated histories, and of classifying and coding the data is described in detail in Chapter 8. There are eight strategies of data evaluation.

Strategy 1: Gender Transposition

Rationale

The function of this initial strategy is to ascertain the proportion of those in the sample who did and did not qualify as manifesting gender transposition, relative to the referral category in which they belonged. In one category, referrals were made initially through the pediatric endocrine clinic for routine, long-term care and follow-up of a birth defect of the sex organs. In the other category, referrals were made from other clinics or hospitals especially for a psychoendocrine and sexological evaluation, because the patient was an applicant for, or was in the process of going through a sex reassignment to begin living as a man. The code terms for these two groups are regular referral and special referral.

A gender transposition can apply to any component of gender-identity/role as female or male. For present purposes, it applies specifically to the erotosexual component as manifested either in imagery and ideation, or in practice, or both. An erotosexual gender transposition encompasses such phenomena, in imagination or actuality, as having a sexual relationship or a love affair with a person living in the same sex as oneself. If each partner lives as a woman, then each is socially defined as lesbian or bisexual. If the hermaphroditic partner becomes sex reassigned from female to male, then the partnership is socially defined as heterosexual. Social, hormonal, and surgical sex reassignment represents the major degree of gender transposition.

Sample and Procedure

The full sample of 32 male hermaphrodites announced as girls and officially registered as girls is used in this strategy. It is subdivided into two referral groups, regular (N = 32) and special (N = 6), as defined above.

Findings

The findings pertain first to the whole range of gender transpositions, namely, lesbian, bisexual, and sex-reassignment; and, second, exclusively to sex reassignment. In both instances the proportion of gender transpositions was heavily biased by the six special patients referred because they were hermaphrodites already undergoing sex reassignment (chi-square = 5.95, $p < .02$; and 14.75, $p < .001$, respectively). Because of this bias the overall findings cannot be used as an estimate of the prevalence of gender transposition in general, and sex reassignment in particular, among the general population of male hermaphro-dites announced and officially registered as girls. The more likely prevalence ratios would be those of the regular clinical referrals, namely 9:23 (39.1%) for all three varieties of transposition, and 3:23 (11.5%) for sex reassignment only.

Comment

The bias in favor of gender transposition created by the special referrals in the present sample is not disadvantageous for present purposes, insofar as it allows for the application of further strategies to investigate the genesis of gender transposition and its culmination, in some cases, in sex reassignment.

Strategy 2: Stigmatization

Rationale

This strategy investigates the possibility that gender transposition in male her-maphrodites assigned as girls is related to the experience of being stigmatized as a hermaphrodite while growing up. Stigmatization may be blatant, as in taunts and insults regarding one's sexually ambivalent status at birth or later; or it may be the more insidious stigmatization of being abnormal because of having a genital defect and being imperfectly a girl. Still more insidiously, it may be the awareness of being a catastrophe in the parents' lives because of an unspeakable something that reaches crisis proportions especially at each clinic visit, and that is associated with the genital examination and the scrupulous avoidance of any explanation of its significance to the child, before or after genital surgery.

Sample and Procedure

All 32 patients are included in this strategy. They are rated as having been stigmatized at home only, in the community only, or both, or neither.

A rating of being stigmatized in the home was given if the hermaphroditic child was treated differently than a sexually normal child in such a way as to signify that she was special, different, or freakish—for example, by elaborately maintaining the privacy of the hermaphroditic genital anomaly, keeping the child at home and forbidding her to play with neighborhood children, placing a veto on communications within the family about the hermaphroditic condition, and telling children in the family to lie or be evasive about the reasons for traveling long-distance for clinic visits. Some hermaphroditic children were additionally stigmatized by the parents' overattentiveness to, and attempted suppression of play that in other girls would have been acceptable, but in them was misread as being too masculine.

A rating of being stigmatized in the community was given if the hermaphroditic child was taunted and teased, irrespective of the degree of her conformity to stereotypes of feminine behavior, because of her genital anomaly, body build, appearance, hirsutism, or voice, as in such remarks as, "She's got a boy's face," or "She's not all girl," or in being ridiculed because of her genital configuration.

Findings

There was a conspicuous tendency for the patients manifesting gender trans-position to have been stigmatized (chi-square = 10.98, p. < .001). Those who were stigmatized were more likely to have been stigmatized both at home and in the community than in only one of the two environments.

Comment

Strategy 2 examines where stigmatization occurs, but not when it begins. The age of its onset is another variable that may be important for the genesis and eventual manifestation of a gender transposition. The age of onset could be as early as the newborn period when stigmatization might have its genesis in the neonatal history of contradiction and confusion regarding the announcement of the baby's sex, entailing in some instances a reannouncement.

Strategy 3: Announced Sex

Rationale

This strategy investigates the possibility that contradiction and confusion concerning the child's neonatal sexual status, and the announcement or reannounce-ment as male or female in the neonatal period contribute to subsequent develop-ment of gender transposition. Typically in male hermaphrodites reared as girls, an abnormality of the external genitalia is recognized at birth. These are the babies for whom a sex reannouncement may occur. Others are announced as female, for their external genitalia are so greatly demasculinized that on casual inspection they appear feminine, and their anomaly is discovered only later.

Sample and Procedure

Only 23 patients are used in this strategy, as their histories alone contained interviews in which the mothers reported information concerning the circum-stances of the child's neonatal diagnosis and declaration of sex. In other cases the mother was deceased or was separated from the patient, in some instances in a foreign country.

There are two classifications, ambivalence and nonambivalence regarding the sex of announcement. Ambivalence means that the parents were confronted with contradiction and confusion in the opinions of different advisors, each using a different criterion for deciding the sex of announcement. The conflicting opinions originated chiefly among physicians, but in some instances included geneticists and other hospital personnel, religious advisors, relatives, and friends. Conflicting professional opinions in some cases led to a sex reannouncement.

Findings

The findings show that ambivalence, contradiction and confusion concerning a male hermaphroditic baby's sex of final announcement did not correlate with the subsequent manifestation of gender transposition (chi-square = 1.32, N.S.).

Comment

It appears from Strategy 3 that most parents were able to abide temporary uncertainty concerning their newborn baby's status as a boy or girl without its subsequently having become, by itself alone, a source of the child's stigmatization. Six of the seven gender-transposed patients did not have a neonatal history of parental ambivalence concerning their announced sex. Some other influence must be presumed responsible for gender transposition. The next strategy examines whether the age of surgical feminization of the external genitalia may be related to stigmatization and gender transposition.

Strategy 4: Surgical Feminization

Rationale

When the decision is made to announce the sex of a hermaphroditic baby as female, the incongruity between the announced sex and the ambiguity of the external genitalia is resolved by means of corrective feminizing surgery. The earlier the surgery, the earlier the resolution of the cognitive contradiction confronting the parents, older siblings, other relatives, friends, and baby-sitters. Early surgery also allows the child to grow up without having to reconcile the contradiction between her assigned sex and genital appearance and tactile perception. Thus, early surgery obviates a potential variable in the genesis of gender transposition as well as of social stigmatization and self-stigmatization.

Sample and Procedure

All 32 of the subjects were eligible for inclusion in this strategy. They were classified into two groups: those who either had early feminizing surgery or did not need it; and those who needed surgery and either did not get it, or got it late. The timing of early surgery was between one month and one year of age. Late surgery was after age three. There were no instances of surgery between ages one and three.

Findings

Strategy 4 examines the relationship between timing of feminizing surgery and the eventual absence or presence of a gender transposition. The chi-square (8.41) shows a connection, significant at the p < .01 level, between surgery that was done late or not at all, and the existence of a gender transposition at the time of adult follow-up.

Strategy 4a examines the relationship between timing of feminizing surgery and a history of stigmatization. The chi-square (4.16) is weak (p < .05), but shows a trend toward increased prevalence of stigmatization when corrective surgery was delayed or not done at all.

Comment

The relationship between late or absent feminizing surgery, on the one hand, and the eventual manifestation of a history of both stigmatization and gender transposition, on the other, suggests the hypothesis of a direct link between stigmatization and gender transposition. Being stigmatized at home and/or in the community as a girl with a masculinized birth defect of the sex organs may become internalized as self-stigmatization, which in turn may lead to a female-to-male transposition of some aspect of the differentiating complex of gender-identity/role (G-I/R). It is likely that the transposition effect takes place before puberty, and that it is not related to hormonal masculinization at puberty.

Strategy 5: Hormonal Puberty

Rationale

A male hermaphrodite announced and reared as a girl needs female hormonal replacement therapy in order to undergo pubertal feminization. Otherwise, if previously gonadectomized, the child develops in teenage as a nonfeminized eunuch. If androgen-secreting gonadal tissue has not been removed, and provided target organs are not androgen resistant, then puberty is masculinizing. Strategy 5 is designed to investigate the possibility that progressive masculinization of the body at puberty is accompanied by a corresponding gender transposition from female to male.

Sample and Procedure

All 32 cases were used in this strategy, subdivided according to whether their puberty was masculinizing or feminizing. Masculinizing puberty was in each instance spontaneous and not clinically induced. No male hormone was administered to induce puberty in a gonadectomized child living as a girl. Feminizing puberty, by contrast was clinically induced in those who had been gonadectomized. Pubertal feminization of the breasts and body shape also occurred spontaneously in some of the patients who had not been gonadectomized.

Findings

The findings show that there is no consistent relationship between the presence or absence of gender transposition, on the one hand, and the feminine or masculine hormonalization of puberty, on the other (chi-square = 3.01, N.S.). Moreover, among the gender transposed with pubertal hormonal feminization, three were on replacement therapy with estrogen; and three developed breast enlargement under the influence of their own gonads.

Comment

On the basis of proverbial wisdom, it has long been assumed that the sex hormones of puberty shape not only the morphology of the body, but also the erotic orientation of the mind as male or female. These present findings, reinforced by a substantial body of evidence from other clinical syndromes (Money, 1974), indicate that erotic orientation of the mind is not preordained by the hormonally regulated morphology of the body. Indeed, the two may be incongruent.

The finding that gender transposition was manifested both in those who feminized at puberty and those who masculinized is in accord with contemporary theory regarding the differentiation of G-I/R (gender-identity/role) as feminine or masculine, namely, that it takes place developmentally and chiefly in the early years, before puberty. Puberty brings the erotosexual component of G-I/R into full bloom, but does not determine its orientation as masculine or feminine.

The prepubertal antecedents of gender transposition, if one interpolates from animal evidence, include juvenile sexual rehearsal play and, before that, the hormonal governance of the development of the sexual brain. In the present study, it was not possible to retrieve evidence from a sufficiently large number of histories for a strategy on the influence of sexual rehearsal play, or its thwarting, on gender transposition and nontransposition. Strategy 6, however, attempts to deal with the issue of early brain-hormonal influence on gender transposition relative to the age of castration.

Strategy 6: Gonadectomy

Rationale

There is an expanding body of experimental brain-hormone research on animals (reviewed in Reinisch et al., 1986) that confirms the hypothesis that sex steroids in prenatal and neonatal life influence the male-female dimorphism of the sexual brain. They do so in such a way as to govern male/female dimorphism of mating behavior later in life.

In human sexology, it is still a matter of speculation and hypothesis as to whether, and to what extent, sex steroid prenatally and neonatally may affect subsequent differentiation of the G-I/R as masculine or feminine. Strategy 6 is designed to examine this hypothesis by comparing the relationship of gender transposition with the age at which a male hermaphrodite assigned as a girl is surgically gonadectomized.

Sample and Procedure

Four cases are excluded from this sample as they were sex reassigned in adolescence to live as men and were not gonadectomized. The remaining 28 cases were arranged in ascending order of age. One of the two oldest individuals, aged 28, had lived half his life as a male when his only testis became malignant with a seminoma and was removed. The other lived her life in hiding as a woman fully hormonally masculinized until she was gonadectomized and given estrogen replacement at age 45.

Findings

Being so widely scattered according to age, the data of Strategy 6 lend themselves to visual inspection rather than statistical treatment. Tentatively, they may be deemed to support the interpretation that the demasculinizing effect of early gonadectomy increases the likelihood that a male hermaphrodite announced and reared as a girl will differentiate a feminine G-I/R without a masculine transposition. This interpretation is, however, confounded by the fact that early gonadectomy was invariably accompanied by surgical feminization of the genital appearance and so may be of cosmetic, not endocrine significance. This interpretation is supported by the fact that the transitional age between early and late gonadectomy is after age two and before age three (chi-square = 6.32, p < .02).

Comment

In normal males, it is known that within two weeks after birth there begins a dramatic rise in the level of the androgen, testosterone, circulating in the bloodstream (Migeon and Forest, 1980). By age three months, it peaks at a level that will not again be reached until puberty. By five months of age it has returned to zero, and remains at that level until the onset of puberty. There is no corresponding hormonal phenomenon in normal female babies. What happens in the case of newborn male hermaphrodites has not yet been ascertained. It is unlikely to be the same in all cases, because etiologically and biochemically, male hermaphroditism is comprised of several different syndromes, some of which have an already identified enzymatic defect in hormonal synthesis, and some not. In the present instance, it was not possible to subdivide the full sample of cases on the basis of their enzymatic or other etiological defect, such as partial androgen insensitivity, for the necessary tests had not been devised in the era when most of them were diagnosed. Thus it is not possible on the basis of the present study to reach a definitive conclusion regarding the influence of a neonatal testosterone surge, nor of its abolition by gonadectomy, on the subsequent differentiation of G-I/R, with or without a gender transposition.

Though it was not possible to subdivide the sample on the basis of hormonal etiology, it was possible to make a subdivision on the basis of whether, during embryonic development, the müllerian ducts had, as in the normal male, been completely vestigiated, or not.

Strategy 7: Müllerian Organs

Rationale

In the embryological differentiation of the male internal reproductive structures, müllerian inhibiting factor [MIF], also known as antimüllerian hormone [AMH] (Josso, 1984; Josso et al., 1977), from the testes vestigiates the müllerian ducts and prevents them from developing into a uterus and fallopian tubes. In some male hermaphrodites this vestigiation effect is either wholly or partly incomplete. Internally they have a uterus and one or both fallopian tubes more or less well developed.

There is no known connection, either direct or indirect, between the effect of MIF in embryonic life and the possibility of gender transposition later in life. Nonetheless, on the off chance that there might be a connection, the sample was divided into those proved to have müllerian organs, and those proved not to have them.

Sample and Procedure

The full sample of 32 is used in this strategy. The presence of müllerian organs (N = 8) was established by surgical exploration: a uterus with fallopian tubes was reported in 5 cases, and fallopian tubes only in 3 cases. The absence of müllerian organs was established by surgical exploration in 19 cases, and by rectal palpation in 5 cases.

Findings

The findings show that the presence of müllerian organs did not preclude the possibility of a gender transposition, any more than did their absence (chi-square = 0.04, N.S.).

Comment

This finding indicates that at the time when MIF is active in embryonic development there is no accompanying or dependent process of differentiation of G-I/R in favor of a subsequent gender transposition, if the male hermaphroditic baby is announced and reared as a girl.

Strategy 8: Family Behavioral Pathology

Rationale

In gender-transposition theory, there are those who continue the outworn tradition of juxtaposing biological against social environmental determinants such as, for example, social and behavioral pathology among family members. For this reason, Strategy 8 compares the presence or absence of gender transposition with three grades of family pathology.

Sample and Procedure

All 32 patients are included. Family pathology was rated as present or absent if information had been obtained in person from family members as well as the patient, and if the evidence was clearcut. When the evidence was not clearcut, especially if the informant had been the patient alone, which happened in the case of some older patients, then the rating was questionable. A rating of present was given when there was clearcut evidence of an extreme degree of psychiatric disability or alcoholic violence in one or more family members, or an excessive amount of abusive feuding within the family; and vice versa a rating of absent.

Findings

The findings show that the relationship between the absence or presence of gender transposition and present, absent, or questionable family pathology was not consistent, but randomly distributed (chi-square = 3.13, N.S.).

Comment

This finding refutes the hypothesis that gender identity in male hermaphrodites assigned to be reared as girls is preordained as a consistent response to any and all varieties of gross behavioral pathology regardless of type, within the child's family. It does not rule out the possibility, however, that gender transposition may be a consistent response to a more subtle variety of behavioral pathology involving the relationship between the child and each parent or other significant figures within the family. The present data on family relationships are not sufficiently detailed to permit a more complex investigation of their role among all the variables that may generate a gender transposition (Money, 1984).

Discussion

As in the present study, any clinical population of male hermaphrodites reared as girls is prone to be biased in favor of those with a gender transposition, particularly those in need of clinical services for a sex reassignment. Elimination of this bias would require a prospective outcome study. Cases would be enrolled neonatally, maintained in followup, and provided with surgical, endocrine, psychological and general health-care services as needed.

Provision of these services would not guarantee elimination of neonatal contradiction and confusion regarding the announcement of sex, since it is not possible to guarantee that all obstetricians, midwives, nurses and consultants have prior specialty training in what to do when a baby is born with a birth defect of the sex organs. However, it is not foreordained that a neonatal period of parental uncertainty regarding the child's sex leads inevitably to later stigmatization of the child as freakish and a source of shame. Stigmatization is more closely related to postponement of surgical feminization until after one year of age, so that the child looks genitally abnormal. She becomes subject not only to stigmatization by others, but also to a self-stigmatization. In a world dichotomized by sex, if she does not look completely like a girl, then the only alternative is that she must look like a boy, or a half-boy, half-girl. Self-stigmatization leads the way to a self-generated development of a gender transposition, masculinizing all aspects of the girl's gender-identity/role (G-I/R).

The developmental genesis of a gender transposition takes place prior to the onset of hormonal puberty. An incongruously masculinizing hormonal puberty does not reverse a feminine G-I/R once it has differentiated, but is subjectively experienced as a mortification, and an error in need of correction. By contrast, if the G-I/R has become transposed and masculine, then the addition of pubertal hormonal masculinization generates a crisis which, in some cases is resolved only by means of sex reassignment.

Because of the age of the patients in this study, the majority were diagnosed prior to the era of diagnostically subtyping male hermaphroditism on the basis of an enzyme deficiency, or of androgen insensitivity. Thus the present study does not lend itself to a statement regarding a possible prenatal or perinatal enzymatic or specific hormonal influence on sexual dimorphism of the brain and of its subsequent governance of G-I/R differentiation.

Prenatal steroid hormonal influences can be manipulated experimentally in animals, but not in human beings. Human perinatal hormonal influences may however, be modified by perinatal gonadectomy. In the present study there were too few cases of very early gonadectomy to provide sufficient evidence one way or the other. Moreover, the possible hormonal effect of early gonadectomy was confounded by the fact that this operation was combined with surgical feminization of the genital appearance, and hence the removal of the genital source of stigmatization.

Clinically, another way to investigate a possible prenatal hormonal influence is by a comparison of patients with and without vestigiation of the müllerian ducts. The findings indicate no influence of MIF (müllerian inhibiting factor), on gender transposition.

A prenatal hormonal determinant and a postnatal social determinant may augment one another. Postnatally, juvenile sexual rehearsal play, if one interpolates from animal studies, is an important social influence in G-I/R differentiation, but present data were too scanty to shed light on this variable. Family relationships constitute another social influence conventionally assigned considerable significance. Whereas subtleties of pathology in parent-child relationships cannot be ruled out as bearing a consistent relationship to gender transposition, the present evidence is that gross behavioral pathology within the family does not.

In a male hermaphrodite assigned as girl, gender transposition during childhood may, when in teenage it expresses itself sexuoerotically, resolve as a lesbian life style, or it may extend to sex reassignment and living as a boy. For hormonal and surgical sex reassignment, the medical profession must be involved. Among physicians, there is traditionally a strong reliance on the sex of the gonads or of the chromosomes as the ultimate criterion of sex. Medical people are, therefore, more likely to condone or prescribe a sex reassignment in a male hermaphrodite assigned as a girl than in a female hermaphrodite assigned as a girl, no matter how completely masculinized the genitalia may appear, nor how extensive the degree to which the body may have become hormonally virilized. The principles and policies of the medical profession are, therefore, an important variable to consider with respect to sex reassignment from female to male in cases of male hermaphroditism, even if the breasts are well developed and the body poorly virilized.

References

Josso, N. (1984) Hormone anti-müllérienne. In *Médicine Reproduction Masculine* (G. Schaison, P. Bouchard, J. Mahoudeau, and F. Labrie, eds.), pp. 7-14. Paris, Flammarion Pub.

Josso, N., Picard, J-Y., and Tran, D. (1977) The antimüllerian hormone. *Recent Progress in Hormone Research*, 33:117-167.

Migeon C. J. and Forest, M. G. (1980) Androgens in biological fluids. In *Nuclear Medicine in Vitro*, 2nd ed. (B. Rothfeld, ed.), pp. 145-170. Philadelphia, Lippincott.

Money, J. (1952) *Hermaphroditism: An Inquiry into the Nature of a Human Paradox*. Doctoral Dissertation, Harvard University. Ann Arbor, University Microfilms.

Money, J. (1955) Hermaphroditism, gender and precocity in hyperadrenocorticism: Psychologic findings. *Bulletin of The Johns Hopkins Hospital*, 96:253-264.

Money, J. (1974) Prenatal hormones and postnatal socialization in gender identity differentiation. In *Nebraska Symposium on Motivation, 1973*, (J. K. Cole and R. Dienstbier, eds.). Lincoln, University of Nebraska Press, 1974.

Money, J. (1984) Gender-transposition theory and homosexual genesis. *Journal of Sex and Marital Therapy,* 10:75-82.

Reinisch, J. M., Rosenblum, L. A. and Sanders, S. A., eds. (1986) *Masculinity/Femininity: Concepts and Definitions,* New York, Oxford University Press (in press).

Note

Written for the International Symposium on Male Sexual Differentiation, organized by Claude J. Migeon, June 15-17, 1985, at the Johns Hopkins University and Hospital; and presented with H. Devore and B. F. Norman as coauthors.

TWENTY-SIX

The Development of Sexuality
and Eroticism in Humankind

Abstract

Sexuality includes eroticism. Though its determinants are multivariate and developmentally sequential, most current biological theories arbitrarily exclude social determinants, and vice versa. Developmentally, masculinization is not necessarily synonymous with defeminization, nor feminization with demasculinization. In the development of brain and behavior, behavior that appears to be either male or female may actually be sex-shared but sex-different in the threshold for its expression. Parent-child bonding is a precursor of subsequent erotosexual pair-bonding. Suppression of erotosexual rehearsal play in childhood is a precursor of postpubertal and adult erotosexual pathology. The criterion defining the heterosexual, bisexual, and homosexual conditions is the sex of the partner with whom a limerent (falling-in-love) pairbond is possible; and there is no evidence that pubertal sex steroids, per se, are responsible for which of the three it will be. The phases of an erotosexual encounter are proception, acception, and conception. The disorders of proception, manifested in both imagery and practice, are the paraphilic syndromes (formerly known as perversions). The disorders of acception may be either hypophilic deficiencies, or hyperphilic increases. The disorders of conception are those of infertility. There is a nonsystematic relationship of erotosexualism to the hormonal cycle of the menses and to gerontological hormonal changes.

Sexuality and Eroticism

Sexuality in animals is usually equated with, and referred to as reproductive behavior or reproductive biology.

Reproduction is more respectable than sex. Except on documents requiring name, sex and age, sex is still a dirty word among many scientists as well as among nonscientists of the new right, and sexology as science is demoted to being bawdry more than scholarship. Reproductive biologists and sexologists seldom attend the same meetings or publish together in the same journals.

Sexuality in human beings may also be equated with reproductive behavior and biology, in which case it has to do chiefly with fertility and infertility, cyclicity, gestation, and delivery; and is evasive with respect to coition, carnal lust, and pairbonded love. Human reproductive biology cannot, however, be divorced from love, carnal pleasures, and coition, except maybe in such a test case as that of donor insemination—and even in that case, imagery may fill the void. In clinical usage, sexuality is the term that, in recent years, has been used to reunite reproduction as respectable science with carnal passion as suspect science. For centuries the church defined passion as sin, even for husband and wife (Boswell, 1980; Bullough, 1976); and to a residual extent, this definition still permeates the law and society. Even today, the term sexuality as used in science excludes much of what is conveyed by the companion term, erotic. Sexuality has as its etymological root the Latin verb meaning to cut or divide—into male and female. Thus, sexuality tends not to be as wide-ranging as eroticism, which has as its etymological root, *Eros,* love. Eroticism embraces sexual union, but much more as well, especially in imagery including verbal ideational imagery, and fantasy. [In this review, the term "imagery" always includes verbal ideational imagery as well as pictorial, tactual, or any other imagery generated through sensory perception directly or retrieved from memory.] For the church, sexual passion in marriage was sin enough, but eroticism ranged far beyond the constraints of marriage and so was even more sinful. Eroticism included all the unconventional expressions of sex, including what are known today as the paraphilias. Formerly they were the perversions. Some of them, particularly the fetishes, may exist independently of a partner.

There is a need for a term that signifies both the sexual and the erotic as a unity. For lack of another, *erotosexual* is that term. It ensures a unity between that which takes place between the ears, and that which takes place between the groins. Developmentally, the two take place as one.

Reductionism vs. Multivariate Complexity

The principle of multivariate sequential determinism is the ultimate and absolutely imperative foundation of any trustworthy theory of the development of human sexuality. Among contemporary theorists, this principle is violated more often than it is obeyed. With ontogenetic single-mindedness of purpose, people all too often follow a reductionist dogma. Theoretically, they reduce the origins and development of human sexuality to a single and usually abstrusely defined determinant which typically belongs on one side or the other of the absolute nature-nurture fence. Foolishly, they juxtapose biology against the socioculturally acquired or learned, unmindful of the fact that there is a biology of learning and memory, albeit mostly undiscovered, as yet. Like the heredity-environment protagonists, they wrongly equate the biological with the fixed and preordained, and the sociocultural with the unfixed and optional. By implication, the preordained is unmodifiable, and the arbitrary modifiable. Herein lurks another implication, a covertly political one. Scientists of the status quo favor a reductionist dogma of the biological unmodifiability of anything in men's and women's sexuality. Scientists of change favor another reductionist dogma, that of the sociocultural and environmental modifiability of everything in men's and women's sexuality.

In the prestige hierarchy of today's science, the biological sciences rate higher than the social sciences. With respect to human sexuality, therefore, there is a deferential attraction among many scientists toward reductionist explanations derived from what is traditionally classified as biology, for example, genetics and endocrinology. Sociocultural explanations are dismissed as non-biological. Quite to the contrary, sociocultural determinants of the development of human erotosexuality are neurochemically mediated through the brain and its peripheral nervous system. Mediation is by way of the transmission of sound and light signals that enter the system by way of the ears and eyes, and chemical, pressure, and temperature signals that enter the nose, mouth, and skin. All are then transmitted as chemical and electrical signals to the brain. There should be no surprise here, for there is, in the development of human beings, an exact parallel with native language. A neonate must be human, and must have a healthy brain, in order to develop a native language. Without the stimulus input, normally auditory, from others who already use a language, the baby will not, however, develop a native language. Sexuality parallels language. A neonate needs to have been born with a healthy human brain in order to develop a human erotosexuality as male or female. The end product is not, however, fully preordained at birth. Its development requires the stimulus input of others who already differentiate and define all the manifestations of erotosexuality as male or female.

The theoretical temptation to neglect sociocultural input into the brain as a component determinant of human erotosexuality is attributable in part to ethical restriction on human experimentation, and in part to the fact that pertinent investigative techniques that are ethically acceptable have not yet been discovered. In addition, there is also the extremely influential fact that the preponderance of laboratory research is done on four-legged rodents and other subprimate species. In these species sexuality and eroticism are governed under a hormonal dictatorship far more rigid than is the case in the primate species with their uniquely hypertrophied cerebral cortices (Beach, 1948). In human beings it need scarcely be said that erotosexualism exists as much between the ears, in the cerebral cortex, as between the groins, in the genitalia. The brain is the organ where erotosexual imagery is learned and remembered, and from which it is retrieved and communicated behaviorally and in words. Other species, no matter how they experience erotosexual imagery, cannot communicate it linguistically. Science lacks the technical expertise, as yet, to read it directly from their brains. Thus it is not possible for a nonhuman species to serve as an animal model for the complete experimental study of sexuality and eroticism as it applies to human beings. Animal models are, to be sure, indispensible. Yet, erotosexual theory derived from animal models alone will be insufficient to parallel and explain human erotosexualism. To illustrate: there is no human counterpart of *Cnemidophorus uniparens* (Crews and Fitzgerald, 1980), a parthenogenic species of lizard in which, though there are no males, a lizard is better able to mature and lay her eggs if first she is mounted by another, nonovulatory lizard who goes through the motions of cloacal copulation typical of the male in other, closely related species.

As applied to selected animal models, a reductionist theory in which hormones are cause, and behavior is effect may suffice, but in human beings more is needed to explain erotosexual masculinity or femininity and also to explain the nonerotic aspects of gender-identity and role (G-I/R).

5α-Reductase

A currently popular reductionist hypothesis argued ad absurdum is that of Imperato-McGinley and coworkers (1974, 1976, 1979) regarding the role of a 5α-reductase as a determinant of human "male sex drive" and "male gender-identity." The hypothesis is based on a three-generation pedigree of 38 hermaphroditic individuals born to 23 interrelated families in two inbred mountain villages in the Dominican Republic. All have the syndrome of 46,XY, 5α-reductase deficiency hermaphroditism. Without 5α-reductase, testosterone is not converted to dihydrotestosterone. Without dihydrotestosterone in fetal life, it is postulated, the external genitalia of a gonadal male fail to differentiate completely as male, and the baby is born with genitalia that appear more female than male. At the time of puberty, 5α-reductase deficiency does not bring about any further feminization, but is responsible for a mild to moderate demasculinization, namely, impairment of secondary sexual virilization. Imperato-McGinley and co-authors (1974), ignoring this impairment, postulated that testosterone without dihydrotestosterone is sufficient for the somatic virilization of puberty; and further claimed that the phallus—clitoridic, hypospadiac, and bound down with chordee—"enlarges to become a functional penis" (p. 1213), which is, in fact, anatomically not possible. These same authors further claimed that testosterone without dihydrotestosterone was sufficient to produce a "male sex drive" and "male gender identity" at puberty. They based this claim on the fact that 19 of the hermaphrodites had been assigned the female status at birth, and that 16 of them later changed to live as men and allegedly changed their gender identities.

To postulate testosterone as the cause of a male gender identity solely on the basis of a hermaphrodite's change of gender status in public is a reductionist folly (Rubin, Reinisch, and Haskett, 1981). There are other factors to be taken into account. In the case of these Dominican hermaphrodites, they were known from birth onward to have a birth defect of the sex organs, and it remained uncorrected. Thus the parents could not assign a hermaphroditic baby as either girl or boy with the same conviction as they could the nondefective brothers and sisters. Likewise with the rearing, there would always be knowledge of the defect; and in fact the hermaphroditic children were raised as "guevedoces" ("balls" at twelve), and not entirely unambiguously as either girls or boys. Hence there is every likelihood that those who had been assigned as girls and were being reared with a girl's name would not differentiate a girl's gender identity (or G-I/R), but an ambiguous or boyish one. Then at puberty, with still no clinical intervention to feminize the body hormonally and surgically, its totally nonfeminine appearance gave further confirmation of nonfeminine status. The child obtained this confirmation both directly from the appearance and proprioception of the body, and directly from the reaction of family members, villagers, and village authorities.

Male and female role stereotypes are rigidly dichotomous in a rural Latin-American culture. To be a mannish-appearing woman without breasts, without menses, and without fertility is to be unmarriageable in a society where the unmarried daughter is a family and community liability. The common-sense conclusion for all concerned, the priest and other village authorities included, is to endorse and legally accept a change of gender status, provided the individual concerned does not repudiate it. Here the social and the hormonal definition of sex both work together congruently. The congruence is all the more favorable when male status begins at birth with assignment of the guevedoce as a boy, except that a man with a defective penis too small for copulation, surgical repair notwithstanding, has a problem in perpetuity that no amount of professional euphemizing can ever euphemize away.

Erotosexualism and G-I/R

Except for some types of hermaphrodite or intersex, people are born with the genital morphology of male or female. That morphology usually dictates the sex of their rearing. Probably the only exception occurs when a baby with a normal penis and empty scrotum is diagnosed as having the adrenogenital syndrome, and is found to be chromosomally 46,XX and gonadally ovarian. In some, though not all such cases (Money and Daléry, 1972), the penis is extirpated, the vagina opened up, and the sex is reassigned as female. Even such a rare case in which the external genitalia are surgically revised serves to reinforce the universal assumption that the morphology of the external genitals of the neonate can be relied upon to prognosticate erotosexual development as male or female, respectively. So confident is this prognostication that folk wisdom has for generations wrongly attributed male and female erotosexualism to the inevitability of preordained instinct.

The prognostication actually encompasses more than erotosexualism. It applies also to the nonerotosexual aspects of being either male or female, masculine or feminine, for the totality of masculinity or femininity is greater than being simply masculine or feminine in the narrow erotosexual sense. The totality includes work and play, legal status, education, manners, etiquette, and grooming. It includes, indeed, all of one's very identity and role as boy or girl, man or woman, for male-female dimorphism perfuses an influence far beyond the narrow confines of the sex organs.

The need for some term to designate this totality I recognized as imperative early in the 1950s, when I tangled with the problem of writing about not only the copulatory roles but also the overall masculine and/or feminine psychology and behavior of hermaphroditic or intersexed individuals whose social and legal sex was, in many instances, discordant singly or severally with their chromosomal, gonadal, or morphologic sex at birth. The need was met by borrowing the term "gender" from its use in philology, to coin the expression "gender role," which was originally defined (Money, 1955) thus: "The term gender role is used to signify all those things that a person says or does to disclose himself or herself as having the status of boy or man, girl or woman, respectively. It includes but is not restricted to eroticism." Eventually it became necessary to divide gender identity from gender role, even though they are two sides of the same coin, because people proved incapable of conceptualizing their essential unity.

The subdivided definition appeared in Money and Ehrhardt (1972), as follows: "Gender Identity: the sameness, unity, and persistence of one's individuality as male or female (or ambivalent), in greater or lesser degree, especially as it is experienced in self-awareness and behavior. Gender identity is the private experience of gender role, and gender role is the public expression of gender identity. Gender Role: Everything that a person says and does, to indicate to others or to the self the degree in which one is male or female or ambivalent. It includes but is not restricted to sexual arousal and response. Gender role is the public expression of gender identity, and gender identity is the private experience of gender role."

Gender identity is not, as commonly misconstrued, a simple assertion of "I am a male," or "I am a female," and it does not exclude, as is also commonly misconstrued, sexual and erotic components.

G-I/R (gender-identity/role) is the acronym that unites the divided halves. It is defined (Money, 1980) as: "Gender-Identity/Role (G-I/R): gender identity is the private experience of gender role, and gender role is the public manifestation of gender identity. Gender identity is the sameness, unity, and persistence of one's individuality as male, female, or ambivalent, in greater or lesser degree, especially as it is experienced in self-awareness and behavior. Gender role is everything that a person says and does to indicate to others or to the self the degree that one is either male or female, or ambivalent; it includes but is not restricted to sexual arousal and response."

The development of G-I/R from infancy onward always has an erotosexual component along with its nonerotosexual components. The degree of concordance among them is variable. Thus, it is possible to speak of a boy who develops a homosexual G-I/R that manifests itself only in erotosexual activity with a partner, and not in behavior at the workplace, whereas another person with a homosexual G-I/R in erotosexual activity with a partner is also a "flaming queen" in public. It is wrong to say of a certain type or homosexual man that he has a masculine gender identity but a homosexual preference or object choice. The correct statement for such a man is that his G-I/R is masculine except in its erotosexual aspects. Counterpart statements apply to lesbianism.

There are many anomalies of the erotosexual component of G-I/R that do not involve the homosexual-heterosexual dimension. Thus one may speak of a sadistic or masochistic G-I/R, and exhibitionistic or voyeuristic G-I/R, and so on through the list of the approximately forty paraphilic G-I/Rs.

Genetics and H-Y Antigen

Formerly, the story of developmental human erotosexuality began with sex-determination by the XX or XY chromosomal constitutions. The newest addition to that process pertains to the H-Y antigen, the Y-chromosome-induced histocompatibility factor (Ohno, 1978; Wachtel, 1978), discovered in 1976. Until 1979, there appeared to be no exception to the rule that the human embryo would fail to differentiate the primitive gonadal anlagen into testes in the absence of H-Y antigen. Conversely, in the presence of H-Y antigen, testes would always differentiate. In 1979 the absoluteness of that rule was questioned by the findings of Eicher and co-authors (1979), namely, that male-to-female transexuals, who are born with testes, are negative for the H-Y antigen. Conversely, female-to-male transexuals, who are born with ovaries, are positive for the H-Y antigen. These findings, provided they are replicated (which has currently proved impossible), will alter the theory of the determinism and development of human erotosexualism in a way not yet ascertained.

Prenatal Hormones

In human beings, there is no evidence that the X or the Y chromosomes which inhabit all of the cells of the body, including those of the brain, have, simply by reason of their presence in the cells, a direct effect on a person's erotosexual status. Rather, they have an indirect and derivative influence by way of their governing the differentiation of the embryonic gonadal anlagen into either testes or ovaries which, in turn, govern the level of testosterone in the fetal blood stream. There is no evidence against this generalization, even when all of the body's cells contain a supernumerary X or Y chromosome, as in the 47,XXX, the 47,XXY (Klinefelter's), and the 47,XYY syndromes, despite the fact that in some patients with these syndromes cerebral cortical function may be pathological.

The situation is somewhat different when one sex chromosome is absent. There is no 45,Y syndrome, a fetus without an X chromosome being nonviable. The converse is the 45,X (Turner's) syndrome, or one of its mosaic or other variants, In Turner's syndrome, one of the embryonic consequences of the cytogenetic anomaly is that gonads fail to differentiate, and without gonads, there are no gonadal hormones, and without gonadal hormones the fetus always differentiates morphologically as female. Thus the erotosexual status of Turner's syndrome in adulthood, which is all but invariably feminine, cannot be attributed to the cytogenetic status alone, without implicating also the antecedent variables associated with a female morphology, female rearing, and female hormonal replacement and rehabilitation in teen-age and adulthood.

Turner's syndrome has importance in experimental ethics insofar as it is a human experiment of nature which is the equivalent of what in animal research would be enforced fetal agonadism or castration. There is one other such experiment of nature, one that affects human pedigrees, namely the androgen-insensitivity syndrome, a syndrome in which a 46,XY fetus differentiates morphologically as a female, there being a permanent intracellular incapacity of all cells in the body to utilize androgen.

These two syndromes raise a question regarding the role of maternal and placental hormones in the development of the mammalian embryo as male or female. In animal experiments, too much estrogen or progestin given to the pregnant mother is incompatible with the maintenance of gestation. The presence of these hormones in normal gestation raises the question of why they do not interfere with the masculinization of the male-differentiating fetus. The answer to this question implicates serum α-fetoprotein. According to the most commonly cited hypothesis (Baum, 1979), which is derived chiefly from experimentation on rodents, this substance captures circulating serum estradiol of maternal, placental, or other origin and protects the fetal brain of either sex from its influence. The fetal male brain, in need of estradiol for its developmental masculinization, is then able to obtain it by converting its own circulating testicular testosterone to estradiol intracellularly (Naftolin et al., 1975; McEwen, 1980). According to an alternative hypothesis (Döhler, 1978), α-fetoprotein captures all but the minimal quantity of maternal estradiol required for feminization of the brain of the developing daughter fetus. This minimal quantity is also supplied to the fetus developing as a son, but its feminizing effect is completely obliterated and transformed into masculinization under the augmenting influence of additional estradiol aromatized, intracellularly, from testosterone of fetal testicular origin (see below). There is little if any evidence that in primates aromatization is necessary for differentiation of the brain or activation of behavior. In human beings the evidence is against α-fetoprotein acting as an estrogen-binding agent. The more favored hypothesis is that progesterone acts as a protective antivirilizing agent in the developing human female fetus.

Abramovich and Rowe (1973) demonstrated that in the human male fetus from the 12th to 18th week of gestation the levels of testosterone (mainly of testicular origin) and of androstenedione (mainly of adrenocortical origin) are higher than in the female fetus. Whether these hormones are, at this period of gestation, used by the brain is not known. The same applies to the postnatal surge of testosterone in males, a surge that peaks between the second and third month of life; then it declines until between the fourth and fifth month it stabilizes at the low level of prepuberty (Forest, Cathiard, and Bertrand, 1973; Forest, Saez, and Bertrand, 1973; Forest, Sizonenko, Cathiard, and Bertrand,

1974). In newborn girls, the low prepubertal level of testosterone is attained by the second week of life.

In the early days of fetal endrocrinology, a simple formula seemed to apply (Money and Ehrhardt, 1972), namely, that with androgen in the proper amount, the fetus differentiates as male; without androgen it differentiates as female. In all of its simplicity, this rule applied across species, and irrespective of chromosomal sex or of gonadal sex. It applied also irrespective of the source of androgen and of the organ system involved, including the brain and its subsequent mediation of sex-dimorphic behavior. The constraints on this formula's applicability applied to the amount of hormone and to its timing, there being a critical developmental period for the induction of a specific androgenic effect. There was one exception to the rule, namely, that suppression of the differentiation of a uterus in a male fetus is dependent on a fetal mullerian inhibiting substance or factor (MIF), of which the biochemical formula still remains unascertained. MIF is a nonandrogenic secretion from the fetal testes.

The nice simplicity of the classification of the sex steroids, on the basis of their biochemical structure, as androgenic, estrogenic, or progestinic, proved not always to correlate with the effects of their activity in vivo. In particular, it has been quite conclusively demonstrated that the effects of experimental injections of the primarily testicular hormone, testosterone, can in some instances be replicated by injections of the primarily ovarian hormone, estradiol (Baum, 1979). The key to this apparent paradox lies jointly in the fact that the biosynthesis of sex steroidal hormones, in vivo, is from cholesterol to progestin to androgen to estrogen; and in the fact that the molecule of one steriod hormone can be taken up intracellularly and transformed to another. One such transformation is the intracellular aromatization of testosterone to the estrogen, estradiol. Another is the 5 α-reductase metabolic reduction of testosterone to dihydrotestosterone (Baum, 1979).

It is now widely recognized that different components of the reproductive system, as widely separated anatomically as the brain and, say, the prostrate, have a different prenatal history of the intracellular transformation and usage of androgen. In fetal life, differentiation of the pelvic genitalia as male is hypothesized to be dependent on intracellular 5α-reduction of testosterone to dihydrotestosterone (Walsh et al., 1974; Maes et al., 1979). By contrast, prenatal differentiation of brain pathways to mediate stereotypically masculine behavior patterns in later life is hypothesized to depend, at least in part, on intracellular aromatization of testosterone to estradiol (Naftolin et al., 1975). For both hypotheses, there is a growing body of mammalian and avian experimental support. Across species, their applicability remains to be ascertained. Within a given species, their applicability still needs to be spelled out in terms of amount, developmental timing, specific organs or structures involved, and synergism with other hormones, neurotransmitters, and related body chemistries. Claims to the contrary notwithstanding (Imperato-McGinley et al., 1974), there is in the case of the human species no evidence to justify, as yet, the application of either the aromatization or the 5α-reductase hypothesis to the brain's differentiation and development of erotosexual status in prepuberty, adolescence, or adulthood as male, female, or mixed.

Masculinized, Feminized; Demasculinized, Defeminized

Embryologically, the process whereby sexual dimorphism differentiates is either unitypic or ambitypic. The ambitypic process applies to the differentiating gonad, which first passes through a corticomedullary phase, after which either the cortex or the medulla becomes vestigial—the cortex yields to the medulla when the organ becomes a testis, and vice versa for an ovary. Subsequently, the ambitypic process applies also to the internal differentiation of sexual dimorphism, which passes through a mullerian/wolffian duct phase after which either the mullerian or the wolffian ducts become vestigial—mullerian duct vestigiation and wolffian duct proliferation characterize male differentiation; and vice versa, for female differentiation.

The next and external phase of dimorphic differentiation as male or female is unitypic. That is to say, there is only one set, not two, of undifferentiated precursors of the external genitalia. They are the same for both sexes, but they develop differently, though homologously, as male or as female. They may differentiate incompletely and appear hermaphroditically ambiguous, but they cannot differentiate as two coexistent sets, male and female. By contrast, it is possible for a gonad to differentiate as an ovotestis, and it is possible for both mullerian and wolffian structures to coexist in the same person.

The next phase of dimorphic differentiation as male or female partly overlaps with the external genital phase and partly extends beyond it into postnatal life. This is the phase that pertains to hormonally induced dimorphism of the brain and its governance of behavior. The theoretical basis of earlier investigation, both experimental and clinical, was naively assimilated from folk tradition, supposing an absolute and mutually exclusive male-female dichotomy. Using the new terminology of this present review, differentiation of the brain was assumed to be unitypic, on the model of the external genitalia. To be masculinized was synonymous with being unfeminized (or defeminized), and to be feminized was synonymous with being unmasculinized (or demasculinized).

The weight of experimental evidence now requires a theoretical change in favor of the ambitypic model. That is to say, there are in the brain two schemas, each one having its own set of neural pathways. Developmental activation of the one does not reciprocally deactivate the other (Ward, 1972; 1977; Baum, 1979). Activation and deactivation are two separate, though possibly linked processes. To illustrate, it is possible for a male animal to mount a female whereas, under changed circumstances, it will get into the lordosis position and be mounted by another male (or possibly by a female). The behavior of such an animal shows that masculinization, does not automatically signify defeminization, and vice versa. Masculinization and feminization may coexist, bisexually. The ratio of masculine to feminine is not a perfect bisexual 50:50. Any ratio may be represented, over the entire range from 100:0 to 0:100.

The bisexual ratio is partly a function of species differences and, within a species, of individual differences in the determinants of sexual differentiation. These differences are well illustrated in the comparison of hamster and rat (Money and Ehrhardt, 1972). Under experimental circumstances, the normal male hamster can readily be induced to manifest both mounting and lordosis, whereas lordosis is seldom observed in the male rat. It is possible, however, to manipulate experimentally the determinants of sexual behavior in selected individuals of either species so as to make the hamster less bisexual and the rat more so. In the hamster, the method is to inject the neonate with testosterone, thus bringing about what must be called a degree of ultramasculinization. In the rat, the converse effect can be produced by deandrogenizing the neonate either by surgical castration or by hormonal antiandrogenization. A similar effect can be experimentally induced prenatally by subjecting the mother to constraint under intense bright light. The disruption of maternal hormone secretion thus produced has a derivative effect on the male fetus and, eventually, on its bisexual behavioral ratio (Ward and Weisz, 1980).

Sex-Shared/Threshold-Dimorphic Response

The influence of hormones, either prenatally or neonatally, on the bisexual ratio is best conceived in terms of a threshold effect, and hormonal alteration as a resetting of the threshold. Sexual dimorphism is a characteristic not of the response, per se, but of the threshold for its emergence under given stimulus circumstances. The response is sex-shared but threshold-dimorphic.

In human beings, the catalogue of sex-shared/threshold dimorphic behavior for which the threshold is determined in part by the influence of prenatal hormones on the central nervous system cannot be established by experimenting on human beings. One must rely instead on animal, predominantly primate, models, and especially on human clinical models. One such model is the congenital masculinizing adrenogenital syndrome in 46,XX gonadal females, some of whom are prenatally so masculinized that they are born without a clitoris and vulva but with a normal penis and an empty scrotum. At the opposite extreme is the congenital feminizing androgen-insensitivity syndrome in 46,XY gonadal males who, when androgen insensitivity is complete, are born with a clitoris and normal vulva and with no penis and scrotum. Between these extremes, there are various other syndromes in which at birth the external genitalia appear neither typically male nor female, but ambiguously hermaphroditic. These are the syndromes in which, because there is no unanimity among either professionals or the laity, some babies may be publicly declared and reared as boys and others, with the very same syndrome, as girls. These are the cases, concordant for prenatal history, but discordant for postnatal history, that constitute a gold mine of comparative information regarding the prenatal versus postnatal components of sex-shared/threshold-dimorphic behavior (Money and Ehrhardt, 1972).

On the basis of comparative animal and clinical models, it is possible to delineate at least nine components of behavior that qualify as sex-shared but threshold-dimorphic (Money, 1980).

First is kinetic energy expenditure, which, in its more vigorous, outdoor, athletic manifestations is typically more readily elicited and prevalent in males than females, even before males reach the postpubertal stage of being, on the average, taller, heavier, and more muscular than females.

Second is roaming and becoming familiar with or marking the boundaries of the roaming range. Whereas pheromonal (odoriferous) marking is characteristic of some small animals, in primates, including man, vision takes the place of smell. The secretion of marker pheromones is largely under the regulation of the male sex hormone and thus is more readily elicited in males than females. The extent of any sex difference in the threshold for visual marking in primates is still conjectural.

Third is competitive rivalry and assertiveness for a position in the dominance hierarchy of childhood, which is more readily elicited in boys than in girls. A position of dominance may be accorded an individual without fighting, or after a victory. Whereas fighting and aggressiveness per se are not sexually dimorphic, despite a widespread scientific assumption that they are, sensitivity to eliciting stimuli may or may not be. An example of the latter is retaliation against a deserter or rival in love or friendship, which is not sex-specific.

Fourth is fighting off predators in defense of the troop and its territory, which, among primates, is typically more readily elicited in males than in females.

Fifth is fighting in defense of the young, which is more readily elicited in females than in males. Females are more fiercely alert and responsive to threats to their infants than, in general, are males.

Sixth is provision of a nest or safe place for the delivery, care, carrying, and suckling of the young. It is possible that this variable is associated with a greater prevalence of domestic neatness in girls than boys, as compared with the disarray that is the product of, among other things, vigorous kinetic energy expenditure.

Seventh is parentalism, exclusive of delivery and suckling. Retrieving, protecting, cuddling, rocking, and clinging to the young is more prevalent in girls' rehearsal play with dolls and playmates than in the play of boys.

Eighth is sexual rehearsal play, in which evidence derived from monkeys is that juvenile males elicit presentation responses from females, and that juvenile females elicit mounting responses from males, more readily than the opposite. The taboo on human juvenile sexual rehearsal play and on its scientific investigation prohibits any present generalization regarding boys and girls.

Ninth is the possibility that the visual erotic image more readily elicits an initiating erotic response in males than in females, whereas the tactile stimulus more readily elicits a response in females. Here again no generalization can yet be made with confidence, because of the effects of the erotic taboo and erotic stereotyping in our society.

Neonatal Bonding

Human postnatal erotosexual differentiation and development as male or female is not prewritten in the genetic code, nor in a hormonal or other prenatal coding process or program. The end of the story is not automatically preordained by its beginning, but is dependent also on postnatal input from the environment in which it is being written. As aforesaid, this same principal applies to the development of native language, which clearly depends on the prenatal development of a brain that is both human and unimpaired, and then on the postnatal input of exteroceptive language signals, usually through the ears.

At its onset, the postnatal phase of erotosexual differentiation is not gender-specific, but gender-shared. It begins neonatally in the bonding of the baby boy or girl to its mother. The bonding of the newborn to its mother begins as soon as the mother establishes eye contact and finger contact with it, and the same applies to the father (see review by Trause, Kennell, and Klaus, 1977, Ch. 57). Parent-infant bonding is essential to survival. Without it, there is a greatly increased risk of parental child neglect and abuse. With it, the baby is cuddled, fondled, kissed, stroked, and rocked, even before suckling is established. The haptic (related to touch) and kinesthetic components of infant-parent bonding are for the baby the prototype of what later in life will become lover-lover bonding. Impaired parent-infant bonding becomes a prototype of impaired lover-lover bonding.

Erection of a baby boy's penis in utero has been demonstrated by sonogram. Postnatally, erections continue spontaneously in sleep, as they will do at least three times a night throughout childhood and into advanced healthy old age (Karacan and coworkers, 1972, 1975). When the baby is awake and being bathed or diapered, more erections occur either spontaneously or in response to tactile or temperature stimulation. Evidence that there is a parallel phenomenon, possibly a vaginal blood-flow change, in the baby girl is uncertain. Whatever the final verdict, it is nonetheless clear that baby boys and girls experience their genitals differently from birth onward. It is what the genitals do, as well as what they look like, that engages the attention of the parent or other observer and elicits a gender-differentiated response. Depending upon whether the latter is positive or negative, it will, in turn, either reinforce or inhibit the baby's response. Either way, the effect will eventually become generalized to encompass far more than the reactivity of the genitalia. This is the interactive way that gender-differentiated behavior becomes built up in boys and girls. It is also the way in which either positive or negative erotosexual foundations are laid and built upon. In the case of boys who are neonatally circumcised an additional complexity is added in so far as their neonatal behavior as boys is partly dictated by parent-baby interaction with respect to the unanesthetized trauma of surgery and the subsequent pain of urine on a raw penis (Richards, Bernal, and Brackbill, 1976).

Freudian Doctrine

It scarcely needs saying that, ever since its enunciation early in this century, Freud's psychoanalytic doctrine of the sequence of oral, anal, and phallic stages has dominated developmental conceptions of psychosexuality in childhood. This doctrine has, in fact, become too dogmatic. The concept of the first stage puts too much emphasis on suckling and the mouth, to the exclusion of the sensuousness of haptic skin contact and body motion, and it also overlooks the specificity of infant-parent bonding. The concept of the second, or anal, stage exaggerates the sensuous significance of elimination and the discipline of training, at the expense of recognizing the maturational and cross-species significance of territorial marking with urinary pheromones, and of finding a private place to defecate and cover the excrement.

In classic psychoanalytic doctrine, the first two phases are together defined as pregenital, as terminating at around age three, and as not being gender-differentiated. In actual fact, however, the differentiaton of gender-identity/role (G-I/R) is well advanced by age three, so that one may conceptualize the differentiation of a core gender identity, as do some contemporary psycho-analysts (e.g., Stoller, 1964), far in advance of the phallic phase and its Oedipus complex, castration anxiety, and penis envy.

The Oedipus complex may well have constituted the imagery of Freud's own adolescent masturbation fantasy, in which case its extension to all of humanity is untenable. In so far as the Oedipal drama is a metaphor of early childhood development, it can be conceptualized in terms of identification and reciprocation in sexual rehearsal play.

Identification/Reciprocation

The differentiation of G-I/R as boyish or girlish is consolidated postnatally by way of the paired principles of identification and reciprocation or complementation (Money and Ehrhardt, 1972). Identification means learning by copying or imitating—doing or saying things the same way as some other person who constitutes the identification model. Reciprocation means learning by doing or saying things in such a way as to reciprocate or complement some other person, who is the reciprocation model. In either instance, the principle applies across a wide age range. Thus, an identification model may be as variable in age as a parent or an age-mate. Identification with a same-sexed parent is axiomatic to many theories of child development, though its exact prevalence and extent are probably overestimated at the expense of identification with other models, especially siblings and members of the peer group. Identification may also take place with models in absentia, for example, with characters in books and on television. The same applies, vice versa, to reciprocation, in which case reciprocating to a character in print or on television takes place in fantasy rather than in actuality.

In the ultimate analysis, gender identification and reciprocation do, of course, take place in the brain. Thus there are two gender schemas in the brain, one typifying or stereotyping masculinity, and the other femininity. In most human beings the two schemas develop with well differentiated gender applicability—the identification schema as mine, and the complementation schema as thine, for the other gender. One governs my gender, and the other prophesies what to expect from those who belong to thy gender.

Developmentally, the brain thus postnatally differentiates as gender ambitypic. The potential for interchangeability between the two schemas is inversely related to age. In rare clinical cases, as in the syndrome of transvestophilia, the potential is never lost, and the person is able to alternate convincingly between identification and reciprocation as male and female in G-I/R, with two names, two wardrobes, two personalities (Money, 1974), and two occupations. Fertility in humans does not alternate as it does in some fish that are able to alternate their sex of breeding (Chan, 1970, 1977; Robertson, 1972; Zupanc, 1980). When alternation involves only the erotosexual component of G-I/R, in synchrony with whether the partner is male or female, then the phenomenon is that of bisexualism.

Flirtatious Rehearsal Play

In human infants of nursery school age, erotosexual identification and reciprocation can be observed in the context of flirtatious behavior between the sexes. A girl at this age can be very coquettish with, say, her father or other men of his generation, as well as with a same-aged playmate. Correspondingly, a boy at the same age can play the escort role with his mother, playmate, or other person. By age five or thereabouts, same-aged playmates in some instances become involved in kindergarten romances or love affairs. Most such bonds are transient, but some eventuate in a full-blown adolescent love affair and ultimately, maybe, in marriage.

Flirtation and romantic pair-bonding are not the only manifestations of early sexual rehearsal play. Rehearsal includes also explicit erotosexuality involving body contact and the sex organs (Martinson, 1973). The best observed and recorded animal model of such rehearsal is the rhesus monkey (Goldfoot, 1977; Goldfoot and Wallen, 1978).

Erotosexual Rehearsal Play in Monkeys

When reared as members of a troop, baby rhesus monkeys typically begin to engage in erotosexual rehearsal play at age 3 months, approximately three to three and a half years prior to puberty. At first they climb on each other in all directions, in pairs or threes or fours, indiscriminate as to the sex of the partner, and as to which sex does the mounting, and which the presenting. At this stage of differentiation, the mounting and presenting behavior qualifies as ambitypic. Eventually it becomes more unitypic, but the sex of the partner depends partly on whether the peer group is sex-segregated or coeducational.

If there are, by experimental design, no males in the peer group, then there develops a hierarchy in which some females are more dominant and do more mounting. The converse happens in an all-male peer group, some being mounted more than they mount. In a mixed-sex group, the moves eventually become sorted out so that males predominantly mount females, and do so with the foot-clasp mount typical of mature mating—that is, with their own feet off the ground and grasping the shanks of the female, who presents in the quadrupedal position.

If totally deprived of erotosexual rehearsal play by being reared without age-similar playmates, a monkey, male or female, grows up unable to assume a position for mating, even with a gentle and experienced partner, and hence unable to reproduce its species. Less than total deprivation of erotosexual rehearsal play reduces the severity of the subsequent impairment. Thus, when male monkeys, permanently separated from their mothers at 3 to 6 months of age, were allowed half an hour of peer group play daily, about 30 per cent of them developed success at foot-clasp mounting, but its appearance was delayed by a year or more until they were 18 to 24 months of age. The remaining 70 per cent remained permanently impaired, unable to mount and breed. Even the successful 30 per cent were less proficient at copulation and breeding than animals reared in the wild.

Erotosexual Rehearsal Play in Humans

The erotosexual rehearsal play of monkeys needs the stimulus of playful age mates, but not, according to present evidence, an actual demonstration of other monkeys in the copulatory position. In human beings at ages 3 to 4 years, spontaneous erotosexual rehearsal play can be observed as pelvic rocking or thrusting movements as children lie side by side at nap time (Money, Cawte, Bianchi, and Nurcombe, 1970). The full range of erotosexual rehearsal play at this age should have been documented and classified in those few ethnic societies that do not prohibit it, but it has not been. Likewise, there is no documentation of whether children at age 5 to 6 years in these societies spontaneously extend their erotosexual rehearsal play to include coital positioning, or whether they copy positioning from the example of others who are older, but they do engage in coital positioning play from time to time. They do so without being socially obtrusive or objectionable.

The great majority of the world's children are raised under the influence of a stringent religious taboo on sex. Their infantile erotosexual rehearsal play, whether alone or with playmates, is subject to severe, often brutal, reprisals if it is discovered. Yet the evidence from rhesus monkeys confirms that copulatory rehearsal in infancy is an age-specific precursor and absolute prerequisite of successful copulation and breeding in adulthood.

Latency

Erotosexual rehearsal play in monkeys begins in infancy and continues in pre-puberty. There is no period of latency. Psychoanalytic doctrine notwithstanding, there is also no latency period in the erotosexual rehearsal play of human children. There is, however, a period when children assimilate the sexual taboo of our society. They collude in obeying the age-avoidancy demands of the sexual taboo, and practice erotosexual privacy, modesty, prudery, and neglect. In accordance with the allosex-avoidancy demands of the taboo, they do the same with age-mates of the opposite sex.

Maximally imposed, the sexual taboo requires not only privacy, modesty, prudery, and neglect, but complete suppression and eradication of erotosexual rehearsal play in prepuberty. The sanctions imposed for disobedience can be very traumatic and abusive. In addition to standard threats, beatings, and depriva-tions, they include bizarre assaults on the genitals with a knife or scissors, threats of amputation, or threats of infibulation with a needle and thread.

The long-term developmental effects of the prohibition, prevention, and punishment of prepubertal erotosexual rehearsal play, which in the so-called latency years includes heterosexual rehearsal play, have received negligible scientific attention. Texts on child development unanimously omit erotosexual development in prepuberty. It is the only aspect of child development that is off limits to empirical science. The subject is totally neglected in pediatric health care and in preventive pediatrics. Parents and professional persons collude in not finding out whether erotosexuality is developing healthily or pathologically in a child. To maintain ignorance is to maintain also the moral myth of innocence and the scientific myth of latency. Contradictory evidence is denied, neglected, or misconstrued—especially misconstrued as having been caught from the con-tagious bad influence of someone else.

Puberty

Proscriptions on erotosexuality in childhood notwithstanding, there are some recorded instances during prepuberty of incongruities that come into full flower only after puberty. For example, in longitudinal study, it has been demonstrated that persistent incongruity of gender role in its nonerotosexual aspects in pre-puberty evolves after puberty into a healthy homosexual G-I/R (Money and Russo, 1979). For the most part, however, it is only after the hormones of puberty lower the threshold for the emergence of erotosexual behavior and imagery (typically known only through the filter of verbal report) that the products of prepubertal development first become observed. The hormones of puberty activate or release patterns of erotosexual behavior or imagery for which the template, the lovemap, already exists. They do not create the template.

In vernacular parlance, one says that the sex hormones of puberty increase the sexual drive. Drive is a motivational concept, too amorphous to define operationally. In the present writing, motivation as an explanatory principle has not been used, and the principle of threshold has been substituted.

The mechanism governing the onset of puberty recently was traced by Wildt, Marshall, and Knobil (1980) to the arcuate region of the mediobasal hypo-thalamus and specifically to its pulsatile release of gonadotropin-releasing hormone (GnRH). In prepubertal female rhesus monkeys, experimental simula-tion of pulsatile GnRH release in pulses of 6 minutes once every hour induced hormonal puberty, complete with cycles of ovulation. To be effective, pulsatile, not tonic, release of GnRH was essential. Upon cessation of the experiment, the animals reverted to a prepubertal hormonal status and stayed that way for several months until, when aged between 24 and 30 months, they became pubertal as normally expected. Only then, apparently, was the biological clock of the mediobasal hypothalamus set to begin its pulsatile function. The governance of the setting mechanism remains, as yet, unknown. Speculatively, the pineal has been implicated.

In human beings, the setting of the biological clock of puberty ranges widely, from as early as the first year of life, at the precocious extreme, to late teenage, at the delayed extreme. In either precocity or delay, there is a dis-crepancy between the age of the physique and the chronological age, while the social age (which includes the erotosexual age) is anchored firmly to neither one, but is closer to the chronological age, and also close to the social age of the friendship peer group. Pubertally precocious children do not become eroto-sexually wild and delinquent (Money and Alexander, 1969; Money and Walker, 1971), and pubertally delayed teenagers are not inevitably erotosexually inert, though they tend to be neglected by their pubertally developed age-mates, except in nonromantic comradeships (Money and Clopper, 1975; Clopper, Adelson, and Money, 1976; Money, Clopper, and Menefee, 1980). Though rare, it is not unknown for an older, pubertally undeveloped youth to have begun his sex life, to have sexual intercourse, and to achieve a dry-run orgasm (Money and Alexander, 1967).

Homosexual/Bisexual/Heterosexual

Hormonal investigations designed to distinguish homosexuals from heterosexuals have in general been directed more to steroidal hormones from the gonads than to peptide hormones from the pituitary, presumably because masculinity is falsely equated with androgen and femininity with estrogen, as aforesaid. Claims to the contrary notwithstanding, the overall verdict is that the hormones of puberty do not cause one's erotosexual status to be heterosexual, homosexual, or bisexual (Parks et al., 1974; Jaffee, McCormack, and Vaitukaitis, 1980).

More information is needed regarding erotosexual status and gonadal-pituitary-hypothalamic interaction, for the weight of evidence from animals points to prenatal hormonal brain effects far more than postnatal ones as holding the key to the homosexual-heterosexual continuum. There are two published studies in which this more sophisticated approach has been utilized. Dörner and co-authors (1975), in a study still not replicated, measured the feedback effect of an injection of conjugated estrogens (Premarin) on the hypothalamic-pituitary governance of LH (luteinizing hormone) release from the pituitary. The subjects were men located in a venereal and skin disease clinic and were homosexual, bisexual, or heterosexual. Homosexual males were said to have first a decrease in serum LH and then a rebound elevation to a higher level than before receiving Premarin. The other men did not have the rebound elevation. Normal heterosexual females have a very high rebound.

Seyler, Canalis, Spare, and Reichlin (1978) test-treated female-to-male transsexual candidates with DES (diethylstilbestrol) administered orally for a week and then gave them an injection of LHRH (luteinizing-hormone releasing hormone). Heterosexual women so treated have an elevation of pituitary LH and FSH (follicle-stimulating hormone). In the female-to-male transsexuals, the elevation response was weak, and close to that of heterosexual men.

Concepts do not exist without terminology, but terminology may entrap and restrict concepts. The term, homosexual, restricts the concept to sex (same sex) at the expense of love (homophilia). So it is that science has long failed to recognize that the defining characteristic of the homosexual person is not sex, but love. The complete homosexual is a person who can fall in love or pairbond as a lover only with a person of the same genital morphology as the self. The complete heterosexual can fall in love only with a person without the same genital morphology as the self. Strictly speaking, the complete bisexual should be able to do both, though usually the bisexuality is not 50:50, but leans at least a little more to one sex than the other.

If the pairbonding experience of falling in love is the criterion of homosexuality and heterosexuality among human beings, then it is naive to expect to distinguish one type from the other on the basis of circulating gonadal steroids, for falling in love is not sex dimorphic but sex unimorphic.

Homosexual pairbondedness has been recorded in birds, for example, in mallard drakes (Schutz, 1965, 1967) and in female western gulls (Hunt and Hunt,

1977). Longterm avian pairbonding may be exclusively homosexual. In sub-human mammals, genital homosexual encounters may occur (Maple, 1977), but they are more sporadic than long-term, and mostly do not exclude heterosexual pairing as well. The animal model most closely approximating the human in this behavior is that of the stumptail macaque (Chevalier-Skolnikoff, 1974). In this species a lesbian relationship complete with orgasm occurring in the female doing the mounting has been photographed (Goldfoot, Westerborg-van Loon, Groenveld, and Slob, 1980).

Limerence

The experience of homosexual or heterosexual falling in love is the same for males and for females. It is the same also regardless of age. The first big love affair is usually after puberty, but it can happen in prepuberty (Money, 1980), or during any other part of the life span, including advanced age.

Limerence is a new word without etymological roots coined by Tennov (1979) to name that state of being that exists in a person who falls in love. When limerence is mutual, a high euphoria ensues. When it is less than mutual, an agony of anticipation and hope flaws the euphoria. Limerence unrequited or abandoned becomes the syndrome of love-sickness. Liebowitz and Klein (1979) have proposed a preliminary hypothesis that this syndrome may be associated with a depletion in the brain of phenylethylamine. There may be a permanent impairment of limerence as a sequel to brain surgery for a pituitary tumor, and also as a deficit accompanying idiopathic hypopituitarism (Money, Clopper, and Menefee, 1980).

The possessiveness of limerence in some people becomes irrational jealousy. Limerent jealousy is a watch-dog on duty to guard against a competitor or rival who might abduct one's partner. If it is too fierce, it may so restrict and alienate the partner it guards as to destroy the relationship. In the so-called crime of passion, it destroys the very partner, a paradox which is the ultimate in irrational self-sabotage and self-deprivation. Such paradoxical irrationality is characteristic of pathological jealousy.

Limerent jealousy and the violence that may accompany it are not sex-dimorphic. They may occur in either sex, in women as well as men, even though violence is culturally stereotyped as male.

Ever since the 12th century, when the troubadours of Provence formulated Europe's new philosophy of romantic or courtly love (Locke, 1978; Valency, 1961), limerence between lovers has become progressively the basis of the marriage contract. Before that time, and especially among European courtiers and the nobility, the marriage contract had been an arranged one—arranged by the two families on the basis of uniting their wealth, lands, and power and maintaining the unity of religion and race.

In troubadour philosophy, later exemplified in Shakespeare's *Romeo and*

Juliet, the lover was forever unattainable in marriage. In fact, the limerent passion of the lovelorn, if discovered in marriage, would bring ecclesiastical punishment, for the church taught either celibacy and chastity, or a minimum of passionless copulation for a maximum of marital reproduction (Valency, 1961). Here are found the historical origins of the split between romantic love and carnal lust—above the belt in public, and below the belt in private. After eight centuries, the split still survives in the "if-you-love-me" formula that unlocks the door to copulation between unmarried companions.

Mismatching

Today's troubadours are the writers of the lyrics of rock and roll and other popular songs. They still sing of the invincibility of limerent love as the touchstone of eternal bliss, erotosexual and otherwise. They are the chief source of love education for the young. Sometimes they sing of love spurned and failed, but they are short on explanations as to why lovers prove to be mismatched.

Lovers are mismatched on love above the belt less often than on lust below the belt. Above-the-belt erotosexualism is less negated in childhood than is lust below the belt. Developmentally, therefore, it is less subject to eccentric distortion and circuitous expression. Lovers can imagine what to expect of one another at the above-the belt stage of their encounter, and usually be correct.

Below-the-belt expectancies are different. They are much more frequently a source of lover mismatching. Below-the-belt erotosexualism, since it is heavily negated and unmonitored in childhood development, cannot be assumed to be uncomplicatedly heterosexual. It is likely to have developed with eccentric distortions and circuitous, paraphilic ways of circumventing the negations imposed on it. Thus the mutual expectancies that two lovers project onto one another, respectively, may not match the actuality of what each can, in fact, live up to. Such mismatching eventually leads to disillusionment regarding erotosexual function and enjoyment. It may induce secondary symptoms. It may lead to estrangement, separation, and divorce. Then, by having a consequent deleterious effect on the developing erotosexual health of the children, it ensures that erotosexual pathology will be transmitted to yet another generation.

Proception/Acception/Conception

The totality of a human erotosexual experience is conveniently subdivided into three phases, each of which has its own health and pathology: proception, acception, and conception. The term *proceptive* was proposed by Rosenzweig (1973) as an antonym for contraceptive (both contrasted with extraceptive or non-genital erotic behavior). Beach (1976) independently recommended the term *proception* with a different nuance, to refer to the interplay, usually highly stereotyped and species-specific, between the male and female prerequisite to intromission, and hence to conception.

In men and women, the proceptive phase is the phase of preparatory arousal. It is comprised of both imagery and practice. Image units (*imagerons* to coin a new term) in sequence become fantasies, usually visual or narrative, as in masturbation fantasies, coital fantasies, and wet dreams. Put into practice, erotosexual imagerons become practice units or *practicons* (to coin another new term). Fantasies become enacted in practices that are variously called courtship rituals, mating games, making-out, and foreplay. They are staged usually with a cast of two, possibly more, and with or without stage properties. There is no one-word generic term for these proceptive enactments.

In some species of animals and birds, the courtship ritual or mating dance of the proceptive phase is highly stereotyped and species-specific, with minimal individual variation. It is an essential prerequisite of copulation, which cannot be completed without it. In human beings, the imagery and enactment or staging of the proceptive phase also is prerequisite to copulation. It is not phyletically sterotyped but is ontogenetically variable. Variability exists between people, however, though not within one person over time. In fact, each person's proceptive imagery and its enactment tends to be stable, personally stereotypic, and habitually reiterated over long periods of time.

There is some evidence for the hypothesis that, relative to women, men are proceptively more dependent on vision and the visual image to release erotosexual arousal and initiative, whereas females are comparatively more dependent on touch and the tactile image. Cross-cultural evidence, particularly from those societies which endorse an erotosexual initiative in females, will be needed to test the possible cultural relativity and validity of this hypothesis.

Should the hypothesis hold across cultures, it would offer support for an explanatory theory that begins prenatally, when androgen prepares the way for erotosexual arousal to be linked with visual imagery. The content of the imagery has its input during the early childhood period of erotosexual rehearsal play. When standard heterosexual rehearsal play is displaced or thwarted, then heterosexual proceptive imagery becomes either deficient or revised. Extensively revised and altered, the imagery becomes that of a paraphilia. The paraphilias are more prevalent in men than women. Men's paraphilias involve visual imagery more often than tactual, women's being more often tactual (and also more subordinate than dominant).

The proceptive phase merges into the acceptive phase in which the two bodies accept or receive one another, mutually. The female is not unilaterally passive and receptive, and the male is not unilaterally active and intrusive. The penis accepts the vagina, and the vagina accepts the penis. In the build-up to orgasm, fantasy imagery that may have been prominent in the proceptive phase, and essential to arousal, typically yields to concentration on only sensory body feeling.

The conceptive phase may or may not follow proception and acception. It is the phase of pregnancy and parenthood and is a sequel to, as well as a component of erotosexualism.

Disorders of Proception

Proception may be subject to simple failure manifested as erotosexual apathy and inertia. Failure may be complete and total. It extends into the acceptive phase. The sex ratio, the prevalence, and the differential etiology of such failure remains largely unknown. Only rarely can a hormonal deficit be implicated. In some instances, erotosexual apathy and inertia are limited to adolescence and subsequently are self-correcting. In youth and young adulthood, they may temporarily mask a paraphilia that eventually manifests itself. Except when a hormonal deficit can be authenticated, there is no syndrome-specific therapy.

Proception may be dependent on paraphilic imagery in fantasy, practice, or both. In the absence of such imagery, erotosexual arousal and performance then fail or are deficient. In everyday speech, the imagery of a paraphilia is eccentric to the point of being bizarre. But there are no fixed criteria of what is eccentric, either statistically in terms of prevalence, or ideologically in terms of nonconformity to an arbitrary standard. There is no graduated scale on which to measure when eccentric becomes bizarre. There are no absolute standards by which to define tolerance of either the eccentric or the bizarre. Some very bizarre paraphilias are playful and harmless, and some are extremely noxious and traumatic. The former include many of the fetishisms. The latter include erotosexual self-strangulation, suicidal masochism, lethal sadism, violent pedophilia (child molestation), assaultive rapism, and lust murderism.

The imagery that makes an erotosexual fantasy or practice paraphilic has both phylographic (species) and idiographic (personal) origins. For example, it is phylographically determined that primates have the brain and peripheral nervous pathways that govern licking the newborn to keep them clean of feces and urine. It is not phylographically but idiographically determined that, in human cases of coprophilia and urophilia, these pathways will be recruited to subserve erotosexual arousal and the release of orgasm.

Coprophilia and urophilia are inclusion paraphilias. Inclusion paraphilias are those in which some image or practice that is not typically included in erotosexualism becomes included, and indeed imperative. There are also displacement paraphilias, of which voyeurism is an example. Looking at one's partner nude is typically included in erotosexualism. In voyeurism, looking, which must be surreptitious, is not simply included but actually displaces penovaginal practice as the trigger of orgasm. The voyeur who has a regular partner for penovaginal coitus builds up his arousal by prior peeping on a stranger, or while having intercourse replays the imagery of peeping as a coital fantasy. Otherwise his orgasm fails to eventuate.

The prevalence of paraphilia in adolescence or later has not been ascertained. It vastly exceeds those cases that are ascertained in clinics and courts. In the United States it almost certainly runs into the hundreds of thousands. The sex ratio is disproportionate, according to all the clinical and legal evidence available for both teenagers and older adults, with males greatly outnumbering females, and also having a wider range of paraphilias represented among them. The differential etiology has scarcely been investigated. In the neurosurgical literature (reviewed by Money and Pruce, 1977, Ch. 78) there are a few cases, no more than a score, in which a paraphilia proved to be associated with a temporal lobe lesion, and was responsive to surgery. Some paraphilic patients have nonoperable epilepsy, and others have clinically documented signs of neurological pathology. Of the vast majority of cases, it can be said only that the paraphilia is developmental in origin. As yet, no uniformity in the developmental biographies of paraphiliacs has been uncovered. The paraphilias do not appear like Athena from the head of Zeus, de novo, in adulthood. They afflict children at puberty and in adolescence, as well as later. They are not copied. They are not contagious. The most successful form of therapy combines hormonal antiandrogenic treatment with counseling therapy which, preferably, should be joint therapy for both the patient and partner (Money et al., 1975; Money, 1980, 1981).

Disorders of Acception

Disorders of the acceptive erotosexual phase are those in which the genitals themselves malfunction. The malfunction may be hyperphilic, that is, in excess, or hypophilic, that is, deficient.

Scientifically, the hyperphilias have for the most part been neglected or, perhaps with bantering envy, jokingly written off as nymphomania, erotomania, satyriasis, and Don Juanism. Behind the names, however, lies the fact that some men and women engage in some form of erotosexual activity with atypical frequency, or with many partners as couples or in groups. Rather than experiencing spaced diversity and variety, they may experience instead a compulsive repetitiousness that, like an addict, they cannot govern. For some the correct term is polyiterophilia, for they reiterate over and over again a limited and stereotyped pattern of behavior, changing only their partners. Hyperphilia includes also such phenomena as priapism, a pathological failure to detumesce; and excessive frequency of orgasm, hyperorgasmia, which can become almost the equivalent of an automatism. Hyperorgasmia is so frequently associated with paraphilia that it is virtually pathognomonic.

Until very recently it was believed that women were hyperphilic and abnormal if they claimed to ejaculate fluid at orgasm. New findings (Sevely and Bennett, 1978; Belzer, 1981; Addiego, et al., 1981; Perry, and Whipple, 1981) indicate that some women do secrete an ejaculatory fluid from the periurethral glands (the female homologue of the prostate); and that these glands engorge to form the Grafenberg spot from which orgasm can be released by either digital or penile pressure.

Recent findings have also confirmed that it is not hyperphilic for a man to be able, prior to ejaculating, to feel several sets of muscular contractions, measurable intraanally, of the same type as occur with ejaculation (Robbins and Jensen, 1978; Bohlen, Held, and Sanderson, 1980). These sets of contractions correspond to multiple orgasms experienced by some women prior to the final, big climax.

The hypophilias constitute the majority of the case load of today's sex therapists. In both sexes, they include coital aninsertia, which may carry over from proceptive fears, or may be a specific phobia of the penis or of the vagina; genital anesthesia; and coital pain or dyspareunia. The additional male hypophilias of impotence and premature ejaculation have, as their female counterparts, lubrication failure and vaginismus.

Prevalence regarding sex-ratio and age statistics for the various hyperphilias and hypophilias have not been ascertained. The hypophilias, especially impotence and premature ejaculation in males, and, in females, coital aninsertia (phobia of penetration) and anorgasmia, have been conjectured to affect up to 50 per cent of the population, regardless of age, though the criteria of evaluation are not standardized. The differential etiology ranges widely and includes: birth defects; prenatal brain hormonal anomaly; hormonal target-organ anomaly; toxic substance, prescribed or unprescribed; infection; neoplasm; surgical or accidental trauma; vascular anomaly; peripheral or cerebral neurologic anomaly; and neuropsychogenic dysfunction.

Recent publications on the etiology of impotence have shown that penile vascular disease and low penile blood pressure (lower at the end of the waking day than after lying down sleeping) are more frequent than has been traditionally believed (Michal and Pospíchal, 1978). Hormonal, especially pituitary, disorder has also been shown to have been too readily overlooked (Spark, White, and Connolly, 1980). Hyperprolactinemia, for example, has recently been implicated in some cases of impotence in men, as well as anovulation in women (Kolata, 1978; Merceron, Raymond, Courreges, and Klotz, 1977). Bromocriptine therapy lowers prolactin levels. Since prolactin is elevated in response to external stress, the differential etiology of hyperprolactinemia must always be established, and not be taken for granted as originating in a pituitary lesion.

The appropriate treatment of hyperphilias and hypophilias is, of course, related to their etiology. For hypophilias, the current vogue is for various modes of behavioral or psychological therapy, which together constitute the new sex therapy.

Erotosexual Cyclicity

The example of animals that copulate only when the female is ovulatory and in heat raises the question of whether there is a copulatory cycle in primates synchronous with the menstrual cycle. There has been a modest amount of human research (see reviews by McCauley and Ehrhardt, 1976; Baum, Everitt, Herbert, and Keverne, 1977; Money, 1980) directed toward the hypothesis of cyclic synchrony between hormones and behavior in women, and a minor amount of research concerning male and female synchrony. A deficiency in all of this literature is methodological. No studies have been designed to be comprehensively multivariate in approach. To illustrate, it is not feasible to investigate the synchrony of human coital frequency with the hormonal phase of the menstrual cycle without taking into account the personal moral and religious concepts and taboos of both partners regarding menstrual uncleanliness, orgasm by digital or oral stimulation, contraception, scheduled pregnancy, fear of pregnancy, and copulation as an enforced marital and reproductive duty. It is necessary to take into account also the partner's knowledge of ovulation and fertility, ovulatory and menstrual cramping, premenstrual symptoms, and the history of coital apathy, phobia, pain or dysfunction, including anorgasmia. There exists also the possibility of seasonal or other cycles superimposed on the menstrual cycle. Rossi and Rossi (1977) showed that menstrual mood patterns vary according to working days versus weekend days off work. Englander-Golden, Chang, Whitmore, and Dienstbier (1980) showed that self-reports on arousal and menstrual synchrony varied according to women's awareness of the purpose of the investigators.

With so many variables likely to influence cyclic menstrual synchrony of both erotosexuality and the general sense of well-being, it comes as no surprise that there is frequent lack of consistency among published findings. Such consistency as can be found indicates (Money, 1980) there may be a cyclic peak of erotosexual arousal in either imagery or practice, or both, as verbally reported, at around the time of the ovulatory peaking of estrogen and LH. This is the time when there is a peak in olfactory acuity (Money and Ehrhardt, 1972) and visual acuity (Diamond, Diamond, and Mast, 1972). Alternatively, or additionally, there may be an erotosexual peak that coincides with the estrogen/progesterone low point of the days of menstrual bleeding. Coincident with the ovulatory phase, plasma testosterone has been found to peak at a level somewhat higher than that of the early follicular phase that precedes it, and that of the late luteal phase that follows it (Persky et al., 1977). This finding needs replication. In women, exogenous testosterone enhances the initiation and prevalence, and possibly the intensity, of erotosexual arousal in imagery (experienced as desire) and practice (Money, 1961).

The erotosexual significance of the relationship between the circulating level of testosterone and the production of testosterone intracellularly by conversion from androstenedione is not known. Androstenedione is partly of adrenocortical origin. In primates, there is an increasing body of evidence (Gray and Gorzalka, 1980) that adrenocortical, as well as ovarian, androgen is essential to erotosexual arousal and practice in females.

Women differ in their reports as to whether they experience a peaking of erotosexualism more as an intaking and receptive yearning or an outgoing initiation of interaction. There is no systematically demonstrated relationship of this difference to either hormonal levels or cyclicity.

Independently of erotosexualism, there tends to be a low point in the sense of well-being synchronized in the luteal phase with the diminished level of estrogen and the build-up of progesterone in the premenstruum. In recent years this phenomenon, commonly referred to as premenstrual tension, has been hyperbolized into the premenstrual syndrome (Dalton, 1964). It is not universal, but ranges all the way from nonexistence to the extreme schizophreniform pathology of the periodic psychosis of puberty. This psychosis synchronizes with the waning of the gonadotropic and estrogenic peak of ovulation and can be controlled by treatment with a progestinic hormone that suppresses the estrogenic peak of ovulation.

The dysphoric phenomena of premenstrual tension are muted in women whose ovulation and hormonal cyclicity are suppressed by the oral contraceptive pill. Whether or not erotosexual arousal is increased or diminished by the pill is individually variable. In addition, arousal varies with the brand-name variations in hormonal content of the pill, so that no overall generalization is justified (Cullberg, 1972; Baum et al., 1977; Adams, Gold, and Burt, 1978).

Premenstrual tension in some women is followed by menstrual cramping induced by an excess secretion of prostaglandin, which brings on uterine contractions (Marx, 1979). Therapy is with an antiprostaglandin medication.

In many nonprimate mammals, mating synchrony between the sexes is mediated pheromonally by way of the nose. The male responds to the scent of the pheromone released from the vagina of the female at the time of ovulation. There is some evidence of a minor role of pheromones in mating synchrony in subhuman primates (Herbert, 1970; Michael, Keverne, and Bonsall, 1971), but for the most part olfactory signals are secondary to visual ones. In humankind, odor has been proposed as playing a role in establishing menstrual synchrony among women (McClintock, 1971; Hopson, 1979; Russell, Switz, and Thompson, 1980); but systematic evidence of pheromonal synchronization of copulation has not been forthcoming (Morris and Udry, 1978). That, of course, does not rule out the possibility that olfactory responsiveness occurs sporadically or in a subgroup minority of human beings, for example, in those who are extremely enthusiastic about oral sex.

There is some preliminary evidence, still awaiting replication, regarding male-female couple synchrony with respect to menstrual-cyclic temperature fluctuations (Henderson, 1976); and also with respect to the minor premenstrual peak in plasma level of testosterone (Persky et al., 1977). In both instances, if the man fluctuates, he does so in synchrony with the woman, when they live together as a couple.

The impact of pregnancy, especially frequent pregnancy, on the erotosexual synchrony of a couple has not been systematically investigated. The pros and cons of coitus during gestation vary according to folk belief or professional doctrine. Lack of systematic investigation also characterizes what is known about the erotosexual synchrony of a couple during lactation.

Erotosexual Gerontology

Inconsistency characterizes research data regarding not only the synchrony of erotosexuality with the menstrual cycle, but also—and for the same reason, namely, multivariate complexity—with the menopause and, in both sexes, the later geriatric years. Most variables have so far been studied singly, through lack of a statistic designed to handle developmental multivariate determinism. Moreover, most studies have been cross-sectional and not longitudinal, for the very obvious reason that longitudinal follow-up studies require logistical and financial guarantees that are extremely difficult to obtain. Inevitably, therefore, there are more questions here than there are answers, and too many answers that are doctrinaire rather than empirically substantiated.

Historically, the relationship between hormones and geriatric erotosexual decline began with Brown-Séquard's famed announcement in 1889 of rejuvenation at age 72 from self-injected *liquide orchitique* (Olmsted, 1946). With a generous assist from the media, the idea of rejuvenation grew into the popular monkey-gland legend of geriatric lechery, and the widely held clinical belief in testosterone as the remedy for impotence and other symptoms of the so-called male climacteric (Marañón, 1929).

Laboratory data do not support the concept of universal geriatric erotosexual decline developing synchronously with a declining level of testosterone. Harman and Tsitouris (1980), for example, in a cross-sectional study of different age groups of healthy men, found no decline in plasma testosterone with age up to the decade of the seventies, and in some men not until the eighties. Earlier studies reviewed by Harman (1978) had similar findings except that, after the age of 50 years, the prevalence of men with low plasma testosterone progressively increased—probably as a function of an increased prevalence of suboptimal health.

The foregoing endocrine measures were not correlated with erotosexual evaluations. The men in Harman's study, however, belong in a longitudinal study that includes an erotosexual history from which Clyde Martin (pers. commun.) was able to demonstrate, in men between 60 and 80 years of age, a statistically significant, but in absolute terms a small, correlation between testosterone level and the current history of sexual activity. Martin has concluded that most men, for most of their lives, function sexually at a level far below what might be predicted on the basis of hormone levels alone.

The most likely hypothesis regarding the relationship of hormonal level to erotosexual function in men, regardless of age, is that after an optimal level of testosterone has been attained, any excess is superfluous and is spilled out in the urine. There is no reasonable hypothesis regarding a direct relationship between either gonadotropins or hypothalamic releasing factors on erotosexuality, but there is growing evidence that elevated pituitary prolactin has a negative effect (see above).

Syndromes of hormonal pathology excepted, it is not possible to attribute the level of erotosexual vigor to the level of any hormone. On the basis of his longitudinal and retrospective studies of men of upper educational and socio-economic status being followed at the National Institute of Aging, Martin (1975, 1977) has found that erotosexual vigor is individually variable but not age-dependent. The earlier and more vigorous the erotosexuality of youth, the later and more vigorous the erotosexuality of aging.

The developmental changes of erotosexual maturity and aging have not been systematically classified in either sex. In the male they appear to be a lessening of the frequency of erection and ejaculation; a lengthening of the time to achieve full erection; an increasing frequency of obtaining an incomplete erection or of reverting to one; a lengthening of the interval betwen erections and/or orgasms; an increasing prevalence of prolonged staying power before ejaculating; an increasing likelihood of nonejaculatory copulation or masturbation, with or without a subjective feeling of climax; a maintenance of the feeling and intensity of climax; and an increasing prevalence of body sensuousness or grooming without copulating. There may be an increasing dependence on the fulfillment of erotosexual imagery and fantasy rather than touch for erotosexual arousal.

Nocturnal penile tumescence is one phenomenon that, according to present evidence, remains relatively stable from young adulthood onward, with 3 or 4 episodes of erection per night and a total mean duration of 2 to 3 hours (Hursch, Karacan, and Williams, 1972; Karacan et al., 1975). At puberty, by contrast, the number of episodes ranges from 3 to 11, with a mean of 7 and a mean total duration of aproximately 3½ hours (Karacan et al., 1972).

Nocturnal penile tumescence occurs chiefly during REM sleep. The corresponding phenomenon in women (Abel, Murphy, Becker, and Bitar, 1979) is an intravaginal decrease in blood volume and an increase in pulse pressure. There have been no investigations of age-related changes of this female phenomenon.

The challenge of multivariate complexity is as great in females as in males, if not greater with respect to erotosexual development at the menopause and subsequently. Some women, though by no means all, are severely afflicted with menopausal somatic symptoms and malaise that have a secondary adverse effect on erotosexuality. Menopausal hot flashes occur in synchrony with pulsatile elevations of LH triggered by pulses of hypothalamic LHRH which are synchronized with pulsatile changes of hypothalamic thermoregulation, both being hypothetically under brain catecholamine control (Tataryn, et al., 1979; Meldrum et al., 1980).

The hormonal changes of the menopause include estrogen depletion (Schiff and Wilson, 1978; Talbert, 1978). Thereafter, the fatty tissues in the labia majora shrink, the vaginal wall shrinks and becomes less elastic, vaginal lubrication lessens, and the uterus may have painful contractions (Masters and Johnson, 1970). However, many erotosexually active women do not find these changes impede their sex lives. Others find relief by treatment with low-dose replacement estrogen (Schiff and Wilson, 1978), though there is a cost-benefit ratio that needs individual evaluation in every case.

There have been no investigations in postmenopausal women of synchronous erotosexual and hormone-level changes. Androgen of either adrenocortical or postmenopausal ovarian origin (Schiff and Wilson, 1978; Judd, 1980), even at a very low level might well be proved significant to postmenopausal erotosexualism, but there are at present no age-related data one way or the other.

Age-related changes in erotosexuality in women, irrespective of hormonal changes, appear on the basis of anecdotal data to include the following: a lessening frequency of lubrication; a lengthening of the time to lubricate sufficiently for penile intromission; an increasing frequency of partial lubrication; a lengthening of the interval between lubrications and/or orgasms; an increasing prevalence of prolonged staying power before climaxing; an increasing likelihood of either genital interaction without intromission, or of masturbation, with or without a subjective feeling of climax; maintenance of the feeling and intensity of climax; and an increasing prevalence of body sensuousness or grooming without copulating. There may be a decreased dependence on imagery and fantasy and an increased dependence on touch for erotosexual arousal. Breast sensitivity is maintained; so also is clitoral sensitivity, which may even be enhanced.

There is no complete explanation of why some postmenopausal women remain erotosexually active, or become more so, whereas others lose interest. Self-image is important—to feel desirable and to be desired leads to being aroused. The impediment to being desired is the shortage of available male partners who are compatible. The search may seem too difficult. The numerical disparity of men and women increases exponentially as, for each age, more men than women die, leaving more and more women alone.

For the lonely ones who do find a partner, the sexual taboo that earlier they obediently imposed on their children in some cases boomerangs. Those same children reimpose the taboo on their parents and, ever mindful of their inheritance, denounce the old people's erotosexual partnership and possible remarriage as immoral or unseemly. Thus does the sexual taboo complete its circle of negating healthy erotosexual function across the entire life span. To create conditions for healthy erotosexual development in our society is an enormous public health challenge; but the very existence of the taboo that produces the challenge itself frustrates attempts to do something about it.

Acknowledgments

This study was supported by USPHS grants HD 00325 and HD 07111.

References

Abel, G. G., W. D. Murphy, J. V. Becker, and A. Bitar. 1979. Women's vaginal responses during REM sleep. *J. Sex & Marital Therapy*, 5:5-14

Abramovich, D. R., and P. Rowe. 1973. Foetal plasma testosterone levels at mid-pregnancy and at term: Relationship to foetal sex. *J. Endocrinol.*, 56:621-622.

Adams, D. B., A. R. Gold, and A. D. Burt. 1978. Rise in female-initiated sexual activity at ovulation and its suppression by oral contraceptives. *N. Engl. J. Med.*, 299:1145-1150.

Addiego, F., E. G. Belzer, Jr., J. Comolli, W. Moger, J. D. Perry, and B. Whipple. 1981. Female ejaculation: A case study. *J. Sex Res.*, 17:13-21.

Baum, M. J. 1979. Differentiation of coital behavior in mammals: A comparative analysis. *Neurosci. Biobehav. Revs.*, 3:265-284.

Baum, M. J., B. J. Everitt, J. Herbert, and E. B. Keverne, 1977. Hormonal basis of proceptivity and receptivity in female primates. *Arch. Sex. Behav.*, 6:173-192.

Beach, F. A. 1948. *Hormones and Behavior: A Survey of Interrelationships between Endocrine Secretion and Patterns of Overt Response*. Hoeber, New York.

Beach, F. A. 1976. Sexual attractivity, proceptivity, and receptivity in female mammals. *Horm. Behav.*, 7:105-138.

Belzer, E. G. 1981. Orgasmic expulsions of women: A review and heuristic inquiry. *J. Sex Res.*, 17:1-12.

Bohlen, J., J. Held, and M. Sanderson. 1980. The male orgasm: Pelvic contractions measured by anal probe. *Arch. Sex. Behav.*, 9:503-521.

Boswell, J. 1980. *Christianity, Social Tolerance, and Homosexuality*. Univ. of Chicago Press, Chicago.

Bullough, V. L. 1976. *Sexual Variance in Society and History*. John Wiley and Sons, New York.

Chan, S. T. H. 1970. Natural sex reversal in vertebrates. *Philos. Trans. R. Soc. Lond.*, B, 259:59-71.

Chan, S. T. H. 1977. Spontaneous sex reversal in fishes. In J. Money and H. Musaph (eds.), *Handbook of Sexology*, p. 91-105. Elsevier/North-Holland, New York.

Chevalier-Skolnikoff, S. 1974. Male-female, female-female, and male-male sexual behavior in the stumptail monkey, with special attention to the female orgasm. *Arch. Sex. Behav.*, 3:95-116.

Clopper, R., J. M. Adelson, and J. Money. 1976. Postpubertal psychosexual function in male hypopituitarism without hypogonadotropinism after growth hormone therapy. *J. Sex Res.*, 12:14-32.

Crews, D., and K. T. Fitzgerald, 1980. "Sexual" behavior in parthenogenetic lizards (*Cnemidophorus*). *Proc. Natl. Acad. Sci. USA*, 77:499-502.

Cullberg, J. 1972. Mood changes and menstrual symptoms with different gestagen/estrogen combinations: A double blind comparison with a placebo. *Acta Psychiat. Scand., Suppl.* 236. Munksgaard, Copenhagen.

Dalton, K. 1964. *The Premenstrual Syndrome*. Charles C Thomas, Springfield.

Diamond, M., A. L. Diamond, and M. Mast. 1972. Visual sensitivity and sexual arousal levels during the menstrual cycle. *J. Nerv. Ment. Dis.*, 155:170-176.

Döhler, K. D. 1978. Is female sexual differentiation hormone-mediated? *Trends NeuroSci.*, 1:138-140.

Dörner, G., W. Rohde, F. Stahl, L. Krell, and W. G. Masius. 1975. A neuroendocrine predisposition for homosexuality in men. *Arch. Sex. Behav.*, 4:1-8.

Eicher, W., M. Spoljar, H. Cleve, J.-D. Murken, K. Richter, and S. Stangel-Rutkowski. 1979. H-Y antigen in transsexuality. *Lancet*, ii:1137-1138.

Englander-Golden, P., H-S. Chang, M. R. Whitmore, and R. A. Dienstbier. 1980. Female sexual arousal and the menstrual cycle. *J. Hum. Stress*, 6:42-48.

Forest, M. G., A. M. Cathiard, and J. A. Bertrand. 1973. Evidence of testicular activity in early infancy. *J. Clin. Endocrinol. Metab.*, 37:148-150.

Forest, M. G., J. M. Saez, and J. Bertrand. 1973. Assessment of gonadal function in children. *Paediatrician*, 2:102-128.

Forest, M. G., P. C. Sizonenko, A. M. Cathiard, and J. Bertrand. 1974. Hypophysogonadal function in humans during the first year of life. I. Evidence for testicular activity in early infancy. *J. Clin. Invest.*, 53:819-828.

Goldfoot, D. A. 1977. Sociosexual behaviors of nonhuman primates during development and maturity: Social and hormonal relationships. In A. M. Schrier (ed.), *Behavioral Primatology: Advances in Research Theory*, Vol 1, p. 139-184. Lawrence Erlbaum, Hillsdale.

Goldfoot, D. A., and K. Wallen, 1978. Development of gender role behaviors in heterosexual and isosexual groups of infant rhesus monkeys. In D. J. Chivers and J. Herbert (eds.), *Recent Advances in Primatology*, Vol 1, p. 155-159. Academic Press, London.

Goldfoot, D. A., H. Westerborg-Van Loon, W. Groeneveld, and A. K. Slob, 1980. Behavioral and physiological evidence of sexual climax in the female stumptailed Macaque (*Macaca Arctoides*). *Science*, 208:1477-1479.

Gray, D. S., and B. B. Gorzalka, 1980. Adrenal steroid interactions in female sexual behavior: A review. *Psychoneuroendocrinology*, 5:157-175.

Harman, S. M. 1978. Clinical aspects of aging of the male reproductive system. In E. L. Schneider (ed.), *The Aging Reproductive System*, p. 29-58. Raven Press, New York.

Harman, S. M., and P. D. Tsitouris. 1980. Reproductive hormones in aging men. I. Measurement of sex steroids, basal luteinizing hormone and Leydig cell response to human chorionic gonadotropin. *J. Clin. Endocrinol. Metab.* 51:35-40.

Henderson, M. E. 1976. Evidence for a male menstrual temperature cycle and synchrony with the female menstrual cycle. *N. Z. Med. J.*, 84:164.

Herbert, J. 1970. Hormones and reproductive behavior in rhesus and talapoin monkeys. *J. Reprod. Fertil., (Suppl.)*, 11:119-140.

Hopson, J. L. 1979. Scent and human behavior: Olfaction or fiction? *Science News*, 115: 282-283.

Hunt, G. L., Jr., and M. W. Hunt. 1977. Female-female pairing in western gulls (*Larus occidentalis*) in Southern California. *Science*, 196:1466-1467.

Hursch, C. J., I. Karacan, and R. L. Williams. 1972. Some characteristics of nocturnal penile tumescence in early middle-aged males. *Comprehen. Psychiat.*, 13:539-548.

Imperato-McGinley, J., L. Guerrero, T. Gautier, and R. E. Peterson. 1974. Steroid 5α-reductase deficiency in man: An inherited form of male pseudohermaphroditism. *Science*, 186:1213-1215.

Imperato-McGinley, J., and R. E. Peterson. 1976. Male pseudohermaphroditism: The Complexities of male phenotypic development. *Am. J. Med.*, 61:251-272.

Imperato-McGinley, J., R. E. Peterson, T. Gautier, and E. Sturla. 1979. Androgens and the evolution of male-gender identity among male pseudohermaphrodites with 5α-reductase deficiency. *N. Engl. J. Med.*, 300:1233-1237.

Jaffe, W. L., W. M. McCormack, and J. L. Vaitukaitis. 1980. Plasma hormones and the sexual preferences of men. *Psychoneuroendocrinology*, 5:33-38.

Judd, H. L. 1980. Reproductive hormone metabolism in postmenopausal women. In B. A. Eskin (ed.), *Menopause, Comprehensive Management*, p. 55-71. Masson Publishing, New York.

Karacan, I., C. J. Hursch, R. L. Williams, and R. C. Littell. 1972. Some characteristics of nocturnal penile tumescence during puberty. *Pediatr. Res.*, 6:529-537.

Karacan, I., R. L. Williams, J. I. Thornby, and P. J. Salis. 1975. Sleep-related penile tumescence as a function of age. *Am. J. Psychiat.*, 132:932-937.

Kolata, G. B. 1978. Infertility: Promising new treatments. *Science*, 202:200-203.

Liebowitz, M. R., and D. F. Klein. 1979. Hysteroid dysphoria. *Psychiat. Clin. N.A.*, 2:555-575.

Locke, F. W. (ed.). 1978. *Andreas Capellanus: The Art of Courtly Love*. Frederick Ungar, New York.

Maes, M., C. Sultan, N. Zerhouni, S. W. Rothwell, and C. J. Migeon. 1979. Role of testosterone binding to the androgen receptor in male sexual differentiation of patients with 5α-reductase deficiency. *J. Steroid Biochem.*, 11:1385-1390.

Maple, T. 1977. Unusual sexual behavior of nonhuman primates. In J. Money and H. Musaph (eds.), *Handbook of Sexology*, p. 1167-1186. Excerpta Medica, Amsterdam.

Marañón, G. 1929. *The Climacteric*. Mosby, St. Louis.

Martin, C. E. 1975. Marital and sexual factors in relation to age, disease, and longevity. In R. D. Wirt, G. Winokur, and M. Roff (eds.), *Life History Research in Psychopathology*, Vol 4, p. 326-347. University of Minnesota Press, Minneapolis.

Martin, C. E. 1977. Sexual activity in the ageing male. In J. Money and H. Musaph (eds.), *Handbook of Sexology*, p. 813-824. Excerpta Medica, Amsterdam.

Martinson, R. 1973. *Infant and Child Sexuality: A Sociological Perspective*. Gustavus Adolphus College, St. Peter.

Marx, J. L. 1979. Dysmenorrhea: Basic research leads to a rational therapy. *Science*, 205:175-176.

Masters, W. H., and V. E. Johnson. 1970. *Human Sexual Inadequacy*. Little, Brown, Boston.

McCauley, E., and A. A. Ehrhardt. 1976. Female sexual response: Hormonal and behavioral interactions. *Primary Care*, 3:455-476.

McClintock, M. K. 1971. Menstrual synchrony and suppression. *Nature*, 229:244-245.

McEwen, B. S. 1980. Steroid hormones and the brain: Cellular mechanisms underlying neural and behavioral plasticity. *Psychoneuronendocrinology*, 5:1-11.

Meldrum, D. R., I. V. Tataryn, A. M. Frumar, Y. Erlik, K. H. Lu, and H. L. Judd. 1980. Gonadotropins, estrogens, and adrenal steroids during the menopausal hot flash. *J. Clin. Endocr. Metab.*, 50:685-689.

Merceron, R. E., J. P. Raymond, J. P. Courreges, and H. P. Klotz. 1977. Sexuality in hyperprolactinemics. *Probl. Actuels Endocrinol. Nutr.*, 21:185-189.

Michael, R. P., E. B. Keverne, and R. W. Bonsall. 1971. Pheromones: Isolation of a male sex attractant from a female primate. *Science;* 172:964-966.

Michal, V., and J. Pospíchal. 1978. Phalloarteriography in the diagnosis of erectile impotence. *World J. Surg.*, 2:239-248.

Money, J. 1955. Hermaphroditism, gender and precocity in hyperadrenocorticism: Psychologic findings. *Bull. Johns Hopkins Hosp.*, 96:253-264.

Money, J. 1961. The sex hormones and other variables in human eroticism. In W. C. Young (ed.)., *Sex and Internal Secretions*, 3rd ed., pp. 1383-1400, Williams and Wilkins, Baltimore.

Money, J. 1974. Two names, two wardrobes, two personalities. *J. Homosexual.*, 1:65-70.

Money, J. 1980. *Love and Love Sickness: The Science of Sex, Gender Difference, and Pairbonding*. Johns Hopkins Univ. Press, Baltimore.

Money, J. 1981. Paraphilia and abuse-martyrdom: Exhibitionism as a paradigm for reciprocal couple counseling combined with antiandrogen. *J. Sex Marital Ther.*, 7:115-123.

Money, J., and D. Alexander. 1967. Eroticism and sexual function in developmental anorchia and hyporchia with pubertal failure. *J. Sex Res.*, 3:31-47.

Money, J., and D. Alexander. 1969. Psychosexual development and absence of homosexuality in males with precocious puberty. *J. Nerv. Ment. Dis.*, 148:111-123.

Money, J., J. E. Cawte, G. N. Bianchi, and B. Nurcombe. 1970. Sex training and traditions in Arnhem Land. *Br. J. Med. Psychol.*, 43:383-399.

Money, J., and R. Clopper. 1975. Postpubertal psychosexual function in post-surgical male hypopituitarism. *J. Sex Res.*, 11:25-38.

Money, J., R. Clopper, and J. Menefee. 1980. Psychosexual development in post-pubertal males with idiopathic panhypopituitarism. *J. Sex Res.*, 16:212-225.

Money, J., and J. Daléry. 1972. Iatrogenic homosexuality: Gender identity in seven 46,XX chromosomal females with hyperadrenocortical hermaphroditism born with a penis, three reared as boys, four reared as girls, *J. Homosexual.*, 1:357-371.

Money, J., and A. A. Ehrhardt. 1972. *Man and Woman, Boy and Girl: Differentiation and Dimorphism of Gender Identity from Conception to Maturity*. Johns Hopkins Univ. Press, Baltimore.

Money, J. and Pruce, G. 1977. Psychomotor epilepsy and sexual function. In J. Money and H. Musaph (eds.), *Handbook of Sexology*, p. 969-977. Elsevier/North-Holland, New York.

Money, J., and A. J. Russo. 1979. Homosexual outcome of discordant gender identity/role in childhood: Longitudinal follow-up. *J. Ped., Psychol.*, 4:19-41.

Money, J., and P. A. Walker, 1971. Psychosexual development, maternalism, nonpromiscuity, and body image in 15 females with precocious puberty. *Arch. Sex. Behav.*, 1:45-60.

Money, J., C. Wiedeking, P. Walker, C. Migeon, W. Meyer, and D. Borgaonkar. 1975. 47,XYY and 46,XY males with antisocial and/or sex-offending behavior: Antiandrogen therapy plus counseling. *Psychoneuroendocrinology*, 1:165-178.

Morris, N. M., and J. R. Udry. 1978. Pheromonal influences on human sexual behavior: An experimental search. *J. Biosoc. Sci.*, 10:147-157.

Naftolin, F., K. J. Ryan, I. J. Davies, A. Petro, and M. Kuhn. 1975. The formation and metabolism of estrogens in brain tissues. *Adv. Biosci.* 15:105-121.

Ohno, S. 1978. The role of HY antigen in primary sex determination. *J. Am. Med. Assoc.*, 239:217-220.

Olmsted, J. M. D. 1946. *Charles-Édouard Brown-Séguard: A Nineteenth Century Neurologist and Endocrinologist*. Johns Hopkins Univ. Press, Baltimore.

Parks, G. A., S. Korth-Schutz, R. Penny, R. F. Hilding, K. W. Dumars, S. D. Frasier, and M. I. New. 1974. Variation in pituitary-gonadal function in adolescent male homosexuals and heterosexuals. *J. Clin. Endocrinol. Metab.*, 39:796-801.

Perry, J. D., and B. Whipple. 1981. Pelvic muscle strength of female ejaculators: Evidence in support of a new theory of orgasm. *J. Sex Res.,* 17:22-39.

Persky, H., H. I. Lief, C. P. O'Brien, D. Strauss, and W. Miller. 1977. Reproductive hormone levels and sexual behavior of young couples during the menstrual cycle. In R. Gemme and C. C. Wheeler (eds.), *Progress in Sexology: Selected Papers from the Proceedings of the 1976 International Congress of Sexology,* p. 293-309. Plenum, New York.

Richards, M. P. M., J. F. Bernal, and Y. Brackbill. 1976. Early behavioral differences: Gender or circumcision? *Developmental Psychobiology,* 9:89-95.

Robbins, M. B., and G. D. Jensen. 1978. Multiple orgasm in males *J. Sex Res.,* 14:21-26.

Robertson, D. R. 1972. Social control of sex reversal in a coral reef fish. *Science,* 177:1007-1009.

Rosenzweig, S. 1973. Human sexual autonomy as an evolutionary attainment, anticipating proceptive sex choice and idiodynamic bisexuality. In J. Zubin and J. Money (eds.), *Contemporary Sexual Behavior: Critical Issues in the 1970s,* p. 189-230. Johns Hopkins University Press, Baltimore.

Rossi, A. S., and P. E. Rossi. 1977. Body time and social time: Mood patterns by menstrual cycle phase and day of the week. *Soc. Sci. Res.,* 6:273-308.

Rubin, R. T., J. M. Reinisch, and R. F. Haskett. 1981. Postnatal gonadal steroid effects on human sexually dimorphic behavior: A paradigm of hormone-environment interaction. *Science,* 211:1318-1324.

Russell, M. J., Switz, G. M. and K. Thompson. 1980. Olfactory influences on the human menstrual cycle. *Pharmacol. Biochem. Behav.,* 13:737-738.

Schiff, I., and E. Wilson. 1978. Clinical aspects of aging of the female reproductive system. In E. L. Schneider (ed.), *The Aging Reproductive System,* Vol. 4, p. 9-28. Raven Press, New York.

Schutz, F. 1965. Homosexualität and Praegung. Eine experimentelle Untersuchung an Enten. *Psychol. Forsch,* 28:439-463.

Schutz, F. 1967. Homosexualität bei Tieren. In *Homosexualität oder Politik mit dem* § 175, p. 13-33. Rowohlt, Reinek bei Hamburg.

Sevely, J. L., and J. W. Bennett. 1978. Concerning female ejaculation and the female prostate. *J. Sex Res.,* 14:1-20.

Seyler, L. E., Jr., E. Canalis, S. Spare, and S. Reichlin. 1978. Abnormal gonadotropin secretory responses to LRH in transsexual women after diethylstilbestrol priming. *J. Clin. Endocrinol. Metab.,* 47:176-183.

Spark, R. F., R. A. White, and P. B. Connolly. 1980. Impotence is not always psychogenic: Newer insights into hypothalamic-pituitary-gonadal dysfunction. *J. Am. Med. Assoc.,* 243:750-755.

Stoller, R. J. 1964. A contribution to the study of gender identity. *Int. J. Psychoanal.,* 45:220-226.

Talbert, G. B. 1978. Effect of aging of the ovaries and female gametes on reproductive capacity. In E. L. Schneider (ed.), *The Aging Reproductive System,* Vol. 4, p. 59-83. Raven Press, New York.

Tataryn, I. V., D. R. Meldrum, K. H. Lu, A. M. Frumar, and H. L. Judd. 1979. LH, FSH and skin temperature during menopausal hot flash. *J. Clin. Endocrinol. Metab.,* 49:152-154.

Tennov, D. 1979. *Love and Limerence—The Experience of Being in Love.* Stein and Day, New York.

Trause, M. A., Kennell, J. and M. Klaus. 1977. Parental attachment behavior. In J. Money and H. Musaph (eds.), *Handbook of Sexology,* p. 789-799. Elsevier/North-Holland, New York.

Valency, M. 1961. *In Praise of Love: An Introduction to the Love-Poetry of the Renaissance.* Macmillan, New York.

Wachtel, S. S. 1978. Genes and gender. *The Sciences,* May-June: p. 16-17, 32-33.

Walsh, P. C., J. D. Madden, M. J. Harrod, J. L. Goldstein, P. C. MacDonald, and J. D. Wilson. 1974. Familiar incomplete male pseudohermaphroditism, type 2. *N. Engl. J. Med.,* 291:944-949.

Ward, I. L. 1972. Prenatal stress feminizes and demasculinizes the behavior of males. *Science,* 175:82-84.

Ward, I. L. 1977. Exogenous androgen activates female behavior in noncopulating, prenatally stressed male rats. *J. Comp. Physiol. Psychol.,* 91:465-471.

Ward, I. L., and J. Weisz. 1980. Maternal stress alters plasma testosterone in fetal males. *Science,* 207:328-329.

Wildt, L., G. Marshall, and E. Knobil. 1980. Experimental induction of puberty in the infantile female Rhesus monkey. *Science,* 207:1373-1375.

Zupanc, G. H. K. 1980. Marine biology: Life underwater with Hans Fricke. *The German Tribune,*
1 June, No. 943:8.

Notes

Originally published in *Quarterly Review of Biology,* 56:379-404, 1981. [Bibliog. #3.69]
    See also Chapter 30, Author's Comment, regarding research on the hypothalmus-pituitary-
gonadal system and homosexuality.

TWENTY-SEVEN
Pairbonding and Limerence

Falling in Love

A "pairbond" is a strong and long-lasting attachment between two individuals. Pairbonding between parent and newborn and between potential breeding partners is known in many species. The conditions governing its onset and duration are widely variable from species to species. In human beings, pairbonding is idiomatically equated with loving.

Pairbonded attachment of an erotic and sexual type in human beings lacked a one-word term in the English language until Tennov (1979), deliberately avoiding etymological antecedents, coined the term "limerence," a noun from which a verb, adjective, and adverb can be derived. Limerence is synonymous with being love-smitten, being in love, having fallen in love, or having a love affair.

Love is both affectional and erotosexual or limerent. Affectional love may be parental, filiative, neighborly, or comradely. Erotosexual or limerent love may be either recreational or procreational, each of which may be either connubial or companionate.

Love of both the affectional and limerent variety by its very nature involves attachment or bonding with a partner. There are four criteria according to which a limerent pairbond varies in degree: speed of onset, intensity, reciprocal matching, and duration. A pairbond may be sudden or gradual in onset, strong or weak in intensity, reciprocally matched or mismatched, and brief or long-lasting, in various combinations and permutations. An intensely strong and well-matched limerent bond of rapid onset may be either casually brief, intermittent, or permanent. The same variations in duration may apply to limerence well-matched but of gradual onset and weaker intensity. Strong limerence does not, ipso facto, guarantee that pairbonding will be long-lasting; conversely, a long-lasting bond may be weakly limerent.

The prevalence of limerence of sudden versus gradual onset is not known. Nor is anything known about who is likely to experience one type or the other, or maybe both. There are some few people who appear to be limerently inert or apathetic during adolescence. Many of these eventually become limerent and have their first limerent love affair in their twenties. In others it does not occur until later, perhaps several years after they have been married. In still others limerence does not occur at all. It is rather common, for example, that men with the 47,XXY anomaly (Klinefelter's syndrome) are limerently more or less inert and do not pairbond. There is some evidence also (Money et al., 1980) that people with a hypopituitary syndrome—of either the idiopathic variety or as a sequel to juvenile brain surgery for a hypothalamic tumor—do not subsequently fall in love and pairbond, although they do establish companionships and marriage. Since those who develop a tumor requiring surgery would, presumably, otherwise have matured to have normal pituitary function and also a love affair, it is fair to conjecture that surgical removal of the tumor resulted in lesions in two sets of pathways in or adjacent to the hypothalamus. One set of pathways governs release of hormones from the pituitary gland, and the other set governs release of the behavior of pairbonding, which works in concert with pituitary hormones governing fertility.

By contrast with limerent inertia, there is also a phenomenon of limerent overactivity, or "ultraertia." People with this condition are unable to exist with a sense of well-being unless they reiterate the experience of limerent pairbonding in periodic love affairs. They may be said to have a syndrome of compulsive multiphilia. Multiphilia is not the same as repetitive promiscuity of the type often known as nymphomania and satyriasis, or jointly as erotomania. The multiple partnerships of the erotomanic condition are coital but *not* pairbonded. They may be compulsively unsatisfactory, or they may be consistent with a sense of well-being.

At the opposite extreme there are shy or schizoid people who become limerent toward a remote and unattainable stranger. This syndrome of the autistic love affair exists unbeknownst to the beloved, from whose image the autistic lover cannot become disengaged.

Signs and Course of Limerence

Whether sudden or gradual in onset, when limerence is at its peak the limerent person undergoes subjective and somatic changes similar to those that signify a state of expectancy or anticipation. The cycle of sleeping and waking is altered, as is food intake, thermoregulation and kinesis. At the approach or thought of the beloved, there are changes in pulse rate, blushing, breathing, swallowing, perspiration, and vocal fluency. Communication with the beloved becomes a prime occupation. Dreams may involve imagery of being together romantically, erotically, and genitally. They may culminate in orgasm with the partner represented *in absentia*. Awake, attention becomes distracted by preoccupation with considerations of the beloved, even to the point of obsessive rumination that adversely affects work and study.

When limerent attachment is not reciprocal but one-sided and unrequited, the limerent person who importunes his or her beloved in vain becomes lovelorn or lovesick. The bodily signs and ideation that typify limerence become pathologically intensified in the syndrome of lovesickness. This syndrome is akin to, though not identical with, grief and depression. Acute lovesickness may be suicidal in intensity. It may also be dangerously homicidal. Liebowitz and Klein (1979) link lovesickness with depletion of phenylethylamine, one of the brain's neurotransmitter chemistries that plays a presumptive part in the governance of pairbonding.

Jealousy

Limerent attachment to the beloved is possesive and, in varying degree, jealous and intolerant of an actual or suspected rival. The possessive jealousy of limerence may be bilateral or, in other words, concordantly shared on a fifty-fifty basis. Pathologically intense, bilateral jealousy may isolate a couple from ordinary socializing, though not break their mutual attachment.

The possessive jealousy of limerence may also be unilateral or, in other words, discordantly shared and unequal in origin. One partner imposes more of it on the other than he or she receives in return. Pathologically intense possessive jealousy suspects, constricts, dominates, abuses, humiliates, and violates the partner. Jealousy permits the mutual attachment to survive only if its victim becomes entrapped and addicted to it; otherwise, the victim becomes disattached and abandons the partnership, either without contest or with retaliation. Hatred is one outcome of unilateral limerence, possessiveness, and jealousy that fails. In various guises the same dynamic applies to divorce: the demands of possessiveness are unilaterally unbalanced in the marriage so that the pairbond becomes unbonded and sometimes culminates in murderous destructiveness.

Limerent, possessive jealousy may be lowgrade or violently acute. An acute attack may be triggered by an inferential suspicion or by witnessing one's actual or suspected rival. The acute reaction is so spontaneous in onset that it may occur despite a prior contract with oneself to have an open, unbinding relationship. The acute reaction may destroy the bond that ostensibly it should save, for it not only drives away the rival but alienates one's own partner as well. In the so-called crime of passion, one's partner and one's rival both may be murdered and the catastrophe completed in suicide.

Freed of jealousy and reciprocated, limerence sustains itself at its highest degree of euphoric agitation for a maximum of approximately 2 years. Thereafter, it tranquilizes into a more quiescent fondness and continuing erotosexual attachment. Nature's timetable is at work here, for 2 years is sufficient time to allow for pregnancy and birth. Then, under conditions of limerent health, the pairbond expands into a threebond. Mother-infant bonding, if the mother is not anesthetized, begins in the delivery chamber with the mother establishing eye contact and finger contact with the baby and talking to it; if the father is present, he may do the same. Expansion of the pairbond into a threebond requires some dilution of the all-possessiveness of the initial limerent bond, for otherwise the baby could not be included. For some parents the transition is smooth; for others it is fraught with difficulty. Either parent may react to the baby as a rival and a threat to their own relationship, and may fail to bond to the baby; or the parent-child bond may, for one or both parents, usurp their own bondedness and become a substitute for it.

Sex, Love, and Commitment

Some birds—wild geese and penguins, for example—pairbond for life and remain exclusive breeding partners. Their pairbonding dictates that they copulate only with one another. The same does not apply to human beings; human pairbonding is associated with copulation, but not permanently and exclusively with one partner only.

Pairbondedness can exist without copulation, and copulation can exist without pairbonding. A relationship that is exclusively physical is elusive, if not downright impossible.

The status of being strangers, near-strangers, or transients seems to be the criterion of a sexual relationship that is decried as only physical. A more accurate criterion would be that one or both of the partners has no responsibility or commitment to the partnership other than in the here and now. A commercial commitment is one type of example. Others are the coerced encounter, or the mutual and highly exuberant brief encounter of two travelers fated never to meet again. In such contexts pairbondedness is either excluded, one-sided, or thwarted, for it requires a future and continuity in order to actualize.

A common custom among young people today is that they declare they should not have sexual intercourse without the man first giving assurance, albeit ritual and contrived, that he loves the woman. Love presumably will guarantee a continuity of commitment that will safeguard her against the exigency of a pregnancy and also safeguard her against the possibility of lovesickness. He is equally vulnerable; but custom decrees his role to be played otherwise in the man/woman relationship.

Pairbonding as Imprinting

The concept of imprinting was first formulated in ethology, and it was applied to the establishment of a pairbond between a newly hatched or newborn animal and its mother. Imprinting circumvents the traditional polarization of heredity/ environment; innate/acquired; and biological/psychological. It introduces instead a concept of critical timing when the organism is phyletically prepared from within to respond to stimuli that reach it from without. When response and stimuli converge and coalesce, a long-lived imprint is laid down in the brain. For example, at a critical age a newly-hatched gosling becomes imprinted to and pairbonded with its mother. If first transferred to the brood of a duck, however, it will imprint to the duck and become permanently pairbonded with her as its mother while it grows up. Excluded from the company of other geese, it will reach the age of mating and pairbond with a duck.

In human beings, mother-infant pairbonding can be conceptualized as a form of imprinting, and so also can lover/lover or limerent pairbonding. The critical age for human limerent pairbonding is not as rigidly inflexible as the critical age for other varieties of imprinting in lower species. The typical age is adolescence, but it may be earlier or later, and it can occur more than once in a lifetime.

In lower mammalian species, the nose is typically the primary organ of pairbonding, and an odor, or "pheromone," is the attractant. The pheromone is released from the vagina at the time of ovulation. When it reaches the nostrils of the male, it stimulates his brain and releases a pattern of behavior that culminates in mating.

In primates, the eye is typically the primary organ of pairbonding, and a visual image is the attractant. Men and women both can be stimulated to pairbonding by what they see. Culturally varied prescriptions dictate whether men or women may initiate an approach, and/or the way in which they do it. The tradition of the man as the initiator is widespread, but there is no proof that this tradition is dictated by phyletic heritage. It is possible that pairbonding in males is dependent more on vision than touch, and vice versa in females.

Childhood Rehearsals

Around the kindergarten age, children go through a developmental phase of rehearsing limerent pairbonding in their play. The first manifestation of this rehearsal is with an older person, as in the coquettish and flirtatious play of the little girl with her father, uncle, or another man. Correspondingly, the little boy play-rehearses the escort role with his mother, aunt, or another woman. Two principles are involved: (1) identification with the parent or another adult of the same sex and (2) complementation or reciprocation to the parent or another adult of the opposite sex.

An early outcome of this first rehearsal is its extension to boyfriend/girlfriend rehearsals in the playmate group. The imagery of these rehearsals may include fantasy of a wedding, honeymoon, and family life. The fantasy may be shared with adults, but it may also be censored, depending on how strongly the sexual taboo is imposed.

In our society, the sexual taboo takes hold strongly enough in most children by age 8 that they may give the misleading appearance of having entered the so-called period of latency. Boys and girls spend significant amounts of time in sex-segregated play groups, perhaps thereby consolidating the nonerotic components of their gender identity/role. They exclude adults from being privy to their juvenile pairbond rehearsals (which may include genital stimulation and rehearsal play of the positioning of coitus).

In some instances pairbonding and genital play at around the age of 8 or later may be a manifestation of prepubertal limerence. Their bonding may carry on through puberty and become a full-blown love affair, culminating in marriage and eventual parenthood. In other instances the juvenile rehearsal of pairbonding may have the quality of a "crush," being experienced in fantasy rather than in the actuality of participation. Some crushes are between partners of the same sex and include genital play. This play makes eroticism a progressively familiar part of one's sense of well-being before extending it to become a familiar part of intimacy with the other sex. In this sense, self-sex and same-sex erotic play serve as a rehearsal for eroticism with the other sex.

A juvenile crush may begin as admiration and hero-worship of an older person. The bond of identification subsequently extends to become eroticised as a bond of limerence. With or without actual genital eroticism, the relationship of hero-worship typically becomes a rehearsal for the limerent bonding of an eventual age-matched love affair in adolescence.

There is an animal model for juvenile erotosexual rehearsal play in rhesus monkeys. When reared as members of a troop, baby monkeys typically begin to engage in erotosexual rehearsal play at age 3 months, approximately 3 to 3.5 years prior to puberty. At first they climb on each other in all directions, in pairs or threes or fours, indiscriminate as to the sex of the partner and as to which sex does the mounting, which the presenting. At this stage of differentiation, the mounting and presenting behavior qualifies as ambitypic. Eventually it becomes more unitypic, but the sex of the partner depends partly on whether the peer group is sex-segregated or coeducational.

If there are no males in the peer group, then there develops a hierarchy in which some females are more dominant and do more mounting. The converse happens in all-male peer groups, with some being mounted more than they mount. In a mixed-sex group, the moves eventually become sorted out so that males mount females, predominantly, and do so with the foot-clasp mount typical of mature mating—that is, with their own feet off the ground, grasping the shanks of the female who presents in the quadruped position.

If totally deprived of erotosexual rehearsal play by being reared without age-similar playmates, a monkey male or female grows up unable to position for mating, even with a gentle and experienced partner, and unable to reproduce its species. Less total deprivation of erotosexual rehearsal play reduces the severity of the subsequent impairment. Thus, when male monkeys, permanently separated from their mothers at 3 to 6 months of age, were allowed one-half hour of peer group play daily, about 30% of them developed success at foot-clasp mounting, but its appearance was delayed by a year or more until they were 18 to 24 months of age. The remaining 70% remained permanently impaired, unable to mount and breed. Even the successful 30% was less proficient at copulation and breeding than animals reared in the wild (Goldfoot and Wallen, 1978).

Romantic Love: The Troubadours

One may conjecture that in ancient Greece, among the wealthy and educated who left written records, pairbonding was institutionalized as homosexual and ephebophilic, and marriage was institutionalized as a procreative service. In

Greek, as in Roman and medieval, times, the pairbonding customs of the masses went chiefly unrecorded. Among the Roman nobility, marriage commonly was an arrangement for the union of property and power, and pairbonding was an extramarital institution that, under some of the emperors, became extravagantly debauched.

Marriage as a union of property and power was perpetuated among the nobility of medieval Europe, and maintains much of that status among today's royalty and nobility. The same tradition permeates many other families as well, especially families that wield great mercantile, financial, and political power. In less powerful families, unions within the same religious faith or race are pressured or arranged by the elders. Even among royalty, however, where the old restrictions are strongest, some allowance is made for romantic love between the prospective bride and bridegroom.

Among European nobility, romantic love as a criterion of being eligible for marriage made its first tentative, recorded breakthrough in the songs of the troubadours of southern France in the 200 years after 1090. This was the age of cultural diffusion by way of the Crusades; the age of the flowering of the Albigensian version of the Manichean heresy in southern France, which the church brutally exterminated with the Inquisition in the 13th century; the age of accommodating Mariolotry into church doctrine; and the age of the Little Renaissance of science and academic freedom.

Some troubadours were educated noblemen and some itinerant entertainers or jongleurs who, with their lutes and songs of love and protest, were the medieval counterpart of today's rock and roll poet-musicians as youth's philosophers and love educators. Four hundred of them are known by name. They sang in their vernacular languages and diffused from Mediterranean France to Paris, Germany, and England in the north, and to Italy and Spain in the south. Though the origin of their art went unrecorded, their songs of love might have derived from the poetry of ancient Greece by way of translation and transformation into Arabic. The love of which they sang was always unrequited and unattainable, for the hand of the lady sung to had invariably already been given in marriage, or would be given, at the decision of her father. The marriage was arranged by the parents, not proclaimed by personal romance. The poet of courtly love had no hope of winning his lady, and he must be satisfied with unfulfilled longing. Even if he fell in love with the bride arranged for him, the passionate consummation of love as carnal lust was condemned and punished by the Church. To be free of sin, marital coitus, as decreed by the Church, must be limited to the bare essentials of procreation—infrequent and without passion. The Church's penitentials spelled out all sexual sins and their penances.

The troubadours avoided being charged as heretics by celebrating love and romance as an unattainable longing never to be consummated in the sinful passion of sexual intercourse. The importunate lover implored a reply and expected silence. Several troubadour poems were paeans to the Virgin Mary. History proved that the songs of the troubadours were the thin edge of the wedge. Petrarch took up the theme of unattainable love with Laura, Dante with Beatrice, and Shakespeare with Romeo and Juliet. Poetry, songs, operas, and novels of the Romantic movement in the 19th century exploited the theme still further, but often as a prelude to resolving it in a happy ending. The triumph of love, waiting for the right one to come along, became an expectation of everyday life.

However, the old juxtaposition between romantic love, the ideal and unattainable, and carnal lust, the inevitable sin of procreation, has not been fully resolved—the compromise protest that sex in holy matrimony is sacred and beautiful notwithstanding. Love still resides above the belt, and lust below. Love, the madonna, is lyrical, clean, pure, and viewed in public; lust, the whore, is bawdy, dirty, obscene, and hidden in private.

This is the tradition that, applied to sex education, decrees both disciplinary neglect and abuse, in order to ensure that love remain above the belt, and lust below.

Lovemaps

The antisexual heritage of childhood is the irreconcilability of love and lust. Lust, the experience of genital joy, is prohibited, prevented, and punished; and juvenile erotosexual rehearsal play of male/female bonding is subverted. Rationalizing, society says that it is preserving the innocence of childhood and that puberty is time enough for lust to incite the instincts of the penis and vagina into performing the original sin in which all of us are conceived.

Children who grow up together manifest remarkable conformity in the way they speak. There is less conformity in the features of their mental lovemaps. The explanation for nonconformity almost certainly lies in the fact that society forbids overt age-mate sharing of rehearsals of erotosexualism in pairbonding. There are on this planet a few ethnic traditions that do not include our own sexual taboo, and in which juvenile erotosexual rehearsal play is not prohibited, prevented, and punished, but expected as normal (Money et al., 1977; Money and Ehrhardt, 1972; Wolman and Money, 1980).

In our culture there is neglect of parental responsibility in ensuring the conditions and knowledge prerequisite to healthy erotosexual development, and abuse of parental authority in imposing threats, deprivations, and punishments when children's rehearsal play, alone or together, transiently or in a pairbond, is discovered to include erotosexual activity.

The outcome of abuse and neglect is a function not only of abuse and neglect, but also of the make-up of the particular organism subjected to abuse and neglect. Some may be more vulnerable than others, and also more vulnerable to certain outcomes rather than others. Whatever the combination of determinants, there are three categories of outcome: hypophilia, hyperphilia, and paraphilia. In all three there is a factor in common, namely a discontinuity between love and lust—between above and below the belt.

HYPOPHILIA. In hypophilia the mental lovemap stabilizes in adolescence and adulthood as erotosexually deficient in some aspect or other, without necessarily being pairbonding-deficient. A couple may fall in love above the belt, but below the belt one or both may be erotosexually apathetic and inert, experiencing a lack or impairment of sexual desire. In the terminology of sex therapy, the couple is sexually inadequate, anorgasmic, impotent, or having premature ejaculation.

HYPERPHILIA. In hyperphilia the juvenile response to thwarting of the development of the mental lovemap is one of compensatory retaliation and defiance. In adolescence and adulthood, the lovemap stays intact, except for limerent pairbonding that is impaired, lacking, or detached from erotosexual activity. Use of the genitals is typically compulsively and excessively reiterative and promiscuously distributed among partners. Another possibility is that of *multiphilia,* a reiterative series of limerent pairbonds that may be either successful or self-sabotaging and wreaking havoc in one's life. Another possibility is to participate erotosexually with several partners contemporaneously, as in group sex and swinging, while having one primary attachment that may or may not survive.

PARAPHILIA. In paraphilia the juvenile response to developmental thwarting of the mental lovemap selectively impairs neither erotosexual function nor pairbonding alone, but imposes new constraints on both. The lovemap is redrawn, or altered and distorted, so that the thwarting effect is circumvented. It becomes no longer a lovemap of the ordinary male/female imagery of pairbonding and its erotosexual component. It is idiosyncratic, and it restricts the number of suitable partners by displacement or inclusion.

Paraphilic displacement is exemplified by exhibitionism. Exhibiting the genitalia is a form of erotic invitation in many primate species. In the paraphilic syndrome of exhibitionism it becomes displaced from the preliminaries and usurps the central place of penovaginal intromission as the chief component of erotosexual participation and gratification. For the male exhibitionist the startle, surprise, shock, or panic reaction of the female stranger to whom he flashes his penis is an essential prerequisite to subsequently becoming aroused and experiencing erection and ejaculation, whether by masturbation or by copulation with a wife or other consenting partner. If the developmental juvenile history of an exhibitonist can be retrieved, one expects to find evidence of early "show me" play in which he displayed his penis to a female playmate and for which he received traumatic punishment or other treatment that exaggerated the significance of exhibiting the penis to a female.

Paraphilic inclusion is exemplified by the syndrome of klismaphilia. For the klismaphiliac, to be given an enema by the beloved is erotogenically superior to ordinary penovaginal intercourse. It is a necessary prerequisite, either as practiced or as replayed in imagery, to intromission and penovaginal orgasm. Giving of an enema stimulates an erogenous response by way of the erogenous sensitivity of the anus and the prostate gland. For the klismaphiliac the imagery or fantasy of being given an enema is erogenously stimulating, secondary to an early history of an emphasis on enemas, the receiving of which became erogenic.

The list of the paraphilias comprises about forty categories. Transvestism and transexualism, which are chiefly gender transpositions, are not included (Money, 1977), though transvestophilia is. Within each category, individual cases may be highly idiosyncratic. It is very unusual for a person to have more than one paraphilic syndrome, either contemporaneously or in sequence. A harmful and dangerous paraphilia manifests itself as harmful and dangerous from puberty onward; a harmless and playful one does the same. Paraphilias that have the legal status of sex offenses can be dealt with by combined hormonal and counseling treatment (Money, 1980). The hormone is an anti-androgenic steroid (in the U.S., medroxyprogesterone acetate). Paraphilias are less prevalent in women than men, and fewer in variety.

Loveblots

Partial correspondence between an actual person and the image of an ideal partner as represented on one's mental lovemap may suffice to set one's limerence in motion. That person is both the uninvited stimulant of limerence and simultaneously its target recipient. This stimulus-target is, by analogy with the Rorschach inkblot test, a loveblot. Onto this loveblot one projects the meanings, expectancies, and hopes of one's own lovemap. The loveblot exists not as an individual self-understood and self-defined, but as one whom one endows, Pygmalion-like, with one's own percepts and meanings.

If two people are loveblots for one another, the match may be either a symmetrical, hand-in-glove fit of complementarity or it may be an asymmetrical and badly-fitting mismatch. When the match is good, the image projected onto each partner by the other is a mirror image of the self-representation of the recipient in his or her own lovemap. When there is a mismatch, the image projected onto each partner by the other is a distorted image of the self-representation of the recipient.

In the case of a good match, there is a high probability that the limerent pairbond will be long-lasting. This rule applies no matter how idiosyncratic, eccentric, or even bizarre the two lovemaps may be.

For those who separate, disillusionment and the erosion of hope may be progressive and the break postponed until, finally, the day of disillusionment dawns. As in possessive jealousy, the reaction then may be destructively punitive, even murderous or suicidal.

The criteria of mismatching are not restricted to the erotic component of pairbonding, but may involve the nonerotic components as well.

For pairbonded health and well-being it is a great advantage if the loveblots projected by each onto the other are reciprocally well-matched, in which case there will be a good fit between the projected image and the actuality of the person, homosexual or heterosexual, onto whom it is projected. The goodness of fit can best be tested if the two partners disclose to one another early in their relationship their respective lovemaps—their fantasy, imagery, and ideation of what the erotosexual and other components of the partnership should be. It is not easy to expose oneself in this way, for intimate details of one's lovemap are easily subject to rebuff, ridicule, and even blackmail. The personal costs of suffering a mismatch are too great, however, to be worth the risk. The correction of a mismatch is difficult and cannot be guaranteed, no matter what the type of intervention. The maximum guarantee of pairbonded well-being is to be well-matched to begin with, and not to have to work at it.

References

Goldfoot, D. A., and Wallen, K. Development of gender role behaviors in heterosexual and isosexual groups of infant rhesus monekys. In D. J. Chivers and J. Herbert (Eds.), *Recent advances in primatology,* Vol. 1. London: Academic Press, 1978.

Liebowitz, M. R., and Klein, D. F. Hysteroid dysphoria. *Psychiatric Clinics of North America,* 1979, 2(3), 555-575.

Money, J. Paraphilias. In J. Money and H. Musaph (Eds.), *Handbook of sexology.* Amsterdam: Excerpta Medica, 1977, pp. 917-928.

Money, J. *Love and love sickness: The science of sex, gender difference, and pair-bonding.* Baltimore: Johns Hopkins Press, 1980.

Money, J., Cawte, J. E., Bianchi, G. N., and Nurcombe, B. Sex training and traditions in Arnhem Land. In J. Money and H. Musaph (Eds.), *Handbook of sexology.* Amsterdam: Excerpta Medica, 1977, pp. 519-541.

Money, J., Clopper, R., and Menefee, J. Psychosexual development in postpubertal males with idiopathic panhypopituitarism. *Journal of Sex Research,* 1980, 16(3), 212-225.

Money, J., and Ehrhardt, A. A. *Man and woman, boy and girl: Differentiation and dimorphism of gender identity from conception to maturity.* Baltimore: Johns Hopkins Press, 1972.

Tennov, D. *Love and Limerence: The experience of being in love.* New York: Stein and Day, 1979.

Wolman, B. B., and Money, J. (Eds.) *Handbook of human sexuality.* Englewood Cliffs, N.J.: Prentice-Hall, 1980.

Note

Originally published in *International Encyclopedia of Psychiatry, Psychology, Psychoanalysis and Neurology.* Progress Volume I (B. B. Wolman, ed.). New York, Aesculapius Publishers, 1983. [Bibliog. #3.70]

Author's Comments: Sex, Love and Commitment

The following comment on the semantic difficulty of defining love in terms of commitment is taken from a brief note published in the *Journal of Sex and Marital Therapy,* 2:273-276, 1976 [Bibliog. #2.203]:

Commitment is an "in" term at the moment. Among counselors and therapists it has, unhappily, joined forces with other "in" terms like *meaningful,* as in meaningful relationship; *emotional,* as in emotional illness; *setting,* as in hospital setting; and false plurals, as in behaviors, homosexualities, and schizophrenias.

"In" terms give the impression of precision where there is none. They are always cabalistic. They always become used by a cabalistic elite to disguise a covert value judgment. They cover for an absence of raw data required for an empirical and operational definition of the phemomena that they purport to denote. They succeed more in giving emblematic prestige to "in" members of the cabal that uses them than in clarifying meaning and contributing to the advancement of science. They are so imprecise and amorphous in connotation that they are, in fact, scientific word garbage. What does it mean, for instance, to have love, sex, and commitment without specifying commitment to what? Love, sex, and commitment to paying the bills? Raising the children? Monogamy and a closed relationship? An open relationship? An obligation to submit to violence, sabotage, treachery, false piety, or any form of noxious behavior from the partner? My own interpretation is that commitment as an "in" term is covertly synonymous with commitment to the Freudian ideal of monogamous genitality, which itself is synonymous with the Judeo-Christian ideal of monogamous marriage.

From the foregoing it is obvious that commitment is a slippery term for sexologists to use. Sex is not so slippery, but it has too many meanings—from civil status to copulation. Love also is not so slippery, but like sex it serves too many purposes—sacred or profane, erotic or patriotic, romantic or carnal.

Sexologists need an international nomenclature congress so that they can agree on basic terminology!

To Quim and To Swive:
Linguistic and Coital Parity, Male and Female

Parity of the sexes in pairbonding, love, and commitment is not automatically concordant with parity in the genitoerotic relationship. The idiom of the language dictates that the sexual act is something that males do to women. Rescued from obsolescence in the vernacular, *to quim* and *to swive* are two verbs that serve very well to distinguish and define the active-assertive practice of, respectively, the female and the male in penovaginal copulation.

The following item from the Adversaria column of *The Journal of Sex Research,* 18:173-176, 1982 [Bibliog. #4.93], presents this new terminology to ensure male-female copulatory parity personally, and in sexological research, education, and therapy:

In neither the standard English vocabulary of literature and science, nor the vernacular vocabulary of uncensored speech, are there terms by which to distinguish what the woman does to the man, in the procreative act, from what the man does to the woman. Terminologically, each is obliged to do the same thing to the other, whether it be poetically making love, politely copulating, metaphorically balling or screwing, colloquially fucking, or evasively "getting some." None of this terminology is, however, truly androgynous. It all carries, in some degree, the implication that the male is the active partner who does something to the inactive, receptive female. He takes, and she gives—or at least passively acquiesces.

In the terminology of the barnyard and animal breeding, the same implication of the male as the active agent also applies. Terminologically, the bull services the cow, not the other way around. A detailed inventory of animal mating behavior, however, reveals a high degree of reciprocity. Thus, whereas the male mounts the female, it is equally true that she crouches or lordoses and presents to the male. In many species, moreover, it is the female that invites the male, for when she is ovulating and in heat, her vagina releases a pheromonal odor that inititates the male's response.

In the mating of human beings, it is not idiomatic to say that the woman presents, crouches, or lordoses. Nor is it in the vernacular idiom to say that the male mounts the female. When he begins thrusting, the female may thrust reciprocally, but that terminology, though not vulgar, is also not a common idiom.

This deficiency of idiom reflects and perpetuates the potency and pervasiveness of the sexual taboo in our social heritage. In addition, it reflects and perpetuates another great premise of our social heritage, namely, that the woman's sexual and erotic role is passive-receptive, and the man's active-assertive.

This male-female disparity permeates deeply into both our social and scientific concepts of male and female. Thus, for centuries, the doctrine of procreation held that only the man, not the woman provided the seed of pregnancy. Her womb was a mere receptacle for his seed, the semen, which formed the fetus. In 1677, in the early days of the microscope, van Leeuwenhoek saw spermatozoa for the first time. Soon thereafter, it became popular to represent a sperm diagramatically with a fetal homunculus as its nucleus, thus assuring the primacy of the male in procreation.

Male-female disparity permeated deeply also into moral, legal, political, and medical concepts of eroticism and sexuality. The doctrine of female erotic passivity in the nineteenth century equated passivity with erotic apathy, inertia, and anhedonia. William Acton (1813-75) was an exponent of this extreme doctrine in his book, "The Functions and Disorders of the Reproductive Organs in Youth, in Adult Age, and in Advanced Life," which, through many editions, was actively influential into the twentieth century. Acton wrote:

> The majority of women (happily for them and society) are not very much troubled with sexual feeling of any kind. . . . Married men . . . or married women . . . would vindicate female nature from the vile aspersions cast on it by the abandoned conduct and ungoverned lusts of a few of its worst examples. . . . The best mothers, wives, and managers of households, know little or nothing of sexual indulgences. . . . As a general rule, a modest woman seldom desires any sexual gratification for herself. She submits to her husband, but only to please him; and, but for the desire of maternity, would far rather be relieved from his attentions. (Quoted from Fryer, 1966, p. 17.)

Acton's doctrine disregarded the evidence of women who did not conform to the anhedonic ideal, but who were sexually active and assertive. To be such a woman was to be wanton and lewd, and tantamount to being a harlot, paramour, or adulteress. The right to their own sexuality and eroticism had for centuries been allowed only to such women and not to the virgins who became wives, cast in the respected and revered role of madonna. The madonna's sexy sister was the whore.

The proverbial disparity between the madonna and the whore is well known to sex therapists. Its male counterpart is the disparity between the provider and the playboy. In both sexes, it is a disparity that afflicts unnumbered thousands of lives with its saint-and-sinner conflict, robs them of their sexual birthright (less than 50 cents to the erotosexual dollar!), and impairs both genitosexual and erotosexual health. Its persistence is reinforced by the lack of an idiomatic vocabulary that endorses active-assertive sexuality and eroticism in women—a vocabulary that would be of equal utility for both sexes.

Ideally, this vocabulary would provide a term for every behavioral unit (behavioron) in the sexuoerotic repertory of both partners. For sexological research the development of such an analytic vocabulary is not simply an ideal, but an absolute necessity, for without it erotosexual practice cannot be properly subdivided and reduced to identifiable units for investigation in research. Beach (quoted in Money & Ehrhardt, 1972) in 1969 developed an analytic vocabulary of dimorphic sexual behavior in the rat, which has influenced all animal sexological research.

The vocabulary for human beings should sound idiomatic so that it will be applicable in daily life and in sex therapy, as well as in sexological research; and it should be endorsed by an international committee on sexological nomenclature.

As a starter, I have conducted an extensive library search for two words by which to distinguish the female component from the male component of penovaginal interaction. The two words that sound the most idiomatic and least neologistic are *quim* and *swive*. Both can be used as either a verb or a noun.

Quim, according to Eric Partridge (1967), though its etymological origin is uncertain, probably derives form the Celtic *cwm,* a cleft or valley. Its usage as a vernacular term for the female pudenda can be traced from the 17th to the 20th century, where it has survived in vernacular verse and humor, along with various derivatives: *quimming* (copulating), *quim-stick* or *quim-wedge* (penis), and *quim-sticking* (intercourse). In its standard usage as a verb, it would mean, as here proposed, to take the penis into the vagina and perform grasping, sliding, and rotating movements on it of varying rhythm, speed and intensity. As a noun, a *quim* would be the name of the aforesaid practice.

Swive, meaning to copulate with a woman, according to Partridge (1967), was in standard English usage as far back as the 14th century. By the early 17th century, its status had changed to that of a vulgarism. Since the early 19th century, it has survived as a literary archaism, in some dialects, and occasionally in vernacular verse and humor. In its standard usage as a verb it would mean, as here proposed, to put the penis into the vagina and perform sliding movements of varying depth, direction, rhythm, speed, and intensity. As a noun, a *swive* would be the name of the aforesaid practice.

The term, *to copulate,* would retain its standard meaning as a reciprocal, two-person, penovaginal practice; but, as here proposed, it would mean only the penovaginal practice, with no other simultaneous embellishments, such as kissing. *Copulation,* the noun, would not be wholly synonymous with coitus (coming together or meeting) or sexual intercourse; both of which, though sometimes given only the penovaginal meaning, sometimes also include associated activities prior to, simultaneous with, or following the penovaginal component. In usage, all three of these nouns are subject to adjectival modification,as in oral or anal copulation, coitus, or intercourse. In standard usage, there is no verb, *to coition,* nor *to intercourse,* though the latter is sometimes used among teenagers who need, as a transitive verb, a polite substitute for the vernacular, *to fuck.*

To quim, to swive, and *to copulate* are very useful words to have in one's sexological and sex-therapy lexicons. Because each is conceptually discrete, they greatly facilitate the precision of communication in talking with fellow professionals and, even more extensively so, in teaching sex education and in giving sex therapy.

References

Fryer, P. *Secrets of the British Museum.* New York: Citadel Press, 1966.

Money;, J., & Ehrhardt, A. A. *Man and woman, boy and girl: The differentiation and dimorphism of gender identity from conception to maturity.* Baltimore: Johns Hopkins Press, 1972.

Partridge, E. *A dictionary of slang and unconventional English* (6th ed.). New York: Macmillan, 1967.

PART IV
Transexualism and Paraphilia

TWENTY-EIGHT

Gender-Identity/Role:
Normal Differentiation and Its Transpositions

Gender-Identity/Role: Differentiation

Most people do not question their own or others' established gender identity and role as male or female. They are readily accepted at face value. What is said and done by men and women in different societies varies and may overlap, since dimorphic norms of gender role are culturally and historically determined. But once an individual's identity and role as a male or a female become differentiated, they remain stable and are unlikely to be shaken even by major crises in life, physiological, social, or accidental.

The greater proportion of gender-identity/role differentiation takes place after birth. It develops on the basis of prenatally programed sex differences in body morphology, in hormonal function, and in central nervous system (CNS) function, but is not preordained or preprogramed *in toto* by prenatal determinants. Prenatal antecedents lay down a predisposition to which postnatal influences are added. A prenatal defect, skew, or bias may be either augmented or counteracted by postnatal influences.

The dimorphism of gender-identity/role as male or female begins with the genetic dimorphism of the sex chromosomes, XY for the male, XX for the female. It is followed by the differentiation of the gonads with H-Y antigen on the Y bearing sperm governing the differentiation of the testes. Fetal hormonal functioning then programs differentiation of the internal reproductive anatomy, and the external genital morphology. Then follows differential sex assignment at birth, rearing as a boy or a girl, and differentiation of the childhood gender role and identity. The differentiation process is continued through the prepubertal and pubertal phases with, in adolescence, a sexually dimorphic response or, more accurately, threshold of response manifested in erotic attraction, falling in love, courtship, mating, and parenthood.

Figure 1 in Chapter 17 provides a framework for a descriptive catalogue of conditions and events necessary for normal gender identity/role differentiation. It also may be used for a descriptive catalogue of biogenic factors and living conditions harmful to the differentiation of an intact, functioning, normal, or healthy gender identity.

Definitions

Gender identity: The sameness, unity, and persistence of one's individuality as male, female, or ambivalent in greater or lesser degree, especially as it is experienced in self-awareness and behavior. Gender identity is the private experience of gender role, and gender role is the public expression of gender identity.

Gender role: Everything that a person says or does to indicate to others or to the self, the degree that one is either male, female, or ambivalent. It includes, but is not restricted to sexual arousal and response. Gender role is the public expression of gender identity, and gender identity is the private experience of gender role.

Gender-identity/role: The term used to express the unity of gender identity and gender role which are opposite sides of the same coin. Gender identity and gender role both belong to the self. One's own gender role is not synonymous with a socially prescribed or conventional gender role stereotype, even though, it in some greater or lesser degree reflects this stereotype.

Gender-identity/role differentiation: The differentiation of gender-identity/ role is the product of the interaction of prenatal (phyletically prescribed) and postnatal (social-environmentally prescribed) determinants or events, the latter outweighing the former in their overall influence.

Psychosexual differentiation: A term which historically antedates the term, gender-identity/role differentiation, and which is sometimes used synonymously, despite the confusion of its also being used as a synonym for gender identity differentiation.

Genotype: An abstract term referring to the hereditary or gene-determined contribution to individual development. The genotype interacts with the envirotype to produce the uniquely individual phenotype.

Envirotype: An abstract term referring to the environmentally determined contribution to individual development. It interacts with the genotype to produce the uniquely individual phenotype. The term recognizes the fact that substances and events from the environment enter the cells of the body, including the cells of the central nervous system. There is an intrauterine, antenatal environment as well as a postnatal, extrauterine one.

Phenotype: The product of the interaction of genotype and envirotype. Both set limits on each other. The genotype, in order to express itself, depends on a favorable envirotype, and the envirotype cannot process what the genotype does not supply.

Critical period: A time-limited phase, specific to a given aspect or phase of individual development, during which a state of sensitivity or readiness of the organism must be met by phyletically specific external stimuli in order to permit that aspect or phase of development to progress optimally. For example, speech cannot be acquired until the sensitive stage is reached, at which time there must be stimulation from hearing other people talk. At the conclusion of the critical period the development which has taken place is likely to remain permanent.

Identification and Complementation: In the differentiation of gender-identity/role, identification signifies that an individual establishes a mental schema in the brain by imitating and copying or modeling the behavior of members of one's own assigned sex. Complementation signifies the mental schema through learning the behavior of members of the opposite assigned sex and through reciprocating with gender-appropriate responses of one's own assigned sex.

Disorders of Gender-Identity/Role

Gender-identity/role disorders occur most frequently in people with normal external and internal reproductive anatomy. Sexual pathways of the central nervous system (CNS) do not show gross morphological changes to which gender-identity/role disorders might be attributed. This is not surprising, since one would expect CNS functions mediating such disorders to be related to the dynamics of neurochemistry, specifically of neurotransmitters, and thresholds of arousal and inhibition in neurosexual pathways. Identification and measurement of these functions is not technically possible at the present time.

Transpositions versus Intrusions or Displacements

Some clinicians use the term disorder in connection with gender-identity/role, to refer only to male-female transpositions. Sometimes known as gender dysphorias, these transpositions contain the syndromes of transexualism and transvestism (transvestophilia). They also may include homosexualism and bisexualism, though neither of these need be considered pathologies or disorders (see below).

Other clinicians include in the category of disordered gender-identity/role all the paraphilias. Paraphilia refers to a condition in which sexual arousal and performance is dependent on highly specific imagery, perceived or remembered, other than imagery of the erotic partner. A paraphilia may be benign or noxious. The imagery of a paraphilia, as in fetishism, for example, may be in the nature of an imagistic intrusion, to be associated with the erotic image of the partner, or it may be rather a displacement or substitute for the erotic image of a partner, in whole or in part. A paraphilia can be regarded as a part of gender-identity/role in that it is essential to the person's masculine or feminine erotic functioning. Thus for the male sadist, his masculine gender-identity/role in its erotic manifestation is dependent on remembered or enacted sadistic imagery.

The list of the paraphilias is long. It includes, for example, masochism and sadism, rape and lust murder, voyeurism and exhibitionism, pedophilia and gerontophilia, amputeephilia (apotemnophilia), zoophilia, klismaphilia, coprophilia, urophilia, necrophilia, fetishism, and so on.

The transposition syndromes generally are classified along with the intrusion or displacement syndromes as paraphilias. There is not total professional consensus, however, especially in those cases of homosexualism (and by extension, bisexualism) in which the perceived or remembered imagery of erotic arousal and performance is concordant with the body and the person of the same-sexed, pair-bonded partner, the latter itself being the only unorthodoxy. The syndrome of transvestism, because of its associated fetishistic dependency on clothing, qualifies as a paraphilia (transvestophilia). So also does transexualism, for the transexual person can function erotically only by reason of having, or imagining having a body reassigned and transformed from that of the sex of birth.

The distinction between transposition and intrusion or displacement paraphilias having been made, the transposition syndromes are the focus of the remainder of this chapter, after the examination of what constitutes pathology.

Harmless versus Noxious, Normalcy versus Pathology

A paraphilia is not, by definition, a pathology. Rather, it becomes pathological when it becomes too severe, too insistent, and too noxious to the partner, or to the self. In mild form, paraphilic imagery and the behavior it engenders may be simply a part of love play. For example, a playful degree of biting, slapping, or pinching qualifies as sadistic but is harmless when the play is between consenting partners.

In medicine generally, and in sexology in particular, there are many occasions when one is confronted with the issue of how to establish criteria of pathology. When, for example, does an elevation in temperature become a fever? Or a shortness of stature, dwarfism? Or an insufficiency of food, malnutrition? The criterion point adopted in answer to such questions may have great practical significance. In Peking, for example, Westerners in the diplomatic corps recently may have been denied a Chinese driving license because their blood pressure, judged normal at home, would be elevated according to the norms of the Chinese who have a lower average blood pressure.

There is always something arbitrary about the choice of a criterion of normalcy. It is arbitrary even to choose the statistical norm—it may be normal to be infested with hookworm or schistosomiasis in certain locales, but it is not healthy. The criterion of health versus pathology involves a chain of logical reasoning that sooner or later brings one into direct confrontation with a value judgment. The personal criterion of pathology may be too much pain, suffering, and loss of the feeling of well-being. The social criterion may be too much harm to, or threat of endangering the health or well-being of others. The well-being of others may be covertly or implicitly defined as their political, legal, moral, spiritual, or religious well-being.

In matters of sexual health, as in behavioral health in general, social criteria have traditionally dominated personal ones. They have been powerfully religious and legalistic, but politically and ethnically arbitrary. This arbitrariness is presently under fire, and to some extent there is today a social reexamination of criteria and standards. In their 1974 referendum, for example, the membership of the American Psychiatric Association confirmed the action of their committee on nomenclature in changing the status of homosexuality from disease to nondisease.

The mood of society today is toward the greater tolerance of the principle of live and let live sexually, provided both partners are consenting adults or, if young, of like age. There is no fixed dividing line between the tolerable and the intolerable, socially, and no criterion for establishing one. A workable criterion, which is both expedient and pragmatic, is the criterion of mutual consent between erotic partners, up to the point of noxious injury to health and well-being. This criterion rules out lust murder, rape, abusive sadism, a masochist's self-arranged torture and death by homicide, enforced amputation of the partner by an amputee fetishist, enforced celibacy or erotic deprivation of the partner by a transexual, and the like. Other forms of erotic expression, subject to the proviso of mutual consent, are not ruled out. Any individual whose form of erotic expression engenders too great a loss of well-being is, however, eligible for whatever therapy sexological medicine may be able to offer.

Greater Vulnerability of the Male

Sexologists agree that the incidence of gender-identity/role disorders is greater in males than in females, though there are as yet no fixed statistics. The embryology of prenatal hormonal regulation of sex differentiation clearly shows that nature's first choice is to differentiate the morphology of a female. The differentiation of male morphology requires that something be added (the "Adam principle"). This something is, for the most part, androgen released by the fetal testes. A second substance, known only as müllerian inhibiting substance, suppresses development of the mullerian ducts which otherwise would form a uterus in the male. By inference from animal experiments to human beings, androgen also influences brain pathways or thresholds that mediate erotic and mating behavior. Apart from some rodent studies, the neuroanatomy and neurochemistry of this influence still must be demonstrated.

It is, by hypothesis, likely that prenatal androgen has a masculinizing effect on brain thresholds subserving the relationship of visual signals and images to erotic attraction and arousal. In lower mammals, including primates, an odor or pheromone from the ovulating female's vagina serves as a sex attractant. In man, the sense of sight overrides smell as a sex attractant. Both sexes respond to visual erotic signals, but woman is more dependent on touch for complete arousal, according to present evidence. In man, the visual stimulus prompts the initiation of an erotic approach. Nature demonstrates the primacy of the visual image in male eroticism in the phenomenon of the pubertal orgasm dream (wet dream) for which there is no exact counterpart in the female.

The actual image that is erotically stimulating is not phyletically programed so as to be identical in all human males. If it were, any two males and females could pair-bond, that is, fall in love with each other. But nature, in its own wisdom, has designed us as a species rich in the diversity of individual differences, erotic individual differences included. Thus, the image of erotic arousal is no more innate than is native language. Like native language, the image of erotic arousal is established in response to early life experience, and it becomes engramed or imprinted. The so-called errors of imagery, manifested as transpositions of gender-identity/role, or as the intrusion or displacement paraphilias, also become engramed or imprinted. The infant and juvenile male appears more vulnerable to such an imprinting error than does his female counterpart, probably because of the greater importance of the visual image to erotic arousal in nature's design of the human male.

Gender-Identity/Role Transpositions

As shown in Table I, gender-identity/role transpositions may be classified in a 3 × 2 scheme of: chronic and episodic versus total, partial, and adventitious. In this scheme, transexualism represents the most extreme transposition in terms of time and completeness, and also of prognosis and therapy. Transvestism (transvestophilia) may appear equally complete, except that the transposition is time-limited, that is, cyclic or episodic, alternating between male and female. Homosexualism in its extreme forms of effeminate homosexuality in the male and virilist homosexuality in the female shows itself not only in erotic but also in nonerotic everyday behavior. The less extreme and more frequent manifestations of homosexualism may not be detectable except in erotic imagery and practice. This type of homosexualism may not, in everyday activities, be distinguishable from bisexualism. Bisexualism as here defined refers to homosexual behavior which alternates with heterosexual behavior as manifest primarily in eroticism and the sex of the partner.

TABLE I

3 × 2 Representation of the Transposition of Gender-Identity/Role

	Total	Partial	Adventitious
Chronic	Transexualism	Homosexualism	Sex-coded work, schooling, and legal status
Episodic	Transvestism (Transvestophilia)	Bisexualism	Sex-coded play, dress, manners, grooming, and decoration

The transpositions classified as adventitious in Table I do not pertain to erotic behavior itself, but to behavior in general that is culturally and historically sex-stereotyped. This applies to vocational sex-stereotyping as related to economic and legal rights of equality. It applies also to recreational and decorational sex-stereotyping. Vocational, recreational and decorational sex-stereotypes represent historically determined options. Nonetheless, many people think of them as eternal verities of sex difference, not subject to personal option and caprice. So great is the conviction of gender-identity/role, once it becomes differentiated and built-in, postnatally!

Transexualism

Transexual, the adjective, means simply going from one sex to the other. Thus one could have a casual transexual thought or dream, one's hermaphroditic baby could have a transexual change of the birth announcement, or as a hermaphrodite, one could undergo a transexual reassignment of one's sex. A person of nonhermaphroditic, nonambiguous genital anatomy may also seek and qualify to undergo a legal, hormonal, and surgical sex reassignment. This is the person who, in today's nomenclature, is known as a transexual.

Definition and Description

The transexual is genitally an anatomical male or female who expresses with strong conviction that he or she has the mind of the opposite sex, who lives as a member of the opposite sex part-time or full-time, and who seeks to change his or her original sex legally and through hormonal and surgical sex reassignment.

The actual demand for hormonal and surgical intervention has been dependent historically on the patient's knowledge of the availability of such procedures. The personal sense and conviction of having the wrong-sexed body, however, predates such knowledge. Typically, a transexual dates in childhood the onset of his or her sense of belonging to the other sex. The age at which sex reassignment becomes an *idée fixe* varies. It may be prepubertal or adolescent, or it may be delayed until, in young adulthood or early middle age, the obsession finally can be postponed no longer.

Incidence

Public health statistics in the United States do not include incidence figures on any sexological problems, including the incidence of birth defects of the sex organs. Voluntary registration of sexological problems would fail statistically, owing to the social penalties of self-disclosure. Therefore, there are no authentic estimates of the incidence of transexualism in the United States or anywhere else. However, it can be said that postoperative transexuals in the United States now number in the thousands, but almost certainly not in the tens of thousands. In a total United States population of just over two hundred and twenty million, the condition is far more common than most physicians might think, but not so common that every physician should expect to treat several cases in the course of his or her career. Some will see no cases, and some will miss cases because the patient is too apprehensive to state his or her chief complaint.

Etiology

In the etiology of transexualism, as of other gender-identity/role disorders, there is no demonstrable evidence of a hereditary factor, either in the family tree or as a spontaneous mutation. Transexualism has been recorded in some males with the 47,XXY chromosomal condition (Klinefelter's syndrome), but most XXY individuals are not transexuals.

By inference from experimental animal studies, prenatal hormonal history may be etiologically significant. There is as yet no directly demonstrable human evidence to implicate a prenatal hormonal effect, chiefly because there are no retrospectively retrievable records of the prenatal hormonal history of transexuals. If hormones do play an etiologic role, however, then it is almost certainly in the prenatal period, and not at puberty or later. It is very rare to find a hormonal abnormality in an untreated postpubertal transexual.

In cases of hermaphroditism with a known prenatal history of hormonal abnormality, transexualism is not a subsequent sequel, except in the presence of ambiguity of gender assignment and rearing postnatally. Such cases indicate that prenatal hormonal history alone is not capable of determining the subsequent differentiation of gender-identity/role. Postnatal history is proportionally more important. It has not yet proved possible to find a formula from which to predict transexualism on the basis of early childhood history, even among children who overtly wish to change sex. These same children have proved to develop as adolescent homosexuals or bisexuals rather than transexuals. In some families, it is possible to recognize a covert collusion of the parents and the child with respect to the child's repudiation of his or her anatomic sex.

Diagnosis

The diagnosis of transexualism is based initially on the presenting complaint, namely the need for sex reassignment. It is necessary for legal and ethical reasons to check the anamnesis against other informants and social records. It is in the nature of transexualism to give a revised or edited biography. The best diagnostic test is the "real-life test" for a minimum of two years, during which time social, emotional, and economic rehabilitation in the new sex role is achieved.

Usually the physical examination yields nothing contributing to the diagnosis, but it should not be omitted. In a few cases, other unrelated pathology may limit the therapy for sex reassignment. Very rarely, the EEG may show a temporal lobe epileptic focus requiring neurosurgery after which the sex problem may remit. Hormonal evaluations, useful for the research information they provide, are typically noncontributory.

Differential Diagnosis

The check list for the differential diagnosis includes:

Temporal lobe epilepsy with transexualism or transvestism as a related symptom.

Schizophrenic disorder with transexual gender-identity confusion as a symptom.

Transvestism (transvestophilia) with a strong element of transexualism that emerges, especially in middle life.

Female impersonation in an extremely effeminate (gynemimetic) male homosexual (drag queen) or male impersonation in a virilistic (andromimetic) lesbian.

The above diagnoses do not, in and of themselves alone, rule out the possibility of rehabilitation by means of sex reassignment, but they do require caution and unhurried decisions. Much the same applies also to transexuals who are pathologically depressed, for sex reassignment alone does not reverse depression.

Therapy

Sex reassignment is a rehabilitative form of therapy, not a cure. It is used because other forms of therapy capable of ameliorating the transexual's suffering have not, to date, been proved effective.

Initially the therapeutic goal is for the patient to achieve success in the two-year, real-life test. During this period, hormonal reassignment is instituted. With the exception of deepening of the voice in the female-to-male transexual, hormonal changes are reversible if the test proves to the patient that his or her transexualism does not warrant further pursuit of reassignment.

The following male-to-female hormone dosages have been found satisfactory: Estinyl (ethinyl estradiol) 0.02 mg. to 0.05 mg. daily, or Premarin (conjugated equine estrogens) 0.6 to 1.25 mg. daily. Before gonadectomy, the treatment would be every day for a minimum of four to eight months. Following surgery, treatment should be cyclic, for the first three weeks of each month, missing the fourth week.

An alternative to the foregoing would be a commercial product combining estrogen and progestin, for example: Lo-Ovral 1 mg. (norgestrel 0.3 mg. and ethinyl estradiol 0.03 mg.), or Ovral (norgestrel 0.5 mg. and ethinyl estradiol 0.05 mg.). The dosage of those preparations is one tablet daily for the first three weeks of each month.

If the patient prefers not to accommodate to a daily oral therapy, but to an intramuscular one instead, then the following could be prescribed: Delestrogen (estradiol valerate) 5 mg. plus Delalutin (hydroxy-progesterone caproate) 62.5 mg. every two weeks. Another intramuscular combined treatment could be: Depo-Estradiol cypionate 1 mg. plus Depo-Provera 25 mg. every two weeks.

After four to eight months of biweekly therapy, the same dosages could be given once every three or four weeks.

If in the preoperative state, the above dosages prove insufficiently effective after four to six weeks, then the dosage could be doubled. Otherwise, the rule is to use the dosage that is thought presently to be replacement therapy for normal women. The lower the effective maintenance dose, the better.

Hormonal feminization of male-to-female transexuals promotes a female appearance insofar as it brings about a feminine redistribution of subcutaneous fat. It also stimulates breast enlargement (gynecomastia), and may somewhat retard the growth of facial and body hair.

Hormone dosage for female-to-male transexuals which has provided satisfactory results is: Delatestrel (testosterone enanthate) 400 mg. intramuscularly once a month or half the dose every two weeks.

Hormonal masculinization of the female-to-male transexual induces suppression of the menses, but breakthrough bleeding may eventually occur. Permanent suppression requires castration (ovariectomy) or hysterectomy, preferably both. Other effects of hormonal masculinization include deepening of the voice and growth of facial and body hair. The shrinking effect on the breasts is minimal. The clitoris enlarges, but not sufficiently to permit masculinizing surgical reconstruction as even a very small micropenis. Its erotic sensitivity increases. The feeling of orgasm is reported as increased with no loss of the female capacity for multiple orgasm.

The above hormonal dosage may not prevent menopause-like symptoms following ovariectomy. Control of such symptoms may require additional estrogenic therapy with gradual withdrawal over a period of three to six months.

During the period of the real-life test, male-to-female transexuals may take voice retraining. They may also begin electrolysis for removal of facial hair and perhaps body hair also. These services are provided by trained and certified experts, usually in private practice, not in a hospital.

In some cases of female-to-male transexualism, mastectomy is necessary during the period of the real-life test, especially if the patient works as a male in a job in which exposure of a female chest contour, however disguised, is incompatible with continued employment.

A few patients need cosmetic and etiquette counseling, but most are masters of these arts without special help.

To a variable extent, local legal advice may be needed during the period of the real-life test, especially if a divorce is necessary, and also with regard to change of name and sex on documents. Complete legal recognition of the change of sexual status, in the form of a reissued birth certificate, varies according to legal jurisdiction. Usually a medical statement is needed for the legal change, after the sex reassignment has been completed.

The amount of counseling needed during the real-life test varies according to individual need and traveling distance. Patients from far away need a local counselor working in collaboration with the main center.

Some transexuals disown their families, and others are disowned by their families. The ideal of rehabilitation is to have the reassigned transexual acceptable to the family, however limited the personal contact. Therefore, family counseling is also a prerequisite. The siblings, especially the young ones, should not be overlooked in the overall plan of counseling. Nonfamily members, including the lover, personal friends, teachers, and employers also may be given information and advice on how to contribute to the transexual's total rehabilitation.

Sex reassignment surgery is too highly technical a procedure to be discussed here in detail. Male-to-female surgery has been reasonably well perfected, though in some cases there are residual problems of contracture and constriction of the vaginal canal requiring an additional operation. The end result can be convincingly feminine in appearance and function. Female-to-male surgery of the external genitalia presents insurmountable problems as great as in the case of congenital aplasia of the penis or accidental amputation of the penis. A plastic surgeon can make a penis of grafted skin, but it requires from five to fifteen surgical admissions, and the end result is a penis that is numb, unable to erect, and subject too easily to urethral constriction and urinary infection. For sexual intercourse, such an organ can penetrate the vagina only if supported, as in a hollow dildo. Thus, there is very good reason for the female-to-male transexual to settle for a strap-on prosthetic penis and to avoid the expense, pain, and poor result of very time-consuming surgery.

Female-to-male transexuals who undergo genital surgery do not lose the clitoris and so retain the capacity for orgasm. In fact, the orgasm is enhanced under the influence of androgen therapy. Male-to-female transexuals lose the kind of ejaculatory orgasm they once knew, but without regret, for it is replaced by a climactic feeling which, even though more diffuse, satisfies them all the more because they are able to satisfy a male partner.

Prognosis

The number of known cases of sex reassignment followed by a second reassignment to the original sex are few (four known and probably no more than ten) and the number of such cases published, fewer still. The transexual with such a history apparently rushes into the initial surgery prematurely, impulsively, and even against psychological advice. In contrast, for those sex-reassignment applicants who pass the two-year real life test, surgery confirms the status they have already achieved, and they continue to do well. They do well according to the criteria of earning a living, not being arrested, settling down with a partner, not needing a psychiatric referral, and saying that they are contented in their new status and do not regret the change.

The surgical prognosis is guarded. Male-to-female transexuals may need follow-up surgery to keep the vaginal canal functional and patent. The end result, however, only rarely is persistently unsatisfactory. Female-to-male transexuals may have problems, eventually correctable, of urethral stricture, and they always have the problem of impotence for which no successful surgical technique has yet been devised.

The hormonal prognosis is satisfactory for both male-to-female and female-to-male transexuals. Some male-to-female transexuals, particularly those few in show business, are unsatisfied with hormonally induced breast growth. They seek and obtain either augmentation mammoplasty or silicone injections. The latter are dangerous to health and are absolutely contraindicated.

Transvestism (Transvestophilia)

Transvestism means cross-dressing, that is, dressing in the clothes of the other sex. On the stage, it may be done as a dramatic device, as in a play by Shakespeare. For Halloween, it may be done as a gag or joke. A professional impersonator may cross-dress for a living, but such a person is likely to have more than a salaried interest in dressing up. He may be a drag queen, or she may be a butch lesbian, or either may be a would-be transexual. In the case of the male, he may be a clinically diagnosed transvestite (transvestophile); clinical transvestophilia has not yet been recorded in the female.

Definition and Description

As clinically defined, transvestism is a paraphilic condition (transvestophilia) in which a male has a sexual obsession for or addiction to women's clothes, such that he episodically experiences intolerable psychic stress if he does not dress up. In addition, he is handicapped in getting erotically aroused and performing sexually, regardless of being either heterosexual or homosexual in partnership, unless he is wearing female garments, as though wearing a fetish, or at least imagining himself as doing so. Some transvestophiles discover their proclivity at puberty by discovering that they can masturbate to orgasm only if wearing or handling some article or articles of female apparel. Many eventually try to find or educate a partner with whom to practice their transvestism. A few, especially as they advance in age, are erotically inert, but cross-dress permanently or as often as expediently possible. They do not request transexual surgery, but they may take female hormones. The typical transvestophile, however, wants no female hormones and no feminizing surgery. He simply dresses and wears makeup episodically as a female, and then returns to his male garb, until irritability, restlessness, and inner agitation demand relief again by impersonating a female and having an orgasm. Almost all transvestophiles have a female name to go with the female wardrobe. There is also a female personality. Like the male personality, it is in the literal sense unwholesome. The two personalities, if they can be put together, would make a whole. The female personality by itself is a travesty of a conventionally stereotypic woman and, correspondingly, the masculine personality.

Incidence

The incidence of transvestophilia is unknown. There are no public health statistics, nor are there satisfactory statistics of transvestites arrested by the police, nor of those seen by psychiatrists. There are some transvestite organizations with their own magazines or newsletters. The syndrome is probably more frequent than is generally assumed.

Etiology

The precise etiology of transvestophilia cannot be formulated on the basis of today's knowledge. Most evidence points to the early years when gender-identity/role is being differentiated as critical to the beginnings of transvestism. A few transvestophiles recall being dressed in girls' clothes as a punishment—the so-called petticoat punishment of the older literature.

Diagnosis

The diagnosis is made primarily from the patient's account of his chief complaint and its history. As in the case of transexualism, it is necessary to get corroborative evidence from family members or others and from available records. The physical examination is a routine necessity, even though it can generally be counted on as being noncontributory.

Differential Diagnosis

The diagnoses to be ruled out parallel those for transexualism (see above). There may be some confusion with transexualism in the case of the patient who wears women's clothes, but with a full unshaven beard, with or without taking estrogen, and with no demand whatsoever for genital surgery. Until the last few years this variant of transvestism was unknown, through lack of public disclosure. A corresponding female condition is that of the woman who wears men's clothes and who requests only a mastectomy, but no other treatment.

A tricky problem of differential diagnosis occurs in those cases of transvestophilic transexualism that sit on the fence, so to speak, of both diagnoses. Typically the patient is fortyish, and has been a covert transvestite throughout adulthood. Finally the compulsion for public appearance as a woman and for total sex change demands expression, despite personal commitments to wife and family. Without a real-life test of two years or longer, such a patient cannot get his affairs in order and himself rehabilitated. Some of them, however, are past masters at clinic shopping. They maneuver from one doctor to another, editing the information given to each, until they finally implement their plans, despite contradictory advice. Some of them become adequately rehabilitated. The burden imposed on their dependents may be excessive.

Therapy

Some transvestophiles live for years before they seek therapy or before an incident with the law requires them to do so. Others undoubtedly never seek therapy. Some associate with other transvestites, sometimes in bars where they congregate, or by joining a society formed for the purpose of sociability and self-help.

Transvestophilia is closely related to the hysterical, dissociative phenomenon of dual personality. It is to be expected, therefore, that the symptom of cross-dressing may in some instances undergo spontaneous remission, or that it may go into remission under the influence of some form of psychotherapy, including hypnotherapy, behavioral modification (aversive conditioning), or even religious exorcism. It has been known also to remit, at a time of formidable personal crisis, under a combined therapy of antiandrogen (medroxy-progesterone acetate) plus counseling. However, since the transvestism is also a form of addiction—addiction to female clothing—it is not surprising that it has proved singularly resistant to today's known methods of therapy.

For the most part, the treatment of transvestophilia is ameliorative and supportive. Often it is necessary as well as wise to include the family in the counseling program. In the case of the married transvestophile effective counseling can ameliorate a separation, if separation is inevitable, and equally well ameliorate continuance of the marital relationship.

Prognosis

The prognosis for complete and permanent remission of symptoms is poor, but not totally negative. The possibility of relapse is such that, in any instance of remission, the patient should be kept in followup at least four to six times a year, indefinitely.

Most patients with transvestophiles will not have a remission of symptoms. They can be helped in rehabilitation, however, to find a modus vivendi as transvestophiles.

Homosexualism

Homosexualism is the same as homosexuality. Professional opinion is currently divided as to whether homosexuality should be considered a syndrome or simply a socially sanctioned erotic alternative analogous to left-handedness. In the American Psychiatric Association the majority opinion, as expressed in the referendum of early 1974, supported a change in official nomenclature, so that homosexuality per se is no longer classified as a mental disease or illness. In the religious law of former times, homosexuality was a crime synonymous with treason and heresy. In the civil law today, in many states, homosexuality is classified as a crime against nature, with penalties that are brutally severe. In other states, homosexuality is considered a matter of private morality, provided it takes place between consenting adults.

Definition and Description

In current usage, there are those who define homosexuality mentalistically as a trait, state, or disposition emanating from the personality, and those who define it behaviorally as something that happens between two people with similar sex organs. The mentalist says that a person can be homosexual even though his or her only sexual practices have been heterosexual, provided the erotic imagery is consistently homosexual. To the mentalist, a single homosexual act by itself does not make the person homosexual, because homosexuality is defined as a continuing state of mind or personality. The behaviorist says that a single homosexual act makes a person homosexual for the duration of that act, but from that one act alone it will not be possible to predict more of the same in the future, nor what the person will say or do to indicate a trait, status, or disposition toward homosexuality.

The only evidence that both a behaviorist and a mentalist have about homosexuality is behavioral, that is, what the ostensible homosexual says or does. Thus, it makes sense to define homosexuality in terms of two people each with a penis, or two each with a vagina in an erotic partnership. Anything further about the fortuitousness of the event versus its replication, and anything about the imagery and thoughts of the partners, will need extra information. Only then can an inference be made about whether either partner is an obligative versus a facultative (situational) homosexual, the latter being in fact a bisexual. Homosexuality is extensively, though quite wrongly, used as a synonym for bisexuality in today's literature.

Extra information, over and beyond that of erotic performance, also is needed before an inference can be made regarding the extent or pervasiveness of the gender transposition in homosexuality. There are some male homosexuals who manifest negligible femininity vocationally and recreationally. Even in erotic performance, they may be more masculine than feminine in what they do, except that it is usually considered a feminine sign to have a male copulatory partner. The same applies, vice versa, in the case of the female homosexual.

A male homosexual who manifests little gender transposition, except for entering into an erotic activity or partnership with a male, is often said to have a male gender identity, but to prefer a male partner. For the sake of precision, one should say more restrictively that his gender-identity/role is predominantly male, though not completely so. Sexual practice and partnership are components of gender-identity/role and must be included in its definition as masculine or feminine in any given case.

Incidence

There are no public health statistics on the incidence of either male or female homosexuality or bisexuality. The figures most commonly quoted are those of Kinsey, since subsequent smaller-scale studies confirm them. Kinsey rated homosexuality on a seven-point scale (0—6). A rating of six signifies exclusive or obligative homosexuality of long duration, most likely a lifetime. A man with a rating of three will have had more than incidental homosexual participation off and on for several years during adolescence or later, not necessarily for a lifetime, and not to the exclusion of heterosexual participation. Kinsey estimated a rating of from three to six for 10% of the adult male population, and of five or six for 3%. The figures for the female population are less definite but are estimated at one-half to one-third those for males. On the basis of these estimates, the predominantly homosexual male population in the United States today is approximately three million plus, and the female, one million or more.

Etiology

There is disagreement, sometimes acrimonious, among experts as to the etiology of homosexuality, as there is also of heterosexuality and bisexuality. Theories range from loose assumptions of voluntary choice, through psychodynamic determinants in the personal biography, to hereditary predestinarianism. There is a good possibility, based on experimental animal studies, that an anomaly in prenatal hormonal function may influence sexual pathways in the central nervous system to remain sexually undifferentiated or potentially bisexual. In human beings, an individual so affected would be vulnerable, or easily responsive to additional postnatal influences, primarily social influences that enter the brain through the eyes, ears, and skin senses, that might favor perpetuation of bipotentiality or its resolution in a homosexual differentiation of gender-identity/role. Once differentiated, a strongly homosexual gender-identity/role tends to persist without changing.

There is not enough knowledge yet to formulate a rational program of prevention. Nonetheless, there is strong presumptive evidence that lifting the taboo on infantile and childhood sexuality, and responding positively to normal heterosexual rehearsal play in the early years, strongly favors heterosexuality at puberty and in adulthood. This evidence comes from anthropological studies and from experimental studies of psychosexual development in nonhuman primates.

Diagnosis

To apply the term diagnosis to homosexuality raises the same problem as applying it to red hair, left-handedness, or limb amputation, all of which are conditions not usually considered syndromes. All are conditions that are self-declared and do not need a diagnostic workup. In consensual homosexuality the evidence may be observed or the person may report it verbally. Without such direct evidence, there may be no way of inferring it from other aspects of behavior.

When homosexuality is not expressed in action, the only evidence may be the person's report of homosexual imagery in dreams, daydreams, and fantasy, or of responding erotically to homosexual images and percepts. In some instances, the only evidence, initially, may be symbolic and disguised; overt homosexual imagery, under the inhibiting pressure of guilt, embarrassment, or shame, may be unable to manifest itself directly. Its place is taken by erotic apathy, inertia, or depression, or by some symbolic sexual substitution.

There are no known or measurable somatic correlates of homosexuality which are important diagnostically. In particular, measures of circulating hormonal levels are noncontributory. However, homosexuality may occur in the presence of other syndromes such as hypogonadism, Klinefelter's (47,XXY) syndrome, and others.

Differential Diagnosis

Extreme cases of effeminate male homosexuality or virilistic lesbianism need to be differentiated from:

transexualism
transvestism

The most common error in differential diagnosis is to confuse homosexuality with:

bisexualism

The next most common error is to confuse homosexuality with accompanying or derivative symptoms or syndromes of behavioral disability such as:

psychosomatic stress reaction
anxiety neurosis
paranoid schizophrenic reaction
body-image neurosis or psychosis
delinquent or criminal character or conduct disorder
masochism, sadism, pedophilia, or other paraphilia

Therapy

The incidence of homosexuality is sufficiently high that, on the basis of the simple logistics of health-care delivery, it is economically nonsensical to declare all homosexuals in need of therapy. It would be impossible to supply enough therapists or to meet the staggeringly high cost. Moreover, there is no known form of therapy that can guarantee to change or regulate homosexuality, or bisexuality or heterosexuality, for that matter.

Pragmatically, it makes good sense to conserve society's therapeutic resources for those homosexuals who lack a sense of well-being in the practice of consensual homosexuality. These are the people who seek and who are able to respond to services offered. The only known effective form of therapy is some form of counseling or psychotherapy. If behavior modification therapy is used, it is preferable to use not punishment for homosexual response, but reward for heterosexual response. The reward may be a permitted homosexual encounter, but rewards are so programed in this form of therapy as to be earned only by an ever-expanding amount of heterosexual involvement.

The goal of therapy should be defined pragmatically, not ideologically. For those homosexuals who are actually bisexual, it may be pragmatic to aim for predominant or exclusive heterosexuality. For others, the goal preferably might be to gain a sense of well-being as bisexual and for still others, a sense of well-being as homosexual.

Prognosis

Provided the goal of treatment is pragmatically set, the prognosis is good, as it is also for those individuals who do not require treatment. Homosexuality is not a debilitating or life-threatening condition, except for secondary symptoms and reactions which may include even suicide and homicide. The severity of secondary symptoms decreases proportionately as family, friends, and society at large decrease their stigmatization and alienation of the homosexual.

In the course of history, homosexuality has been consistent with the highest levels of achievement and creative originality in the professions of science, art, religion, government, law, and business.

Bisexualism

Bisexualism and bisexuality are synonyms. In established usage, one may speak of the morphologic bisexuality of the embryo or of psychosexual bisexuality of the child or adult. In the Freudian and psychoanalytically derived theory of bisexualism, it is implied that a bisexual tendency lurks covertly, if not overtly, in all people. However, by analogy with embryonic development, it is more accurate to conceptualize an undifferentiated stage of gender-identity/role which, in the course of a critical developmental period, becomes permanently differentiated as either masculine or feminine, or as a combination of both.

Definition and Description

The bisexual person has traditionally been stigmatized as homosexual, since specialists as well as society at large overlook the heterosexual component in favor of penalizing the homosexual component.

As in the case of homosexuality, bisexuality can be defined either mentalistically or behaviorially. The most workable definition is that a bisexual person is one with a history of performing sexually with a person of either genital sex, separately or in a threesome or group. More broadly, the definition may also include those who have not actually performed but have experienced overt imagery of doing so. The transitoriness or regularity of either the practice or the imagery needs to be ascertained separately. The definition can then be appropriately augmented or qualified. The qualification may include an estimate of whether the degree and frequency of involvement with each sex is approximately the same (50:50) or disproportionate. Usually it is disproportionate. Falling in love, for example, is usually more intense and less perfunctory with one sex than the other.

Ambisexual, a term not widely used, refers to characteristics shared by both sexes—kissing, for example, as a form of erotic expression.

Incidence

The incidence of bisexuality in American men and women is currently unknown. Except among those who constitute a community of bisexual interest, bisexuality is stigmatized by society and the law. Many people cannot, therefore, admit their bisexuality, even if it occurs only in imagination. Others are not so inhibited, but are among those who can actually practice bisexuality, though only when the homosexual component of their bisexuality is situationally evoked—as among teenaged boys reared in a neighborhood in which hustling with older homosexual teenagers or young men is an acknowledged source of spending money, quite independently of affairs with girlfriends—or among men and women who are able to be homosexual while in sex-segregated jails, camps, or schools, but are heterosexual once released.

In some ethnographically reported societies, sequential bisexuality is a universally prescribed way of life. That is to say, young people at puberty and adolescence are sex-segregated and expected to interact homosexually together until, in young adulthood, their families can negotiate a bride price. After the marriage, the predominant, and usually exclusive form of sexual expression is heterosexual.

In America today, optional bisexuality among consenting adults is openly discussed as a viable and legal life style. In consequence, an increasing number of people admit their bisexuality. Some may also dare to express it for the first time. There is no evidence, however, that social permissiveness regarding erotic expression actually increases bisexuality. If such were the case, permissiveness would have to encourage a bisexual differentiation of gender-identity/role from infancy onward. In actual fact, permissiveness in the spontaneous sexual rehearsal play of infancy and childhood, and permissiveness in sex education, appear to encourage the differentiation of a heterosexual gender identity.

Etiology

The etiology or developmental differentiation of bisexuality follows the same general principles as apply to homosexuality. The evidence from embryonic anatomy and neuroanatomy is that nature's primary plan is to differentiate a female. Whereas the female pattern differentiates because the male pattern is not activated by something added (the Adam principle), the male pattern is differentiated by the active suppression of the female pattern. For bisexual behavior, one may speculate on the basis of animal experiments, that the female more than the male retains some of the original bisexual potential. The male, by contrast, may become either totally masculinized, or only partially so. If this speculation is correct, then it is easier for women than men selected at random to enter into a casual bisexual encounter—for example at a swinging, group-sex party. Some men will be impotent and erotically unable to respond to any stimulus from a person of the same sex. Others will be erotically versatile with both sexes.

There is no known single determining factor, prenatal or postnatal, that leads to the differentiation of a potentially bisexual erotic component in the gender-identity/role. The first bisexual experience may be preceded by bi-erotic fantasy and desire, a decision for sexual experiments, a change of sexual politics as in the women's movement, an awareness and admittance of previously covert bisexual orientation, or an alleviation of some traditional taboos among members of the "swinging" and "group sex" subculture.

Diagnosis

As in the case of homosexuality, bisexuality per se is a condition or way of behaving erotically, not a syndrome. Therefore, in the strict sense, there is no diagnosis. The condition is identified by the history either of sexual practice or imagery, or both. In its most covert form, bisexuality may not be identifiable as such, being manifest only as a failure of complete heterosexual abandon. Physical signs are noncontributory.

Differential Diagnosis

The issues are the same as in the differential diagnosis of homosexuality (see above).

Therapy

Of and by itself alone, bisexualism is not a disease and does not require therapy. The vast majority of individuals with a bisexual history never see a therapist. If bisexualism is associated with a lack of well-being, however, or if it is experienced as a source of distress to the person or partner, then either or both will benefit from some form of psychologic counseling or therapy. The goal of treatment most often is to restore a sense of bisexual well-being. Less often and in selected instances, the goal may be one of predominant heterosexual eroticism.

Prognosis

Bisexuality as an optional life style, equally acceptable to consenting partners, is like a vocational life style in not requiring a diagnosis. If a prognosis is required, it is for the sequelae of the life style. For some, overt bisexuality represents a compounding of problems, with a prognosis that is guarded, but not necessarily negative.

With less social stigmatization, bisexualism could become therapeutically accepted as a variant of human sexuality. For some individuals who otherwise might be victimized by social pressures into becoming patients, bisexuality enlarges the range of their behavioral options in eroticism and love so that they need not become patients.

References [Recommended Reading]

Green, R., and Money, J., eds. 1969. *Transexualism and sex reassignment.* Baltimore: Johns Hopkins Press.

Laub, D. R., and Green, R., eds. 1978. *The fourth international conference on gender identity dedicated to Harry Benjamin, M.D.: Selected proceedings. Volume 7, Number 4, Archives of Sexual Behavior.* New York: Plenum Press.

Money, J., 1970. Use of an androgen-depleting hormone in the treatment of male sex offenders. *Journal of Sex Research* 6:165-72.

Money, J., 1971. Prefatory remarks on outcome of sex reassignment in 24 cases of transexualism. *Archives of Sexual Behavior* 1:163-65.

Money, J., and Ambinder, R., 1978. Two-year, real-life diagnostic test: Rehabilitation versus cure. In *Controversy in Psychiatry,* ed. J. P. Brady and H. K. H. Brodie. Philadelphia: W. B. Saunders.

Money, J., and Ehrhardt, A. A., 1972. *Man and woman, boy and girl: The differentiation and dimorphism of gender identity from conception to maturity.* Baltimore: Johns Hopkins University Press.

Money, J., and Musaph, H., eds. 1977. *Handbook of Sexology.* Amsterdam/New York: Excerpta Medica.

Money, J., Wiedeking, C., Walker, P., Migeon, C., Meyer, W., and Borgaonkar, D. 1975. 47,XXY and 46,XY males with antisocial and/or sex-offending behavior: Antiandrogen therapy plus counseling. *Psychoneuroendocrinology* 1:165-78.

Notes

Originally published in *Handbook of Human Sexuality* (B. B. Wolman and J. Money, eds.). Englewood Cliffs, N.J., Prentice-Hall, 1980, with C. Wiedeking as coauthor. [Bibliog. #3.67]

The hormone dosages recommended in the text are presently still applicable in 1986.

Transvestophilia, the contemporary term, is synonymous with what used to be called the syndrome of transvestism as distinguished from the act of cross-dressing. In Chapter 29, which follows, the older term, transvestism, is used.

TWENTY-NINE

Two-Year, Real-Life Diagnostic Test: Rehabilitation versus Cure

Transvestism and Transexualism: Historical

In the Middle Ages anomalies of sexual behavior, including transvestism and transexualism, were considered to be manifestations of demonic possession, and those who exhibited such anomalies were subject to torture and imprisonment. Unusual sexual behavior was generally considered to be outside the realm of medicine, for since antiquity the boundaries of medicine had been defined in terms of the complaints of pain and suffering which patients brought to physicians. Transvestism and transexualism may bring secondary pain and suffering whereas, primarily, in and of themselves alone they are pain relievers.

After the Middle Ages the notion of disease expanded to include much of what had previously been regarded as demonic possession and sin. In the late 1700s modern psychiatry was born with the reclassification of certain of the behavioral anomalies as mental illness. By the twentieth century, the sexual behavioral anomalies were among those so reclassified.

As the definition and etiology of disease were being broadened in the nineteenth century, the role of the physician underwent profound change. A growing knowledge of germ theory and the spread of disease served as the impetus for society to mandate medical treatment in the interests of public health. In many instances, the prerogative for the initiation of medical treatment shifted from patient to physician, government official, or lawmaker. This shift underscored a discrepancy of therapeutic goal between patient and physician, especially with respect to enforced quarantine or immunization against infection. Eventually the same discrepancy affected gender identity transpositions. Psychiatrists defined these transpositions—homosexualism, bisexualism, transvestism, and transexualism—not as demonic possessions, sins, or crimes, as had formerly been the case, but as diseases. In the interest of public social health, they required treatment—treatment aimed at altering gender identity so as to match the genitalia. Viewing such therapy as a threat to their personal identity and possibly destructive of their sexual pleasure, patients who were coerced or cajoled into treatment often covertly protested, but they did not find the voice of overt political protest until very recently.

With the advent of modern plastic surgery, and the synthesis and commercial manufacture of sex hormones, in the first half of the twentieth century, persons with extreme gender identity transposition increasingly made their demands known to the medical profession. They sought surgical and hormonal alteration of their genitalia and secondary sex characteristics so as to give them the somatic appearance of the opposite sex. These people, with a conviction of belonging to the opposite sex and a compulsion to have their bodies changed, have since come to be known as transexuals.

Despite the failure of conventional psychotherapy in the treatment of transexualism, many physicians feared that honoring the request of self-proclaimed transexuals for genital surgery was little more than playing along with a psychosis, analogous to amputating the limbs or enucleating the eyes at a patient's request. However, some gave consideration to the alternative view that the wisdom of the body is such that the organism tries to heal its own prior injuries and traumas, psychic or somatic, and that there are occasions when medicine does best to respect that wisdom.

The proponents of this point of view hypothesized that by bringing about a resolution of the disparity between the mind of the transexual and his or her body and public image, hormonal and surgical sex reassignment would ameliorate the plight of the transexual. This rationale is analogous to that for the cosmetic surgical reconstruction of the breasts, nose, or face, or congenital or traumatic deformity. In all such instances, one recognizes the importance of the body image in promoting personal and social well-being, and undertakes rehabilitative therapy accordingly. Since the 1960's, the worldwide census of sex reassignments numbers in the thousands. Some few follow-up data have been published, but extensive follow-up has been prevented by the widespread disapproval of requests for the funding of any type of research pertaining to sexuality in human beings. The available evidence indicates that in authentic cases, sex reassignment does indeed prove to be rehabilitative.

Etiology

In the final analysis, the etiology of transexualism and related gender identity transpositions is unknown. However, a brief outline of the process of gender identity and gender role differentiation provides some insights into possible etiology. Chromosomes begin the process of gender differentiation, but do not preordain the end result. Their effects must be mediated by prenatal hormones, the effects of which in turn are mediated by cellular receptors. When these receptors are nonfunctional, as in the androgen insensitivity syndrome, it is possible for a normal female external physique and subsequently a normal female gender identity to differentiate in a body that chromosomally would otherwise would have been male.

The prenatal hormones are known to influence the central nervous system (CNS), as well as the rest of the body. Animal researchers have demonstrated that the sex hormones control the differentiation of sex-dimorphic neural pathways in the hypothalamus. Research in humans is constrained by ethical considerations. Clinical studies do, however, permit one to infer similar CNS effects. Particularly instructive are cases of prenatal adrogenization. In an earlier era, a few cases of prenatal androgenization occurred when a synthetic progestin, now known to be metabolized to an androgen, was administered to women in hopes of preserving an endangered pregnancy. More frequently, prenatal androgenization results from an adrenocortical metabolic error which leads to the endogenous production of excess androgen (the adrenogenital syndrome).

Girls thus androgenized *in utero* are more likely than their female age mates to spurn doll play, cosmetics, and jewelry in favor of vigorous outdoor athletic activity. They have a tendency to become competitive, and in later life are likely to give higher priority to career than to family. Such personality traits, although shared to a greater or lesser extent by members of both sexes, have traditionally been regarded as sex different.

It is still speculative that an unusual prenatal hormonal history makes one especially variable with respect to the differentiation of the erotic aspect of gender identity. None of the androgenized girls has ever evidenced desire for sex reassignment, though a large proportion is bisexual in fantasy or, less so, in practice.

The importance of the postnatal determinants of gender identity is indicated by studies of children matched for various characteristics, but differing in sex of rearing. Pairs of infants born with ambiguous genitalia and matched for karyotype and clinical diagnosis have been raised as members of opposite sexes and followed into adulthood. In virtually all of these cases romantic and sexual interests as well as general behavior patterns have differentiated predominantly in accord with assigned sex. This finding suggests that gender identity is in large part differentiated postnatally and is subject, like native language, to social learning.

The sort of learning which takes place is in many ways akin to the learning of language: tenacious and largely irreversible. And like the acquisition of language, the acquisition of gender identity and gender role are facilitated during a critical period which begins at about 18 months of age. While further learning can occur in later life, the critical period experience will continue to exert a strong influence. Just as an accent is a linguistic manifestation of critical-period learning, sexual idiosyncrasies may be the manifestations of critical-period, gender-identity learning.

The child differentiating gender role and identity mentally codes behavior as being masculine or feminine. This coding is a product of identification, that is of imitating or copying the behavior of one sex, and of complementation of the behavior of the other sex. Similarly, the natively bilingual child encodes words and other utterances as belonging to one language or another. In the same way that a bilingual child may have difficulty learning to speak when one speaker uses two languages, so too gender identity confusion may result when the gender-dimorphic expectancies of the parents and other important models are ambiguous and inconsistent.

Confusion may also develop when the distinctions between the sexes are clear enough, but the brain mechanism serving to differentiate the identification schema from the complementation schema becomes impaired. Just as in senility a more recently learned language may give way to the language of childhood, so too senile men and women may show traits formerly coded as belonging exclusively to the opposite sex. In some cases a brain lesion may result in a loosening of differentiation. Thus, extremely rare cases of temporal lobe epilepsy have been reported in which the epileptic focus induced not only seizures, but compulsive transvestism as well. Both the seizures and the transvestism remitted following successful neurosurgery. A similar but currently undetectable neural phenomenon may be associated with many of the gender-identity transpositions.

Developmental factors in the etiology of gender-identity transpositions range from covert and unidentified genetic programing, to possible effects of hormones, drugs, foodstuffs, and infections, to neonatal trauma, to inconsistencies and ambiguities in the child's social experience of gender, to gender-unrelated traumas which impair the differential coding of sex signals and/or retrieval of sexual behavior patterns.

Diagnostic Procedures

The physical examination is typically contributory only insofar as it may reveal unrelated pathology contraindicating surgery. In rare instances an EEG may indicate, in association with transexualism, temporal lobe epilepsy subject to pharmacological or neurosurgical control.

Psychologic tests may reveal associated syndromes, such as depression, schizophenia, or character disorder (psychopathic delinquency with lying and stealing). Though they do not rule out the possibility of rehabilitation through sex reassignment, these syndromes are not relieved by sex reassignment per se.

The primary source of initial diagnostic information is the standai.ized, objective interview with the patient, augmented by interviews with close kin. In order to insure that all pertinent topics are discussed a standard schedule of inquiry is imperative (Money and Primrose, 1969). Tape recording and transcription of the interviews insures an accurate record and facilitates the cross checking of information with family members and others necessary to minimize the patient's editing and/or misrepresentation, deliberate or otherwise, of his or her own history.

No diagnostic test that can be carried out within a hospital clinic or physician's office substitutes for the two-year, real-life test prior to the final and irreversible step of surgical sex-reassignment. This is a difficult test. It requires that the patient become socially, vocationally, economically, and emotionally rehabilitated in the sex of reassignment prior to surgical change of the genital anatomy. During the two-year test, hormonal reassignment is permitted, for its effects can be reversed, even in the most difficult instance of surgically reversing vocal cord masculinization in the female-to-male transexual.

The two-year, real-life test allows both the patient and the physician to monitor from waking to sleeping, week by week and month by month, the experience in the new sex status as he/she habituates his/her responses to other people. Without this test of how other people react, and how he/she reacts to other people, the patient knows only his/her private convictions and fantasies of being a member of the opposite sex.

Convictions and fantasies can be notoriously unreliable. They may include a covert and magical proposition in which the reassignment operation is equated with being born again, fully accommodated, as a member of the new sex, to the gender-dimorphic expectancies and responses of other people. Such accommodation does, however, require time. It should be accomplished prior to the irreversible step of surgery. Sex-reassignment surgery should occupy a place in a person's life that corresponds rehabilitatively to hysterectomy in the life of a woman, or prostatectomy in the life of a man.

Differential Diagnosis

Effeminate homosexuality, masculinate or "butch" lesbianism, and episodic transvestism are conditions which should be considered in the differential diagnosis of transexualism. These variable manifestations of gender identity transposition may be regarded as constituting either a statistical typology, or as marking idealized points on a continuous distribution. One of the problems of differential diagnosis is that some diagnosticians postulate a typology, whereas the clinical phenomena are not polymodal, but statistically continuous in distribution. Confusion on this issue leads to unnecessary argument and dissent with regard to differential diagnosis.

The idealized type of erotically effeminate homosexual male derives his erotic pleasure from giving orgasmic satisfaction to another male. He simulates the receptive female and withdraws attention from his own penis. He may avoid orgasm with his male partner, and in the partner's presence may even be impotent. Stimulated by a replay of his sexual encounter in imagery, he may later masturbate alone to orgasm.

His affectations, mannerisms, carriage, interests, and attitudes may be effeminate. Although he may cross-dress as a drag queen routinely or only occasionally at parties, he is without a compulsion to do so. He often reports an aversion to vigorous competitive games and rough outdoor activities dating from childhood and recalls being labelled "sissy" by his playmates. In adulthood he has been able to make his peace with life as an effeminate homosexual; he does not have a compulsion to become a woman, and does not detest his genitals. In fact they are an integral part of his sexual identity.

The female counterpart of the effeminate male homosexual is the masculinate lesbian. In the idealized case her mannerisms, movements, speech, and attitudes are typically masculine. She may dress as a man and seek to be a husband to her female lover. She often repudiates her breasts as a source of erotic pleasure and binds them as flat as possible.

The idealized type of male transvestite is heterosexual with respect to erotic partner. He is fetishistically dependent on dressing in feminine attire, or on the imagery of it for erotic arousal. He discovered his proclivity before or at puberty when he could masturbate to orgasm only while wearing or fondling women's clothing. In adulthood his cross-dressing may have come to involve a change in name and personality as well as wardrobe. Each cross-dressing episode is in response to an overpowering tension that builds up in the intervals between episodes, and which ideally is relieved by intercourse with a woman while wearing female garments. In the absence of partner consent, the male transvestite may have to rely on fantasy alone in order to have a coital orgasm. He cannot erotically divorce himself from either his penis or his transvestite wardrobe.

Bona fide transvestism either does not occur in females or is extremely rare, for it has not been reported in the sexological literature. Indeed it is a general rule that errors of psychosexual development leading to a paraphiliac image or object of sexual arousal are more frequent in the male. Most are virtually unheard of in women.

The idealized transexual is someone who in early childhood differentiated an incongruous gender identity, and has always felt that nature made an anatomical mistake. The possibility of sex reassignment and the label "transsexual" are discovered later. The idealized male-to-female transexual gets erotic pleasure from giving orgasmic satisfaction to the partner. In coitus and sex play he assumes the receptor role, receiving the partner's penis rectally, interfemorally, or orally. Preoperatively, the idealized male-to-female transexual's penis does not penetrate any orifice of the partner's anatomy, and penile stimulation is regarded as unpleasant and undesired.

The male-to-female transexual's fantasy may conform to the popular stereotype of the female as being sexually passive and accepting, slowly aroused, less prone to the initiation of sexual activity, and able to gain satisfaction from pleasing a partner. Adherence to this misconception is perhaps a function of the fact that many male-to-female transexuals have not experienced intercourse with a woman, and are, therefore, reliant on popular stereotypes. Many sex-reassigned male-to-female transexuals have had, and continue to have a sexual life with multiple male partners. A few establish themselves, in sex reassignment, as lesbians.

The idealized female-to-male, sex-reassigned transexual is erotically attracted to females. Like many ordinary women, he finds satisfaction in fidelity, and his sexual relationships are not too often casual or multiple. Also, like many women, he is dependent on intimate closeness for genitopelvic arousal. If he masturbates at all, it is infrequently. Presurgically, he regards penetration of his own vagina by a finger, a penis, or prosthetic device as intolerable, and is desirous of having male genitalia. Surgically, mastectomy has priority over genital plastic surgery. The breasts are a constant negative reminder of natal sex. Breast fondling either negates sexual arousal or is erotically unimportant. Coital imagery is of the self as male, without breasts, and usually complete with a penis, regardless of the sex of the partner.

In the idealized case, the conviction of transexualism dates from early childhood, although it also may evolve over the course of an individual's lifetime. For instance, in the fourth or fifth decade of life an apparent transvestite may find his episodes of femininity occurring with greater frequency and greater duration. The increasingly demanding female personality may come to insist on permanent repudiation of male clothing, and removal of the offensive male genitalia.

Effeminate homosexuality and butch lesbianism, as well as transvestism, may all be way stations en route to transexualism. If so, the differential diagnosis may be extremely difficult. Such people, above all others, owe it to themselves to live the real-life test for two years or more before surgery.

Social, Recreational, and Cosmetic Rehabilitation

A transexual beginning the real-life test may find it expedient in terms of earning power not to change the way he/she dresses at work, but only during off-work hours, until ready to embark on vocational rehabilitation.

Although the majority of patients are past masters at impersonating the other sex, a few exaggerate sexually dimorphic behavior patterns and require special counseling. For the female-to-male transexual this may mean toning down a macho swagger, and for the male-to-female transexual it may mean tutoring so that the daytime appearance is not that of a midnight whore.

The male-to-female transexual may begin electrolysis for the removal of facial and body hair. If carried out gradually and not completed until just prior to surgery, some hair follicles will remain should the real-life test be failed.

The female-to-male transexual may undergo mastectomy in order to flatten the chest. Should a return to the female role later be indicated, implantation mammoplasty will be possible.

Social rehabilitation may continue long after surgery, but prior to surgery the transexual must at the very least be comfortable and convincing in the sex of reassignment.

Establishing a New Public Identity

Early in the real-life test the transexual should establish a new public identity. Initially, this is a rather simple procedure since, by common law, any citizen of the United States has the right to change his/her name by personal decision, provided there is no intent of fraud or prejudice to others. Then the new name may be used on applications for library cards, credit cards, bank accounts, and various other items of identification.

When the transexual's public appearance as a member of the opposite sex becomes convincing, he/she will need a legal certificate of name change prior to applying, in most jurisdictions, for an amended or reissued birth certificate. In some jurisdictions, bureaucratic regulations constitute no obstacle, whereas in others it still is not possible to get a change of sexual status on the birth certificate. In such a case, the help of an attorney is advisable in getting other documentary changes, as for example, passport or academic certificates.

Financial and Vocational Rehabilitation

Vocational and financial rehabilitation usually, though not always, begins before a new public identity has been established. Since work is gender-coded in our society, many transexuals begin their work career in an occupation suited to their transexual personality. Some of these people will arrange to declare their new public identity and remain in their place of employment. Others will decide to break with the past and change to a type of employment which they like better and find more in keeping with their sex of reassignment. Still others will change employment as part of a total program of breaking with the past so as to avoid stigmatization as a transexual.

It is enormously complicated for any person, transexual or otherwise, to live in total alienation from his/her prior personal history, constantly evading the chance of discovery. Most transexuals are well-advised not to make the attempt. If they are tutored in the public relations of transexualism, and how to explain their situation medically and psychologically, then they will probably be surprised at how well they are publicly accepted. Some transexuals experience a sense of triumph and achievement at "going public," and being not stigmatized but congratulated at work.

In those instances in which the patient does not expect to be financially autonomous, but to rely upon a parent or benefactor for support, it is necessary to familiarize this third party with sex-reassignment procedures and to secure assurance that support will indeed be forthcoming following surgery.

Familial Rehabilitation

At the time the transexual makes known his or her plans for sex reassignment, it is good policy to offer family counseling regarding the medical and rehabilitation aspects of transexualism. Younger siblings especially need to be included. So counseled, family members are better able to reintegrate the transexual into the kinship as a member of the opposite sex. The family can be an important source of psychological support during the progress of sex reassignment. If, even with professional counseling, no reconciliation proves possible, the transexual will have the opportunity to accommodate himself or herself to the lack of familial support or to rethink the reassignment decision.

In those cases in which the obsession for sex reassignment develops in later life, the transexual may be a spouse and parent. If so, reassignment is not indicated until the necessary personal, legal, and financial arrangements have been made. Counseling of the spouse and children is obligatory.

Hormonal Reassignment: Male-to-Female

Endocrine reassignment of the male-to-female transexual with estrogen and progestin results in hormonal castration which is reversible. The patient thus gains first-hand acquaintance with impotence and reduced libido, before the irreversible steps of surgical castration, penectomy, and vaginoplasty. Should the patient find the effect of hormonal treatment to be anything other than desirable, he should not be considered a candidate for reassignment surgery.

Hormonal feminization promotes a female appearance insofar as it brings about a feminine redistribution of subcutaneous fat. It also stimulates breast enlargement (gynecomastia), and may retard the growth of facial and body hair. If a return to the male role is indicated, the breasts may be flattened surgically, and the other effects may be reversed upon withdrawal of hormonal therapy.

Hormonal Reassignment: Female-to-Male

Hormonal masculinization of the female-to-male transexual with androgen induces suppression of the menses. Since breakthrough bleeding usually will eventually occur, permanent suppression requires castration or hysterectomy, preferably both.

The effects of hormonal masculinization include deepening of the voice and growth of facial and body hair. The effect on the breasts is minimal. The clitoris enlarges, but not sufficiently to permit masculinizing surgical reconstruction as even a very small micropenis. Its erotic sensitivity increases. The feeling of orgasm is reported as increased, with no loss of the female capacity for multiple orgasm.

Should a return to the female role be indicated after a trial of hormonal masculinization, the menses will return upon withdrawal of androgen therapy. Masculine hair growth may be reversed by electrolysis. An expensive and difficult procedure also makes possible the restoration of a feminine voice.

Associated Psychopathology

Psychopathic delinquency with lying and stealing may occur in association with transexualism. Less frequently, hallucinations, delusions, or suicidal depression may also occur. All such symptoms require therapy in their own right. It is preferable that they be brought under control prior to embarking on sex reassignment, as they are not relieved by reassignment per se.

Explanation of Surgical Procedures

Informed consent is a necessary prerequisite of surgery. This entails an explanation of the surgical procedures involved, and possible outcomes. Because sex-reassignment surgical technique is not yet standardized, the approach varies from surgeon to surgeon. Explanations must be individually tailored. However, a few generalizations are possible.

The male-to-female transexual can expect that the surgical admission will require approximately two weeks and, in the case of a two-stage procedure, an additional surgical admission for a week or longer. The body of the penis will be excised, the urethral tube shortened and implanted in the feminine position, and a vaginal cavity created in the musculature of the perineum and lined with penile skin augmented with skin grafted from the thigh. Postsurgically the patient must wear a form in the vagina for at least several months in order to ensure its patency.

The postoperative capacity for erotic sensation will depend on how the skin of the penis and scrotum are utilized in feminization and on the particular hormonal regimen. The experience of orgasm may be a warm glow throughout the body or an orgasm of spasmodic intensity. The artificial vagina will supply a male partner with satisfying sexual feelings.

Surgical masculinization of the female-to-male transexual involves mastectomy (already discussed), and panhysterectomy, a relatively simple procedure in which the ovaries and uterus are removed. Should phalloplasty be decided upon there are two general procedures. Both are much more difficult than vaginoplasty for the male-to-female transexual, and produce a much less satisfactory end result. One involves the creation of a penis complete with urinary tube from abdominal skin grafts. As many as 15 surgical admissions over several years may be required in order to get a completely satisfactory urinary tube. In this procedure the clitoris is preserved intact, and retains its capacity to produce orgasm, but the numb roll of skin in which it is embedded is too flabby to effect sexual penetration, unless supported inside a hollow prosthetic penis.

The surgical alternative is to create a copulatory rather than a urinary organ. This procedure involves fashioning a hollow tube from an apron of skin peeled downward from below the navel. It also requires multiple hospital admissions. The clitoris is embedded in the base of the hollow tube as in the former procedure. For intercourse a prosthetic device must be fitted into the hollow tube.

Since sexual intercourse will be impossible without a prosthetic device regardless of the surgical procedure performed, the female-to-male transexual should be counseled as to the wisdom of making-do with a strap-on prosthetic penis, and forgoing the lengthy and complex procedures involved in phalloplasty.

A Promise to Cooperate in Follow-up Studies

Having embarked on the real-life test, some patients will decide that reassignment is not the solution they've been seeking to life's problem. Others will require a longer test period. For these, as for those who have passed the real-life test, and are still convinced in favor of sex-reassignment surgery, one final prerequisite remains. The patient must guarantee to cooperate in long-term follow-up studies. Transexuals eager to forget their preoperative past may balk at this requirement, but it is imperative if the procedure of sex reassignment is to remain acceptable as a proven form of therapy.

Outcome of Surgical Sex Reassignment

Though rare, it does happen that sex-reassigned individuals decide to revert to their original sex assignment. We have had personal interviews with three such individuals, and had correspondence from a fourth. In each instance, the patient planned his own timetable of sex reassignment so as to evade the two-year, real-life test.

Because the criteria of selection for sex reassignment have varied from institution to institution in the absence of proven standards, it is difficult to interpret much of the follow-up data in the literature. However, it is clear that when the two-year, real-life test is a prerequisite for sex-reassignment surgery, virtually 100 per cent of the patients benefit from surgery according to both subjective and objective criteria of evaluation. Thus, following surgery, job status stays the same or improves, sexual relationships tend to be more stable and longer lasting, and patients do not become psychotic. A history of arrests for solicitation may continue, but there is no increased incidence of law-breaking behavior. Patients report subjective satisfaction with sex reassignment, and indicate that if they had it to do over again they would make the same decision, even though the surgical outcome may have been a disappointment and, by the coital criterion, a failure.

Conclusion

By next century, research into the etiology of gender identity transposition may suggest new and better therapeutic approaches to transexualism. Insofar as sex reassignment provides the opportunity for the medical profession to maintain contacts with transexuals, and stimulates the systematic collection of data about transexuals, it will facilitate such research. In the interim, sex reassignment is the only demonstrable effective treatment—rehabilitative treatment, not curative. Truly preventive and/or curative treatment still awaits discovery.

Summary

Transexualism, once considered to be a sin and outside the realm of medicine, is now classified as an illness. Prenatal endocrine and postnatal social factors may be important determinants of gender identity transposition, as in transexualism, but in the final analysis the etiology is unknown. Whereas psychotherapeutic attempts to cure transexualism by altering gender identity so as to conform to the body have been unsuccessful, alteration of the body so as to conform to the gender identity through sex-reassignment surgery has proved to be an effective rehabilitative therapy. In the differential diagnosis of transexualism an important source of information is the tape-recorded, transcribed, and tabulated diagnostic interview. The differential diagnosis includes effeminate homosexuality, masculinate lesbianism, and episodic transvestism. The most important diagnostic test is the two-year, real-life test during which time the candidate for sex-reassignment undergoes social, recreational, vocational, economic, familial, and hormonal rehabilitation in the new gender role. The final prerequisite for the irrevocable step of surgical reconstruction is the patient's informed consent and agreement to cooperate in follow-up studies. When the real-life test is required prior to surgery, the outcome is positive according to both objective and subjective criteria.

Reference

Money, J., and Primrose, C.: Sexual dimorphism and dissociation in the psychology of male transexuals. In Money, J., and Green, R. (eds.): *Transexualism and Sex Reassignment.* Baltimore, Johns Hopkins University Press, 1969.

Note

Originally published in *Controversy in Psychiatry* (J. P. Brady and H. K. H. Brodie, eds.). Philadelphia, Saunders, 1978, with R. Ambinder as coauthor. [Bibliog. #3.52]

Author's Comment: Transexualism and the Philosophy of Healing

Medicine has a venerable and continuing history of controversy regarding methods of treatment. It came as no surprise that controversy surrounded Harry Benjamin's pioneering book, *The Transsexual Phenomenon* (New York,

Julian Press, 1966) and, that same year, the inception of the program of surgical sex reassignment at Johns Hopkins. In defense of that program, which I had been instrumental in founding, I wrote the following policy statement for the *Journal of the American Society of Psychosomatic Dentistry and Medicine*, 18:25-26, 1971 [Bibliog. #4.24], at the request of its editor, Leo Wollman:

> Some illnesses are acute, time-limited, and subject to therapeutic arrest or reversal, followed by return to health. These, in the Hippocratic tradition, the physician aims to cure. Other illnesses are chronic, progressive, and deteriorative. For these, the physician is less ambitious. He aims to ameliorate or palliate, with whatever treatment available, the suffering they engender. Still other illnesses or conditions are chronically, though not progressively disabling. For these, the physician's goal is ameliorative plus rehabilitative.
>
> Transexualism is not a reversible condition, judging by today's therapeutic techniques. Nor is it a progressively deteriorative condition, but it does represent a chronic disability, requiring a patient's life to be rehabilitated.
>
> Sex reassignment—social, hormonal, surgical, and legal—is an ameliorative and rehabilitative treatment for transexualism. It is not a cure. There cannot be a clearly formulated cure for this condition in the absence of a clearly formulated etiology so far not discovered.
>
> In the wisdom of nature, the organism's attempt to defend itself against either traumatic or developmental insult may be less than ideal, but superior to total failure. Dwarfed stature, for example, may be a less than ideal reaction to malnutrition, but it obviously has survival value. Years later, after the critical growth period has passed, no known treatment will bring about increase in height. Treatment, to be of any help, must be of the rehabilitative type, based on the assumption of short stature forever. Here in stunting of growth is a parallel to transexualism, which is the end product of maldifferentation of gender identity relative to sexual anatomy.
>
> In transexualism, sex-reassignment therapy not only endorses the organism's own attempt at self-healing, but also furthers it by the administration of hormones and performance of surgery. Except for those already familiar with intersexuality and related disorders, such therapy represents a radical departure from tradition. It is small wonder, therefore, that the legalistic mind, trained to rely on precedent, should be hesitant to legitimate the new procedure. Eventually, however, the law catches up with history.
>
> What is amazing is the extent to which the law has already accepted transexual sex-reassignment, even when it does not accept change of the birth certificate. Even the birth certificate is not a stumbling block in many states of the U.S.: the decision for their reissue was made by administrative order, not by legal decision. Whereas legal decisions generate publicity and make headlines, administrative orders seldom attract attention. Yet they may, in the long run, be more effective in establishing precedent.

THIRTY

Endocrine Influences and Psychosexual Status Spanning the Life Cycle

I. Psychosexual Differentiation and Development

In developmental psychosexual theory, it is no longer satisfactory to utilize only the concept of psychosexual development. Psychosexual differentation is the preferential concept, for the psychodevelopment of sex is a continuation of the embryonic development of sex. The embryonic reproductive system is sexually dimorphic. So also is subsequent behavioral and psychic development. The purpose of this chapter is to review and integrate research findings on endocrine influences on psychosexual differentiation of man and woman from conception to maturity.

II. Essential Variables for Understanding Hormone-Behavior Interactions

Variables that need to be distinguished in analyzing endocrine influences on behavior are: phase of the life cycle; hormone involved; quantity of hormone and its diurnal and other rhythmic fluctuations; biologic activity of the hormone measured; timing or duration factor; and method of measurement used. It is also necessary to be alert to exogenous interference and factors that change hormonal secretion and necessitate the use of multivariate statistics.

Phase of the Life Cycle

The same hormone may have different effects on behavior, dependent on whether it is present during the prenatal, neonatal, childhood, pubertal, adult, or senescent stage of the life cycle. Prenatally, for example, androgen has an organizing effect, which it later will not have on developing neural tissues that eventually will mediate sexual behavior. The critical fetal period for this effect differs according to species. Briefly stated, the principle is that the addition of androgen masculinizes (the Adam principle) and absence of androgen feminizes (the Eve principle).

At puberty and subsequently, the role of androgen in relation to behavior is not to program or organize, but to activate brain pathways that subserve sexual behavior. Otherwise stated, androgen lowers the threshold for the emergence of sexual imagery and behavior, either spontaneously or in response to a sensory stimulus. It is highly probable that androgen is the hormone responsible for this threshold-lowering effect in females as well as males.

Hormones Involved

According to present knowledge, the hormones directly involved in human psychosexual differentiation and development are the gonadal steroids, especially androgen. The function of estrogen and progesterone in the developmental differentiation of human female psychosexuality is obscure. The psychosexual issue is rendered more complex because the route of steroid biosynthesis is from progesterone to androgen to estrogen and because target cells may take up one hormone and transform it into another. Prenatally, for example, there is some evidence that testosterone converted to estradiol may be the active hormonal agent in cells of the central nervous system (McDonald and Doughty, 1973; Reddy et al., 1974). Intracellular conversion of testosterone to dihydrotestosterone is also known to be of widespread occurrence.

The pituitary hormones—the gonadotropins, follicle-stimulating hormone (FSH) and luteinizing hormone (LH); and growth hormone and prolactin—so far as is known do not directly influence psychosexual differentiation and development, though a positive role for them has not been clearly ruled out. The possible role of hypothalamic hormones as directly affecting psychosexual status remains also to be investigated.

Two or more hormones may act either independently, antagonistically, or synergistically. The antiandrogenic action of estrogen in the male is a prime example of an antagonistic effect, with consequent psychosexual repercussions, for estrogen diminishes psychosexual as well as genital functions in the male.

Quantity of Hormone

The quantity of the various hormones in target cells influences psychosexual differentiation and development. Prenatally, for example, females may be exposed to different amounts of fetal adrenal androgen, with resultant different degrees of psychosexual masculinization. At and after puberty, androgen deficiency in the male induces a psychosexual deficit.

Not just the level of hormones, but also the rate of secretion of a hormone may be influential. For example, the psychologic distress experienced by some women during the premenstrual phase of the cycle has been attributed to the rapidity of the change, prior to the onset of the menses, in the quantity of estrogen and progesterone secreted (Dalton, 1964).

Biologic Activity

Not all biochemical precursor or derivative variants of a hormone—androgen, for example—are equally potent in biologic activity; and not all target cells respond equally to the same variant. Thus, brain cells may respond more avidly to one variant of androgen, and prostate cells to another. The actual hormonal variants most contributory to the regulation of human psychosexual development and differentiation in the brain still cannot be identified, for the technique of choice, using radiolabeled hormones, gives no guarantee that the body's cells take up labeled hormone at the same rate as they do the unlabeled hormone from the body's own endocrine glands.

The level of a hormone circulating in the bloodstream can be measured by radioimmunoassay of a blood sample. The actual level as usually measured, however, is not the level of the hormone that is actually free for biologic activity. Only that fraction which is free or unbound is available for cellular uptake and use. A special laboratory procedure is needed to separate the free from the protein-bound fractions. Routine radioimmunoassy does not separate the two fractions. Thus it is necessary to go through the procedure of ascertaining the unbound level of a circulating hormone in order to make any hormone-behavior correlation valid. This precaution is not always adhered to in studies attempting to correlate blood hormone level with some aspect of psychosexual status or function.

Timing Factor

Fluctuations in the circulating level of a hormone in the bloodstream vary from one hormone to another according to different biological clocks: circadian, monthly, or seasonal, and sleeping or waking. Levels vary also in response to specific stimuli, e.g., suckling, or life experiences, e.g., starvation. Sophisticated studies of hormone-behavior interrelationship control for these fluctuations, as when minute quantities of blood are withdrawn continuously for a 24-hr. period through an indwelling catheter operated by a miniaturized blood pump.

Blood hormone levels fluctuate also according to the phase of the life cycle. Developmentally, if hormone secretion is premature, on time, or delayed, there is a parallel scheduling effect on either the precursor of the actual phases of psychosexual differentiation or development or both. The correlation is not perfect, however. This is in part due to the fact that psychosexual status is governed by the brain to some extent independently of sex steroids. Thus, penile erections occur in prepuberty. Their prevalence increases under the influence of hormonal puberty. Nonetheless, it is possible for a youth of nineteen with no gonads and no hormonal replacement therapy to copulate, to have a subjective experience of climax, and even to establish a pair-bond (Money and Alexander, 1967).

Psychosexual maturation parallels general social maturation as well as hormonal maturation. Statural maturation, independently of hormonal and secondary-sexual maturation, indirectly parallels psychosexual maturation, as when statural dwarfism elicits infantilizing reactions from other people.

Method of Measurement

The radioimmunoassay technique for determining the circulating level of a hormone dates from the mid-1960s. It permits a degree of accuracy and precision previously undreamed of, and can be carried out on a minute sample of blood. Studies using the earlier techniques of hormone determination render obsolete all earlier attempts to correlate hormones and behavior.

There has been no corresponding advance in technique with respect to behavioral study. The most trustworthy studies are those in which the primary data are tabulated from real-life observations and recordings, not from second-hand reports. The least trustworthy studies are those employing questionnaires that purport to measure abilities, powers, traits, attitudes, or motivations of the mind.

III. Hormonal Measurements over the Life Cycle and Psychosexual Differentiation and Development

Prenatal Phase

It has long been known that the external genitalia differentiate as masculine or feminine between the 12th and 16th week of gestation. In the absence of any gonadal steroid, the genitalia assume a female appearance. The presence of androgen is absolutely necessary if differentiation is to produce male genitalia. In the normal course of development, the androgen needed for male differentiation is supplied by the fetal testis. Testicular secretion of testosterone, the most potent form of androgen, can be detected as early as 8 to 10 weeks after conception (Siiteri and Wilson, 1974). The maximum output of fetal testosterone is reached at approximately 20 weeks, and then declines until parturition (Taylor et al., 1974).

During this same period of human fetal life, specifically from the 12th to the 18th week of gestation, levels of testosterone, mainly from the testes, and androstenedione, mainly from the adrenal cortices, are higher in the male than the female fetus (Abramovich and Rowe, 1973). No one has yet devised a method for correlating the midtrimester surge of testosterone in the human male fetus with dimorphic differentation of sexual pathways in the brain's hypothalamus and limbic system. In subprimate animal studies, however, it has been demonstrated that during the peak period of fetal androgenic activity, when the external genitalia are masculinized, there is a corresponding masculinization of the neural pathways that will subsequently subserve sexually dimorphic pituitary rhythm, and the associated dimorphism of copulatory reciprocity.

The extensive literature on this subject is reviewed in Harris (1964), Whalen (1968, 1974), Gorski (1971, 1973), Money and Ehrhardt (1972), Reinisch (1976), and Dörner (1976). The principle of brain differentiation is the same as for the external genitals, namely, the Adam principle; which signifies that female differentiation takes priority and requires neither fetal gonads nor their hormones, whereas male differentiation requires the addition of androgen which in the usual course of events is supplied by the fetal testes.

From human clinical studies of hermaphroditism (reviewed in Money and Ehrhardt, 1972) it is evident that sexually dimorphic behavior later in postnatal life is to some degree influenced by prenatal androgenization. A parallel effect can be induced experimentally in rhesus monkeys by injecting a pregnant mother carrying a female fetus with testosterone during the critical period of fetal brain differentiation. The daughters are born with a penis and develop behaviorally in a tomboyish way. That is to say, fetal androgenization induces a threshold-masculinizing effect.

Conversely, fetal deandrogenization of chromosomal males induces a threshold-deandrogenizing effect morphologically synonymous with a feminizing effect. Fetal deandrogenization occurs as a feature of some human syndromes of hermaphroditism. It can also be induced experimentally in animals by either surgical or hormonal (antiandrogenic) castration. The effect of fetal deandrogenization subsequently manifests itself in behavior that is erotic or procreative, like copulatory positioning, and in behavior that is not erotic, like urinary positioning and activity cycles.

In the males of some species, e.g., hamster, an excess of prenatal or neonatal androgen induces a degree of behavioral ultramasculinization, abolishing what would otherwise be normal for the species, namely, bisexual or sex-shared behavior. The significance of such a finding for the human species is not known; however, it does generate the hypothesis that individual difference in bisexual, as compared with exclusively heterosexual or homosexual capacity, is in some way related, or partly related to prenatal hormonal history.

The effect of fetal androgenization on behavior is to create not an absolute male-female dichotomy, but to set a behavioral activator or biostat at a different level for males and females, so that behavior which is, in fact, sex-shared is also threshold-divergent in males and females. Thus, the readiness with which it is evoked by its eliciting stimulus, and its overall prevalence, is sex-different.

From the study of experimental androgenization and deandrogenization of animals and corresponding clinical syndromes in humans, it is possible to make a provisional list of at least nine components of behavior that are sex-shared, but threshold-dimorphic.

The first sex-shared behavior is general kinesis, a high level of organized energy expenditure. This is not reminiscent of the behavior of a hyperkinetic child. It is expressed in outdoor athletics or team-sport activities or in muscular work. It is more prevalent in males than females.

Second, competitive rivalry and assertiveness to elevate one's rank in the dominance hierarchy is more prevalent in males than females. It is more transparently evident in childhood than adulthood, when it may take more covert and symbolic form as a power struggle. It is associated with a preference for utility clothing and disregard of adornment.

Third, roaming, appears to be related to territorial mapping or marking. It is more prevalent in boys than girls, and may, by a stretch of the scientific imagination, indirectly have something to do with space-form perception and praxic ability. In many lower species, marking is done with special scent glands that, under the influence of androgen, secrete pheromones.

Fourth, defense of the troop against intruders and predators, is also related to boundary maintenance. It is more prevalent in males than females. It does not mean that males are more aggressive than females, but rather that the stimulus that triggers aggression in the two sexes is threshold-different.

The fifth sex-shared behavior is guarding and defense of the young. It is more prevalent in females than males and demonstrates the potential aggressiveness of females as well as males.

Sixth, nesting and homemaking, is explicitly under hormonal, especially progestinic, control in lower species. It is more prevalent in females than males, but even in lower species it can also be evoked in the hormonally untreated male.

Seventh, prenatal care of the young, includes the rehearsal of parentalism in doll play and other forms of playacting. It is more prevalent in females than males. It may be associated with a more sensitive threshold for detecting distress sounds of the young, especially in sleep. Thus, by another stretch of the scientific imagination, it may indirectly have something to do with the linguistic achievement of girls, especially in reading.

Eighth, sexual mounting and thrusting, is more prevalent in males, as vs. presenting or spreading and containing, more prevalent in females. Observation of the play of juveniles among lower primates suggests that there may be some degree of prenatal programing of these sexual positionings in humans.

The ninth behavior is dependence on visual stimuli for erotic arousal, especially with respect to initiating an erotic engagement. This is more prevalent in the male, vs. dependence on tactual or haptic stimuli, more prevalent in the female. There is no good animal model against which to test this hypothesis, and the insufficiency of comparative, human cross-cultural data permits no firm conclusion. If the hypothesis is correct, males are prenatally hormonally programed to be developmentally more sensitive in infancy and childhood to establishing a connection between genital arousal and a visual image, including an atypical image. The main evidence in favor of this hypothesis is that more males than females develop a paraphilia, that is to say a disorder in which sexual arousal is dependent on an atypical or bizarre image (either benign or noxious); and that the more rare and bizarre paraphilias are not recorded in females. Evidence of the greater prominence of visual imagery in male than female eroticism is the pubertal occurrence of the wet dream, in which the sleeping boy is confronted with a visual spectacle of whatever it is that is his personal erotic turn-on, be it hererosexual or otherwise. There is no corresponding experience for the pubertal girl, who is also less likely than the boy to have a masturbation fantasy or to masturbate, according to current evidence.

Neonatal Phase and Infancy

Endocrine function in the fetus is not autonomous but is tied to the hormonal secretions of the placenta and to the mother's own endocrine secretions. In neonatal life, hormonal measurements reflect the change-over from prenatal endocrine symbiosis to postnatal autonomy (Mitchell and Shackleton, 1969). Normative values are being established by Bertrand, Forest and their co-workers at Lyons, France (Forest, et al., 1973a; Forest et al, 1973b; Forest et al., 1974). According to the findings of these workers, the level of testosterone in cord blood obtained at the time of birth was significantly higher in males than in females. In male infants, the concentration of testosterone increased from birth, reaching a peak between 2nd and 3rd month of life, followed by a gradual decrease until between the 4th and 5th month, when the concentration was down to the level found in prepubertal boys. In females, the cord level of testosterone was high at birth, though less so than in males. There was no neonatal peaking, and by the 2nd week of life testosterone had reached the low level maintained throughout female prepuberty.

In both sexes, the level of androstenedione from the adrenal cortices fell neonatally, but more rapidly in girls than boys. Throughout the first year, the mean level of LH was lower in girls than boys, whereas the reverse held true for FSH.

The significance of the foregoing hormonal dimorphism in neonates with respect to either somatic or behavioral and psychosexual development is presently unascertained.

Even though no correlations have been established between neonatal and early infantile androgen levels, on the one hand, and psychosexual function, on the other, there is evidence that psychosexuality, broadly construed, is present from birth onward. The most comprehensive source of literature on childhood sexuality is Martinson's 1973 volume.

Erection, like thumb-sucking, is possible in utero. A boy may be born with an erection. Erections in male infants may occur as frequently as once or twice an hour (Halverson, 1940). Throughout boyhood, and until senility, erections occur during sleep. The corresponding phenomenon in girls has not yet been studied in any detail.

The neonatal phase of psychosexuality appears not to be exclusively a matter of male or female differentiation; it is similar for both sexes. At least, there have not yet been any reports of sex differences that might be correlated with neonatal sex-hormone levels. At the outset neonatal psychosexuality appears to be intimately associated with the infant's pair-bonding to the parents. It involves very strongly the haptic sense (grooming, cuddling, rocking, and clinging). In the mother-infant interaction, it includes nursing at the breast. The haptic phase begins at delivery, and the oral phase joins it soon thereafter. When the mother breastfeeds, the haptic phase becomes associated more with the mother's than the father's body. If the infant is bottle-fed, either parent can become the mediator of the haptic-oral phase. Deprived of neonatal haptic experience, an infant becomes permanently impaired behaviorally and psychosexually, as is evidenced in extreme child-abuse-deprivation cases, and in the experimental model of the same phenomenon in rhesus monkeys.

In both sexes, genital self-touching occurs early in infancy (Galenson, 1975), especially if not punished. It precedes not only what in classical Freudian doctrine is known as the genital phase, but also the pregenital, anal phase. Strictly speaking, the anal phase is less a phase of psychosexual development than of the establishment of urinary and fecal continence. In the same way, various animals capable of being housebroken reach a phase of development when they are neurally mature enough to seek a special place to eliminate—as when kittens scratch a hole in dry earth or sand.

The differentiation of what is now coming to be known as the core gender identity and role—the self-identity and self-role as male or female—parallels developmentally the establishment of native language. It is established on the basis of identification with, usually though not exclusively, the parent of the same sex and of complementation to, usually though not excusively, the parent of the opposite sex. Gender-identity/role differentiation takes place apparently without dependence on circulating hormones, though it may be indirectly sex-differentially influenced by predispositions hormonally programed in the central nervous system in prenatal life (see above).

The establishment of core gender-identity/role precedes the era of the oedipus complex as defined in classical psychoanalytic doctrine. In recognition of this fact, Freudian oedipal theory is currently undergoing revision. As originally formulated, oedipal doctrine applied to disturbed development. It is now thought that in normal development the oedipal phase is simply a continuation of the process of identification and complementation that began earlier.

Probably because the sexual taboo in our society affects scientists as much as parents and other observers, there are no firm data as to when pelvic thrusting first becomes manifest as a type of sexual rehearsal play, but it is clearly present in the 3- and 4-year-old. So far as is known, these thrusting movements are not different in boys and girls to begin with, though more information is needed before a definitive statement can be made. Later on they become differentiated; the mounting role becomes more prevalent in the male and the spreading role more prevalent in the female. It is not yet known to what extent such play is copied from older children and/or adults rather than being a spontaneous developmental emergence, as it may well be, according to evidence of lower primates.

Psychosexual differentiation during the period of late infancy and early childhood is rather easily disruptable, if one judges by the evidence of primate experiments and the evidence of clinical syndromes in childhood or their later manifestations in adolescence and adulthood. It is highly likely that the foundations of all the paraphilias (formerly referred to as the perversions) and of the male-female transposition syndromes are set at this early stage. The nature of the programing, or misprograming, involved in the genesis of these conditions is open to dispute that cannot be settled on the basis of present developmental evidence. The most likely hypothesis is that, if there is a hormonal component to such misprograming, it belongs to prenatal and not to postnatal life and exerts its effect by creating a predisposition to difficulty in the later differentiation of an uncomplicated psychosexual status, unencumbered by paraphilic imagery. Postnatally, psychosexual differentiation, plus or minus errors, resembles the establishment of native language. That is, it is heavily dependent on input from the social environment and may be adversely influenced by disturbances in the social environment, including disturbances that are not themselves clearly related to sexuality but evoke widespread disturbance in the developing organism. Parental abandonment or traumatic proximity to death and dying are examples.

Prepuberty and Onset of Puberty

The prepubertal phase of childhood is neither endocrinologically nor psychosexually so dormant as the doctrine of latency once formerly claimed. As compared with the neonatal and pubertal phases of development, the ovaries and testes are hormonally relatively dormant in prepuberty, though not totally so. Their own hormonal production is negligible, but they maintain a sensitive responsivity to pituitary and hypothalamic stimulation, as can be tested experimentally.

The biological clock that regulates the timing of puberty still has not been discovered (Grumbach et al., 1974). It is something of a mystery that the age of puberty has been decreasing by an average of 4 months every 10 years for the last century and a half. No explanation, including improved nutrition, or change in the dark/light ratio after candles were replaced by kerosene lamps, gas, and electricity amounts to more than a speculative hypothesis.

Though it does not always hold up in cases of extreme precocity or delay in the onset of puberty, there is a correlation between body size and the ratio of fat to lean body weight and the onset of puberty. The correlation itself does not clarify which is cause and which effect. In cases of child abuse dwarfism (also known as reversible hyposomatotropic dwarfism or psychosocial dwarfism) not only growth hormone but also, at the age of puberty, gonadotropic secretion from the pituitary may be suppressed. In one extreme case (Money, 1977; Money and Wolff, 1974), a 16-year-old boy had the stature and nonpubertal development of an 8-year-old. Rescued from the home of abuse, he grew rapidly and became pubertal in less than a year.

The most likely localization of the biological clock of puberty is in the central nervous system. There is some clinical and experimental evidence to implicate the pineal gland, especially when early puberty occurs in conjunction with a pineal tumor. Today's evidence, however, points primarily to the hypothalamus and its nearby connections in the limbic system of the brain. The hypothalamus secretes its own neurohormones or neurotransmitters which signal the endocrine system via the pituitary gland. The pituitary, in turn, signals the gonads to secrete their own sex hormones.

Today's favored endocrine hypothesis of pubertal onset is formulated in terms of gonadal-pituitary-hypothalamic feedback, but without an explanation of how the "gonadostat" is changed at puberty. From a purely logical viewpoint, this pubertal change of the gonadostat could be formulated in terms of either the activation of a previously dormant biological clock or in terms of the deactivation of a biological clock phyletically programed to inhibit puberty, perhaps by way of a juvenile hormone or neurotransmitter substance. The existence of a juvenile hormone has been demonstrated in the endocrinology of insect metamorphosis. It is not fashionable, however, to entertain the analogous hypothesis of a juvenile hormone in vertebrates, or to search for one. The most parsimonious explanation of the anomalies of pubertal onset, either precocious or delayed, would be in terms of an as yet unidentified juvenile hormone or hormonal substance. Hence, the possibility cannot be discarded a priori.

The hormonal change from prepuberty to puberty begins earlier than the visible body signs of the onset of puberty, and it correlates with physiologic age (physique age) rather than chronologic age. In the female the change begins approximately a year earlier than in the male, that is to say at some time between age 7 and age 11 vs. between age 8 and age 12. In the female, the first measurable hormonal change is an elevation of FHS, which eventually stimulates the ovarian follicle to produce estrogen. In the male, the first measurable increase is in LH, which stimulates testicular growth and, eventually, the secretion of tesicular androgen. In both sexes, FSH and LH secretion from the pituitary greatly increase as puberty progresses. In the female these two hormones are secreted cyclically, to regulate the menstrual cycle, whereas in the male their secretion is acyclic.

As the gonads respond to FSH and LH by secreting their own puberty-inducing hormones, the body undergoes its progressive pubertal changes (see reviews by Forest et al., 1973b; Root, 1973; and Visser, 1973). Without these body changes, the psychosocial maturation of puberty is severely restricted, for the juvenile-looking person, regardless of chronological age, is treated as juvenile by other people. Conversely, the child with somatically precocious puberty is expected by others to be socially and psychosexually more mature than chronologic age permits (see Money and Mazur, 1977).

The sex difference in the timing of the onset of puberty as gauged by the rise in gonadotropin release, with accompanying changes in testicular size in boys and breast budding in girls, is approximately a year, not the two years conventionally cited. The earlier onset of puberty gives the typical girl a temporary statural advantage over her typical male counterpart, the implications of which are speculative, since there have been no studies that attempt to correlate behavior with physique age rather than chronologic age. The same applies to the somewhat earlier advent in girls of the sexual maturity of the body. In human beings the heightened eroticism of puberty is not automatically expressed in sexual behavior as it is in lower mammals but is regulated in part by cultural norms. Cases of precocious somatic puberty illustrate this point well, for affected children may be able to procreate by 8 or 9 years of age, but they do not establish procreative relationships with older teenagers as they are socially inexperienced and immature. In content, the erotic behavior and imagery of the somatically precocious child parallels social age which in turn parallels chronologic age, and, coincidentally, the dental age, more closely than hormonal age.

A normally pubertal girl may be well advanced into somatic puberty before a romantic interest in boys shows itself. Conversely, in a culture that does not prohibit childhood sexuality, romantic rehearsals may be in evidence before, or at, the onset of puberty. In our own culture, it is widely taken for granted that the female will be shorter and younger than her male partner. Thus not only at the time of the onset of puberty, but throughout the life cycle, there is a strong bias in favor of a disparity in the ages of heterosexual partners. This is reversed in the geriatric age group as there are not enough surviving older men to be partners for the women who, because of their greater longevity, will be forced to turn to younger men or live a second spinsterhood.

The sex difference in the onset of the somatic maturation of puberty has generated some speculation on a parallel difference in mental maturation, to which is added the further speculation that the relative delay in males may have permanent sequelae on cerebral lateralization and the greater prevalence of praxic and mathematical achievement in boys than in girls. Such speculation has not yet been substantiated. It could be pure science fiction, for there is currently no way of disproving that the sex disparity in praxic and mathematical reasoning is anything more than an educational artifact derived from an earlier era of history in which it was considered unladylike for a female to receive any education except in the domestic and decorative arts.

Adolescence and Adulthood

In mammals, the hormones of puberty do not bring about as great a change as is seen, for example, in the metamorphoses of insects. Rather, they activate and proliferate tissues and organs already present. The same principle applies to psychosexuality: the hormones of puberty activate already-programed sexual and erotic patterns of behavior and imagery but they do not originate them. They also increase the frequency with which these patterns of behavior and imagery manifest themselves either spontaneously, as in dreams, or in response to a triggering stimulus. That is to say, the sex hormones lower the threshold for erotic responsiveness.

This threshold effect may tempt one to endow hormones with a mystical aphrodisiac quality and to expect a quantitative correlation between hormonal level and frequency and/or intensity of erotic behavior and imagery. In actual fact, there is an upper limit to how much hormone the cells of the body can use. When the saturation point is reached, any excess of hormone is excreted in the urine. Below that point, a deficiency state exists, both somatically and psychosexually, and may be corrected by hormonal supplementation. When a deficiency state has its onset subsequent to pubertal maturation, as in cases of postpubertal castration, the psychosexual and behavioral effects range over a wide degree of individual variation in animals as well as humans. In some individuals, sexual function may fade rapidly and completely, whereas in others modified sexual interaction may persist for years. In men, castration is followed by a return to prepubertal sexuality which may include erection and build-up to an emissionless climax. In women, the effects of castration pertain more to the physiology of the vagina, especially lubrication, than to sexual performance and orgasm. In both sexes there is an astonishing lack of systematic information on the effects of castration, despite the ancient history of male castration to produce eunuchs.

There are some syndromes with a history of pubertal delay or insufficiency in which a hormonal deficiency state in adulthood can be ascertained on physical examination. In the majority of cases of psychosexual deficit, however, there is no endocrine deficit and no permanent defect of target organ responsivity. The only way to be sure whether to implicate a hormonal deficiency in psychosexual deficiency syndromes is to take a blood sample and measure the actual levels of available hormones circulating in the bloodstream. This is particularly true in cases of erotic apathy and in such instances of erotic unresponsiveness as impotence, failure to lubricate, and anorgasmia. It is malpractice and potentially dangerous to prescribe hormones that are not needed. In the treatment of sexual dysfunctions, this rule applies not only to the sex steroids, androgen, estrogen and progestin, but also to other hormones, notably thyroid hormones, which in the past have been prescribed faddishly.

Though there are some sex-hormonal deficiency states requiring replacement therapy to bring psychosexual function up to par, the converse is not known. That is to say there is no correlation of sexual behavioral excess with excessively high hormonal levels. In rapists, for example, plasma testosterone levels were found to be within the normal range (Rada et al., 1976), and the same holds true for other sex offenders who get into trouble with the law. Above average frequency of masturbation or coitus does not correlate with elevated hormone levels, though such a correlation may be wrongly inferred from the fact that low-frequency, hormone-deficient people may increase their sexual activity after hormonal supplementation.

Another mystical quality with which many people are tempted to endow sex hormones is an absolute and dichotomous sex specificity. That is to say androgen is equated with maleness and estrogen with femaleness, with progesterone set to one side, reserved for pregnancy. This faulty absolutism is the product of careless etymology, whereby androgen was named for the Greek word for "male," estrogen was named for the phenomenon of estrus or sexual heat in female animals, and progesterone was named for the phenomenon of gestation or pregnancy. The three hormones are, in actual fact, all sex-shared. All three are part of the healthy functioning of both sexes and are sex-different only in their ratios, not their presence or absence.

The proportionate level of estrogen in males as compared with females varies according to the female's menstrual phase, and ranges from an average 30% postmenstrually to 2% at the peak period of ovulation, when the female's estrogen secretion is at its maximum. The corresponding proportions for progesterone are 100% premenstrually and 6% at the female's progestinic peak period, which is after ovulation and before the premenstrual decline in preparation for menstruation. The average level of androgen in females as compared with males is 6%, though it has been calculated to be as high as 20%.

For all three hormones, the ratios given do not discriminate between bound and free blood levels of the hormone, but they do indicate the relative amounts secreted.

In the female, the function of estrogen and progesterone in the regulation of the menstrual cycle is well understood and is the basis of the contraceptive pill. The function of the two hormones in regulating pregnancy is also rather well understood, though not so perfectly as to allow totally predictable control of the course of pregnancy, either for the purpose of terminating or maintaining it. By contrast, the function, if any, of the two hormones in relation to human psychosexual function and erotic behavior in the course of either the menstrual cycle or pregnancy is still pretty much a mystery, masked by taboo and superstition. In subprimate species, reproductive behavior in females can be experimentally and predictably controlled by manipulation of the two hormones, whereas in women the corresponding behavior is not tied to the hormonal and menstrual cycle, nor to its cessation at the menopause, and attempts to prove otherwise have yielded inconsistent results (see below). There is no adequate animal model of sexuality in women, and the same is true of sexuality in men.

The amount of androgen that circulates in the female bloodstream is not sufficient to compete with estrogen and progesterone and bring about masculinization. In much larger amounts, however, androgen will masculinize the female in the same way as it does a pubertal boy, as can be readily demonstrated in the androgenic treatment of a female-to-male transexual. A similar effect occurs spontaneously in women who produce an excess of their own androgen, as from an androgen-producing tumor, hyperplasia of the adrenocortex, or from malfunctioning ovaries in the Stein-Leventhal syndrome. The normal adrenal cortex secretes sufficient androgen to induce the growth of pubic and axillary hair, even in girls who have no ovaries to secrete ovarian androgen.

It is likely that the nonvirilizing level of androgen found in normal women plays a role in the maintenance of woman's sexuality, that is, in her sexual behavior and imagery, and in her personally reported subjective experience of sexual drive or desire. The clinical evidence from women with an excess of androgen is that they experience what they may interpret as an increase of sexual feeling. Female-to-male transexuals under treatment with androgen get some enlargement of the clitoris and report an increased intensity in the feeling of orgasm, without losing the female capacity for multiple orgasm. The pertinent human and animal literature (reviewed in Money, 1961a,b, and Money and Ehrhardt, 1972) suggests the hypothesis that androgen is the libido hormone for both sexes.

The amount of estrogen circulating in the male bloodstream is not sufficient to compete with androgen and bring about feminization, in particular, growth of the breasts, nor is there any known competitive action of progesterone with androgen in the normal male. Either hormone, however, if administered in high enough dosage, temporarily has a "chemically castrating," antiandrogenic effect, which can be reversed upon withdrawal of the hormone. Only estrogen induces breast growth. Evidence in proof of these statements comes from the treatment of prostatic cancer with estrogen, from the treatment of male-to-female transexuals with estrogen and progesterone or a progestinic synthetic substitute, and from the temporary treatment of male sex offenders with either of two antiandrogens, medroxyprogesterone acetate (a progestin) and cyproterone acetate, a chemically related steroid. Antiandrogenic effects include suppression of ejaculation, reduction or suppression of erection, decrease or abolition of the subjective feeling reported as sexual drive, suppression of erotic imagery, and suppression of fertility.

Antiandrogens are used as adjunctive therapy along with counseling to help adult men, paraphilic sex offenders, regulate their own behavior in order to keep out of jail. They have proved beneficial in the treatment of sex offenders who proved otherwise untreatable (Money, 1968, 1970b; Laschet, 1973; Money et al., 1976). The length of treatment is variable on an individual basis.

From the effects on behavior of therapeutically high levels of a hormone in the bloodstream one cannot extrapolate the effects of physiologic levels. For human sex hormones, detailed information on their relationship not only to explicitly erotic behavior but also to other sex-attributed behavior, including pair-bonding (falling in love), ranges from negligible to zero.

That special case of pair-bonding known in humans as falling in love has its counterpart in some animal species. Usually it is manifested not as partner exclusivity, but partner preference or favoritism that persists even after a long separation. Among humans, pair-bonding associated with falling in love usually occurs for the first time in adolescence but is not restricted to that age. A new love affair may have its onset in the years of adulthood, up through old age.

The prototype of the first love affair begins as a kind of play rehearsal of courtship during the kindergarten age. This is also the age when little girls continue to flirt with their fathers, and little boys play the protective escort role with their mothers. Though it is not the rule, a love affair that lasts long into adulthood may have its beginnings in middle childhood, at around age 8, and it may include copulatory rehearsal play, including intromission.

In some cases of prolonged delay of puberty or failure of puberty secondary to anorchia or prepubertal castration, romantic and erotic pair-bonding, complete with coitus, may be established; in some few cases, this has been authenticated. Despite their rarity, such cases support the hypothesis that the biological clock in the brain responsible for awakening the pituitary's hormonal program of puberty is not the same clock that programs readiness for pair-bonding in a love affair. Further support for the independence of the two clocks comes from patients with a juvenile history of brain surgery for pituitary tumor (Money and Clopper, 1975). In the teens, the postsurgical deficit in hypothalamic-pituitary hormonal function can be partly, though not fully, compensated for with hormonal replacement therapy. Hormonal therapy, however, has no effect in compensating for what must be assumed to be a surgical impairment of hypothalamic pathways associated with the pair-bonding of falling in love. Not only postsurgical hypopituitary patients, but also those with idiopathic hypopituitarism, manifest a high degree of adult apathy and inertia with respect to romantic and erotic pair-bonding (Clopper et al., 1976). In every-day terminology, they do not fall in love. Some eventually marry, but the relationship has the quality of an arranged, nonerotic companionship.

The relative independence of hormonal puberty and the maturation of the ability to fall in love is further illustrated in cases of somatically precocious puberty. In such cases, the first love affair commonly does not occur until the late teens, even when puberty begins as young as 5 or 6 years of age. The earliest love affairs recorded in precocious puberty began in girls around age 11 (Money and Walker, 1971) and around age 12 in boys (Money and Alexander, 1969).

In the majority of cases, the sequel to the pair-bonding of a love affair is pregnancy and parenthood, which means the enlarging of the pair-bond to a three-way bond. The hormonal component of pregnancy and parenthood is not, however, the topic of this chapter, requiring as it does a chapter of its own.

Menstrual Cycle and the Pill: Premenstrual Tension

As is true of puberty, the menstrual cycle is programed by a biological clock situated in the hypothalamus but with connections elsewhere. By inference, it is the existence of these connections that allows, at least in some women, personal life experiences to interfere with the hormonal rhythms that govern menstrual regularity and to suppress ovulation for various periods of time. Releasing hormones (RH) from the hypothalamus program the cyclicity of pituitary gonadotropic hormones which, in turn, program the cyclic hormonal functioning of the ovaries, which program the endometrial cyclicity of the uterus.

There are different starting points for counting the days of the menstrual cycle. One convention is to begin with the first day of bleeding as day one. At the conclusion of the menstrual flow, the preovulatory or follicular phase begins; this culminates in midcycle with the day of ovulation. Then ensues the postovulatory or luteal phase, lasting about two weeks, though this varies according to whether the total cycle is longer or shorter than 28 days. The premenstrual phase that terminates the luteal phase is loosely defined and has no fixed duration. It ends abruptly with the onset of the next menstrual flow. Apart from the beginning and ending of the menstrual flow, the only other fixed point in the menstrual cycle is ovulation, the occurrence of which can be determined by a rise in body temperature, if a daily temperature chart is kept; or by the viscosity of the cervical mucus if it is tested.

Figure 1 shows the fluctuations of estrogen and progesterone during the course of the menstrual cycle (androgen is not represented). Estrogen and progesterone are low at the beginning of the follicular phase. Then estrogen and androgen both rise in the preovulatory phase. Ovulation is precipitated by a dramatic rise of LH and a lesser rise of FSH. Then there is a rapid decline in estrogen level as progesterone rises, soon to be joined by a midluteal increase in both estrogen and androgen. Before estrogen reaches the same high level that heralds ovulation, it begins to decline, along with the levels of progesterone and androgen, to the low levels that precede the onset of the next menstrual flow. The level of ovarian androgen is highest during the luteal phase; it is mostly androstenedione, which is also secreted by the adrenal cortices. About 10% of androstenedione is converted to testosterone intracellularly, and the remainder is secreted in the urine.

Knowledge of the sex-hormonal concomitants of the menstrual cycle, still not complete, dates from the 1920s, when the gonadal steroids were first isolated, and from the 1930s, when they were first synthesized. One of the earliest attempts to establish a behavioral endocrinology of the menstrual cycle is the 1931 paper, "The Hormonal Causes of Premenstrual Tension," by Robert T. Frank. "It is well known," Frank wrote, "that normal women suffer varying degrees of discomfort preceding the onset of menstruation. Employers of labor take cognizance of this fact and make provision for the temporary care of their employees. These minor disturbances include increased fatigability, irritability, lack of concentration and attacks of pain."

It was not these normal women with whom Frank was concerned however, but a group of patients in whom pain played a predominant role, requiring a day or two of bed rest; and another group in whom grave systemic disorders, including epilepsy, were exacerbated during the menstrual period. These latter were so disabled that Frank put to use the new ovarian hormonal knowledge of

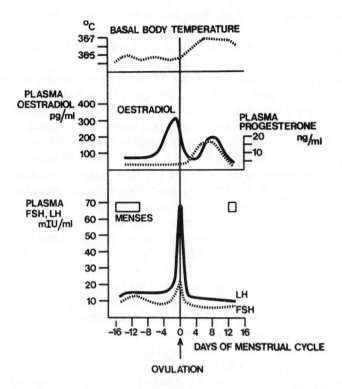

FIG. 1. Schematic representation of hormonal and temperature fluctuations in the course of the menstrual cycle. (Reproduced courtesy of H. K. A. Visser, 1973.)

his day by "applying a sterilizing dose of roentgen rays to the ovaries," so as to suppress their endocrine output, prevent menstruation, and successfully dispel the symptoms that had become premenstrually exaggerated.

Since 1931, not much progress has been made toward understanding the etiology of the phenomena of premenstrual tension. In an imprecise way, they have been ascribed to the increased secretion of progesterone in the luteal phase of the menstrual cycle and to edema associated therewith. The severity of symptoms in extreme cases is ascribed to neurotic augmentation but the ascription remains vague and has not been spelled out psychoneuroendocrinologically. It is not known why severe symptoms may be age-related, though in an unpredictable and unsystematic way. Short-term remission may occur if a cycle is anovulatory.

In the past, therapy for severe premenstrual symptoms was ameliorative at best, and was based, like contraception by means of the pill, on the hormonal principle of ovulation suppression. In the absence of ovulation, there is no post-ovulatory surge of progesterone. More recently prostaglandins (see review by Marx, 1979) have been implicated in menstrual cramping. Excessive release of prostaglandin from the uterus can be controlled by medications that inhibit prostaglandin synthesis, for example, naproxen, the use of which is still under clinical investigation. The medication controls not only menstrual cramping and pain but also the prostaglandin-related symptoms of nausea, vomiting, diarrhea, and headache, if they occur.

The diagnosis of premenstrual tension has become immensely fashionable since the 1930s, even to the point of achieving syndrome status. As in the case of other fashionable diagnoses, dyslexia, for example, or minimal brain damage, the medical popularity of the syndrome has outstripped the capacity of research to define it. Thus, the premenstrual syndrome has become something of a medical grab-bag, its meaning stretched to include the ills of menstruation itself, of the week preceding it, and even of the days surrounding ovulation. The behavioral correlates of the syndrome have been extended to include not only subjectively experienced mood changes but also an increased prevalence of poor judgment, delinquency, violence, accidents, hospital clinic visits for self and children, acute psychiatric illness (the periodic monthly psychosis of puberty can be dramatically prevented with exogenous progestin), suicides, and calls to a suicide prevention center (see review by O'Connor et al., 1974).*

Correlations intrinsically fail to tell anything about etiology. Sampling bias distorts the truth about the population at large. Faulty research design or method masks the complexity of multivariate determinism. Established maxims become enshrined as dogma. Nonetheless, the premenstrual syndrome does exist in some women. It is variable in degree of severity. Other women have it not at all. It occurs across cultures and classes and so almost certainly is not simply an artifact of cultural taboo. However, it is not culture free. Even in its mildest manifestation, better known simply as premenstrual tension, it is multidetermined. A. S. Rossi and P. E. Rossi (1977) found, for example, among other individual differences, that the subjective feeling of a negative mood swing varied not only according to the premenstrual phase of the cycle, but day of the week. On weekends, the premenstrual phase brought a less negative mood swing than when it fell at midweek.

From the point of view of sexual politics, there is no doubt that the concept of the premenstrual syndrome has been misused, and the adverse effects of premenstrual tension on both work efficiency and mood have been exaggerated. It is time to call a halt to the misrepresentation of premenstrual behavioral endocrinology, and time to study groups of men as well as women as did Dan (1976). In a study of 24 couples, Dan found that mood variations of women and their husbands were comparable, over a given period of time, regardless of menstrual cycling. In women, fluctuating mood change may coincide with the

---

*Other reference sources for the menstrual cycle and fluctuations of mood and behavior are: Benedek and Rubenstein (1939a,b); Coppen and Kessel (1963); Dalton (1959, 1964); Glass et al. (1971); Gottschalk et al. (1962); Ivey and Bardwick (1968); Janowsky et al. (1969); Kane et al. (1967); Lamb et al. (1953); MacKinnon et al. (1959); Mandell and Mandell (1967); May (1976); McCance et al. (1937); Moos (1968); Moos et al. (1969); Morton et al. (1953); Shainess (1961); Smith and Sauder (1969); Stenn and Klinge (1972); and Wetzel et al. (1971).

premenstruum but, according to May (1976), in only 50% of cases. This percentage changes if the information is ascertained retrospectively.

Proceptivity and Acceptivity

The behavioral endocrinology of the menstrual cycle includes what is variously known as woman's sexual life, her eroticism, or her libido, or her sex drive. More precisely and operationally, the terminology should be woman's proceptivity [a term applicable to both sexes and recently introduced by Beach (1976)], acceptivity or receptivity, and conceptivity. Scientific progress has been in the reverse order, for knowledge of the relationship of the menstrual hormonal cycle to the ability to conceive, which is the basis of hormonal contraception, is more advanced than in the case of either acceptivity or proceptivity. Acceptivity and proceptivity are not distinguished in research on women's sexuality to date, and only the last two years have articles begun to appear in which the two phases are distinguished in research on other mammalian females. Acceptivity (receptivity) refers to the readiness of the female to accept or receive the approaches of the male and eventually of the vagina to accept the penis. Proceptivity has two components: the female's attractedness to the male so that she presents herself and solicits his sexual attention, and the attractiveness of the female to the male, usually by reason of her sexual appearance, sexual smell (pheromonal odor), or in some instances her courtship ritual. There are, of course, many factors that may inhibit or interrupt proceptivity and acceptivity as well, not least of which is insufficient privacy, auditory or visual, especially when there are young children in crowded living quarters and the parents are erotically prudish and secretive. Regardless of hormonal levels, the frequency of coitus during the course of one menstrual cycle in young adult couples screened for psychologic normalcy varies widely. In the study of 11 couples by Persky and co-workers (1977), the range per cycle over a total of three cycles was from 3 to 18 occasions of coitus, with a mean of 11.

In subprimate animals, the three behavioral phases of sexuality correlate closely with the hormonal cycle of estrus, regardless of whether estrus is continually cyclic or governed by climatic seasons. In primates the cycle is menstrual, not estrual, and the menstrual behavioral cycle is less strictly enchained to the hormonal cycle than is the estrual cycle. In subhuman primates living in the wild, according to the available evidence, the female's sexual interaction with the male is more enchained to the hormonal cycle of the menses than is the case among human females in their interaction with males.

The present state of knowledge concerning menstrual fluctuation of estrogen, progesterone, and androgen and their effect on proceptivity and receptivity (acceptivity) in monkeys is updated in an exceptionally well-informed review by Baum et al. (1977). The review concludes with a statement about human beings.

The methods currently being used for studying human sexual behavior make it very difficult to distinguish between proceptivity and receptivity and hence to ascribe individual roles to various hormones in the way now possible for monkeys. Rhythmic changes in sexual interaction in humans during the menstrual cycle have been reported, although contradictory reports continue to appear and maximum levels are as commonly found early in the follicular phase as at mid-cycle. It has been suggested that the human female's attractivity may decline during the luteal phase (as in monkeys) and that this can be counteracted in women taking contraceptive steroids.

The consequence of withdrawing endocrine secretion, or treatment with steroids, have usually been assessed in terms of loss or gain of "libido," although some studies have used other criteria such as incidence of orgasm or "coital satisfaction." It is not clear whether loss of libido indicates changes in receptivity, proceptivity, or both. Furthermore, changes in libido may occur secondarily to those in attractivity, as in monkeys.

Ovariectomy is generally agreed not to diminish the human female's libido consistently, and the same conclusions have been reached in studies of menopausal women. Insofar as comparisons are justified, this correlates with findings on ovariectomized monkeys described above. Adrenalectomy, however, [which diminishes androgen] has been found to diminish promptly the human female's libido, whereas giving intact women testosterone stimulates their sexual interest in many cases. This suggests that there may be a role for androgens in the human female's sexuality comparable with that experimentally determined for the rhesus monkey, although exact correspondence awaits further clinical investigation.

Oral Contraception

The foregoing statement continues with a summing up of today's all too sparse knowledge concerning the effect of the hormonal changes induced by the contraceptive pill on woman's sexual function (Bulbrook et al., 1973).

The most common steroid therapy given to women is the contraceptive pill, usually a variable mixture of an estrogen and a progestagen. A number of investigations on the effect of this treatment on libido have been made, with conflicting results. In some cases, libido has been depressed, and this has been a major factor in women's discontinuing their use of the pill. In others, little change has apparently occurred, or libido has even seemed to increase. The way in which such data are collected may have a crucial effect on the apparent change in behavior. Furthermore, effects on behavior, if they occur, may be attributed as much to social factors as to endocrine factors. There are other complications. Clinical depression, of which diminished libido is one symptom, sometimes occurs in women taking contraceptive steroids; the converse, euphoria, may also occur . . . women taking the pill excrete less androgen metabolites and have no midcycle peak in either testosterone or estrogen, which may provide an endocrine explanation for some cases of decreased libido.*

*Other reference sources for the menstrual cycle and fluctuations in women's sexuality, including effects of the contraceptive pill, are: Davis (1929): Frölich et al. (1976); Hamburg et al. (1968);

There has been much inconsistency in findings on the effect of the contraceptive pill on mood and sexuality. A large part, if not all, of the inconsistency can probably be attributed to the fact that mood and sexuality are multidetermined, and few studies have been designed for multivariate analysis. This is not so in the case of the study by Cullberg (1972). The summary of his monograph may prove enlightening.

Three different hormone preparations and one placebo preparation were given to a sample of 322 women volunteers. The hormone preparations contained a constant dose of estrogen (.05 mg ethinyl oestradiol) in combination with varying gestagen (progestin) doses (1.0 mg, .5 mg, and .06 mg norgestrel respectively). The compounds could be characterized as strongly gestagenic, medium gestagenic (identical with a commercial oral contraceptive) and estrogenic, according to the dominant physiological effects. The placebo was identical in shape and taste. The medication was given in a double blind, randomized order and taken during a two-month time period.

Overall mental reactions: The mental effects of the hormones showed (themselves) to be low. In the interview ratings, 14 per cent more individuals of the gestagen dominated medication groups reported adverse mental change in comparison with the placebo group. The estrogen dominated group showed 18 per cent more negative reactions than did the placebo group. The differences from placebo are significant at the .05 level. The mental symptoms were generally mild and mostly of a depressive-dysphoric type.

The self-rating questionnaire for mental change did not show any conclusive evidence of mental change except for the estrogen dominated group which showed a negative change (irritability) in comparison with the placebo group.

Specific somatic and mental symptoms: There are signs of a direct link between gestagen induced weight increase and adverse mental changes, as well as between estrogen induced nausea and mental changes. The subjective reactions towards these physiologic effects of the hormones have some importance for the reporting of mental symptoms, but there is also evidence that hormonally induced mental symptoms appear independently of the somatic reactions. Headache has often been reported as a side effect of oral contraceptive treatment. In the present study no difference was seen in any of the hormone groups as compared with the placebo group.

Nor were any differences found regarding increase or decrease of sexual drive in comparison with the placebo group. There is however an association between adverse mental change and lowered sexual interest. These findings could be interpreted as indicative of the absence of any direct negative effects on sexual functions of the hormones used.

Change of menstrual symptoms: Dysmenorrhea was clearly relieved by the gestagen dominated preparations in a dose related response. Estrogen dominated treatment showed no difference from placebo treatment in this respect. Pre-

Hart (1960); James (1971a,b); Janiger et al. (1972); Kane et al. (1969); Luschen and Pierce (1972); Markowitz and Brender (1976); Masters and Johnson (1966); McCance et al. (1937); McCauley and Ehrhardt (1976); Michael (1972); Morris and Udry (1978); O'Connor et al. (1974); Perksy et al. (1977); Spitz et al. (1975); and Udry and Morris (1968).

menstrual tension, as defined by the presence of premenstrual irritability prior to medication, differed in response according to type of medication. Here one could observe only nonsignificant trends towards symptom relief with the gestagen dominated medication and impairment with the estrogen dominated medication.

These results have a practical implication in questioning the frequent use of oral contraceptive treatment in cases of premenstrual tension. They also elucidate the different clinical views held on the causes for premenstrual tension. In the present material the premenstrual tension group could be divided into subgroups. There is one relatively small, more purely hormone-responding group, which reacts positively to gestagen dominated medication and negatively to estrogen dominated medication. The majority of the premenstrual tension subjects, however, seem to be dominated by signs of general emotional problems and thus do not respond better to hormone than to placebo treatment.

Signs of endogenous estrogen sensitivity and mental effect of exogenous hormones: On subdivision of the material into those with and those without premenstrual irritability it was shown that estrogen dominated treatment exerted an adverse mental influence on the group with premenstrual irritability before medication while those without premenstrual irritability did not show a higher frequency of adverse mental effects than the placebo group. On the other hand, the individuals without premenstrual irritability reacted adversely to the gestagen dominated treatment in comparison with the placebo group.

These relationships have not been shown before. However, as was the case with the somatic responses towards female hormone treatment, it seems reasonable to postulate some kind of competition between the two kinds of hormones regarding their mental effects. If we hypothesize that premenstrual irritability among other things is due to some kind of sensitivity towards endogenous estrogen, estrogen treatment would tend to produce similar symptoms during the medication period, while gestagen given concurrently would tend to abolish that reaction.

Contrarily, absence of premenstrual irritability may point to the fact that some individuals are endogenously progesterone dominated (or otherwise progesterone sensitive) and thus react negatively towards exogenous gestagen. Such a gestagen mechanism is, however, not as clearly shown as the estrogen reaction, since we do not as yet have any positive evidence for mental symptoms related to endogenous gestagen dominance in untreated women, analogous to the premenstrual irritability with estrogen dominance.

Couple Synchrony

There are no known cyclic rhythms, circadian, seasonal, or of other duration that influence men's sexuality. The few attempts that have been made to correlate men's orgasmic activity and frequency with circulating testosterone level, irrespective of cyclic regularity, have been inconclusive and inconsistent. The same applies to the possibility that defeat or the stress of competition with or obedience to more authoritarian or dominant males may lower both the testosterone level and the mating activity of the subordinate male (see reviews by Rose, 1972, 1975).

It is only very recently that research attention has been directed to the possibility that proceptivity and receptivity in men may fluctuate in synchrony with the hormonal cycle of the woman partner. Persky and co-workers (1977) found a strong trend for a husband's blood level of testosterone to peak at its maximum value at around 7 days after his wife's ovulation, at which time the wife's testosterone level reached its second or postovulatory peak in the menstrual cycle. The behavioral concomitants, if any, of this conjunction of testosterone peaks remain to be investigated.

Another phenomenon of sexual synchrony, still preliminary and unconfirmed, was reported by Henderson (1976). In a study of married couples, she found that, at the time of the female's midcycle temperature low point and subsequent postovulatory rise, the male's basal body temperature underwent a synchronous change, though the elevation was maintained for fewer days in the male than the female. Henderson obtained data also on one homosexual male couple, and found that if their basal body temperatures fluctuated, they did so in synchrony. This finding resembles that of McClintock (1971) who found that college women living in the same dormitory established menstrual synchrony. It was not necessary for two roommates to know each other's menstrual timetable for synchronization to occur. Axillary odor is the responsible agent of menstrual synchrony.

The most likely hypothesis of erotic synchronization is that it is mediated, possibly subliminally, through the sense of smell by way of pheromones or odors. In subhuman primates and other mammals it is well established that the female, at the time of ovulation, emits a vaginal odor or pheromone which is for the male an erotic attractant. It is also established that the human female emits an ovulatory pheromone which chemically is the same as that emitted by the rhesus monkey female, and is an attractant for the rhesus male. There is a dearth of information and no definitive investigation on the role of the vaginal pheromone in human male sexuality. Morris and Udry (1978) conducted a properly designed study on 62 young adult couples, all university students, and were not able to demonstrate a pheromonal effect on the frequency of intercourse. They suggested that males may be differently responsive to pheromone. If so, then some way of identifying those who are responsive will need to be found and further studied.

Menopause and Postmenopause

The hormonal transmutation of the menopause varies from rapid to gradual. It takes place typically in the fifth or sixth decade of life, at the latest by around age 60. The mechanism of the biological clock that regulates the menopause is not known. In all probability, the process begins in the brain, as the neurotransmitter cells of the hypothalamus change from a cyclic to an acyclic schedule of secreting their neurotransmitter substances—biogenic amines among others.

When the hypothalamus goes on any acyclic schedule, it programs the pituitary to do likewise, with an ensuing steady state of gonadotropin secretion which results in an elevation particularly of the gonadotropin, FSH, in the bloodstream. When pituitary gonadotropins are secreted on an acyclic schedule, then the ovary becomes acyclic also, with a resultant disappearance of cyclic ovulation and menstrual bleeding. With the further passage of time, ovarian function diminishes, and the blood level of ovarian estrogen decreases until only a small amount can be detected. According to Eisdorfer and Raskind (1975), quoting Grodin and associates (1971), urinary estrogen in the elderly postmenopausal woman reflects peripheral conversion of steroid precursors and the continued production of estrone from adrenal androstenedione.

Sudden onset of ovarian insufficiency as, for example, in the wake of surgical castration, or of sudden withdrawal of estrogen replacement therapy, induces symptoms of vasomotor insufficiency, experienced as hot flashes, sweating, vertigo, headache, fatigue, and insomnia. These same symptoms accompany the onset of menopause in an estimated 25% of women. Eventually they go into spontaneous remission, though they can, if too uncomfortable, be helped by treatment with estrogen. This effect of estrogen on symptoms of vasomotor instability has led to an extensive lay and medical folklore regarding a putative menopausal syndrome of anhedonia, somatic complaints, and hypoeroticism. Eisdorfer and Raskind (1975) reviewed the published evidence regarding this so-called syndrome and reached the conclusion that, if it occurs, only the vasomotor symptoms can be attributed to estrogen insufficiency. The prevalence of the syndrome has not been ascertained and almost certainly has been highly exaggerated through lack of adequate statistics. In those whom the syndrome hits, however, it may hit very hard, creating an intense subjective lack of well-being which is in no way helped by the change from spontaneity to perfunctoriness in erotic response to the partner. The return to well-being following replacement therapy with cyclic, low-dose estrogen is dramatic.

There is no universal correlation between estrogen insufficiency and hypoeroticism before, during, or after the menopause. There may be an indirect association after a prolonged period of estrogen insufficiency, secondary to changes in the reproductive anatomy of the type tallied by Masters and Johnson (1966): shrinkage of fatty tissue in the labia majora, involution and loss of elasticity of the vaginal wall, reduced vaginal lubrication, and possible painful uterine contractions. In most things pertaining to human sexuality normative data are nonexistent. Thus there are no normative data as to how many postmenopausal women encounter copulatory difficulty secondary to the foregoing somatic changes. Nor is it known whether, or to what degree, these changes accelerate or decelerate in relation to erotic inactivity or activity, respectively.

Estrogen replacement therapy in low dosage prevents postmenopausal somatic changes in the genitalia, the restoration of vaginal lubrication being of particular significance to the maintenance of erotic activity when vaginal dryness has become a problem. Clinical opinion is divided as to whether the erotic benefits of estrogen replacement are outweighed by suspected adverse side effects, notably hormone-dependent cancer. At present, there is a suspected positive relationship between estrogen and increased risk of heart attack in both sexes.

When vaginal dryness hinders coital activity and estrogen is not taken, an exogenous vaginal lubricant is adequate to permit intercourse without discomfort. There are no statistics with respect to the use or nonuse of vaginal lubricants in the postmenopausal era. There are also no statistics relating prevalence of sexual activity to circulating hormone levels in the aged. Prevalence statistics are additionally inadequate insofar as they commonly omit information with respect to masturbation and also the relationship of masturbation frequency to the availability or unavailability of a partner and the relationship of the psychosexual status of her husband to a wife's sexual frequency.

Prevalence statistics are lacking also with respect to the frequency of orgasm in postmenopausal women. It is well established, however, that in women who continue an active sex life, the menopause does not interfere with the experience of orgasm. Whether or not they continue an active sex life depends more on the availability of a partner than anything else. In keeping with the mores of their upbringing, unpartnered elderly women are less likely to find a new partner than are their male counterparts. Moreover, men have a shorter life expectancy than women, thus leaving a surplus of lonely older women. For women with a partner, the frequency of sexual intercourse diminishes gradually with each advancing decade. Whether it fades altogether or not, sexual frequency depends more on factors that are individually variable than on those that are specific to aging alone. Cross sectional and follow-up facts and figures on sexuality and aging are documented in Pfeiffer et al. (1968, 1969) and in Verwoerdt et al. (1969a,b).

Sexual Gerontology in Males

There are two doctrines regarding psychosexual and psychoendocrine aging in the male. One is the doctrine of gradual and progresssive diminution or winding down and the other is the doctrine of the male climacteric (Marañon, 1929). It is not possible at the present time to arbitrate between these two doctrines, because there are no longitudinal studies in which hormonal and sex-behavioral age changes have been recorded in parallel.

There are also no longitudinal studies in which sex-hormonal age changes have been recorded independently of behavior. The only information presently available is cross sectional, as for example in the study by Vermeulen et al. (1971).

Male senescence is characterized by a decrease in plasma testosterone levels, an increase in testosterone binding and binding capacity, a decrease in metabolic clearance rate, a decreased testosterone production, and a metabolic pattern of testosterone suggestive of hypogonadism, with decrease of the androstanediol formation and preponderance of the 5β over the 5α pathway.

The youngest group in which the foregoing changes first appeared was between 50 and 60 years of age. More men between 60 and 70 had undergone the same changes, but a good proportion of men between 70 and 80 still had not manifested them, and even by age 90 there was still an occasional man whose hormonal levels were at the same level as the lower limit of the norm for men of 40 or 50.

In the absence of progressive measurements in a longitudinal study, there is no way of knowing whether, in individual men, the hormonal transition of aging is relatively abrupt or gradual. There is also no way of knowing whether the transition is subjectively perceived or not, and if it is perceived, what the perceptions are. According to the doctrine of the male climacteric, the transition represents something of a crisis, though there is no way of differentiating a neuroendocrine crisis from a crisis in career achievement or in the relationship with spouse and offspring, except in a prospective, longitudinal study.

Because of the imperfections and falsifications of memory, retrospective investigations of developmental sexuality in older men are less satisfactory than prospective investigations. The Duke University gerontology studies of sexuality have already been mentioned in connection with women. In men, they showed that the availability of a partner is a prime determinant of an older man's sex life, but that the older male, conforming to the stereotype of our culture, is more likely than the older female to find a new partner. In addition, they showed a gradual thinning of the frequency of sexual encounters with advancing age.

The longitudinal gerontology studies of sexuality by Clyde E. Martin (1975, 1977, and personal communication) at the National Institute of Aging have used both retrospective recall and longitudinal developmental data. On the basis of these two sources of information from subjects in the upper educational and socioeconomic bracket, it appears that the earlier and more vigorous the sexuality of youth, the longer and more vigorous the sexuality of aging. In addition, it appears that lessening frequency of erection and/or ejaculation, with or without a partner, is not experienced as a traumatic deprivation in probably the majority of men who are healthy in body and mind.

From anecdotal clinical reports, it appears likely that the psychosexual concomitants of aging comprise lessened frequency of erection and ejaculation; longer time to achieve full erection; greater likelihood of incomplete erection; shorter duration of complete erection; longer refractory period between erections and/or orgasms; greater likelihood of ejaculatory delay; greater likelihood of non-ejaculatory copulation (or masturbation) with or without the subjective feeling of orgasm; and continued appreciation of erotic sensuousness despite the foregoing changes. Hypothetically, there is also a possibility that, with advancing age, genital performance in the acceptive phase becomes more dependent on performance with a partner during the proceptive phase of the erotic drama that has always been the person's secret or semisecret fantasy of the ultimate erotic experience. If correct, this hypothesis—popularly formulated as "life begins at forty"—would account for sexual behavior in some older men that seems out of character with respect to their earlier and more moralistic erotic orthodoxy.

The wide range of individual variability in geriatric eroticism exists independently of partner availability and does not depend on prior history and/or quality of a long-term erotic relationship.

There is no conclusive evidence presently available as to the effectiveness of androgen supplementation therapy on sexual function in old age, nor of potentially adverse side effects. However, there are individual reports of positive sex-organ response to such therapy in terms of improved sexual performance. Without statistical evidence from a group of cases, however, it is not possible to distinguish the effects of hormonal supplementation from the effects of stimulus novelty and the effects of visual or imagistic arousal from those of tactual arousal. The effects of hormonal supplementation on the occurrence and frequency of erotic imagery in old age are unknown.

IV. Hormones and Dimorphism of Pair Partnerships

When techniques for measuring sex steroids in the bloodstream and/or urine first became available to clinical case management in the 1930s, the very names of the hormones made it inevitable that some investigators would hypothesize a lack of male or female hormone as the cause of male or female homosexuality, respectively. Attempts to prove this hypothesis (see reviews by Money, 1961a,b and 1970a) gave inconsistent, inconclusive, or contradictory evidence. Likewise, correlative attempts on the basis of trial and error to treat homosexuality hormonally failed. Androgen given to male homosexuals either had no effect or, possibly, increased the frequency of homosexual activity. Lesbians, always ignored by both law and medicine as compared with male homosexuals, were seldom treated with estrogen but, when they were, there was no effect on their having a partnership with a female.

The precision techniques of blood-hormonal measurements in the mid-1960s ushered in a new flurry of attempts to correlate hormones and homosexual behavior. None has been so designed as to take account of multivariate determinism but simply to prove a rather naive assumption that the sex of the partner is hormonally ordained. The sample size and criteria of selection have varied, as have the procedures for determining hormonal levels, the hormones measured, and the precautions to safeguard against diurnal fluctuations in hormone secretion.

To date, there is only one study that has addressed itself to the possibility that prenatal hormonalization of the hypothalamic-pituitary-gonadal system may be different with respect to homosexuality. This is a study (Dörner et al., 1975; Dörner, 1976) of the feedback effect of an injection of conjugated estrogens (premarin) on the hypothalamic-pituitary regulation of the release of LH. The subjects were heterosexual, bisexual, and homosexual males admitted to a hospital for venereal or skin disease. Homosexual males were reported to manifest a primary decrease in serum LH level, followed by a secondary rebound effect to levels above the initial values. A similar, though stronger, rebound occurs in heterosexual females, whereas in heterosexual males and bisexuals the rebound that followed the primary decrease did not exceed initial values. This finding still awaits replication.

In a somewhat similar experiment, Seyler et al. (1978) in New England test-treated female-to-male transexual applicants with oral diethylstilbestrol followed by an injection of the hypothalamic luteotropin releasing hormone (LRH). The expected feminine elevation of the pituitary gonadotropins, LH and FSH, did not occur, which suggests the hypothesis that the hypothalamic pathways of these transexuals may have been subject to a prenatal masculinizing influence. If so, then this finding may link up with the most recently discovered anomaly in transexuals (Eicher, 1979), subsequently unconfirmed, namely that H-Y antigen is present in female-to-male transexuals and missing in male-to-female transexuals. H-Y antigen is a male-determining factor normally present in the Y-bearing sperm and transmitted by it to all other cells in the XY (male) progeny.

In other studies of pituitary function in male homosexuality, there has been no test-dosage of an injected hormone, but simply a blood-plasma measurement of the pituitary's own spontaneously secreted gonadotropic hormones, LH and FSH. Kolodny and his associates (1972) reported elevated LH levels in some volunteer homosexual subjects who rated as 5 or 6, the predominantly or exclusively homosexual ratings on the Kinsey scale of heterosexuality/bisexuality/homosexuality. The exact number of subjects was not specified, but four received special mention because they had, in addition to high LH, high FSH and azoospermia—which suggests that they represent an as yet unrecognized psychoendocrine syndrome. In two cases only, pituitary prolactin level was also elevated.

Increased prevalence of elevated LH was found also by Doerr and associates (1976) among homosexuals given ratings of 4, 5, or 6 on the Kinsey scale. By contrast, Tourney and associates (1975) found no significant difference in gonadotropin (LH and FSH) levels in a homosexual as compared with a heterosexual group. The same applies to a meticulous study reported by Parks and coauthors (1974), in which they took blood samples every day for a month, thus eliminating as a source of error the potentially distorting effect of day-to-day fluctuations in hormonal output (which were of great magnitude). They also tested youths institutionalized as juvenile offenders, which eliminated the potential distorting effect of unreported medications, illicit drugs, and alcohol.

The foregoing findings indicate that many homosexuals cannot be differentiated from heterosexuals on the basis of tests of pituitary function, but they do permit the speculation that there may be some differential in hypothalamic-pituitary programing before birth that expedites, though does not preordain, the differentiation of a homosexual, a bisexual, or a heterosexual gender identity or psychosexual status in the postnatal developmental years. By contrast, the findings from measurements of the gonadal hormones, the sex steroids themselves, invite no theoretical speculation, for they are inconsistent. Their levels in homosexuals as compared with heterosexual controls have variously been found to be the same, lower, or higher. Such inconsistency may be secondary to sample size, method of sample selection, differences in laboratory technique, the difference in hormonal products that are measured in urine as compared with blood, diurnal fluctuations in the amount of steroid hormone released into the bloodstream from the gonads and from the adrenal cortices as well, the time period and frequency with which blood samples are drawn, recency of sexual experience, and the possible intrusion of effects of recent sleeplessness, toxic drugs, and so on.

The inconsistent findings regarding steroid hormones in homosexuals are as follows. A below-average level of testosterone was reported by Loraine and coauthors (1971) and for a subgroup of their homosexual volunteers by Kolodny and coauthors (1971). Evans (1972) confirmed a finding first reported by Margolese (1970) of a lower ratio of androsterone to etiocholanolone, both of which are urinary metabolites of steroid hormones from the adrenal cortice^r as well as the gonads. They do not give information about the levels c the biologically active hormones of which they are the waste product. Another measure of urinary hormonal waste, total 17-ketosteroids, was at the same level in both homosexuals and heterosexuals.

An above-average level of plasma testosterone in homosexuals was reported by Brodie and coauthors (1974) and by Tourney and coauthors (1975). Plasma estrogen (estradiol and estrone) were reported higher by Doerr and coauthors (1973, 1976), who also found the levels of dihydrotestosterone and of free testosterone (both utilizable intracellularly) to be higher in homosexuals than heterosexual controls, though total testosterone levels (free and bound) as determined in the 1973 study did not differentiate the two groups.

Other studies that failed to differentiate homosexuals from heterosexuals on the basis of testosterone levels are those of Birk and coauthors (1973), Barlow and coauthors (1974), Parks and coauthors (1974), and Pillard and coauthors (1974). Tourney and coauthors (1975), in the same study in which they found plasma testosterone higher in homosexuals than heterosexuals, found no difference between the groups with respect to androstenedione (a precursor of testosterone) and dehydroepiandrosterone.

Hormonal studies of female homosexuals have been fewer than those of male homosexuals, perhaps because of the empirical difficulties engendered by the hormonal fluctuations of the menstrual cycle. Loraine and coauthors (1970), on the basis of four cases, suggested that the urinary levels of LH and testosterone may be higher, and the level of estrogen lower in lesbians than controls. Griffiths and coauthors (1974) studied the urinary output of estrogenic, androgenic, and adrenocortical steroids in 42 lesbian subjects, and found that no consistent pattern emerged.

The most likely conclusion to be drawn from the foregoing findings is that the attempt to correlate the sex of a person's erotic partner with urinary or blood levels of the person's steroids in adulthood is naive and doomed to failure. The hormones of adolescence and adulthood activate programs of sexual-erotic behavior, but they do not originate them. To understand their origins, it is necessary to take account of the hormonal programing of fetal life and of the subsequent developmental learning experiences of childhood which have as profound an influence on psychosexual status and gender identity as they do, in another context, on native language.

V. Summary and Conclusions

Inconsistencies and contradictions in published findings on hormones and psychosexual status may reflect disparities in research design that pertain to phases of the life cycle; the biochemical variants of the hormones under study and their quantities; the amount of free (vs. bound) hormone available and its biologic potency; a circadian, seasonal or other timing factor; and the method of measurement.

In humans, the sex steroids play an active role in prenatal sexually dimorphic differentiation. They influence sexually dimorphic pathways in the brain according to "the Adam principle," but only to program predispositions toward behavior, not to preordain the finished product of behavior. For the latter, the postnatal phase of psychosexual differentiation is a prerequisite, and it is predominantly stimulus-and-response programed, socially.

The levels of gonadal hormones and gonadotropins in the bloodstream are higher in the neonatal period than later infancy and childhood, until they begin to rise again in prepuberty, ultimately to adult levels. There is no known correlation between hormone levels and either amount or dimorphism of sexual rehearsal play in childhood, nor in the childhood differentiation of gender-identity/role in its psychosexual aspects. Psychosexual status, paraphilias included, is differentiated prepubertally, mostly in early childhood. The hormones of puberty activate erotic activity and imagery, increasing its prevalence and strength, but they do not determine its content as either masculine, feminine, or unorthodox.

The precise relationship between hormones and behavior, erotic and non-erotic, in the menstrual cycle still has not been formulated; and there is no explanation for the vast range of individual differences. The same applies to the effect of hormonal oral contraceptives. A man's behavior may cycle in synchrony with the cycle of his woman partner, at least in some respects. Attempts to relate the heterosexual-bisexual-homosexual continuum to gonadal hormonal levels have failed, except that further discoveries remain to be made regarding dimorphism of the hypothalamic hormones or releasing factors and their possible correlations with behavior.

Acknowledgments

Supported in part by U.S. Public Health Service Grants HD 00325 and HD 07111.

Much preliminary assistance was given by Sue Blair, Mark Piasio, B.A., Mary Puckett, B.A., and Mark Schwartz, B.S.

References

Abramovich, D. R., and Rowe, P. (1973). Foetal plasma testosterone levels at mid-pregnancy and at term. Relationship to foetal sex. *J. Endocrinol.* 56, 621-622.

Barlow, D. H., Abel, G. G., Blanchard, E. B., and Maviffakalian, M. (1974). Plasma testosterone levels and male homosexuality. A failure to replicate. *Arch. Sexual Behav.* 3, 571-575.

Baum, M. J., Everitt, B. J., Herbert, J., and Keverne, E. B. (1977). Hormonal basis of proceptivity and receptivity in female primates. *Arch. Sexual Behav.* 6, 173-192.

Beach, F. A. (1976). Sexual attractivity, proceptivity, and receptivity in female mammals. *Horm. Behav.* 7, 105-138.

Benedek, T., and Rubenstein, B. B. (1939a). The correlations between ovarian activity and psychodynamic processes. I. The ovulation phase. *Psychosom. Med.* 1, 245-270.

Benedek, T., and Rubenstein, B. B. (1939b). The correlations between ovarian and psychodynamic processes. II. The menstrual phase. *Psychosom. Med.* 1, 461-485.

Birk, L., Williams, E. H., Chasin, M., and Rose, L. I. (1973). Serum testosterone levels in homosexual men. *N. Engl. J. Med.* 289, 1236-1238.

Brodie, H. K. H., Gartrell, N., Doering, C., and Rhue, T. (1974). Plasma testosterone levels in heterosexual and homosexual men. *Am. J. Psychiatry* 131, 82-83.

Bulbrook, R. D., Hayward, J. C., Herian, M., Swain, H. C., Tong, D., and Wang, D. Y. (1973). Effects of steroidal contraceptives on levels of plasma androgens, sulphates and cortisol. *Lancet* 1, 628-631.

Clopper, R. R., Jr., Adelson, J. M., and Money, J. (1976). Postpubertal psychosexual function in male hypopituitarism without hypogonadotropinism after growth hormone therapy. *J. Sex Res.* 12, 14-32.

Coppen, A., and Kessel, N. (1963). Menstruation and personality. *Br. J. Psychiatry* 109, 711-721.

Cullberg, J. (1972). Mood changes and menstrual symptoms with different gestagen/estrogen combinations. A double blind comparison with a placebo. *Acta Psychiatr. Scand. Suppl.* 236.

Dalton, K. (1959). Menstruation and acute psychiatric illness. *Br. Med. J.* 1, 148-149.

Dalton, K. (1964). *The Premenstrual Syndrome.* Thomas, Springfield, Ill.

Dan, A. J. (1976). Behavioral variability and the menstrual cycle. Unpublished preprint. Paper presented at the Annual Convention American Psychological Association, Washington, D.C.

Davis, K. B. (1929). *Factors in the Sex Life of 2,200 Women.* Harper and Row, New York.

Doerr, P., Kockott, G., Vogt, H. J., Pirke, K. M., and Dittmar, F. (1973). Plasma testosterone, estradiol, and semen analysis in male homosexuals. *Arch. Gen. Psychiatry* 29, 829-833.

Doerr, P., Pirke, K. M. Kockott, G., and Dittmar F. (1976). Further studies on sex hormones in the male homosexuals. *Arch. Gen. Psychiatry* 33, 611-614.

Dörner, G. (1976). *Hormones and Brain Differentiation.* Elsevier, New York.

Dörner, G., Rohde, W., Stahl, F., Krell, L., and Masius, W.-G. (1975). A neuroendocrine predisposition for homosexuality in men. *Arch. Sexual Behav.* 4, 1-8.

Eicher, W., Spoljar, M., Cleve, H., Murken, J-D., Richter, K., and Stangel-Rutkowski, S. (1979). H-Y antigen in trans-sexuality. *Lancet* 2, 1137-1138.

Eisdorfer, C., and Raskind, M. (1975). Aging, hormones and human behavior. In *Hormonal Correlates of Behavior*, Vol. I, B. E. Eleftheriou and R. L. Sprott (eds.). Plenum, New York, pp. 369-394.

Evans, R. B. (1972). Physical and biochemical characteristics of homosexual men. *J. Consult. Clin. Psychol.* 39, 140-147.

Forest, M. G., Cathiard, A. M., and Bertrand, J. A. (1973a). Evidence of testicular activity in early infancy. *J. Clin. Endocrinol. Metab.* 37, 148-50.

Forest, M. G., Saez, J. M., and Bertrand, J. (1973b). Assessment of gonadal function in children. *Paediatrician* 2, 102-128.

Forest, M. G. Sizonenko, P. C., Cathiard, A. M., and Bertrand, J. (1974). Hypophyso-gonadal function in humans during the first year of life. I. Evidence for testicular activity in early infancy. *J. Clin. Invest.* 53, 819-828.

Frank, R. T. (1931). The hormonal causes of premenstrual tension. *Arch. Neurol. Psychiatry* 26, 1053-1057.

Frölich, M., Brand, E. C., and van Hall, E. V. (1976). Serum levels of unconjugated aetiocholanolone, androstenedione, testosterone, dihydroepiandrosterone, aldosterone, progesterone and oestrogens during the normal menstrual cycle. *Acta Endocrinol.* 81, 548-562.

Galenson, E. (1975). Discussion (Early sexual differences and development, P. B. Neubauer). In *Sexuality and Psychoanalysis*, E. T. Adelson (ed.). Brunner Mazel, New York, pp. 103-106.

Glass, G. S., Heninger, G. R., Lansky, M., and Talan, K. (1971). Psychiatric emergency related to the menstrual cycle. *Am. J. Psychiatry* 128, 705-711.

Gorski, R. A. (1971). Gonadal hormones and the perinatal development of neuroendocrine function. In *Frontiers in Neuroendocrinology*, L. Martini and W. F. Ganong (eds.). Oxford University Press, New York, pp. 237-290.

Gorski, R. A. (1973). Perinatal effects of sex steroids on brain development and function. In *Progress in Brain Research*, Vol. 39, E. Zimmerman, W. H. Gispen, B. H. Marks, and D. de Weid (eds.). Elsevier, Amsterdam, pp. 149-163.

Gottschalk, L. A., Kaplan, S. M., Gleser, G. C., and Winget, C. M. (1962). Variations in magnitude of emotion: A method applied to anxiety and hostility during phases of the menstrual cycle. *Psychosom. Med.* 24, 300-311.

Griffiths, P. D., Merry, J., Browning, M. C. K., Eisinger, A. J., Huntsman, R. G., Lord, E. J. A., Polani, P. E., Tanner, J. M., and Whitehouse, R. H. (1974). Homosexual women: An endocrine and psychological study. *J. Endocrinol.* 63, 549-556.

Grodin, J. M., Siiteri, P. K., and MacDonald, P. C. (1971). Extraglandular estrogen in the post-menopause. In *Menopause and Aging*, K. J. Ryan, and D. C. Gibson (Eds.). Department of Health, Education, and Welfare, Washington, D.C., pp. 15-35.

Grumbach, M. M., Grave, G. D., and Mayer, F. E. (eds.). (1974). *Control of the Onset of Puberty*. Wiley, New York.

Halverson, H. M. (1940). Genital and sphincter behavior of the male infant. *J. Genet. Psychol.* 56, 95-136.

Hamburg, D. A., Moos, R. H., and Yalom, I. D. (1968). Studies of distress in the menstrual cycle and the postpartum period. In *Endocrinology and Human Behavior*, R. P. Michael (ed.). Oxford University Press, New York, pp. 94-116.

Harris, G. W. (1964). Sex hormones, brain development and brain function. *Endocrinology* 75, 627-648.

Hart, R. A. (1960). Monthly rhythm of libido in married women. *Br. Med. J.* 1, 1023-1024.

Henderson, M. E. (1976). Evidence for a male menstrual temperature cycle and synchrony with the female menstrual cycle. *Aust. NZ J. Med.* 84, 164.

Ivey, M. E., and Bardwick, J. M. (1968). Patterns of affective fluctuation in the menstrual cycle. *Psychosom. Med.* 30, 336-345.

James, W. H. (1971a). Coital rates and the pill. *Nature* 234, 555-556.

James, W. H. (1971b). The distribution of coitus within the human intermenstruum. *J. Biosoc. Sci.* 3, 159-171.

Janiger, O., Riffenburgh, R., and Kersh, R. (1972). Cross cultural study of premenstrual symptoms. *Psychosomatics* 13, 226-235.

Janowsky, D. S., Gorney, R., Castelnuovo-Tedesco, P., and Stone, C. B. (1969). Premenstrual-menstrual increases in psychiatric hospital admission rates. *Am. J. Obstet. Gynecol.* 103, 189-191.

Kane, F. J., Jr., Daly, R. J., Ewing, J. A., and Keeler, M. H. (1967). Mood and behavioral changes with progestational agents. *Br. J. Psychiatry* 113, 265-268.
Kane, F., J., Jr., Lipton, M. A., and Ewing, J. A. (1969). Hormonal influences in female sexual response. *Arch. Gen. Psychiatry* 20, 202-209.
Kolodny, R. C., Masters, W. H., Hendryx, B. S., and Gelson, T. (1971). Plasma testosterone and semen analysis in male homosexuals. *N. Engl. J. Med.* 285, 1170-1174.
Kolodny, R. C., Jacobs, L. S., Masters, W. H., Toro, G., and Daughaday, W. H. (1972). Plasma gonadotrophins and prolactin in male homosexuals. *Lancet* 2, 18-20.
Lamb, W. M., Ulett, G. A., Masters, W. H., and Robinson, D. W. (1953). Premenstrual tension. EEG, hormonal and psychiatric evaluation. *Am. J. Psychiatry* 109, 840-848.
Laschet, U. (1973). Antiandrogen in the treatment of sex offenders. Mode of action and therapeutic outcome. In *Contemporary Sexual Behavior. Critical Issues in the 1970s,* J. Zubin and J. Money (Eds.). Johns Hopkins University Press, Baltimore, pp. 311-319.
Loraine, J. A., Ismail, A. A. A., Adamopoulos D. A., and Dove, G. A. (1970). Endocrine function in male and female homosexuals. *Br. Med. J.* 4, 406-408.
Loraine, J. A., Adamopoulos, D. A., Kirkham, K. E., Ismail, A. A. A., and Dove, G. A. (1971). Patterns of hormone excretion in male and female homosexuals. *Nature* 234, 552-555.
Luschen, M. E., and Pierce, D. M. (1972). Effect of the menstrual cycle on mood and sexual arousability. *J. Sex Res.* 8, 41-47.
McCance, R. A., Luff, W. L., and Widdowson, E. E. (1937). Physical and emotional periodicity in women. *J. Hyg. (Camb.)* 37, 571-611.
McCauley, E., and Ehrhardt, A. A. (1976). Female sexual response: hormonal and behavioral interactions. *Primary Care* 3, 455-476.
McClintock, M. K. (1971). Menstrual synchrony and suppression. *Nature* 229, 244-245.
McDonald, P. G., and Doughty, C. (1973). Androgen sterilization in the neonatal female rat and its inhibition by an estrogen antagonist. *Neuroendocrinology* 13, 182-188.
MacKinnon, I. L., MacKinnon, P. C. B., and Thomsen, A. D. (1959). Lethal hazards of the luteal phase of the menstrual cycle. *Br. Med. J.* 1, 1015-1017.
Mandell, A. J., and Mandell, M. P. (1967). Suicide and the menstrual cycle. *JAMA* 200, 792-793.
Marañon, G. (1929). *The Climacteric.* Mosby, St. Louis.
Margolese, M. S. (1970). Homosexuality. A new endocrine correlate. *Horm. Behav.* 1, 151-155.
Markowitz, H., and Brender, W. (1976). *Patterns of Sexual Responsiveness during the Menstrual Cycle.* Audio cassette (76-S-29) of paper read at the 2nd International Congress of Sexology, Montreal, October 1976. Hallmark Films and Recordings, Baltimore.
Martin, C. E. (1975). Marital and sexual factors in relation to age, disease, and longevity. In *Life History Research in Psychopathology,* Vol. 4, R. D. Wirt, G. Winokur, and M. Rolff, (eds.). University of Minnesota Press, Minneapolis, p. 327.
Martin, C. E. (1977). Sexual activity in the ageing male. In *Handbook of Sexology,* J. Money and H. Musaph (Eds.). Excerpta Medica, Amsterdam, pp. 813-824.
Martinson, F. M. (1973). *Infant and Child Sexuality, A Sociological Perspective.* The Book Mark (Gustavus Adolphus College), St. Peter, Minnesota.
Marx, J. L. (1979). Dysmenorrhea: Basic research leads to a rational therapy. *Science* 205, 175-176.
Masters, W. H., and Johnson, V. E. (1966). *Human Sexual Response.* Little, Brown, Boston.
May, R. R. (1976). Mood shifts and the menstrual cycle. *J. Psychosom. Res.* 20, 125-130.
Michael, R. P. (1972). Determinants of primate reproductive behavior. *Acta Endocrinol. Suppl.* 166, 322-361.
Mitchell, F. L., and Shackleton, C. H. L. (1969). Investigation of steroid metabolism in early infancy. *Adv. Clin. Chem.* 12, 141-215.
Money, J. (1961a). Components of eroticism in man. I. The hormones in relation to sexual morphology and sexual desire. *J. Nerv. Ment. Dis.* 132, 239-248.
Money, J. (1961b). The sex hormones and other variables in human eroticism. In *Sex and Internal Secretions,* 3rd ed., W. C. Young (ed.). Williams and Wilkins, Baltimore, pp. 1383-1400.
Money, J. (1968). Discussion on hormonal inhibition of libido in male sex offenders. In *Endocrinology and Human Behavior,* R. P. Michael (ed.). Oxford University Press, London, p. 169.

Money, J. (1970a). Sexual dimorphism and homosexual gender identity. *Psychol. Bull.* 74, 425-440.

Money, J. (1970b). Use of an androgen-depleting hormone in the treatment of male sex offenders. *J. Sex. Res.* 6, 156-172.

Money, J. (1977). The syndrome of abuse dwarfism (psychosocial dwarfism or reversible hyposomatotropinism). Behavioral data and case report. *Am. J. Dis. Child.* 131, 508-513.

Money, J., and Alexander, D. (1967). Eroticism and sexual function in developmental anorchia and hyporchia with pubertal failure. *J. Sex. Res.* 3, 31-47.

Money, J., and Alexander, D. (1969). Psychosexual development and absence of homosexuality in males with precocious puberty. *J. Nerv. Ment. Dis.* 148, 111-123.

Money, J., and Clopper, R. R., Jr. (1975). Postpubertal psychosexual function in postsurgical male hypopituitarism. *J. Sex. Res.* 11, 25-38.

Money, J., and Ehrhardt, A. A. (1972). *Man and Woman, Boy and Girl: The Differentiation and Dimorphism of Gender Identity from Conception to Maturity.* Johns Hopkins University Press, Baltimore.

Money, J., and Mazur, T. (1977). Endocrine abnormalities and sexual behavior in man. In *Handbook of Sexology,* J. Money and H. Musaph (eds.). Excerpta Medica, Amsterdam, pp. 485-492.

Money, J., and Walker, P. A. (1971). Psychosexual development, maternalism, nonpromiscuity, and body image in 15 females with precocious puberty. *Arch. Sexual Behav.* 1, 45-60.

Money, J., and Wolff, G. (1974). Late puberty, retarded growth and reversible hyposomatotropinism (psychosocial dwarfism). *Adolescence* 9, 121-134.

Money, J., Wiedeking, C., Walker, P., and Gain, D. (1976). Combined antiandrogenic and counseling program for the treatment of 46,XY and 47,XYY sex offenders. In *Hormones, Behavior and Psychopathology,* E. J. Sachar (ed.). Raven, New York, pp. 105-120.

Moos, R. H. (1968). The development of a menstrual distress questionnaire. *Psychosom. Med.* 30, 853-867.

Moos, R. H., Kopell, B. S., Melges, F. T., Yalom, I. D., Lunde, D. T., Clayton, R. B., and Hamburge, D. A. (1969). Fluctuations in symptoms and moods during the menstrual cycle. *J. Psychosom. Res.* 13, 37-44.

Morris, N. M., and Udry, J. R. (1978). Pheromonal influences on human sexual behavior: An experimental search. *J. Biosoc. Sci.* 10, 147-157.

Morton, J. H., Additon, H., Addison, R. G., Hunt, L., and Sullivan, J. J. (1953). A clinical study of premenstrual tension. *Am. J. Obstet. Gynecol.* 65, 1182-1191.

O'Connor, J. F., Shelley, E. M., and Stern, L. O . (1974). Behavioral rhythms related to the menstrual cycle. In *Biorhythms and Human Reproduction,* M. Ferin, F. Halberg, R. M. Richart, and R. L. Vande Wiele (eds.). Wiley, New York, pp. 309-324.

Parks, G. A., Korth-Schutz, S., Penny, R., Hilding, R. F., Dumars, K. W., Frasier, S. D., and New, M. I. (1974). Variation in pituitary-gonadal function in adolescent male homosexuals and heterosexuals. *J. Clin. Endocrinol. Metab.* 39, 796-801.

Persky, H., Lief, H. I., O'Brien, C. P., Strauss, D., and Miller, W. (1977). Reproductive hormone levels and sexual behavior of young couples during the menstrual cycle. In *Progress in Sexology.* Selected papers from the Proceedings of the 1976 International Congress of Sexology, R. Gemme and C. C. Wheeler (eds.). Plenum, New York.

Pfeiffer, E. Verwoerdt, A., and Wang, H. S. (1968). Sexual behavior in aged men and women. I. Observations on 254 community volunteers. *Arch. Gen. Psychiatry* 19, 753-758.

Pfeiffer, E., Verwoerdt, A., and Wang, H. S. (1969). The natural history of sexual behavior in a biologically advantaged group of aged individuals. *J. Gerontol.* 24, 193-198.

Pillard, R. C., Rose, R. M., and Sherwood, M. (1974). Plasma testosterone levels in homosexual men. *Arch. Sexual Behav.* 3, 453-458.

Rada, R. T., Laws, D. R., and Kellner, R. (1976). Plasma testosterone levels in the rapist. *Psychosom. Med.* 38, 257-268.

Reddy, V. V. R., Naftolin, F., and Ryan, K. J. (1974). Conversion of androstenedione to estrone by neural tissue from fetal and neonatal rats. *Endocrinology* 94, 117-121.

Reinisch, J. M. (1976). Effects of prenatal hormone exposure on physical and psychological development in humans and animals. With a note on the state of the field. In *Hormones, Behavior and Psychopathology,* E. J. Sachar (ed.). Raven, New York, pp. 69-94.

Root, A. W. (1973). Endocrinology of puberty. I. Normal sexual maturation. *J. Pediat.* 83, 1-19.

Rose, R. M. (1972). The psychological effects of androgens and estrogens. In *Psychiatric Complications of Medical Drugs*. R. I. Shader (ed.). Raven, New York, pp. 251-293.

Rose, R. M. (1975). Testosterone, aggression, and homosexuality. A review of the literature and implications for future research. In *Topics in Psychoendocrinology*, E. J. Sachar (ed.). Grune and Stratton, New York, pp. 83-103.

Rossi, A. S., and Rossi, P. E. (1977). Body time and social time. Mood patterns are affected by menstrual cycle phase and day of week. *Soc. Sci. Res.* 6, 273-308.

Seyler, L. E., Jr., Canalis, E., Spare, S., and Reichlin, S. (1978). Abnormal gonadotropin secretory responses to LRH in transexual women after diethylstilbestrol priming. *J. Clin. Endocrinol. Metab.* 47, 176-183.

Shainess, N. (1961). A re-evaluation of some aspects of femininity through a study of menstruation: A preliminary report. *Compr. Psychiatry* 2, 20-26.

Siiteri, P., and Wilson, J. D. (1974). Testosterone formation and metabolism during male sexual differentiation in the human embryo. *J. Clin. Endocrinol. Metab.* 38, 113-125.

Smith, S. L., and Sauder, C. (1969). Food cravings, depression, and premenstrual problems. *Psychosom. Med.* 31, 281-287.

Spitz, C. J., Gold, A. R., and Adams, D. B. (1975). Cognitive and hormonal factors affecting coital frequency. *Arch. Sexual Behav.* 4, 249-264.

Stenn, P. G., and Klinge, V. (1972). Relationship between the menstrual cycle and bodily activity in humans. *Horm. Behav.* 3, 297-305.

Taylor, T., Coutts, J. R. T., and MacNaughton, M. C. (1974). Human foetal synthesis of testosterone from perfused progesterone. *J. Endocrinol.* 60, 321-326.

Tourney, G., Petrilli, A. J., and Hatfield, L. M. (1975). Hormonal relationships in homosexual men. *Am. J. Psychiatry* 132, 288-290.

Udry, J. R., and Morris, N. M. (1968). Distribution of coitus in the menstrual cycle. *Nature* 220, 593-596.

Vermeulen, A., Rubens, R., and Verdonck, L. (1971). Testosterone secretion and metabolism in male senescence. *J. Clin. Endocrinol. Metab.* 34, 730-735.

Verwoerdt, A., Pfeiffer, E., and Wang, H. S. (1969a). Sexual behavior in senescence. I. Changes in sexual activity and interest in aging men and women. *J. Geriatric Psychiatry* 2, 163-180.

Verwoerdt, A., Pfeiffer, E., and Wang, H. S. (1969b). Sexual behavior in senescence. II. Patterns of sexual activity and interest. *Geriatrics* 24, 137-154.

Visser, H. K. A. (1973). Some physiological and clinical aspects of puberty. *Arch. Dis. Child.* 48, 169-182.

Wetzel, R. D., Reich, T., and McClure, J. N., Jr. (1971). Phase of the menstrual cycle and self-referrals to a suicide prevention service, *Br. J. Psychiatry* 119, 523-524.

Whalen, R. E. (1968). Differentiation of the neural mechanisms which control gonadotropin secretion and sexual behavior. In *Perspectives in Reproduction and Sexual Behavior*, M. Diamond (ed.). Indiana University Press, Bloomington, pp. 303-340.

Whalen, R. E. (1974). Sexual differentiation. Models, methods and mechanisms. In *Sex Differences in Behavior*, R. C. Friedman, R. M. Richart, and R. L. Vande Wiele (eds.). Wiley, New York, pp. 477-481.

Note

Originally published in *Handbook of Biological Psychiatry, Part III, Brain Mechanisms and Abnormal Behavior — Genetics and Neuroendocrinology* (H. M. van Praag, M. H. Lader, O. J. Rafaelsen and E. J. Sachar, eds.). New York, Marcel Dekker, 1980. [Bibliog. #3.62]

Author's Comment: Sex Hormones and Homosexuality

Section IV of this chapter, Hormones and Dimorphism of Pair Partnerships, reviews the research literature on sex hormones in the bloodstream and homosexuality/heterosexuality. Since its publication in 1980, there have been three new studies of note.

One is a particularly well designed study by Sanders, Bain and Langevin (1985). For attention to details of sampling and experimental design, it is rivaled only by the 1974 study of Parks et al. (see above). In both studies the data showed no difference in the blood-hormone levels of homosexual men and their heterosexual controls.

Another study, by Gladue, Green and Hellman (1984) was designed to replicate the 1975 study of Dörner et al (see above) on the estrogen feedback effect on the release of luteinizing hormone. The data were, in fact, confirmatory. More recently, however, another study produced nonconfirmitory data. This is a study, still awaiting publication, by L. J. G. Gooren in Amsterdam. The data of Gooren's study did not differentiate between homosexual men and their heterosexual controls with respect to the estrogen feedback effect on LH. When the effect did appear, it was in either homosexuals or heterosexuals who shared in common a low testosterone response to the chorionic gonadotropin stimulation test. Thus, the estrogen feedback effect could be attributed to neither homosexuality nor heterosexuality, but to a presumed impairment of the function of the steroid-secreting Leydig cells of the testes in response to gonadotropic stimulation. In a second experiment, this Leydig cell impairment was found absent in untreated male-to-female transexual candidates, despite their ultrafeminine identity/role. In a third experiment, male-to-female transexuals were retested after they had been castrated and, therefore, had no Leydig cells. They then did show the estrogen feedback effect on the release of LH from the pituitary.

References

Gladue, B. A., Green, R., and Hellman, R. E. Neuroendocrine response to estrogen and sexual orientation. *Science,* 225:1496–1498, 1984.

Gooren, L. J. G. Estrogen positive feedback effect in heterosexuals, homosexuals, and transexuals. Preprint, July, 1985.

Sanders, R. M., Bain, J., and Langevin, R. Peripheral sex hormones, homosexuality, and gender identity. In *Erotic Preference, Gender Identity and Aggression in Men: New Research Studies* (R. Langevin, ed.). Hillsdale, NJ, Lawrence Erlbaum, 1985.

THIRTY-ONE
Paraphilias: Phenomenology and Classification

Abstract

DSM-III incorrectly designates the majority of paraphilias as atypical. Only eight are named, and those because of their forensic history, rather than their pathology and therapeutic need. In this paper, thirty-odd paraphilias are subdivided into six categories on the basis of their phenomenological dynamics. The new concept of the developmental lovemap is introduced for the first time. A new treatment originated by the author in 1966 combines an androgen agonist with counseling therapy.

Lovemaps

The most conclusive evidence concerning the importance of sexual rehearsal play in human childhood comes from the study of tribal people whose ancient tribal ways have not been overly Westernized.[1-4] In some cases, the tribal tradition of childrearing does not require that children be punished when they engage in sexual rehearsal play, which they do from time to time, though without being obtrusive about it. Because anthropologists themselves have typically been too prudishly Victorian to have recorded sexual rehearsal play in children, there is not as much evidence as one would like. However, from the evidence available, the conclusion is that heterosexual rehearsal play in childhood lays the foundation for uncomplicated heterosexuality in adulthood.

Children get their native language by practicing it. Similarly, they get a native lovemap by engaging in sexual rehearsal play. When their play is not interfered with, the basic geography of the lovemap develops typically as heterosexual. At puberty and thereafter, when the lovemap is heterosexual, the erotic fantasies, daydreams, and nightdreams are heterosexual. So also is the fantasy of the ideal love affair and the ideal lover.

The features and requirements of the ideal lover may be fairly generalized and nonspecific, or they may be very detailed and personalized, so that only relatively few people in everyday life will qualify as perfectly matching the specifications of the lovemap. For example, the lovemap may specify that the ideal lover be a stand-in for a childhood sweetheart, or a popular hero or heroine, idolized in the early years.

It goes without saying that, in the human species as in any other species, most individuals in each generation have an inbuilt determinant to have young ones, and so to replace themselves with a new generation. This built-in determinant is phyletically programed. That is to say, it exists simply because an individual is a member of the species. Like a cluster of wild mushroms that can push through the paving of an asphalt court, it cannot easily be sealed over. However, it can encounter abuses that interfere with its normal expression. The normal heterosexual play of childhood, for example, may be hampered by too much prohibition, prevention, and punishment. In that case the standard heterosexual lovemap does not develop properly in the brain.

In consequence, the lovemap may become defaced in such a way that parts are missing, thus impairing in adulthood the functioning of the sex organs in genital intercourse. This is the hypophilic solution. By contrast, the hyperphilic solution is one in which the lovemap defies defacement, so that the sex organs, in adulthood, are used with exaggerated defiance, frequency, and compulsiveness, and/or with great multiplicity of partners, in pairs or in groups.

There is a third solution in which the lovemap is not completely defaced, but redesigned with detours that include either new elements, or relocations of original roles. In some, if not all, instances, the new elements or relocations may derive from a history of atypical sexual rehearsal play and/or erotosexual experience in childhood. Or they may derive from some other childhood encounter or series of encounters in which the sexual organs become stimulated, for instance, receiving an enema, or a whipping. Whatever the reason, overt or covert, the further development of the lovemap becomes compromised and distorted, perhaps to the extent of being changed almost beyond recognition.

A lovemap carries the program of a person's erotic fantasies and their corresponding practices. Distortions, therefore, get carried over into fantasies and practices. A teenage boy's erotic murder/suicide is an example of what can happen when a lovemap is programed to end in disaster and self-destruction. In such a case, the penalty written into the boy's lovemap is that forbidden lust must be followed by the supreme sacrifice, death.

This deadly sequence illustrates the basic formula of both a distorted lovemap, and also of the paraphilia* for which it is responsible. Two terms of the formula, love and lust are irreconcilable, and the solution is to find a third term, which in the present instance is sacrifice, with which to reconcile them.

Love is undefiled and saintly. Lust is defiling and sinful. The sinful act of lust, therefore, defiles those who participate in it. It turns the saint into a sinner—the madonna into a whore, and the provider into a playboy.

In the joint sacrifice of suicide/murder, both partners are victims of a paraphilic act of atonement for the degenerate sin of carnal lust.

Paraphilias

The erotic fantasies and their practices or animations that are programed in

---

*An erotosexual condition of being recurrently responsive to, and obsessively dependent on, an unusual or unacceptable stimulus, perceptual or in fantasy, in order to have a state of erotic arousal initiated or maintained, and in order to achieve or facilitate orgasm. For examples, see Table I.

TABLE I

Paraphilias

ACROTOMOPHILIA*	MYSOPHILIA (Filth)
(Amputee Partner)	NARRATOPHILIA (Erotic Talk)
APOTEMNOPHILIA*	NECROPHILIA (Corpse)
(Self-Amputee)	PEDOPHILIA (Child)
ASPHYXIOPHILIA	PICTOPHILIA (Pictures)
(Self-Strangulation)	PEODEIKTOPHILIA*
AUTAGONISTOPHILIA* (On Stage)	(Penile Exhibitionism)
AUTASSASSINOPHILIA	RAPISM or BIASTOPHILIA*
(Own Murder Staged)	(Violent Assault)
AUTONEPIOPHILIA* (Diaperism)	SADISM
COPROPHILIA (Feces)	SCOPTOPHILIA (Watching Coitus)
EPHEBOPHILIA (Youth)	SOMNOPHILIA (Sleeper)
EROTOPHONOPHILIA*	STIGMATOPHILIA*
(Lust Murder)	(Piercing; Tattoo)
FETISHISM	SYMPHOROPHILIA* (Disaster)
FROTTEURISM	TELEPHONE SCATOPHILIA
(Rub Against Stranger)	(Lewdness)
GERONTOPHILIA (Elder)	TROILISM (Couple + One)
HYPHEPHILIA (Fabrics)	UROPHILIA or UNDINISM (Urine)
KLEPTOPHILIA (Stealing)	VOYEURISM or
KLISMAPHILIA (Enema)	PEEPING-TOMISM
MASOCHISM	ZOOPHILIA (Animal)

*New term formed from Greek root (in collaboration with Diskin Clay, Professor of Greek, Johns Hopkins University).

distorted lovemaps are popularly known as kinky or bizarre. In law and the criminal justice system, they are known as perversions. In science and medicine, perversions are today known as paraphilias.[4, 5] Paraphilia means love (philia) beyond the usual (*para*). There are more than thirty different paraphilias, the exact count depending on whether overlapping ones are separated or not (Table I). Each paraphilia has its own lovemap.

A paraphilic lovemap may not unfold itself fully at puberty, although it commonly does. Instead, the complete extent of its imagery may remain in hiding for some years, until eventually it reveals itself from beginning to end as a complete fantasy. It may first appear as a wet dream or as a masturbation fantasy. Or it might be a copulation fantasy, without which the penis will not erect (or the vagina lubricate), and the orgasm will not occur. The fantasy may be played or replayed silently in the imagination, or enacted as a paraphilic practice.

The lovemaps of the paraphilias can be understood in terms of six strategies. Each strategy, in its own roundabout way, is a certificate of permission to enter what would otherwise be the inaccessible city of lust and ecstasy. The price of the certificate is that the saint is sold into sin. The six strategies comprise, by type, the sacrificial paraphilias, the predatory paraphilias, the mercantile paraphilias, the fetish paraphilias, the eligibility paraphilias, and the allurement paraphilias.

In individual cases, a paraphilia of one type may share characteristics of another type. It is rare, however, for a person to have more than one paraphilia, or to change from one to another. A lovemap, once it has formed, is rather uniquely personalized. It tends to be remarkably stable throughout life—quite the opposite of what degeneracy theory[6] would lead one to believe.

According to the evidence available today, paraphilias occur more often and in more varieties in boys and men than they do in girls and women. This inequality may derive from the fact that nature has designed males more than females to be dependent on their eyes for erotic turn on, and females to be more dependent than males on skin feelings. Lovemaps get into the brain mostly through the eyes, in contrast with language, which gets in through the ears.

More boys than girls have difficulty in getting their native language, and in learning to read it. It appears that they also have more difficulty in getting their lovemaps. It is easier for misprints to occur. In some boys it may be easier than others. Their brains may be geared in such a way that they are more vulnerable to misprint errors. Vulnerable or not, the brain does not program a misprint into its lovemap without getting instructions coming into it from the eyes and ears and the other senses. These instructions come in during the critical map-making years of early childhood. These are the years when sexual degeneracy theory, outmoded but still socially influential, lurks in a child's life like a polluted smog in biological warfare and sabotages the lovemap instructions that the brain receives. Consequently, the lovemap program gets misprinted, and the misprinting may turn out to be a paraphilia.

The same paraphilic misprintings may occur regardless of whether the partner relationship will prove to be, over the long term, homosexual, or heterosexual, or bisexual. The programing of the part of the sexual brain that governs the sexual matching of the partnership is another story, most of the details of which remain to be discovered—including the details that might relate to the covert influence of degeneracy theory.

Some of the paraphilias are playful and harmless. Some are an unwelcome nuisance to a partner who does not share their fantasy content.[7] Some are dangerous and destructive, even to a consenting partner.[8] Some of those that are legally classified as sex offenses are violently dangerous, and some, like exhibitionism are harmless offenses against modesty.

The Sacrificial Paraphilias

The sacrificial paraphilias are those in which one or both of the partners must atone for the wicked and degenerate acts of defilng the saint with ecstatic lust by undergoing an act of penance or sacrifice. The penalty ranges from humiliation and hurt to a blood sacrifice and death. Self-sacrifice is masochism; partner-sacrifice is sadism. Either may be consenting or enforced.

Masochistic death may be autoerotic (masturbatory) suicide, or the finale of a self-staged murder of oneself enacted in collaboration with a sadistic partner. Sadistic death, in all probability, is rarely invited. More likely, it is violent and imposed without forewarning. The victim may be either spouse, companion, or stranger. There may be many victims. Multiple lust murder is the most gruesome of the paraphilias, and one that provokes the most public outrage, and the most severe criminal punishment.

The repertory of sadomasochistic sacrifice varies in degree of harmfulness and playfulness. At one extreme are the acts of a merciless Dracula: horror, shock, assault, brutality, and torture. At the other extreme are the acts of a velvet dragon: games of humiliation, bondage, punishment, and discipline. At either extreme the participants may have been previously acquainted or not. They may participate by mutual consent. There is one sadistic scenario, however, in which it must be an unsuspecting partner or stranger who is subjected to unprovoked outrage, suffering, and abuse.

The sadomasochistic sacrifice is not, of necessity, directed at the sex organs. Either the sadist or the masochist may find erotic arousal from other afflictions of the body, and of the mind. But there are some instances of direct mutilation of the sex organs, some of them by consent of the victim. The sex organs may be bound, beaten, squeezed, stretched, penetrated, pierced, or cut.

In some, if not all cases of erotic masochism, the first pain that a procedure produces fades and becomes transformed into sensuous ecstasy. In religious and penitential masochism, such as flagellation and being harnessed to flesh hooks, a similar transformation may also be experienced.

Sadomasochistic partner matching is difficult to achieve, as it requires that the fantasies of the two people match hand-in-glove. There is an insufficiency of sadistic women to match up with the excess of men who may be brokers of immense political, business or industrial power by day, and submissive masochists begging for erotic punishment and humiliation by night.

A special form of sacrificial paraphilia, for which a suitable name is symphorophilia (being erotically turned on by accidents or catastrophes), culminates in an arranged disaster, such as an automobile crash. Like a game of Russian roulette, it may end in death—alone or with the partner. However, flirting with disaster, rather than suicide and murder, is the trigger responsible for erotic arousal and excitement. Being the daredevil who will live to risk a love-death again is an essential part of this paraphilia.

As a photographic print is the positive made from its negative, so also the positive of self-crashing is arranging for a disaster to occur on the highway, and then watching the carnage from a preselected observation post. Disasters other than on the highway can be arranged—catastrophic fires, for example. For those members of the general public who have a touch of sadomasochism in them, disaster as an unrehearsed event is often a large part of the appeal of entertainment stunts and sports, from the circus to stock-car racing.

The Predatory Paraphilias

The predatory paraphilias are those in which the wicked and degenerate ecstasy of the sinful act of lust is so defiling that it can be indulged only if it is stolen, or taken from the saint by force. The person experiencing one of this group of paraphilias may have the fantasy of being either predator or prey. Though it is not known for sure, it is probably fairly rare for predator and prey to match up with one another, except by setting themselves up in mutually consenting play acting.

The most notorious of the predatory paraphilias is biastophilic rapism or raptophilia. The biastophilic lovemap prescribes that the partner, typically a stranger, should be unsuspecting of what is about to happen, and should be maximally terror-stricken and resistant, until the fantasy enactment has run its course.

Biastophilia may include breaking and entering, and stealing things as well as stealing sexual intercourse by force. The things stolen may be of value, or they may be more in the nature of tokens. In some cases, stealing alone takes place as a substitute for genital intercourse.

In the "sleeping-princess syndrome" (somnophilia), the sexual approach is a gentle and nonviolent stealing of caresses after breaking and entering, not necessarily followed by genital intercourse. Of course, it is generally mistaken for rape.

Stealing as a paraphilia may also manifest itself as kidnapping or elopement. Though wholly unprepared for the event, the victim may become devotedly bonded to the abductor in a way that totally bewilders those unacquainted with this paradoxical phenomenon (the so-called Stockholm syndrome).

The Mercantile Paraphilias

In the mercantile paraphilias the wicked and degenerate ecstasy of the sinful act of lust is the social vice practiced only by whores and hustlers for pay. Saintly people do not defile themselves with lust. Therefore, if a saint does become sexual from time to time, the act is equated with taking on the role of a sinful whore or hustler, or of one of their customers. The mercantile paraphilia is not necessarily actual prostitution, for it may be the impersonation of prostitution with an orthodox partner in a conventional home life.

In some mercantile paraphilic fantasies, there are elaborate ruses and pretenses of prostitution. In troilism for example, it is a third person, maybe a stranger, whose role is to create an illusion of prostitution. Thus a husband leaves a phone number and invitation in a public place for another man to have intercourse with his wife. He watches, and while watching is enabled to get an erection. Then he achieves penetration and orgasm, which is not possible except that his wife first play the role of a whore.

In a related paraphilia, a man is able to have the same success if he talks to his partner as if she were a whore, and if she responds in character. A woman, by contrast, may have the fantasy that her husband is a casual pickup, or gigolo. The enactment of this fantasy may in either partner include paying, or having money demanded.

Another prostitution fantasy that has widespread male appeal is that of two women involved in wicked and degenerate lust together. Not only is the stimulus in duplicate, but the two Jezebels cry out for rescue from themselves, and he of course is the male who can do it.

The Fetish Paraphilias

The fetish paraphilias are those in which a compromise is made with the saintliness of chastity and abstinence not by trafficking with prostitution, but by including in the sexual act a token that symbolizes the wickedness and degeneracy of the sinful act of ecstatic lust. The token symbolically permits the partner to remain as if saintly, pure, and undefiled. The token is a fetish, and it is the fetish which is the sinful agent of erotic and sexual excitement and arousal. For example, undergarments, especially brassieres and panties or garter belt and stockings, are a fetishistic turn-on for countless American males. In some cases they are stolen from laundry lines. Erotically, they may be more important than the woman who wears them. In the case of the transvestophilic male, they must be worn by the man, himself, before he can perform genitally. If his partner objects, then he must fantasize that he is wearing them in order to perform successfully.

Fetishistic inclusion objects are, with great frequency, sexy because of their texture (hyphephilias; the feely fetishes) or their smell. A rubber fetish combines feel and smell. Its origin is almost certainly traceable, at least in part, to the rubber training pants formerly popular for infants. Plastic will presumably take the place of rubber in the future. A diaper fetish (autonepiophilia) has a similar early origin, presumably, and so has an enema fetish (klismaphilia).

Like the sexual act itself, many fetishes are related to the tabooed parts of the body and their functions—crotch smells, for example, and soiled underclothing or articles of menstrual hygiene; and the products of elimination that are ingested and smeared in urophilia and coprophilia.

The Eligibility Paraphilias

The eligibility paraphilias are those in which self-abandonment to the wicked and degenerate ecstasy of the sinful act of lust can be achieved only if the partner qualifies as eligible by reason of being beyond the pale, that is, beyond the limits, privileges, and protection of being saintly and undefilable. By some criterion or other, the partner must qualify as an erotic heathen, not at all resembling the likes of one's own righteously god-fearing parents who, in the proverbial wisdom of many children, would never do anything so dirty as genital intercourse. The criterion may quite literally be that of belonging to another religious faith.

Interfaith marriage, by itself alone, need not be a paraphilia, for one of the yardsticks by which a paraphilia is measured is that it is addictively repetitious and compulsive. This same yardstick applies to all of the eligibility paraphilias.

Instead of religious affiliation, the criterion of being an outsider may be that of racial or nationality type and color. The specifications of what the partner should look like may be extremely detailed—blue-eyed and blond, facially lop-sided with a crooked smile, or with a wash-board furrowed brow, and so on.

The entire physique may be involved, as when the specification requires that the partner be diminutive or towering in stature; fat or skinny; disfigured, deformed or crippled, and so on. The ultimate extreme of erotic eligibility distancing is in necrophilia: the partner must be dead.

Social or occupational status, rather than physique, may be the criterion that establishes an erotic eligibility distance between oneself and a partner. The eligibility status that is probably the most prevalent in this type of paraphilia is that of paramour. A paramour relationship exists outside the institution of marriage, and is legally defined as adultery or fornication. It may be long term or short term, living together or living apart. Only a thin line divides this type of relationship from a paid one with a courtesan or gigolo, especially if, in both instances, the relationship is a continuing one with one person. Marriage ruins such a relationship, because it endows it with respectability, and robs it of the ecstasy of lust which is stigmatized as defiling, naughty, and illicit, as well as wicked and degenerate.

Rough and sweaty labor as compared with cultured and perfumed leisure is another example: occupational and social-class disparity serve to establish an erotic eligibility distance between the self and partner. Uniforms as insignia of occupation may play an important, almost fetishistic ancillary role.

Along with, or in place of a uniform, body tattoos may be insignia of tough occupational status. For some people, the eroticizing of tattoo is accompanied by erotic piercing (stigmatophilia), and the wearing of gold rings and rods in the nipples and genitals, as well as in other parts of the body.

In some paraphilias alterations of the body go far beyond tattoo and piercing and involve mutilation and/or surgical amputation, amateur or professional, of the genitalia or limbs. In the paraphilia of acrotomophilia, erotic eligibility requires that the partner be an amputee, or a person born with a birth defect of missing limbs. Erotic turn-on is to the stump. The counterpart is apotemnophilia,[9] a paraphilic compulsion to get oneself amputated. In some cases the person stage-manages an injury, by means of a planned hunting accident, for example, so as to require a professional amputation in a hospital.

Surgical alteration applies in some instances not to the limbs but the genital organs. In males only rarely is genital amputation not associated also with a more pervasive transposition of gender status, namely, the compulsion to be reassigned to live as a member of the other sex. In either sex, surgical and hormonal reassignment completes a male/female or female/male transposition of erotic eligibility. Some individuals are highly responsive to a sex-reassigned partner, more so than they are to a nonreassigned man or woman. In the same vein, among men, there are some whose ideal fantasy is fulfilled by a lady with a penis, that is, a surgically unreassigned transexual who takes female hormones to feminize the body from male to female, and who lives full time as a woman.

Age matching, like male/female matching, is a routine social norm of erotic eligibility. Discrepancies, when they exist, are yet another circumvention of the conventional norm. They effect a social distancing that serves to circumvent the wickedness-depravity conception of lust and to preserve its ecstasy. The age-discrepancy paraphilias are gerontophilia, ephebophilia, and pedophilia (including infantophilia).

In gerontophilia, a young adult is inwardly compelled always to seek a partner old enough to be either a parent or, in some instances, a grandparent. In ephebophilia, an older person is inwardly compelled always to have a partner who is in the adolescent age range. In pedophilia, an adolescent or adult is inwardly compelled to have a partner who is pubertal or juvenile. The mathematician, Charles L. Dodgson (1832–1898), better known as Lewis Carroll, author of *Alice's Adventures in Wonderland,* and other books for juveniles, was a pedophilic lover of prepubertal girls. Sir James Barrie (1860–1937), author of *Peter Pan,* was a pedophilic lover of prepubertal boys.

The pedophile is a Peter Pan whose erotic age does not advance with birthday age. Likewise the age of the partner always stays in childhood, so that the relationship is a mixture of parent-child and lover-lover bonding. Often the adult pedophile had, in childhood, a relationship with an older partner. A pedophile relationship wanes and breaks up when the younger partner gets to be adolescent. Similarly, an ephebophile relationship may wane and break up, as adolescence advances into the maturity of young adulthood. Some divorces occur on this account, if one or both of the partners is an ephebophile. Erotically, they are unable to advance in age together, for the ephebophile is compulsively driven to have a new partner of nubile age.

A pedophile and ephebophile relationship within the family, even when there is no blood relationship, is a particularly disruptive double-bind. The sanctions of the incest taboo are so threatening and devastating that those involved are almost inevitably damned if they do, and damned if they don't disclose the existence of the relationship and try to leave it.

All the foregoing specifications and provisos that dictate a degree of erotic distancing between the self and an eligible partner apply to human beings. In zoophilia, the distance that separates is the distance between species. Pets are for petting, and so are lovers. No one knows the prevalence of genital-genital contact between species, but it is not restricted to human-animal contacts. It may happen between other species also.[10] Among human beings, especially the erotically isolated, nonpenetrating stimulation of the crotch by a pet may be a more prevalent comfort than is generally believed.

The Allurement Paraphilias

The allurement paraphilias are displacement paraphilias, whereas those in the foregoing five categories are inclusion paraphilias. The inclusion is some more or less extraneous ritual, participant, or artifact not typically a component of heterosexual mating practices. A displacement paraphilia is one that involves a segment of the preparatory phase of an erotic and sexual activity before genital intercourse begins. This is the phase of eye-talk and finger-talk, when the partners give signals or invitations to one another. They flirt, coquet, woo, or lure one another. It is sometimes known as the phase of courtship or, in animals, of the mating dance or display.

In a displacement paraphilia, some part of the preparatory or courtship phase pushes its way onto center field, instead of remaining on the sidelines. It displaces the main event, which is genital intercourse, and steals the spotlight. In this way, the wicked and degenerate ecstasy of the sinful act of lust is disconnected from the sacred act of genital union, and displaced onto a substitute act. The saint is thus redeemed from defilement. This strategy of disconnection is a rather sneaky one, for the build-up of ecstatic lust can be brought back to the marriage bed and used to power the sexual organs into a successful performance. Without this auxiliary power, they might fail. Exhibitionism is an example.

The paraphilia of exhibitionism has its origins in the primate courtship or allurement ritual of displaying the genitalia as an invitation to copulation. The paraphilic male exhibitionist is compulsively driven to display his penis (peodeiktophilia) in erection so as to elicit from a stranger a startle response ranging from curiosity or surprise to alarm or panic. A neutral response, for example, telling him that his penis should be covered in public, will bring the episode to a docile end.

In some instances, it is possible to retrieve and authenticate information of early childhood erotic pleasure associated with showing the penis in erection, and with defiance in response to being chastised for doing so. In adulthood, the peak intensity of ecstatic feeling associated with exhibitionism, even without ejaculation, surpasses that of orgasm in sexual intercourse. Punishment and imprisonment do not prevent recurrence. It is extremely rare for exhibitionism to include any other activity than display of the penis, even though many people fear that it will lead to an attempt at genital intercourse, perhaps by coercion.

The opposite of showing is looking, which in paraphilic terms means voyeurism or being a Peeping Tom. The voyeur learns from experience where he is likely to find lighted and uncurtained windows, and where, at night, he may glimpse a female occupant undressing. His erotic excitement is in the forbidden act of looking at her. It is rare that he will attempt to meet with or communicate with her. He may make noise that attracts attention to his loitering and gets him arrested. If a woman sees him through the window and continues to appear naked, he may exhibit his penis, and masturbate, though it is not usual for one person to be both an exhibitionist and a voyeur.

The erotic distancing achieved in both exhibitionism and peeping is achieved also in explicitly erotic telephone calling. The recipient may be a stranger, or a consenting listener. Professional consenting listeners, trained to take part in erotic telephone fantasies, make a charge for their play-acting role on the telephone.

The erotic telephone caller has counterparts in those whose primary sexual turn-on is not genital sex with a partner but erotic narrations or readings. Similarly there are those who look at erotic burlesque shows, picture books or movies, and those who take erotic pictures, videotapes or movies of themselves (autagonistophilia). All of these entertainments when they are paraphilias, occupy center stage instead of being preliminaries. When shared with a partner, they augment arousal and genital performance. The contents of the entertainments do not necessarily match what happens with the partner. In one case, for example, a man's maximum turn-on was from sermons, from which he could ejaculate, without masturbating, in church.

Erotic distancing is achieved despite body contact in frotteurism. This is the paraphilia in which erotic arousal, and maybe orgasm also are achieved anonymously by rubbing and pressing against a stranger in a crowded public place, like a subway car or bus. The stranger sometimes may reciprocate.

Tragedy into Triumph

The fantasies of paraphilia are not socially contagious. They are not preferences borrowed from movies, books, or other people. They are not voluntary choices. They cannot be controlled by will power. Punishment does not prevent them, and persecution does not eradicate them, but feeds them and strengthens them. They are an addiction, or the equivalent of an addiction, and they are defiantly persistent. They are theatrical and showy; their vanity leads to self-incrimination. The paraphilic person is a survivor of catastrophe who repeatedly goes on camera or stage, so to speak, to tell the story of how he turned tragedy into the triumph of survival. The tragedy that deprived the paraphiliac of heterosexual normality was the neglect and/or abuse of the rehearsal play and development of early life, and the paraphilic substitute that took its place. The triumph was that lust and its arousal was saved from total wreckage or extinction by being transferred to some other less prevented and at the time less censored, but paraphilic rehearsal. It was a hollow triumph, alas, for in later years, it would bring more tragedy, as paraphila so often does.

Knowing the developmental history of a paraphilia is not the same as knowing the whole explanation of its cause. There is no final certainty as to how one particular paraphilic fantasy instead of another gets personalized, though it seems to be related at least in part to a personalized experience of early genital arousal. For example, it is often possible to pin down an early history of too much fussing with enemas in the infancy of those who as adults have klismaphilia—an obsession with getting an enema as a substitute for genital intercourse.

Apart from the issue of the personalization of a particular paraphilia, there is the larger quesiton of why there should be as many as there are, and no more. The brain may be species-limited as to how many paraphilias it can invent. That is to say, there may be a limit to how many types of behavior not specific to the reproductive act can become attached to erotic arousal.

Once a paraphilia gets lodged in the brain, it is like an addiction that firmly resists dislodging. It is additionally like an addiction in that it needs a new "fix" or repetition, every so often. In between fixes, an outsider would not even suspect its existence. But when it is in action, then it may put the person who has it into what resembles a spell, or a trancelike fugue state, making him do things that he normally would not. As aforementioned, in the case of an exhibitonist flashing his penis to a stranger, if the woman, instead of being startled or scared, would tell him that this was no place to have his penis showing, and that it should be in his pants, then the spell would be broken, and the compulsion to exhibit would cease for the time being.

Many paraphilic men are able to have several ejaculations, as many as ten, on a daily basis. To do so, they must either carry out, or replay in imagination, while masturbating or having genital intercourse, the personalized scenario of the paraphilic fantasy.

Paraphilic fantasies and behavior are not caused by social contagion. A person who does not have klismaphilia can look at five, fifty, or five hundred enema movies of someone getting erotically and genitally turned on by getting an enema, and never be able to get turned on that way himself or herself. Klismaphilic movies are a turn-on only for people who have klismaphilia. For other people they are a curiosity, though to see more than one is uninteresting and a chore.

Treatment of Paraphilic Sex Offenders

The most prevalent treatment of the paraphilias that are legislatively defined as sex offenses is penal incarceration and, in some instances, the death sentence. The rationale for defining paraphilias as crimes instead of illnesses derives from the philosophy of the Inquisition and demon possession, for which offenders were burned at the stake. In the eighteenth century, demon-possession theory was replaced by degeneracy theory. This theory, first published by Tissot[6] in 1758, was used to explain both social and individual ills on the basis of personal responsibility, for the cause of degeneracy was attributed to loss of vital fluid in masturbation, or promiscuity, and also to indulgence in concupiscent thoughts and fantasies.[12] After the advent of germ theory in the 1870s, degeneracy theory rapidly became outmoded in most branches of medicine, except in sexual medicine.[13] It is still resorted to as an explanation of why explicit depictions of erotic sexuality, for education or for entertainment, are dangerous to the individual and society. It surfaces in the media when a paraphilic sex offender is stigmatized as a sexual degenerate, and his degeneracy is attributed to the influence of pornography. Degeneracy theory thus allows the paraphilic offender to be held responsible for his condition, and for his offense, since he is held responsible for having exposed himself to the explicit sexual depictions of pornography. In consequence, punishment as a treatment is held justified.

Castration as a punishment for the male sex offender, though historically vindictive in nature, carried also the implication of asexualization as a way of preventing further offenses. Despite the lack of outcome studies, castration treatment did sow the seeds of the idea that sex offenders might be treated by other than penal methods. By and large, however, medicine, including psychiatry, in the 20th century directed only desultory attention to the treatment of paraphilias. In the recent past, the practitioners of behavior modification have staked out a claim to effective treatment, but they have promised more than they have presently proved. Practitioners of the new sex therapy have not included paraphilias in the catalogue of sexual dysfunctions for which they offer treatment.

In the mid-1960s, the new synthetic steroid hormone, cyproterone acetate, was first used at the Hamburg Institute for Sex Research, West Germany, for the treatment of offenders. Cyproterone acetate, having not been approved for use in the United States, an alternative hormone, medroxyprogesterone acetate, was used when in 1966 the first patient was treated.[15,16] This patient was successfully relieved of sex-offending behavior for which he would otherwise have been given a long prison sentence. He has maintained his nonoffending status until the present.

In males, medroxyprogesterone acetate, injected in its long-acting form, Upjohn's Depo-Provera® is an androgen-depleting antiandrogen.[4] It is probably also an erotic tranquilizer that has a direct effect on erotosexual pathways in the limbic brain. Its hyposexual effects are reversible upon discontinuance of treatment, except that the paraphilic fantasy and the behavior it dictates no longer have the same tyrannical, addictive quality.[17,18]

Antiandrogenic hormonal therapy has increased effectiveness, if it is given jointly with counseling therapy, and preferably couple-counseling therapy.[7] The combination enhances the possibility of a successful realignment not only of sexual life, but also of all those other aspects of occupational and domestic life and relationships that are affected by the time-consuming and tyrannical pathology of the paraphilia.

Summary

In biomedical usage, the perversions are now known as the paraphilias. A paraphilia exists in imagery as a fantasy and, animated, as an erotosexual practice. Developmentally, paraphilic imagery constitutes a lovemap that goes awry during the juvenile period of erotosexual rehearsal play by either the inclusion of new elements, or the displacement of original elements. Each paraphilia has its own paths on the mental lovemap which is a strategy for circumventing the individually encountered incompatibility of the saint and the sinner, the sacred and the profane, in erotosexualism. There are six strategies of circumvention according to which the paraphilias may be classified as the sacrificial, predatory, mercantile, fetish, eligibility, and allurement paraphilias, respectively. Knowing the developmental history of a paraphilia does not explain its existence as an addiction, its phenomenology as a fugue-like syndrome, and its sometimes evident association with central nervous system pathology. The prevalence and variety of paraphilias is greater in males than females. In males, paraphilia is often associated with hyperorgasmia, and its mental representation is typically a prerequisite of orgasm and/or erection. Paraphilias are not socially contagious. Therapeutically, they have a history of being resistant to traditional treatments. Since 1966, an innovative form of treatment combines counseling therapy with hormonal therapy. The hormone is medroxyprogesterone acetate (in Europe, cyproterone acetate) which is a synthetic progestinic steroid. It resembles progesterone, the biological precursor of testosterone. Unlike testosterone, it is biologicaly relatively inert. It diminishes the subjective experience of sex drive and, in addition, may have a direct erotically tranquilizing action on erotosexual pathways in the brain. Its effects are reversible. It has value for the treatment of paraphiliacs who are harassed by their paraphilia, or who, by following the medical route, are able to avoid the penal route.

References

1. Malinowski, B. *The Sexual Life of Savages in North-Western Melanesia.* Halycon House, New York, 1929.

2. Marshall, D. S. and Suggs, R. C., eds. *Human Sexual Behavior: Variations in the Ethnographic Spectrum.* Basic Books, New York, 1971.

3. Money, J. and Ehrhardt, A. A. *Man and Woman, Boy and Girl: The Differentiation and Dimorphism of Gender Identity from Conception to Maturity.* Johns Hopkins Press, Baltimore, 1972.

4. Money, J. *Love and Love Sickness: The Science of Sex, Gender Difference, and Pairbonding.* Johns Hopkins University Press, Baltimore, 1980.

5. Money, J. Paraphilias. In *Handbook of Sexology,* Money, J. and Musaph, H., eds. Excerpta Medica, Amsterdam/New York, 1977.

6. Tissot, S. A. *A Treatise on the Diseases Produced by Onanism.* Translated from a New Edition of the French, with Notes and Appendix by an American Physician. New York, 1832 (reprint edition in *The Secret Vice Exposed! Some Arguments Against Masturbation,* Rosenberg, C. and Smith-Rosenberg, C., advisory eds.). Arno Press, New York, 1974.

7. Money, J. Paraphilia and Abuse-martyrdom: Exhibitionism as a Paradigm for Reciprocal Couple Counseling Combined with Antiandrogen. *J. Sex Marital Ther.*, 7:115-123, 1981.

8. Money, J. and Werlwas, J. Paraphilic Sexuality and Child Abuse: The Parents. *J. Sex Marital Ther.*, 8:57-64, 1982.

9. Money, J., Jobaris, R. and Furth, G. Apotemnophilia: Two Cases of Self-demand Amputation as a Paraphilia. *Journal Sex Res.*, 13:115-125, 1977.

10. Maple, T. Unusual Sexual Behavior of Nonhuman Primates. In *Handbook of Sexology*, Money, J., and Musaph, H., eds. Excerpta Medica, Amsterdam/New York, 1977 (Chapter 95).

11. Money, J. Paraphilias: Phyletic Origins of Erotosexual Dysfunction. *Int. J. Mental Health*, 10(2-3):75-109, 1981.

12. Graham, S. *A Lecture to Young Men* (1834). Arno Press, New York, 1974.

13. Kellogg, J. H. *Man the Masterpiece or Plain Truths Plainly Told about Boyhood, Youth, and Manhood*. Signs Publishing Assn. Ltd., Warburton, Victoria, Australia, London, Capetown, and Calcutta, 1906.

14. Bremer, J. *Asexualization: A Follow-up Study of 244 Cases*. Macmillan Company, New York, 1959.

15. Money, J. Discussion on hormonal inhibition of libido in male sex offenders. In *Endocrinology and Human Behaviour*, Michael, R. P., ed. Oxford University Press, London, 1968.

16. Money, J. Use of an Androgen-depleting Hormone in the Treatment of Male Sex Offenders. *J. Sex Res.*, 6:165-172, 1970.

17. Money, J. and Bennett, R. G. Postadolescent Paraphilic Sex Offenders: Antiandrogenic and Counseling Therapy Follow-up. *Int. J. Mental Health*, 10(2-3):122-133, 1981.

18. Money, J., Wiedeking, C., Walker, P., et al. 47,XYY and 46,XY Males with Antisocial and/or Sex-offending Behavior: Antiandrogen Therapy plus Counseling. *Psychoneuroendocrinology*, 1:165-178, 1975.

Note

Originally published in *American Journal of Psychotherapy*, 38:164–179, 1984, and adapted from an erstwhile orphaned manuscript that became *The Destroying Angel: Sex, Fitness, and Food in the Legacy of Degeneracy Theory, Graham Crackers, Kellogg's Corn Flakes and American Health History* (Buffalo, Prometheus, 1985). The six-fold classification of the paraphilias, original to this paper, became the basis of chapter six through eleven of *Lovemaps: Clinical Concepts of Sexual/Erotic Health and Pathology, Paraphilia, and Gender Transposition in Childhod, Adolescence and Maturity* (New York, Irvington, 1986). [Bibliog. #2.287]

Author's Comment: Opponent-Process Theory

The paraphilic strategy whereby tragedy is converted into triumph is one of converting negative into positive, or aversion into addiction. The first psychologist to name this conversion was Richard Solomon (*American Psychologist*, 35:691-712, 1980). The name is opponent-process learning. An example of opponent process would be the conversion of a terror or phobia of skydiving into euphoric ecstasy and addiction to the thrill and risk of the dive. Opponent-process learning takes place quite rapidly and is remarkably resistant to change, which accounts for the resistance of paraphilias to change.

THIRTY-TWO

Paraphilias: Phyletic Origins
of Erotosexual Dysfunction[1]

Phenomenology

A paraphilia is an erotosexual syndrome in which a person is reiteratively responsive to and dependent on atypical or forbidden stimulus imagery, in fantasy or in practice, for initiation and maintenance of erotosexual arousal and achievement or facilitation of orgasm.

Paraphilic syndromes may be either harmless or noxious. In either case they belong to the first two of the three-phase sequence of mammalian pair-bonding and erotosexuality, namely, proception and acception. Proception is the phase of mutual arousal, attraction, solicitation, and courtship. Acception is the phase of mutual participation in body contact, especially contact with the sex organs. Acception may be followed by conception, the third phase, which includes pregnancy, parturition, and parenthood.

There are paraphilias of displacement and paraphilias of inclusion. In a displacement paraphilia, a stimulus image that is typically a phyletic component of the erotosexual sequence of arousal and orgasm usurps the place of other components and assumes inordinate or exclusive power. For example, in frotteurism the stimulus of fondling, rubbing, and stroking a partner is displaced from being a component of a relationship with a known, or at least compliant, partner and instead is directed to a stranger in an anonymous crowd and becomes of paramount importance, in imagery and/or practice, in the achievement of arousal and orgasm. In an inclusion paraphilia, a stimulus image that is typically not a phyletic component of the erotosexual sequence of arousal and orgasm intrudes and assumes inordinate or exclusive power. The erotosexual sequence in klismaphilia, for instance, is atypical in that taking an enema intrudes and becomes of paramount importance, in imagery and/or in practice, in the achievement of arousal and orgasm.

In phyletically typical heterosexual matching, it is phyletically preordained that if the male and the female reciprocate, erotosexual pair-bonding will occur relatively easily. It is far more difficult for pair-bonding to occur in paraphilia, though it is not impossible. For example, in acrotomophilia, it is imperative that the partner be an amputee or, possibly, a congenital phocomeliac, such as a Thalidomide baby grown up. Since there are many amputees, and many who were born with missing limbs, an acrotomophiliac can indeed find a partner with whom to become firmly pair-bonded, erotosexually. The same person, if forced into a relationship with an able-bodied partner, would be only perfunctorily pair-bonded—erotosexually there would be a gap, a psychic distance, between them, because the acrotomophiliac's idealized imagery of an amputee partner would never be fulfilled. The partner, all limbs intact, would inchoately recognize herself (or himself) as superfluous to the acrotomophiliac partner's erotosexual imagery: "He wants me only for my body," she might well complain; to which he might well reply that coitus with her was for him the equivalent of masturbating himself in her vagina.

In some paraphilias the phenomenon of psychic distance is manifested literally as a split personality, one the partner in a conventional marriage, and the other the partner to a paraphilic ritual. One example that always appalls the public is that of lust murderism. The mass murderer, a subject of sensational stories in the press, is known in his community as a model citizen—usually a husband and often a father. What the community does not know is what his wife also does not know, namely, that he is able to copulate with her by replaying the imagery of one of his lust murders. Eventually such replay loses its power of erotosexual arousal and induction of orgasm, either alone in masturbation or with a partner, and the compulsion to seek another victim, usually an unsuspecting stranger, reasserts itself.

Etiology

The vogue in contemporary theory is to explain the erotosexual pathology of a paraphilia in an adult man or woman as the end product not of the individual's entire personal or ontogenetic developmental program, but more narrowly of the postnatal and social segment of that program. Yet humankind is also the product of its species heritage, its phylogeny. The range of paraphilic pathologies is not infinite, despite the extent of their variety. The limit is set by phyletic inheritance. It is therefore to phylogeny as well as to ontogeny that one turns in order to understand more about the paraphilic pathologies recorded in human behavior.

In the final analysis, the neural pathways that mediate paraphilic pathology may be presumed to belong to the limbic system or paleocortex, where they are phyletically rather than ontogenetically programed. Phyletic programing does not exclude the super-imposition of an ontogenetic or learned component programed in the neocortex.

Learning, insofar as it is relevant to the paraphilias, applies not to the existence of basic and phyletically programed components of behavior, but to their enlistment in the service of erotosexual arousal and to their overlay with secondary or tertiary details. Thus, the way in which a phyletic component is associated with erotosexual arousal is by addition of ontogenetic determinants in the life history, but the brain mechanism responsible for its existence in the first place is phylogenetically determined in the history of the species. For example, whereas the bowel discharges its contents when overloaded, as from the water of an enema, the events of an infantile history in which the giving of enemas becomes associated with genital arousal are responsible for the development of klismaphilia. The klismaphiliac in adulthood is addicted to receiving an enema in order to achieve erotosexual arousal and orgasm.

The ontogenetic events or mechanisms that permit or cause a particular phyletic component of behavior to be released in an erotosexual context are still too poorly understood to be predicted or prevented. Presumably they are variable and complex. In some individuals a genetic factor may give rise to an unstable erotosexual differentiation that is readily subject to impairment by relatively minor stresses, with a resultant erotosexual behavior disorder. Phenotypic males with the XYY genetic constitution would appear to fall into this category.

In other individuals instability of erotosexual differentiation that is too easily subject to impairment may not be genetic in origin, but the ultimate product of a fetal hormonal anomaly. In such a case the anomaly of fetal hormonal function would occur at that time in prenatal life when pathways and nuclei that will ultimately govern sex and pair-bonding are being formed in the hypothalamus and adjacent limbic system of the brain. This aspect of the governance of erotosexual behavior is new to research, and a rapid increase in knowledge of it can be expected within the foreseeable future.

Developmental impairment is one source of error in brain functioning. Its converse is deteriorative impairment some time after development has taken place, including the deteriorative impairment that may accompany senility. Before senility, lesions of the brain's temporal lobe are known in some instances to be specifically associated with changes and disorders in sexual behavior. In cases of temporal lobe epilepsy that respond to surgical intervention, a successful operation may relieve the patient not only of epileptic seizures but also o abnormal sexual behavior. Because paraphilic behavior, even in the absence ι electroencephalographic (EEG) abnormalities, often has a paroxysmal and trance-like quality, increased knowledge of erotosexual functioning in the brain and in paraphilic behavior may be anticipated to go hand in hand.

Gross brain lesions, as in temporal lobe disease, undoubtedly account for only a small minority of anomalies of erotosexual behavior. One can fairly safely assume that the majority of such anomalies represent functional anomalies that become established in the brain partly according to regular principles of conditioning—especially operant conditioning—and imprinting. Empirical knowledge of how these principles function and malfunction during the early developmental years when erotosexual differentiation is taking place is still deplorably sparse, despite all that has been written in the psychodynamic and psychoanalytic literature. For example, there is no incontrovertible empirical evidence as to whether erotosexual behavior disorders are more or less frequent when the rearing of infants and young children permits copulatory rehearsal games, such as one sees in the young of other primates, or when erotosexual prudery and taboo are overtly encouraged. The evidence of comparative anthropology and primatology suggests that deprivation of childhood sexual rehearsal play correlates with increased erotosexual pathology in adulthood.

Like most diseases and disorders in general, the paraphilic behavior disorders have an affinity for males rather than females. There may be a general principle at work here, for in many ways nature seems to have more difficulty producing males than females: conception, birth, and mortality rates are all higher for males. Sexual differentiation of the fetus operates on the principle that something is added, chiefly the male hormone, to differentiate a male morphology; otherwise, nature's choice is to make a female, anatomically, even of a genetically male conceptus. Perhaps this same principle holds with respect to erotosexual differentiation. If so, then male erotosexual differentiation is more complex than that of the female, and subject to more errors. Whatever the explanation, not only are paraphilic sexual behavior disorders recorded more often in males than in females, but the more bizarre among them occur, according to available statistics, exclusively in males, or almost so.

Paraphilias in females are related chiefly to tactile sensation and to bondage and subjugation. This male/female disparity may be related to the fact that females, in the proceptive erotosexual phase, apparently are more dependent than males on the sense of touch for erotic and genital arousal and orgasm. The male appears more often responsive to imagery of the sense of sight to induce erotosexual initiative and as an adjunct to genital arousal and orgasm. The paraphilic syndromes can all be viewed as errors of imagery: the paraphiliac is "turned on" erotosexually by a wrong image.

Territoriality, Dominance, and Erotosexual Aggression

Territoriality is the marking and defense of territory or breeding space. It serves the function of preventing overcrowding of a species in relation to resources. Territory is typically marked and/or defended by males. Marking in some species is by means of boundary odors deposited in urine or feces or as glandular substances from special odoriferous glands. Intruders are attacked and chased away.

In the human species, warnings to intruders on territorial boundaries are, as in other higher primates, visual and vocal rather than odoriferous. Among human beings, territory marking per se, as distinct from fighting and attack on intruders, does not seem to occur as a substitute manifestation of sexual arousal. One should possibly expect this manifestation to be negative rather than positive—that is to say, human erotosexual behavior may be sensitive to impairment and inhibition when adequate breeding boundaries cannot be marked, owing to overcrowding of the species. Though human beings can copulate in public, copulation in safe privacy is a widespread tradition.

Odors and excretions may enter into human erotosexual syndromes, but by way of phyletic mechanisms other than territory marking (see below). By contrast, the phyletic connection between territorial defense and mating is close, so that fighting or attack is fairly readily transposed from defense against intruders and competitors to the partner in erotosexual arousal and pair-bonding. The link between the two relates closely to the fact that human beings, like their closest primate relatives, typically live in troops. But unlike these relatives, we are capable, by means of symbolic and long-distance allegiance, of extending troop membership from the person-to-person group to the impersonal nation state. Phyletically, the typical primate troop is small enough so that each member will be personally identified as having a given status in the social organization of the troop. Two principles underlie this organization: hierarchical pair-bonding of mates, whether briefly or for a long time, and hierarchical responsibility for territorial and troop defense, both of which are closely interlinked.

Hypothetically, in any primate troop regeneration and expansion of the species depend more on females than males, to the extent that a single male can impregnate many females. The optimal ratio of males to females will depend on the male-unassisted food-getting ability of the females and their young and, above all, on their ability to protect themselves from competitors and predators. The primate troop typically needs a proportion of males as warriors in excess of those needed for breeding alone.

A common phyletic arrangement in primate troops is one in which the responsibilty for the first line of defense against competitors and predators is composed of the young adult males, one of whom will be sacrificed to any predator from which escape is impossible. Older and socially more dominant males, who have survived the perils of youth, close ranks nearer to the females. This position is consistent with their responsibility for breeding: dominant males are accorded favored coital status and, depending on their position in the dominance hierarchy, are accorded deference with respect to partner-bonding and to the number of mates with whom they may expect to breed. The dominant leader has priority in choosing which female will share his superiority, thus defining which others will be subordinate to her in his favors.

Polygamy among the older males guarantees group cohesiveness in a primate troop that is more or less constantly exposed to loss of males, with a consequent excess of females. The phyletic mechanism by which polygamy does this is that of erotosexual jealousy. This jealousy phenomenon ensures that, by being jealously possessed, a female is also guarded and protected by a male who does not casually and indifferently abandon her. In return, the female must be responsive to her protector, but not to other males, except with his acquiescence; otherwise, she will be threatened or punished. Males that approach her will also be threatened and punished.

Erotosexual jealousy is a two-edged sword; for unless the possessive jealousies of males and females are exactly reciprocal, hostility will ensue. Such balanced reciprocity, being in part a matter of the male/female ratio, is difficult to achieve. Even with polygamous mating in a primate troop, it is seldom likely that the attrition rate of unattached young males will exactly counterbalance the claims of the older, more dominant males for more than one mate. Moreover, even the dominant males can fight over mates as they jockey for increased power.[2]

One possible solution to fights resulting from sexual jealousy is a partial degree of promiscuity. In a chimpanzee troop, for example, an unattached young male may be allowed sexual access to the partners of his more dominant superior except at the time when the partner is ovulating. Then the more dominant male, in all probability, claims his prerogative, and may even take off alone with his mate for a "honeymoon" in the jungle.

Such solutions notwithstanding, sexual jealousy demonstrates the phyletic link between aggression and erotosexual arousal. Witness the fighting between rivalrous males over a mate, the attacks on errant female partners to force obedience, and attempts to subjugate unwilling females whose noncompliance is based on deference to their own more dominant males. Such aggressive erotosexual behavior occurs in man as well as in the lower primates. In some instances it may become so intense, reiterative, and essential to erotosexual arousal and orgasm as to constitute a form of paraphilic pathology.

It is possible that a female which is attacked may not be the one toward which the attacking male initially directed his erotic attention. Displacement of aggression onto a surrogate, all too familiar in human beings, has been observed in a chimpanzee troop (D. Hamburg, personal communication): An adult male was barred from access to an ovulating female in full estrus because of his inferior status in the dominance hierarchy. She rejected his attempts to approach her. Eventually he turned desperately on a cowering, unguarded, young mother and her baby and savagely killed them both.

This type of displacement onto a surrogate, often with a time lag of years, and perhaps as a sequel to juvenile incest, may account for the savagery of repetitive rapes and/or lust murders among human beings, including lust murders that may not involve actual genital contact. In such cases the sexual orgasm of the murderer may be subject to postponement until such time as the scene can be replayed in imagery while he masturbates or copulates with a nonvictim. In the case of the mass murderer, the offender is compelled to repeat his deed and renew the stimuli of his erotosexual imagination. The pattern of his brutality then tends to be highly stereotyped, if not actually predictable.

The act of brutality itself may in some instances be bypassed. The corpse of a person dead of another cause may be the sufficient and necessary stimulus to erotosexual arousal. This is the condition of necrophilia. It is by no means always the case that necrophilia is a substitute for lust murder, however: it may, for example, represent an intense preoccupation with death as a sequel to intense terror, as in warfare when a comrade is blown to pieces at one's side.

Sadism and Masochism

Within the ordinary person's subjective awareness, the fact that murder and corpses can be erotosexually arousing seems extremely bizarre, to say the least. The same holds true for acts of sadistic aggression, in which a person's erotosexual stimulation is dependent on dominating and humiliating a partner by binding, whipping, burning, cutting, piercing, or the more symbolic injury of smearing or soiling. A particular sadist may be dependent for his erotosexual stimulation on the fact or fiction of initiating a partner for the first time. Another will find himself equally stimulated if he has as a partner a masochist experienced in knowing that his erotosexual arousal is dependent on surrendering to domination. The image of injury then stimulates the inflictor and the inflicted alike.

In addition to being held in physical bondage and submitting to injury, which may be general or specific to the genitals, nipples, or other parts of the body, the masochist may also get erotosexual stimulation by being held in contempt, humiliated, and forced to do menial, filthy, or degrading service. For example, a man of some prestige, accomplishment, and social status may have an erotosexual compulsion requiring him to be dressed as a child, a woman servant, or a slave. Mercilessly and cruelly dominated, he abjectly complies.

The masochist's stimulation from being subjugated may include submission to being urinated upon or smeared with feces, with or without oral ingestion of these products. The phyletic mechanism to explain this particular masochistic association of eroticism and excretion may be associated with infant care or with a modification of the primate territory-marking trait seen, for example, in the squirrel monkey of displaying the penis and challenging an intruding male by urinating at or on him.

Whatever the form of subjugation, extreme masochism is akin to suicide, just as extreme sadism is to homicide. There are some few masochists whose cumulative wounding finally kills them, and some who stage manage their own murder. Though planned acts of death are probably seldom staged, death may occur as a sequel to miscalculation, for example, from asphyxiation in simulated strangulation or hanging. This point is well illustrated by such rare cases of asphyxiophilia as that of the adolescent transvestite's suicide by hanging, in which the victim has miscalculated that the rope will break at the critical moment or will be just sufficiently loose not to kill him. The erotosexual connotation of the venture is indicated by the fact that the boy first dresses up in women's clothes, perhaps his mother's. He is thus able to give expression to his transvestite and/or incest compulsion and, at the same time, to indicate that he despises and punishes the offending compulsion in a tense, exciting act of orgasmic do-or-die. Some adolescents have been known to repeat this performance several times before being discovered, alive or dead.

The person planning suicide has his attention focused on himself and his demise, to the exclusion of anyone or anything else. Thus, the manifestation of erotosexual masochism as an accompaniment of suicide can be ascertained only from those people who survive the attempt or leave notes—on which basis it would seem to be rare. Masochism in general, like sex in general, seems to need a partner for its fulfillment.

In cases of repeated masochistic near-encounters with death, the person presumably experiences arousal of the genital organs and orgasm at the time of each attempt. The erotosexual part of the experience may also be subject to temporal dissociation and be postponed until the experience can be relived in imagery as a masturbation or possibly a coital fantasy climaxed by orgasm.

Ingestion and Excretion

Phyletically there are two ways in which biting and sex are functionally connected. One is via maternalism, in the manner in which a mother retrieves her young. She holds them in her mouth and carries them to where she wants them. The other is via copulation, in the manner in which a male of some species may grasp his mate by biting on a fold of the nape of the neck. To the female the bite itself may then be an erotic stimulus. Neither of these mechanisms occurs in primates, so they are probably not too significant in man. Love bites or "hickeys," which are part of the human lovemaking repertory, are likely to have their phyletic origin in licking and sucking rather than in biting. Biting to induce pain or injury may be a part of sadistic behavior, but it does not appear to be a common technique of sadism that exclusively, by itself alone will induce erotosexual arousal.

Ingestion of urine in urophilia, feces in coprophilia, or possibly other excrement or filth in mysophilia may serve as a stimulant to erotic arousal perhaps in connection with a voyeuristic tendency to watch these natural functions performed. Ingestion of urine and feces bears witness to the fact that the caudal and facial orifices of the body are functionally closer than one might, from first impression, think. One functional connection occurs in territory marking by way of odors secreted from the tail end and scented by way of the nose. A similar functional connection occurs in species in which the fertile phase of the female's sexual cycle is signaled to the male by means of odoriferous secretions from the vulva, which he may smell or lick. Here, probably, lies the phyletic basis of fellatio and cunnilingus, which do not qualify as paraphilias unless they become the sole erotosexual expression, and a displacement of genital-genital contact.

The closest phyletic connection between excretion and the mouth occurs in species in which the mother licks her new baby clean of the excrement it discharges. This method of sanitation occurs as high in the primate scale as the chimpanzee. It has also been reported to be a former Eskimo custom. Thus, it appears that the requisite brain mechanism governing such behavior may well be present in all human beings, though functionally vestigial, except when paraphilically evoked in connection with erotosexual arousal.

The functional connection between the mouth and the genitals is also close in those species, including the higher primates, in which parturition entails licking the young and eating the placenta. The circumstances under which a mother not only licks her newly born offspring but goes on to devour it, as she would the placenta, are not very well defined, species by species. Cannibalism of the young would appear in general, however, to represent a form or product of disorientation. It has been recorded in primate species as high as the squirrel monkey and pigtail monkey. There is widespread doubt that human cannibalism of the newborn occurs, with or without erotic stimulus value, except, perhaps, under rare conditions of psychosis. Cannibalism of any type would seem to be negligible as a source of erotosexual arousal. The same can be said of ingesting any substances except those containing a pharmacologic principle that enhances erotosexual arousal. Urine and feces also constitute an exception in the cases of those few individuals subject to erotosexual arousal by them.

Visual, Narrative, and Sexual Image

The phenomenon of replaying an erotosexual experience from memory as a prerequisite to later erotosexual arousal indicates that the imagery of what is done may be as important, erotosexually, as the act of coitus itself. Imagery assumes great prominence in the fantasies of narratophilia and pictophilia, and also in exhibitionism and voyeurism (peeping-Tomism). Both of the latter paraphilias may, on occasion, go so far as to include an overt attack on the involuntary partner, but this is quite atypical. Sadism or rape is not a usual or inevitable feature of exhibitionism and voyeurism; rather, aggression takes the attenuated form of suddenly surprising and shocking the victim, whose reaction is more likely to be an important ingredient in the exhibitionist's than in the voyeur's erotosexual arousal.

The exhibitionist or voyeur, like other paraphiliacs, feels a buildup of tension driving him to a repeat performance of his erotosexual ritual after a variable period of abstinence. His own capacity for erotosexual release in orgasm is dependent on the excitement of an additional act (or binge) of shocking a woman by, respectively, the display of his own penis, or peeping, unsuspected, on her nudity. His own release may be masturbatory or, if he has a regular sexual partner, coital. If he has a wife or girl friend, then his capacity to perform in intercourse will depend on the preliminary excitement level he is able to build up, either by replaying in fantasy an illicit act of exhibiting or prowling, or by repeating such an act anew. While engaged in his paraphilic activity, he may have had an erection and may or may not have masturbated to the point of orgasm. In either case, the reliving of the experience in imagery will be integral to his ability to perform in intercourse. Some experiences will have more erotosexual stimulus value to him than others, especially those in which the woman to whom he exhibited his penis was aghast with shock or fascination or those from which he barely escaped without being apprehended. Exhibitionists, like voyeurs, individually develop preferred routines and haunts, and so entail an obvious risk of being eventually apprehended.

Although their activities are different, the exhibitionist and the voyeur are alike in that each is addicted to a visual image—the exhibitionist to the image of the nonconsenting observer's surprise, shock, or horror when he flashes his penis in order to be "turned on" sexually himself; and the voyeur to the image of a nonconsenting person's nudity or copulation. Unlike sadism and masochism, in which the same person may, on occasion, play alternate roles to some extent, exhibitionism and voyeurism typically are individually distinct, though not invariably so. Both tend to be heterosexual only, the offenders being men. Perhaps because men customarily have easy access to each other's nudity, exhibiting and peeping among men who are homosexually oriented has either never been reported or does not occur. Lesbians also are not known as exhibitionists or voyeurs. Sadists and masochists may be homosexually or heterosexually oriented, but seldom both.

The element of the unexpected or shocking, as in exhibitionism and possibly in peeping, also appears in other paraphilias. A man may, for example, hire a decoy to make a male or female sexual pickup for him, so that he himself can hide in readiness to startle or horrify the unsuspecting stranger with his weird appearance or a strange noise. A parallel paraphilia occurs in, and is capitalized on, by men who obtain employment in the police force as decoys to pick up prospective sexual partners for the purpose of confronting them with a surprise arrest. In both instances there is only a thin dividing line between surprise and horror or sadism.

An image created by a narrative can evoke pictures in the imagination. Exclusive dependence for erotosexual arousal on narrative (narratophilia) or pictorial (pictophilia) imagery constitutes a paraphilia. Typically, the content of such narratives and pictures is subject to restrictive legislation by society as obscene or pornographic. Converse phenomena, such as narrating sexy stories or displaying sexy pictures or movies to one's sexual partner, have no special name.

A special variant of narratophilia is telephone lewdness—calling a woman (or man) anonymously and making erotosexual propositions and references in lewd talk. This type of paraphilia is the auditory counterpart of gestural exhibitionism. It succeeds in erotosexual arousal partly because of the visual image the male builds up of his respondent shocked or intrigued by his audacity.

Scoptophilia is akin to pictophila: the person is aroused specifically by observing the copulation of others, but with their awareness and consent. The converse is putting one's own copulation on display.

The phyletic mechanism that underlies the various paraphilias in this section is that of the capacity of the male to be aroused erotosexually by the distant sensory receptors, especially the eyes. When erotosexually stimulated by what he sees, the male's arousal is genital. The woman's arousal, by contrast, is more likely to be tactile, though vision plays its part as well. The etiology of this sex difference remains unknown. There certainly is a secondary if not a primary cultural determinant. There may well be a primary phyletic determinant also, ontogenetically transmitted in the course of fetal androgenization of the brain.

The fact that boys at puberty experience visual erotosexual imagery in wet dreams, for which there is no counterpart phenomenon in girls, bears witness to sex differences in visual erotosexuality. Whatever the explanation, genuinely voyeuristic and exhibitionistic paraphilias have not been authenticated in women—that is to say, the occurrence of female orgasm does not become imperatively linked to "peeping" or "flashing."

Fetishism, Feels, and Smells

The fetishistic group of paraphilias has its phyletic basis chiefly in the functional connection between copulation, grooming, and pheromones. There may be a visual reinforcement as well. The clinging of the infant to the mother is the developmental precursor of feel-fetishes. The function of grooming in primates has to date been only cursorily explored scientifically. It is rather obviously connected with licking, preening, and cleaning in some species. In primates below man it is a function of infant care, and also of friendly attentiveness, often to a superordinate individual. To an erotosexually suitable partner, grooming is phase-related to estrus, at least in the rhesus monkey. Thus, it is an indicator of sexual intent or, after copulation, of sexual contentedness. In human beings, grooming has been professionalized as massage, with or without erotic overtones. Some erotosexually responsive couples find that each is highly tuned to touching, stroking, scratching, nibbling, licking, and puffing of warm breath. By contrast, there are some human beings who are made edgy and irritable by skin sensations other than those centered on the genitals.

Smell is related to paraphilia phyletically by way of sexual pheromones, that is, odoriferous substances that act as erotosexual signals or attractants. In mammals these substances are secreted in the vagina at the time of ovulation or estrus. Those who have a cat or dog as a domestic pet are well aware of the sensitivity of the male's nose, even at considerable distance, to the smell of the female in heat. Pheromones that act as sexual attractants have been isolated from the vaginal secretions of ovulating female rhesus monkeys. They attract the attention of the male. The same attractant substance exists in the human vagina at the time of ovulation. Even though the human male's eyes dominate his nose erotosexually, it is likely that some males, if not all, are affectd by vaginal pheromones, possibly subliminally. Smell fetishism is in some cases directly related to crotch odors, and seldom to odors other than those produced by the human body.

Regardless of the specificity of a fetish, the fetishist's erotosexual arousal is contingent on something less than a complete sexual partner. It may be her shoes, hair, or some of her garments, for example. Even if the partner is present and having intercourse with him, the fetishist will be dependent on the fetish object, or at least the memory image of it, in order to perform successfully. He may also use the fetish when alone, masturbating, as a substitute for coitus. As a general rule, the texture and feel of the fetish object are erotosexually more important than its visual shape. Its smell may also be important, as in the smell of hair, shoes, and undergarments.

A fetishist may be unable to get access to his fetish object except by stealing it. It may be a matter of embarrassment, as, for example, in asking a woman for her shoes or soiled underwear. Or it may be a matter of love at a distance and inability to declare oneself, in which case the theft is itself symbolic, since it represents the taking of a love token or gift as well as a fetish object as a substitute for the lover's full attention. This kind of symbolic, erotosexual stealing is kleptophilia, which is akin to kleptomania, though not all kleptomania is erotosexual in its symbolism. For a sterile woman such a theft may be symbolic stealing of a baby, for example, or for a lonely girl, stealing a friend. Kleptophilia may be indiscriminate or promiscuous in its manifestation, as when a youth steals all the brassieres he can find on neighborhood clotheslines.

Akin to the touch fetishist is the frotteur—one whose special erotosexual satisfaction is obtained from being able to rub against other people, usually strangers. The contact of body or limbs is the only form of communication, for words would spoil everything for the frotteur. The frotteur may lean against or touch limbs with someone who is sleeping (one form of somnophilia), perhaps a sleeping child, or a fellow passenger in a night train or bus. Frotteurs are probably rarely from socioeconomically underprivileged classes in which children are habituated, from infancy, to sleeping in close proximity to someone else.

A fetishist may be an erotosexual addict to clothing. It may be sufficient for him simply to manipulate and feel the garments himself, with or without someone wearing them. Thus, there are fetishes for rubber garments, or leather, silk, fur, and so forth. The fetishistic addiction may involve the person's wearing these garments himself, for example, impersonating a baby in diapers or rubber pants, or impersonating a woman in silky lingerie. The dividing line between a fetish for female clothing and nonfetishistic transvestism in a male is often too thin to distinguish. A man's fetish for male clothing is an apparent contradiction in terms, except possibly in the case of a homosexual male who either dresses like a caricature of a truck driver, a sailor on shore leave, or a police-barracks captain, or is attracted to those who wear such uniforms.

Fetishistic attachment to clothing seldom, if ever, occurs in females as it does in males—not even in the lesbian impersonator or the female-to-male transexual[3] who lives full time as a husband and earns a living as a male mechanic or heavy-machinery operator. For such a person male clothing is a utility, not a stimulus to erotosexual arousal. Cross dressing is secondary to the female-to-male transexual's masculine compulsion and conviction, not primary to his erotosexual functioning and orgasm. His primary problem is one of a transposition of gender-identity/role.

Transpositions of Gender-Identity/Role (G-I/R)

People with a normally developed sense of G-I/R have no secret inner urge or compulsion to engage in activities that are generally judged eccentric, bizarre, or pathological in order to experience sexual arousal and orgasm. In a sense, therefore, all the paraphilic disorders might be classified as disorders of G-I/R as well. This latter term tends, however, in today's usage to be reserved for disorders in which there is ambivalence, confusion, or male/female transposition relative to one's personal sense of masculinity or femininity. Such a condition may occur in association with ambiguous genetic or morphologic sex, known as hermaphroditism or intersexuality; but somatic ambiguity is rare, and seldom is found in conjunction with G-I/R ambiguity. The latter typically occurs in people who are normal in gross anatomy. Whether or not they may have some built-in, prenatal, neurosexual ambiguity of the brain is likely to be masked by postnatal sources of ambiguity. On the basis of present knowledge, the G-I/R disorders would appear to be disorders chiefly of postnatal erotosexual differentiation of the brain and, therefore, developmentally subject to influence from social determinants.

Erotosexual differentiation, like the differentiation of language from infantile babbling, requires exposure to social stimulation and interaction for its completion. Human development is probably more dependent on the social determinants of erotosexual status than is that of the other primates. Recent evidence, however, including that of the now famous experiments of Harlow and associates with the rhesus monkey, shows that the erotosexual development of the lower primates is not exempt from social influences. The infant monkey raised in total social isolation, with no mother to cling to and respond to and with no other young ones to play with as it grows up, is permanently impaired erotosexually in adulthood—unable to position itself for successful intercourse and pregnancy. The female, if she does become pregnant, is neglectful and abusive as a mother.

Designed experiments, like those of Harlow, have not yet been carried out on the chimpanzee. Young animals brought in from the wild and raised alone in barred cells, as in a prison barracks, do, however, manifest subsequent erotosexual impairment. For example, one male from the colony at White Sands, New Mexico, was reported to be unable to respond to a willing and interested female in estrus by copulating with her: he was able only to sit beside her, touching the swollen sexual skin of her vulva as he himself masturbated.

The experimental conditions necessary to ensure that a chimpanzee will develop a homosexual rather than heterosexual G-I/R have not been formulated. Therefore, the possibility of producing a homosexual status cannot be predicted. The attempt would be feasible, since sporadic sexual activity between members of the same sex as well as with members of the other sex has been recorded for several different mammalian species. Though such bisexual activity is more prevalent as play in childhood than later, it also occurs in maturity. In adult rams, for example, it may include anal penetration and ejaculatory discharge (D.F.L. Money, personal communication).

The phyletic mechanism that governs G-I/R differentiation in humankind is one that in some instances also allows a discrepancy between breeding capability as a member of one sex and proceptive and acceptive erotosexual behavior more typical of the other sex. This mechanism would appear to have its origins in the sexual bipotentiality of the embryo. The fertilized egg is chromosomally either male or female, but the sexual morphology of the individual remains bipotential for some time after conception. Morphologic sex is hormonally regulated in embryonic and fetal life. Under special circumstances, the hormonal regulators may either fail or contradict chromosomal sex.

Sexual dimorphism in the differentiation of the fetus applies not only to gross anatomy but also to sexual brain functions, notably in the pathways of the hypothalamus and nearby structures of the limbic system. The extent to which prenatal hormones influence the human brain is a matter for conjecture at the present time. The influence is certainly not so great as either to terminate bipotentiality in relation to subsequent development invariably or to dictate it inexorably. Erotosexual differentiaionn after birth is still bipotential in early childhood.

In most individuals the embryonic period of bipotentiality of anatomic sex resolves itself on an all-or-none basis, and the infant is anatomically either male or female. Only a few are born as hermaphrodites with their morphologic bipotentiality incompletely resolved. Analogously, after birth, erotosexual bipotentiality is developmentally resolved on an all-or-none basis for probably the majority of human beings. In most cases this means that, at the conclusion of the developmental years of childhood and adolescence, the adult will have a heterosexual G-I/R. A few will have the opposite, namely, a conviction that their genitals are telling a lie about their G-I/R as subjectively experienced. Such people may ultimately resolve their dilemma by living full time as socially reassigned to the other sex and seeking legal, hormonal, and surgical transexual reassignment.

Some individuals will reach adolescence and adulthood with their bipotentiality of G-I/R not completely resolved. There are many degrees of nonresolution, from trivial to severe, and a variety of circumstances, from transient to permanent, under which nonresolution may show itself. To illustrate: Some men under conditions of complete sexual segregation, as in jail, are able to perform as a male in homosexual relations, and even to commit homosexual rape; but when they have been released from their detention, their sexual activity is completely heterosexual. Their homosexuality is situational and transient, and they themselves are bisexual. By contrast, there are other homosexual males whose erotosexual activity is never heterosexual; their relationships with women are exclusively comradely and sisterly. For them, homosexuality is of the obligatory or essential, not the faculative, type, and it is constant throughout life.

Obligatory male homosexuality is not uniform with respect to erotosexual behavior. Rather, it tends to be distributed over its own spectrum, from most feminine to least feminine homosexuality. The most feminine obligatory male homosexual conforms to the man-in-the-street's stereotype of an effeminate "queen" who betrays his G-I/R status in his speech, gait, and often exaggerated feminine mannerisms and etiquette. His clothing and hair style also may betray his unmasculine G-I/R. He may at times dress as a "drag queen" in women's attire, especially for parties and gay occasions. In bed, he may or may not receive maximum erotosexual pleasure in the insertee, but not the insertor, role, preferring the anal orifice to the oral, though not inevitably so. There may well be a phyletic basis for the anal preference, since presentation of the hind parts is, among primates, not just a female's coital invitation: it is also a male's display of submission when challenged by another, more dominant male.

While engaged in an effeminate coital role, a male homosexual may, despite the intensity of his sensuous satisfaction, have no erection of his own penis, and no ejaculation. His own erection and orgasm will be subject to postponement until he can relive the ecstasy of his experience in a masturbation fantasy. For the homosexual whose own orgasm is delayed in this way, the masculinity of his own erect penis is incompatible with the imagery of his providing a coital orifice for his partner's penis.

In certain, probably rare, cases, overall gratification from the effeminate homosexual role and from the ideal of femininity in general is so incompatible with morphologic masculinity that the individual finds only one resolution of the disparity: he should be the female that he has always felt himself to be. This is one existential route to the eventual status of transexual. Other transexuals reach the same end point with no history of homosexual experience. For them homosexuality is a concept repugnant to their system of moral values. They may have had no sexual life—not even an urge to masturbate. Alternatively, they may have tried to resolve the ambiguity of their G-I/R by getting heterosexually married.

The transexual male who arrives at his sex-assignment decision by way not of homosexual, but of heterosexual, activity almost always has a history of transvestism—an obsession with being able to dress as a female and pass in public as a female. It is likely that there was a strong fetishistic element in his wearing of female garments, so that he could get an erection only by imagining himself as a woman. Conversely, as they engaged in intercourse, he might have imagined his female partner as the man.

Transvestism is not inevitably a way station en route to transexualism, but sometimes is the end of the road itself. The paraphilic transvestite, it might be said, is one who has a fetish for women's garments. Either he must wear female garments in order to get an erection and perform sexually, or he must be able to recall in imagery a recent experience of wearing them either in private or in public. For some transvestites the experience of impersonating a female and passing in public is essential to their fantasy in genital performance. Their actual performance may be either exclusively heterosexual or bisexual. Unlike the case of a heterosexual or bisexual transvestite, it is uncommon to find an exclusively homosexual male who, even though he may wear female clothing, is dependent on it in either reality or fantasy for his erotosexual arousal—because his fantasy dictates that he himself, not his clothing, is feminine.

The transvestite's addiction to female clothing may be highly specific with respect to style: his compulsion may be to dress as a diapered baby, a little girl, a uniformed waitress, a prostitute, an aging matron, or a teen-age ingenue, for example. His fixation may be on underwear rather than outerwear or, fetish-like, on a particular material, especially rubber, leather, fur, or silk. His eroto-sexual arousal may be contingent not only on cross dressing but also on an element of masochism, as when the little girl is spanked, the waitress bullied, or the prostitute whipped.

Transvestism of the type in which clothing is an essential ingredient of erotosexual arousal is a paraphilia of males. Females who habitually wear men's garments exclusively are lesbians or lesbian-transexuals. They despise women's clothes and feel at ease only in men's clothes, which alone is consistent with their masculine self-image. Among female transvestites there are as yet no known fetishistic or sadomasochistic associations with men's wear.

Some lesbians, in the argot of their own gay world, differentiate "butches" from "fems." The latter behave in bed more after the manner of ordinary females, whereas the former are more dependent, for their erotosexual excitation and orgasm, on an image of the self as a male in sexual performance. The actual techniques of erotosexual stimulation may include all the maneuvers of ordinary heterosexual foreplay. Some butch lesbians have an aversive repugnance to their own breasts and forbid their being seen or touched. This breast phobia corresponds to the phobia that some male homosexual transexuals have for their own genitals. There may be a corresponding genital phobia in lesbian transexuals; but it is more likely that the clitoris will, in fantasy, be idealized as a penis. The lesbian with this fantasy will be highly aroused by genital friction when she lies atop her partner in the common male position. She may be even more intensely aroused if she wears an artificial penis and thrusts it, male fashion, in and out of her partner's vagina. She has a revulsion to anything being inserted into her own vagina.

In such a partnership the more feminine of the pair is more likely than the other to have a bisexual history and/or potentiality—but this is by no means invariably the case. The same holds true, in reverse, for male homosexuals. In a male homosexual pair the one whose erotosexual behavior is contingent on his being in the masculine insertor role in bed may or may not be as much an obligatory and exclusive homosexual as is his partner.

Among either male or female homosexuals there is no fixed, positive correlation between predominant role in the sexual act and general work-a-day presentation as masculine or feminine in gender role. Thus, feminine-appearing women, according to today's stereotypes, may be masculine in bed, and masculine-appearing men, feminine in bed. Moreover, there are many homosexuals, male and female, who are versatile in erotosexual practices—or, to quote one young homosexual, "vice-reversible."

The phyletic common denominator in all the varieties and manifestations of homosexuality—from full-time transexualism to a casual, trivial encounter—is the incompletely differentiated erotosexual state of the infant at birth. For reasons that in the present state of knowledge are not specifiable *in toto,* it is possible for some individuals to differentiate a G-I/R that in some degree contradicts their anatomic sex. Once having differentiated this contradiction, these individuals may remain imprinted with it, so that it is resistant to change or unchangeable by presently known methods. The same resistance to change is characteristic of the full-fledged paraphilias, not just of the G-I/R transpositions.

In the postnatal phase of its development, G-I/R is differentiated chiefly between the ages of 18 months and 4 to 5 years. Thus, it is not possible to induce a paraphilia or G-I/R transposition in adult life. These conditions are not acquired in late childhood or adolescence, and the popular dogma that adolescents can be recruited as homosexuals (or as paraphiliacs) by social contagion is therefore wrong.

Species, Age, Group, and Other Disparities

The phenomena of a person's being dependent on an atypical or a fetishistic image for erotosexual arousal—or on a homosesxual or heterosexual one—can be fitted into a theory of imprinting. Just as the following-behavior of the newly hatched duckling may become imprinted to the stimulus image of a squat-shaped moving object that is not its mother, so also the erotosexual response of a human being may become imprinted to a stimulus image other than one emanating from a member of the opposite sex.

Imprints in birds are established with amazing rapidity at the appropriate critical period in the life cycle and are extraordinarily tenacious in their effect. For example, it is possible for a male duckling to become imprinted to another male so that in adult life it will try to mate only with a male, to the total neglect of available females; in like fashion the bird can become imprinted to a human being, and subsequently will restrict its mating endeavors to a member of the human species.

Not only birds but also mammals of various types can establish mating relationships with human beings, so that they become customary and anticipated by the animal. Hence, a dog may service a woman or a homosexual man, and a bitch may be serviced by a man. The human being involved in such a zoophiliac relationship may himself (or herself) become imprinted to the animal, especially if it is a pet. Zoophilia may also, however, be experimental and transient in young people to whom a sexual partner is inaccessible or forbidden. It may be an expediency for those who are isolated from human company, or in burlesque for the exploitation of financial gain.[4]

There are no accurate incidence figures on zoophilia; and the when and how of erotosexual imprinting to an animal are conjectural, not proved. Probably a majority of adults would find it impossible to function sexually with an animal, regardless of any inducement to do so, even though they possess the phyletic mechanism that, earlier in life, may have permitted the establishment of such a relationship.

The mechanism of imprinting may also be invoked to explain cases of a fixation on age disparity—cases in which erotosexual arousal is contingent upon one's partner being either older or younger than oneself.

One extreme of this disparity occurs in pedophilia, in which a person's erotosexual arousal and performance is contingent on having a prepubertal or newly pubertal child as a partner. Strictly defined, in pedophilia the young partner is a prepubertal juvenile. When the partner is already adolescent, the relationship is one of ephebophilia. Pedophilia may be homosexual or hetero- sexual. It may be exclusive, in the sense that no older partner will be satisfactory, or it may exist as a secret and partially suppressed temptation in the context of a conventional sexual relationship or marriage, as when a man who is basically a pedophiliac marries to try and cure himself. People who are basically attracted erotosexually to others of like age seldom if ever are capable of finding any erotosexual attraction to juveniles. Pedophilia is therefore rare. Whereas it may seem to those affected by it a natural outgrowth of parental affection toward children, to those not so affected pedophilia is a confusion of parental and erotic affection. It is not, as most people believe and fear, usually associated with violence or murder. It may or may not frighten the children involved, and may or may not leave a long-term traumatic aftereffect, depending partly on how it is handled at the time of disclosure.

At the other extreme of the age scale is gerontophilia, the condition in which a teen-ager or young adult is "turned on" erotosexually only by an older person. Quite often the older person is old enough to be a parent, and may be explicitly recognized as of such an age. The older person may have some inhibition or shyness in love and may, therefore, be especially responsive to the more active solicitations of the younger person. Legally, there is not the same condemnation as there is with pedophilia.

In addition to disparity in age, disparity in group membership or allegiance may constitute an erotosexual contingency for some people. For instance, a person may be unable to fall in love or to be maximally and ideally eroto- sexually responsive within his (or her) traditionally prescribed racial or religious group—which may perhaps be politically and morally advantageous in the long run and for the larger society. In some cases a person's response to the customs and pressures of membership within his own group is to react against them. In a white society that is traditionally prejudiced against blacks, the response of some of its members to the segregation and prejudice imposed upon them is to be maximally and ideally erotosexually satisfied by blacks. The same phenomenon is found in reverse among blacks: there are some blacks whose erotosexual fulfillment is maximally and ideally achieved only with whites, or those with lighter skins than their own.

Social groups from which the selection of a sexual partner is proscribed are variously defined according to time and place. The criterion may be ethnic, tribal or totemic, religious, or on the basis of family and blood relationship. Restriction of a sexual partner to someone outside the immediate bloodline constitutes the widespread, though not universal, incest taboo. The incest taboo is broken more often than is generally believed, and more often by brothers and sisters and fathers and daughters than by mothers and sons, according to available evidence. It is commonly held that mother-son incest occurs chiefly in association with overt psychosis, whereas such is not so in brother-sister or father-daughter incest. The mental-health outcome of father-daughter relationships is variable, and is complicated by the fact that the mother is often a silent partner to the relationship, even contriving behind the scenes to permit it by not taking notice of its obvious evidence. Similarly, parents may connive not to notice continuing postpubertal brother-sister affairs. Their mental-health outcome, not invariably bad, is also influenced by other contributing interpersonal conditions emanating from the home life.

In addition to disparities of species, age, and social group, disparities of other, more personal features and traits may constitute an erotosexual contingency or "hang-up" for a particular person. In fact, there is probably no limit to personal idiosyncrasy in this respect, however rare the phenomenon. For example, a man may report that he is fully "turned on" only by an amputee as a partner (apotemnophilia), or by a person of different size, shape, or physiognomy, to say nothing of personality and disposition. The latter is exemplifed by the man who is attracted only to a motherly managerial type of girl friend or, conversely, to a whimpering baby doll who tyrannizes him with feigned incompetency, or a deprived and destitute girl for whom he can be the romantic redeemer. Women may have similar specificities.

Transient and Uncompleted Partnerships

As already suggested, nature's basic design for the social organization of the primate troop appears to be that of a dominance hierarchy. A few males, those highest in the order of dominance, are each responsible for several breeding females, thus freeing other males to be warriors and to be sacrificed to carnivorous predators, if need be, to save the rest of the troop.

Establishment and maintenance of dominance entail aggression against competitor males and also against one's own nonacquiescent females, thus providing an easy connection between sex and aggression. Conversely, the dominance of the few entails the submission of the others. These others, if they are females, are not sexually deprived, for they share the dominant males polygamously.

What happens to the nondominant others who are males? Some of them may feud for a place in the dominance hierarchy; but to have all the males of a troop feuding would soon render the troop nonviable. An alternative might be that all nondominant males would, somehow or another, become sexually quiescent, as though sexually hibernating. There is some evidence in partial support of such a phenomenon among higher primates. A second alternative might be some sort of interim homosexuality among nondominant males. The most likely evidence for this hypothesis comes from men, though other primates have not been investigated thoroughly in this respect. A third alternative might be some durable shared relationships between several nondominant males and one female (the prostitute hypothesis). Institutionalized as the whorehouse or public harem, prostitution permits promiscuity for both sexes involved and redresses the imbalance in the availability of copulatory partners when many women are segregated in the private harems and polygynous relationships of a lesser number of males. A fourth alternative might be some sort of general or promiscuous sharing of the troop's females by the nondominant males, perhaps seasonally or cyclically (the consensual adultery hypothesis). Universal promiscuous sharing might be incompatible with primate group cohesiveness, however, since it would not entail the long-term male-female bonds of protectiveness that ensure the safety of breeding females and their young. A certain amount of sexual partner sharing within the dominance system is known to occur among some primate species in addition to humankind. It occurs especially when the female is receptive but not in full estrus, and with the tacit consent of her dominant male. Rhesus monkeys are known to have seasonal visits of males between troops.

Here, in this sharing, is the phyletic mechanism that underlies the opposite of sexual jealousy, namely, versatility in sexual partnerships.

Casual encounters or brief love affairs in human sexual relationships are, phyletically speaking, as much to be expected, at least in some people, as are long-term, jealously possessive relationships in which the couple are strongly bonded together on the basis of genuine falling-in-love. Casual and more or less brief relationships do not, in and of themselves, warrant being classified as pathological. In fact, it is as tenable to view human beings as creatures of episodic monogamy as of a single constant relationship.

It is only when casual and brief affairs become an endless, compulsive merry-go-round and the only kind of relationship of which a person is capable that one speaks of pathology. In the male such a condition is satyriasis or Don Juanism; in the female, it is nymphomania. In both sexes there is also the condition of multiphilia, in which there is a compulsion to have not many casual encounters, but a series of intense love affairs. Despite the generally ribald and envious attitude that is taken toward these conditions, individuals affected by them are not particularly happy and do not necessarily consider themselves enviable. Behind the mask of euphoria may lie a disposition toward loneliness, depression, and even suicide.

A primate male or female whose position in the dominance hierarchy is securely established is guaranteed regular access to a mate and is assured a regular sex life. In the human being this means that there is an opportunity for at least one love relationship to mature to the stage of joint parenthood and child rearing. The Don Juan and the nymphomaniac, always on the run, are deprived of the rewards of one constant relationship.

Inconstancy in erotosexual partnerships is sometimes associated with a more general inconstancy, unreliability, and unpredictability in human relationships, namely, in the so-called psychopathic personality or character disorder. The antithesis is sometimes found in the schizoid type of personality when a person has a secret love affair, autistic and undeclared, or, having experienced a broken heart, lives forever after on the memory of the former lover.

A special variant of pluralism in sexual relationships is, in the very literal sense, sharing, since one of a pair, usually the man, may have his erotosexual arousal contingent on sharing his partner with another man or men. He may actually be erotosexually compelled to watch and join in a threesome (troilism) or foursome, or it may be sufficient for him to know that his wife goes with another man or men. By contrast, the erotosexual arousal of a man living as the husband of a prostitute may not necessarily depend on the image of her prostitution, but rather on his role as her redeemer. Not all couples who are "swingers" and engage in consensual serial adultery and/or group sex of three or more participants are directly dependent on these activities for their erotosexual satisfaction when together in private.

In the early years of childhood when G-I/R differentiation is actively taking place, there is probably a very close link between development relative to sexuality and development relative to dominance, the entire issue being extremely complex. Insecurity in dominance may lead to insecurity erotosexually, and vice versa, with various possible pathologic outcomes in both sexuality and aggression, ranging from assaultive heterosexuality, to promiscuous loving and leaving, to timid homosexual subdominance.

Another possible outcome of failure to achieve a confident position in the hierarchy of dominance is inability to perform confidently in the sexual relationship when a partner is acquired. In men this failure may manifest itself as functional impotence, which may be total failure of the penis to achieve and maintain an erection. Alternatively, though there may be no difficulty in obtaining an erection, it may be precipitously lost by failure to restrain a premature ejaculation. In a few rare instances the malfunction or the impotence of the penis may pertain not to its coital but to its fertility function, for it may always fail to reach a climax and to ejaculate, except in masturbation.

In females who fail developmentally to achieve a confident position in the hierarchy of dominance the failure may manifest itself as incomplete erotosexual responsiveness when a partner is finally acquired. Such erotosexual apathy, or hypophilia, may take the form of overall sexual phobia, with inability to relax the body in erotosexual abandon and build up to sexual climax. If sexual intercourse takes place, it is perfunctory, an obligation to the man, without enjoyment or orgasm for the woman. In some cases hyposexuality may take the form of total inability to have the vagina penetrated. The woman may be so phobically panicked that she is unable to allow anything to penetrate her vagina, even for a medical examination; her vagina may contract in a tight muscular spasm (vaginismus) that renders entry impossible; or her legs may temporarily become paralyzed in a scissors lock that denies any access to her vagina.

In cases in which hypophilia manifests itself as an inhibition against vaginal penetration there may be no phobic avoidance whatever in all the preliminaries of the proceptive phase. The woman may, in fact, be unusually seductive, since sex for her means romantic courtship and body contact above the belt, not coitus. In popular parlance, she is the perpetual teaser.

Complaints of hypophilia are not as simple to understand as would appear at first sight, for the incompletely responsive woman or man may have an uncanny ability to find a partner with an erotosexual problem that in some collusive way complements her or his own. Thus, each member of the couple will have a vested interest in maintaining the *status quo*, despite ostensible pleas for much-needed help.

Specificity of Arousal

Throughout a person's life, the type of erotosexual stimulus on which his/her erotosexual arousal and orgasm are contingent tends to be remarkably stable, except for special interventions. Once conventional, always conventional seems to be the rule; and once hung up, always hung up—hung up always on the same thing. This is not to deny erotosexual versatility, but simply to point out that the amount of variety to which a particular person is capable is circumscribed. To illustrate: If a married couple joins a swingers' club for group sex, the man may be perfectly capable of changing female partners, but may become suddenly impotent should one of the other men begin to touch him. A man capable of responding homosexually to many men of his own age group, even promiscuously, may be totally nonresponsive to juveniles or the aged. A man whose erotosexual arousal is governed by a primary compulsion as a peeping-Tom may be completely incapable of exhibitionism, assault, sadism, homosexuality, or pedophilia. A lewd telephone caller may panic if the woman who responds invites him to a bondage and discipline sex party. And so on.

The specificity of the erotosexual arousal pattern of most people who qualify either as paraphilic or as merely erotosexually eccentric resembles in its delimitation that of the so-called normal person. There are, however, some few people who have a relative developmental lack of erotosexual specificity and who experience a relatively wide range of erotosexual activity indiscriminately and perfunctorily. These are the people who also, in the nonsexual aspects of their lives, tend to be indiscriminate and perfunctory in trying out anything and everything; they are developmentally less regulated than the majority of people by personal rules of conformity and self-governance.

Developmental nonspecificity of erotosexual activity is, for the most part, of unknown etiology. It differs from the unexpected and sometimes sudden loss of specificity that may accompany a brain lesion of adult onset or the cerebral deterioration of certain types of senility, or drug reaction. There is some incompletely confirmed evidence that developmentally impaired erotosexual specificity may be a function of an abnormality in the genetic code. Generally speaking, however, the detailed etiology of the condition in which a number of phyletic mechanisms are enlisted in the service of erotosexuality in one and the same person remains to be ascertained. When this problem is scientifically solved, then the full etiology of all erotosexual behavior will no doubt have been determined.

References

Gebhard, P. H., Gagnon, J. H., Pomeroy, W. B., & Christenson, C. V. (1965) *Sex offenders—An analysis of types.* New York: Harper & Row (Bantam Books, 1967).

Parker, T. (1969) *The hidden world of sex offenders.* Indianiapolis: Bobbs-Merrill.

Money, J. (1980) *Love and lovesickness: The science of sex, gender difference and pair-bonding.* Baltimore: Johns Hopkins University Press.

Money, J., & Ehrhardt, A. A. (1972) *Man and woman, boy and girl: The differentiation and dimorphism of gender identity from conception to maturity.* Baltimore: Johns Hopkins University Press.

Money, J., & Musaph, H. (eds.) (1977) *Handbook of sexology.* Amsterdam/New York: Excerpta Medica (paperback edition, New York: Elsevier/North Holland, 1978—5 vols.).

Appendix

A GLOSSARY OF INCLUSION AND DISPLACEMENT PARAPHILIAS

Acrotomophilia (amputee partner)	Mysophilia (filth)
Apotemnophilia (self-amputee)	Narratophilia (erotic talk)
Asphyxiophilia (self-strangulation)	Necrophilia (corpse)
Autassassinophilia	Pedophilia (child)
Coprophilia (feces)	Pictophilia (pictures)
Ephebophilia (youth)	Rapism or Raptophilia (assault)
Exhibitionism	Sadism
Fetishism	Scoptophilia (watching coitus)
Frotteurism (rubbing)	Somnophilia (sleeper)
Gerontophilia (older partner)	Telephone scatophilia (lewdness)
Kleptophilia (stealing)	Troilism (couple + one)
Klismaphilia (enema)	Urophilia or Undinism (urine)
Lust murderism	Voyeurism or Peeping-Tomism
Masochism	Zoophilia (animal)

Acrotomophilia: the condition of being dependent on the appearance or fantasy of one's partner as an amputee in order to initiate and maintain erotosexual arousal and facilitate or achieve orgasm.

Apotemnophilia: the condition of being dependent on being an amputee, or fantasying oneself as an amputee, in order to initiate and maintain erotosexual arousal and facilitate or achieve orgasm. It is accompanied by obsessional scheming to get one or more limbs amputated.

Asphyxiophilia: the condition in which a person, usually an adolescent male, is dependent on partial asphyxiation, as by hanging, or by restaging of it in fantasy, in order to initiate and maintain erotosexual arousal and facilitate or achieve orgasm. Death may inadvertently result. Some victims have been found cross-dressed.

Autassassinophilia: the condition of being dependent on the masochistic staging one's own murder in order to initiate and maintain erotosexual arousal and facilitate or achieve orgasm.

Coprophilia: the condition of being dependent on the smell or taste of feces in order to initiate and maintain erotosexual arousal and facilitate or achieve orgasm.

Ephebophilia: the condition in which an adult is dependent on the actuality or fantasy of erotosexual activity with an adolescent boy or girl in order to initiate and maintain erotosexual arousal and facilitate or achieve orgasm.

Exhibitionism: the condition of being dependent in fantasy or actuality on the surprise, debasement, shock, or outcry of a stranger (usually female) unexpectedly exposed to the sight of one's genitalia in order to initiate and maintain one's erotosexual arousal and facilitate or achieve orgasm.

Fetishism: the condition of being dependent in fantasy or actuality on a talisman or fetish object, substance, or part of the body in order to initiate and maintain erotosexual arousal and facilitate or achieve orgasm.

Frotteurism: the condition in which a person is dependent on rubbing against and feeling the genital or other region of the body of a stranger, especially in crowded places, in order to initiate and maintain erotosexual arousal and facilitate or achieve orgasm.

Gerontophilia: the condition in which a young adult is dependent on the actuality or fantasy of erotosexual activity with a much older partner in order to initiate and maintain erotosexual arousal and facilitate or achieve orgasm.

Kleptophilia: the condition in which a person is dependent on the actuality or fantasy of the stealing of something in order to initiate and maintain erotosexual arousal and facilitate or achieve orgasm.

Klismaphilia: the condition in which a person is dependent on the actuality or fantasy of being given an enema, in order to initiate and maintain erotosexual arousal and facilitate or achieve orgasm.

Lust murder (homicidophilia): the very rare condition in which a person is dependent in fantasy or actuality on sadistic homicide of the partner in order to initiate and maintain erotosexual arousal and facilitate or achieve orgasm.

In the recorded cases the individuals are either heterosexual or homosexual, but not bisexual.

Masochism (adjective, masochistic): the condition of being dependent on being the recipient of punishment and humiliation in order to initiate and maintain erotosexual arousal and facilitate or achieve orgasm.

Mysophilia: the condition in which a person is dependent on something soiled or filthy, for example, sweaty underwear or used menstrual pads, in order to initiate and maintain erotosexual arousal and facilitate or achieve orgasm.

Narratophilia: the condition of being dependent on reading or listening to erotic narratives in order to initiate and maintain erotosexual arousal and facilitate or achieve orgasm.

Necrophilia: the condition of being dependent on sexual activity with a cadaver in order to initiate and maintain erotosexual arousal and facilitate or achieve orgasm. In necrophilia there is an obsession with death, not with killing, as there is in sexual homicide.

Pedophilia: the condition in which an adult is dependent on the fantasy or actuality of erotosexual activity with a prepubertal or early pubertal boy or girl, in order to initiate and maintain erotosexual arousal and facilitate or achieve orgasm.

Pictophilia: the condition of being dependent on erotic pictures in order to initiate and maintain erotosexual arousal and facilitate or achieve orgasm.

Raptophilia: the condition in which a person is dependent on the terrified resistance of a nonconsenting stranger, under conditions of unexpected assault and threats of further violence, in order to initiate and maintain erotosexual arousal and facilitate and achieve orgasm. True rape is not the same as coercion or the imposition of coitus on an unwilling acquaintance or spouse.

Sadism (adjective, sadistic): the condition of being dependent on punishing or humiliating one's partner in order to initiate and maintain erotosexual arousal and facilitate or achieve orgasm.

Scoptophilia: the condition in which a person is dependent on looking at sexual organs, and watching their coital performance, in order to initiate and maintain erotosexual arousal and facilitate and achieve orgasm.

Somnophilia: the condition in which a person is dependent on the fantasy or actuality of intruding upon and fondling a partner who is a stranger asleep, in order to initiate and maintain erotosexual arousal and facilitate or achieve orgasm.

Telephone scatophilia: the condition in which a person is, in order to initiate and maintain erotosexual arousal and facilitate or achieve orgasm, dependent on making an anonymous telephone call to a known or unknown party, addressing her (him) in language that he expects will be erotosexually crude, offensive, or shocking and a violation of privacy.

Troilism: the condition in which a person is dependent in fantasy or actuality on being the third member of a sexual partnership, in order to initiate and maintain erotosexual arousal and facilitate or achieve orgasm. Typically, a husband arranges that his wife has another male partner, so that he can fantasy her in the role of a whore, without which he cannot become aroused.

Urophilia: the condition of being dependent on the smell or taste of urine, or the sight and sound of someone urinating, in order to initiate and maintain erotosexual arousal and facilitate or achieve orgasm.

Voyeurism: the condition of being dependent on illicitly peeping at an individual (usually female) or a couple undressing or engaged in sexual activity, in order to initiate and maintain one's own erotosexual arousal and facilitate or achieve orgasm.

Zoophilia (bestiality): the condition of being dependent on sexual activity with an animal in order to initiate and maintain erotosexual arousal and facilitate orgasm. Sexual contact (oral or genital) with an animal may occur sporadically in the course of human development without leading to long-term zoophilia.

Notes

1. An earlier version of this paper was written for *Introduction to psychiatry and the behavioral sciences—Readings V: Sexual behavior.* Baltimore: Department of Psychiatry and Behavioral Sciences, The Johns Hopkins University School of Medicine, 1970. Somewhat revised, it appeared as here reproduced in a special issue of the *International Journal of Mental Health,* 10:75-109, 1981. Extensively revised, both conceptually and terminologically, it was expanded into chapters twelve, thirteen, and fifteen of *Lovemaps* (New York, Irvington, 1986). [Bibliog. #2.249]

2. In a recent discussion (January 1986) with Frans de Waal of the Wisconsin Regional Primate Center, I learned of another phyletic connection between antagonism and the use of the genitals, as observed in the bonobo or so-called pygmy chimpanzee (Pan paniscus). After two males quarrel and fight, they restore the social tranquility of the troop in a mutual reconciliation ceremony. The winner leans or lies back and exposes his erect penis. Then the loser wraps his hand around the winner's penis, and slides his hand up and down on it in the manner of masturbation—but not to the point of ejaculation.

3. D. O. Cauldwell in 1949 published a short article, "Psychopathia transexualis," in *Sexology* magazine (Vol. 16, pp. 274-80). This is the earliest known usage and spelling (with one *s*) of the concept of the transexual. Subsequently, Harry Benjamin settled on the alternative spelling, transsexual. In an exchange of correspondence, on November 22, 1971, he replied to me: "I believe you are right in spelling transexual with one 's', provided you consider the word of a nontechnical or semi-technical nature, like transcribe, transect, transistor, etc. If, however, transsexualism is considered a technical, medical, scientific term, comparable to transsternal, transsegment, transsacrum, etc., the two 'ss' would be correct."

There is no absolute dividing line between nontechnical, semitechnical, and technical terms (e.g., transect and transsect). I do not think it necessary to have a nontechnical (transexual) and a technical (transsexual) version of the same term. I strongly endorse simplified English spelling which, in the case of transexual (with one *s*), has also priority status.

4. On the Caribbean coast of Colombia, South America, there is an ancient ethnic tradition of zoophilia dating from the days of the Incas. It prescribes that adolescent youths should practice having sexual intercourse with a donkey or other animal, so as to prepare themselves for marriage. This tradition serves also to prevent premarital pregnancies.

THIRTY-THREE

Use of an Androgen-Depleting Hormone in the Treatment of Male Sex Offenders

Historical Background

In the early 1960s, Neumann and his colleagues in West Berlin, working experimentally with rats, discovered the antiandrogenic properties of cyproterone and cyproterone acetate (Neumann, Elger, Steinback and von Berswordt-Wallrabe, 1968). Shortly thereafter, clinical application of the new drug to human beings was begun investigatively on a small scale in selected clinics in West Germany and Switzerland (Laschet, 1969; Laschet and Laschet, 1968; Laschet *et al.*, 1967; Hoffet, 1968; Seebandt, 1968). Among the patients chosen for treatment were sex offenders, that is men whose self-regulation of publicly and legally unacceptable sexual behavior was so severely impaired that their only alternative was long-term incarceration. In a parallel investigation with another drug, méthyloestrénolone (19-nor-17a-methyltestosterone), Servais (1968) in Belgium also obtained therapeutic results. See also Hubin and Servais (1968). In women the drug has an antiovulatory effect.

In the United States at that time, as now, cyproterone was not released by the Federal bureaucracy of the Food and Drug Administration (FDA) for behavioral research. It has been possible, however, to substitute medroxyprogesterone acetate (Provera®, Upjohn), a synthetic steroid most widely known for its progestinic effect, but known also to have a counteractive effect on the sex hormones in cases of idiopathic sexual precocity.

Claude Migeon, M.D. and his assistant Marco Rivarola, M.D., and I made a decision to try therapy with Depo-Provera® when a bisexual transvestite patient under long-term followup study underwent a crisis of pedophilia, fellatio and incest with his six year old son (Money, 1969; and Case Illustration, below).

In the meantime, the case load of patients for investigative therapy has been modestly expanded, consistent with time available and the demands of prior commitments. The series now comprises eight cases. It has been built up in continuing full-collaboration with Claude Migeon in endocrinology, and also in part-collaboration with Dietrich P. Blumer, Joseph H. Stephens and Thomas B. Vaugham, in psychiatry. The cases range diagnostically and in terms of behavioral response to therapy as indicated in Table I.

Endocrine Aspects

The endocrinology of therapy with Depo-Provera will be reported separately

TABLE I

Behavioral Response in Eight Male Sex-Offenders Treated with
Medroxyprogesterone Acetate

Type of Case	Behavioral Response
1. Bisexual transvestite with pedophilic homosexual incest (see Case Illustration).	Longterm (3½ year) remission of paraphilic behavior and urges.
2. Adult exhibitionist with extensive police record	Rapid reduction of exhibiton to zero from as much as 10 times daily; but some residual obsessive sexual ideation continues after 7 months.
3. Teenaged homosexual and homosexual pedophiliac.	No further sexual behavior with juveniles, but fantasies are occasionally activated. Occasional consensual homosexual acts. Felt relieved after 1st mo. on treatement—and subsequently (8 mo.).
4. Teenaged homosexual drag queen, too flagrant in public; epileptic.	Dropout from treatment in favor of resumption of sex life, but less of a public nuisance.
5. Estrogenized and depilated transexual physician with bisexual history.	Temporary postponement of plans for transexual surgery and brief heterosexual affair after cessation of treatment. Transexual plans resumed.
6. Heterosexual transvestite and transexual army sergeant, twice divorced.	Increase of feeling feminine; eventual postponement of sex-reassignment plans until due to retire in 3 years.
7. Alcoholic transvestite and dropout physician, twice married.	Haphazard self-treatment. Neglected followup. Alcoholism worsened, transvestism remained.
8. Young adult homosexual masochist, stage-managing his own murder.	Slow to respond to medication with functional castration effect; behavior barely modified after 3 weeks of treatment; after 10 weeks drug was withdrawn.

by Claude Migeon. Still another separate report will be that of Dietrich Blumer on the investigative use of the drug to regulate uncontrollable paroxysmal rage in certain temporal lobe epileptics. Suffice it to say here that the effective dosage, dependent on physique and body weight, appears to be between 300-400 mg, intramuscularly every seven to ten days. Within approximately a month, this dosage radically lowers plasma testosterone levels to those typical of the female, or lower. Concurrently, potency and ejaculation are radically reduced, and may become zero. Both of these effects are reversed when the treatment is gradually tapered-off and terminated. There are no known permanent adverse side-effects. While on treatment, patients undergo a weight gain of between 10 and 20 lbs., which is visible especially around the waistline.

Whether or not some patients may have a systemic resistance or partial resistance to the drug is not presently known. The indications are that it is singularly effective in producing a time-limited and reversible hormonal castration effect.

The length of time for which medication should be continued is another unknown, at the present time. Some patients undergo sufficiently dramatic improvements that they can be weaned from treatment in a matter of months. Others may need a repeat series of "booster" injections, if their behavior subsequently deteriorates. Therapeutic risk, if any, is justified, for the alternative, in many cases, is sexual homicide, a life-sentence imprisonment, death in the gas chamber, or a masochistic stage-management of one's own murder.

Behavioral Aspects of Therapy

There appear to be two factors to be taken into account concerning the behavioral-psychologic outcome of therapy. 1). On the basis of evidence to date, an effective dose of Depo-Provera produces a predictable effect (see above) on genital function: the penis becomes unable to have an erection, semen is not produced, and orgasm does not occur. If this loss of function is not total, then it is nearly so, as for example when erections are reduced from more than one a day to only one every couple of weeks, and then perhaps without ejaculation, 2). A man embarks on therapy at a point of crisis in his life, either self-engendered or precipitated by law-enforcement procedures. He more or less articulately formulates for himself an expectancy or hope of what should be achievable, behaviorally, as the genital effects of the medication make themselves manifest.

Loss of erection and ejaculation is accompanied by a concomitant reduction of the feeling of sexual urge or lust. This change is appreciated cognitively. It may be reported as loss of drive, or as a lessening of tension and "nervousness". It is not reported as unpleasant or anxiety-producing, though it may seem strange. Dependent on personal circumstance, there may be regret that a partner is deprived of intercourse. Recognition of personal deprivation is offset by knowledge that the effect is reversible, and by the feeling of release from an erstwhile nagging sexual compulsion that brought too much suffering in its wake as the complement of the pleasure of ejaculation.

Loss of the feeling of lust does not entail automatic loss of ability to be attentive to stimuli formerly associated with sexual arousal. It is rather that the frequency of attentiveness is diminished, and the carry-through to behavior is impeded or inhibited. The same may be said of sexual imagination and fantasy.

What actually happens to the behavior that the individual formerly manifested in a sexual context depends partly on what that behavior was. Behavior requiring an erect penis, as in oral, anal or vaginal penetration, obviously disappears if the penis no longer erects. Other activities of love-making are not lost, but are optional. Whether they are put into practice or not will depend on the ratio of apathy to interest in sexual opportunities and circumstances. Apathy tends to dominate over interest, as potency and lust-feeling wane.

The personal meaning and significance of a waning of erotic interest in favor of erotic apathy is subject to individual variation, dependent on the life situation in which the person finds himself. A man legally on probation from jail, with a wife who resents his program of therapy, is different from a non-bisexual, nonhomosexual man in jail, and both are different from a man, self-referred on a voluntary basis, with a problem that is not likely to get him in trouble with the law.

It is possible also, and remains to be ascertained, that the personal meaning and significance of drug-induced erotic apathy varies according to the type of psychosexual disorder. Thus one already has suggestive evidence that in a transexual person, or a homosexual or transvestite with a strong transexual component, erotic apathy is equated with feminine passivity and is consistent with continuance of the transexual symptom or way of life.

In other cases, the period of drug-induced erotic apathy may be viewed as being in the nature of a respite or reprieve from a sex life that has become too demanding and trouble-producing. While the respite lasts, something else may happen which, for want of a better term, may be called psychic realignment. Psychic realignment means that forbidden components of sexual behavior become "recoded" as unforbidden, and vice versa, as is illustrated in the following case.

Case Illustration

In this case of bisexual male transvestism culminating symptomatically in pedophilic homosexual incest, the component of sexual behavior that had, before treatment, been forbidden expression in the marriage (and throughout life) was in fact the component that most people carry unforbidden, namely, romance, tenderness, love, and surrender of oneself to one's partner's erotic needs, with trust that his or her surrender to one's own needs will take place reciprocally. In the patient's own words, he had formerly used his wife's vagina selfishly to masturbate in, whereas after treatment he made love to her and had intercourse with a feeling of valuing her for herself, as a whole person.

Before treatment, the unforbidden component of this man's sexual behavior, namely his transvestism, would, by the majority of people, have been coded as forbidden. In the place of trust and surrender to a woman, he developed throughout a highly disturbed childhood and adolescence with a compulsion to be episodically a woman, himself, in periods of impersonation. His ability to function sexually was contingent on his cross dressing. His ideal was to be able to dress up as a woman for an evening and then have intercourse with his wife, preferably while still wearing feminine negligee. Since his wife was rendered sexually inert by his cross-dressing, he usually had to resort to the substitute of imagining himself as a woman, this being necessary if he were to obtain an erection for intercourse. The same imagery was a necessary adjunct to masturbation, to which he felt driven two or three times a day, in the manner of an addiction or compulsion, in order to relieve an intensely unpleasant "empty feeling inside." Eventually his impersonation expanded to include anal intercourse as a "pick-up drag queen," though if he were homosexually approached when in men's clothes, he would be repelled, and became assaultive. The culmination of his impersonation was its expansion to include his son, aged six, first of all by playing "television games" in which they both got dressed up, and then by introducing fellatio. It was not the disclosure of the dressing up but of this latter "secret" that finally provoked the wife to take action.

With the knowledge of hindsight, one recognizes that it was good that the wife used her husband's professional contacts with me as her first guide, instead of immediately phoning the police, late at night. As a result, it has been possible to spare the child both the emotional chaos of court testimony and the personal responsibility of putting his daddy, whom he likes, in jail. Instead he has had the positive experience of participating, as a "boy policeman", in his father's successful rehabilitation. The boy gave weekly progress reports by telephone for a few weeks after his initial counseling interviews.

There was an interval of a couple of months before the father's treatment with Provera was decided upon and actually begun. In the meantime, he had passed through a brief period of bragging defiance to a state of abject penitence. His wife told him she would put him on probation for six months, after which she would divorce him, had he not changed. He very strongly wanted to be able to hold on to his family life and marriage. During the probationary period, the wife had no desire for sexual intercourse, and so was not adversely affected by her husband's drug-induced impotence.

Therapy with Depo-Provera began with 300 mg intramuscularly every 10 days for one month. The level of circulating testosterone was supressed from 550 mμg per 100 ml of plasma (normal for a male) to 50 mμg (normal for a female). This amount of treatment was sufficient to induce complete impotence and also to suppress the feeling of libido. In addition, the patient had no further experience of either incestuous or cross-dressing urges. It was not a case of suppressing or disregarding such urges, but of not having them.

After one month, the dosage was reduced to 200 mg every 15 days, and after another two months to 150 mg every 15 days. On this latter dosage, plasma testosterone tended to return to normal by the end of each 15-day period. It became possible for the patient to have an erection again, and he and his wife resumed intercourse, on an infrequent basis.

After a total of two years, treatment was discontinued. There was no return of paraphiliac impulses. Intercourse continued on a 2-3 times a week basis, and without the addictive type of masturbation formerly experienced. The life style and the weekly round of activities manifested an about-face, into an almost idealized mold of the suburban husband and father.

The change maintained itself for a further 9 months at which time the patient and his family made a vacation visit in the home of a former transvestite friend who claimed to be reformed. There were several visible signs to the contrary. Upon returning home, the patient began to feel his old feeling of "emptiness inside," his old insomnia, and his old masturbatory compulsion. He was much afraid that he would lose all that he had gained, and wondered whether he should return to Depo-Provera therapy preventively. After two injections of 300 mg ten days apart, his symptoms were in remission. He discontinued treatment and has remained symptom free for 10 months, as of the present writing. The total time elapsed since his first injection is now 3½ years.

During these 3½ years, the patient did not receive regular psychotherapy, but he has been given ad hoc counseling, on an infrequent basis, as issues have arisen. While receiving medication, he came to the hospital every ten days for an injection and gave a brief progress report to his physician, Dr. C. Migeon. At spaced intervals, a longer interview giving a summary progress-report was taped. Subsequently he has phoned to request an interview when he believed he needed it, or to give a progress report, if he had a new development in his life to record.

At the outset of treatment, the patient put his female wardrobe in storage. He did not want to dispose of it, since he had no feeling of guarantee that he could permanently quit his habit. Actually, he has never returned to his clothes. More importantly, he has not felt the urge to cross dress, and has not had to carry on an inner battle of resistance against temptation. In like fashion, there has been no temptation toward his son. In sum, there has been a psychic realignment so that bizarre eroticism, once expressed, is now negatively coded in the mind and brain, and its expression vetoed. In its place are those manifestations of love in the heterosexual relationship that were formerly prohibited, but now are positively coded and expressed.

Mode of Action

The mode of action whereby medroxyprogesterone acetate could have influenced psychic realignment in the foregoing case cannot yet be precisely specified. The measurable and dramatic fall in plasma testosterone level indicates that the medication shuts off testicular production of the male sex hormone most probably by breaking the cycle of feed-back between gonadotropin release from the pituitary and testosterone release from the testicle. The result is a temporary functional castration. It is still an open question as to whether the therapeutic benefit to behavior is by reason of the castration effect alone. An additional possibility is that medroxyprogesterone acetate has a direct effect, at the cellular level, on brain cells in the hypothalamic and limbic-system nuclei that are directly contributory to the governance of sexual and erotic functioning. Initial support for this conjecture may be found in the fact that the drug is known to have effect as an anesthetic, and in the evidence gathered by Dr. Dietrich

Blumer as to its efficacy in controlling rage attacks in some temporal lobe epileptics.

Conclusion

The use of medroxyprogesterone acetate as an androgen-depleting hormone offers some promise, where none formerly existed, in the treatment of sex-offender disorders. The beneficial effect may well be greatest when the onset of treatment coincides with a life crisis, arising from sexual behavior, for which there is no acceptable alternative resolution.

References

Hoffet, H. Ueber die Anwendung des Testosteronblockers Cyproteronazetat (SH 714) bei Sexual-delinquenten und psychiatrischen Anstaltspatienten. *Praxis,* 7:221-230, 1968.

Hubin, P. and Servais, J. Comparaison des effets inhibiteurs de la méthyloestrénolone et du 6α-methyl-lynestrénol sur la libido de l'homme normal. *Acta Neurologica et Psychiatrica Belgica,* 68:407-415, 1968.

Laschet, U. Die Anwendbarkeit von Antiandrogenen in der Humanmedizin. *Saarlaendisches Ärzteblatt* (No. 7, July 1969).

Laschet, U. and Laschet, L. Die Behandlung der pathologisch gesteigerten und abartigen Sexual-ätt des Mannes mit dem Antiandrogen Cyproteronacetat. In, *Das Testosteron. Die Struma. 13. Symposion der Deutschen Gesellschaft für Endokrinologie.* pp. 116-119. Berlin: Springer, 1968.

Laschet, U., Laschet, L., Fetzner, H.-R., Glaesel, H.-U., Mall, G., and Naab, M. Results in the treatment of hyper- and abnormal sexuality of men with antiandrogens. *Acta Endocrinologica,* Suppl. 119, p. 54, 1967.

Neumann, F., Elger, W., Steinbeck, H., und von Berswordt-Wallrabe, R. Antiandrogene. In *Das Testosteron. Die Struma. 13. Symposion der Deutschen Gesellschaft für Endokrinologie.* pp. 78-101. Berlin: Springer, 1968.

Money, J. Discussion, Chapter 9, p. 169, in *Endocrinology and Human Behavior* (R. P. Michael, ed.). London: Oxford University Press, 1969.

Seebandt, G. Gedanken und Überlegungen zur Behandlung sexualtriebabartiger Psychopathen mit Antiandrogenen. Das öffentliche Gesundheitswesen. *Monatsschrift für Gesundheitsver-waltung und Sozialhygiene,* 30:66-71, 1968.

Servais, J. Etude clinique de quelques cas de troubles psychosexuals chez l'homme, traités par un inhibiteur de la libido: la méthyloestrénolone. *Acta Neurologica et Psychiatrica Belgica,* 68:407-415, 1968.

Note

Originally published in *The Journal of Sex Research,* 6:165-172, 1970. This paper reports the first use in the United States of a hormone, medroxyprogesterone acetate, for the treatment and rehabilitation of a syndrome of paraphilia and sex offense. [Bibliog. #2.124]

THIRTY-FOUR

Clinical Frontiers and the Three Phases of Sexuality: Proception, Acception, and Conception

Academic and Clinical Sexology

Enlargement of today's knowledge of the differentiation and development of human sexuality most certainly should bring with it a new academic tradition, namely, the establishment of an independent department of sexology in most, if not all, medical schools. Today there is a new trend to match gynecology with andrology, at least in divisions, if not full departments. That is not enough, for sexuality is a mutual, not a solo, phenomenon. The sexual system of the body is dimorphic, male and female, and the other systems are not. Disorders of the sexual system are disorders of a partnership, involving and affecting each partner. That is why sexology needs to be its own discipline, specializing in the partnership.

Sexology as a discipline, while taking the sexual partnership as its center of focus, will integrate with other specialties involved in sexual functioning. Thus there will be various components of sexology: genetic, endocrine, neuroendocrine, neurological, vascular, surgical, pharmacologic, psychologic, psychiatric and sociocultural, as well as one relating to reproduction and fertility. Sexology will be also a developmental discipline subdivided so as to represent the prenatal, pediatric, adolescent, adult and geriatric phases of the life span.

Each of the specialty components of sexology will undoubtedly be responsible for uncovering new knowledge, some of it applicable to the stopping or reversal of maldevelopment or malfunction at any phase of the life cycle. Endocrine and neuroendocrine sexology are the most rapidly expanding subspecialties at the present time, producing in particular new knowledge with respect to the prenatal and adult phases of development.

Most new knowledge in sexology is generated by way of experimental studies of animals. Some new knowledge is generated directly through investigation of humans. The heavy weight of our society's sexual taboo still hangs over investigators of human sexuality, however. They are least threatened when they deal with matters of fertility and sterility, though contraception, donor insemination, and abortion are still subject to litigious threat. Investigators directly concerned with erotic and sexual behavior are subject not only to legal threat, but also to academic and research sanctions. Committees concerned with ethical rights and informed consent now have dictatorial power to disapprove any research project, irrespective of the criterion of disapproval which may be blind prejudice against any form of sexual explicitness. One is still ill-advised to include the word, sex, in the title of an application for a research grant. If giving expert testimony regarding human sexuality in a court of law, one must be prepared to answer, under oath, questions regarding one's own sexual history. They are asked by the prosecution solely for the purpose of establishing the possibility of guilt by accusation, in order to mobilize a negative response in the jury.

The sexual taboo, and the antisexual ideology of our society are nowhere stronger than with respect to the developmental sexuality of children. To get research funding for a longitudinal study of childhood sexuality is almost unthinkable. Antagonism is reinforced by official doctrine which maintains that the middle years of childhood are latency years, whereas even cursory cross-cultural observations reveal that that is not true.

The loss of information from longitudinal studies of childhood sexuality is particularly regrettable in view of the bits and pieces of evidence pointing to the extraordinary importance of childhood experience with respect to adolescent and adult sexuality—at least as important as is childhood experience to adult language usage. I refer here to my own studies of matched pairs of hermaphrodites. Two individuals concordant for genetic sex and prenatal hormonal biography can differentiate, postnatally, the one into a masculine and the other into a feminine gender identity and role, dependent on divergent sex assignment, rearing, and rehabilitation.

In addition to the evidence of such extraordinary cases, there is also a growing body of evidence, some of it retrospective, some prospective, to indicate that the major psychosexual anomalies, the paraphilias, have their genesis in the years of late infancy and early childhood. This is the developmental period when the major features of gender identity are laid down. It is also when errors or distortions are built in. The stimulus to such error or distortion need not be itself recognizably sexual. The process of gender-identity differentiation and psychosexual development is apparently quite delicate and easily deflected by, for instance, such traumata as separation from, or loss of loved ones with whom close pair-bonding exists. Here then is a fruitful field of study, though one that will probably be left unstudied while the etiology of a new generation or two of psychosexual crippling remains unascertained.

To some degree, primate animal studies may be able to fill the gap in human studies. There is already evidence from rhesus monkeys that infants deprived of contact with a live mother, and of all play contact with their peers, forever fail to copulate in adolescence and adulthood. In infancy they are deprived of normal sexual rehearsal play, and they are not able to compensate for this deprivation later, even when put with a gentle, experienced mate.

This observation puts a heavy burden on us human beings eventually to ascertain the extent to which we neglect and fail to prevent detrimental psychosexual development in our children, by reason of the severity with which we deprive them of the natural rehearsal play of infancy and the juvenile years. It is an old adage that prevention is better than cure. The likelihood is that a program for preventing psychosexual anomalies will be developed sooner than a program to modify or eradicate anomalies already developed.

Developmental Proceptivity

The rationale for this claim is as follows. The human sexual experience progresses through three phases (Table I): the proceptive, the acceptive, and the conceptive. The proceptive phase is the phase of "eye talk" and body language, of each knowing that the other is interested, arousable, and "turned on." It is the phase of solicitation and presentation, of being both attracted and attractive. It may happen between strangers or lovers. The time lag between proception and acception may be months, as in courtship, or minutes, as in an established partnership.

In human beings, the attractant may be an odoriferous or pheromonal stimulus from the partner, though nature uses the nose as an organ of attraction chiefly in lower animals. The attractant may be also a tactual stimulus of body contact. It is more likely, however, that it will be a visual stimulus, for we human beings are designed to be turned on at a distance by what reaches us through the eyes—males perhaps more so than females. Males, by tradition, are then more likely to take the initiative in moving closer.

TABLE I

Three Phases of Eroticism and Sexuality

	Activity	Organs	Disorders
Proception	Solicitation, attraction, courtship	Eyes, nose, skin	Gender transpositions; paraphilias of inclusion or displacement; apathy
Acception	Erection, lubrication, copulation	Mouth, genitals, anus	Hypophilias, hyperphilias
Conception	Pregnancy, delivery, childcare	Internal reproductive, mammary	Sterility, anovulation miscarriage, nonlactation

In terms of phyletic development, one would expect that human males would always be turned on erotically by the sight of the human female, especially when nude, and vice versa for human females. But the clinically observed fact is that human beings are quite restricted as to what visual image will be erotically stimulating to them. For some, there are restrictions as to physique, physiognomy, age, race and sex. Sex restrictions may involve the self in a gender-identity transposition as transexual, transvestite or homosexual.

The restrictive specificity as to what images will be erotically arousing may to others seem kinky or bizarre. The resultant conduct constitutes, in technical parlance, a paraphilia. Thus there are those for whom genital performance (acception) successfully follows arousal (proception) only in the presence of imagery, in fantasy or perception, of a fetishistic type. Or the imagery may be of a sadomasochistic type, a voyeuristic or exhibitionistic type, a coprophilic or urophilic type, and so on. The paraphilic list is long. Some are gruesomely harmful as in violent rape, lust murder, and erotic self-strangulation by hanging (often associated with transvestism in young males).

Regarding paraphilic etiology, it does not make sense to postulate that a fetish, say for rubber training pants, garter belts and silk stockings, or for women's shoes, is innate. Nor does it make sense to assume that a man who needs his partner to give him an enema (klismaphilia) before he can get an erection was born that way. Likewise in the case of apotemnophilia, which requires that a man get himself amputated, or his partner amputated, because he cannot be aroused erotically except by the stump. In fact, it does not make sense to claim that any of the paraphilias are preprogramed into the system, independently of various experiences of socialization, though there may be a prenatal component or disposition that permits developmental psychosexual errors to be more readily programed into some children than into others. Such malprograming presumably takes place early in life—probably prior to the eighth year.

Once malprograming has taken place it is no easy matter to bring about deprograming, psychotherapy and behavior modification therapy notwithstanding. When the science of the neurotransmitters of learning is more complete, then it may become feasible to deprogram the paraphilias by pharmacologic means. Today, such an hypothesis is pure science fiction.

Differential Diagnosis

In their more spectacular forms, the paraphilias are probably pretty rare. Not so the hypophilias (Table II), the failures of the sexual organs to function properly during the acceptive phase, which includes copulation. Quite often it transpires that hidden behind a hypophiliac failure, for example impotence in the male or vaginismus in the female, lurks a paraphilia. In other words, the fantasy imagery of erotic arousal is inhibited; it is too threatening and guilt provoking, and the perceptual imagery of the partner has no arousal power of its own. Even the ordinary imagery of arousal through perception of the partner, considered normal by others, may be too anxiety provoking, so that genital

TABLE II

Hypophilias, Male and Female
(Partial or Complete)

Male	Female
erotic apathy	erotic apathy
penile anesthesia	vulval anesthesia
anorgasmia	anorgasmia
erectile impotence	vaginal dryness
premature ejaculation	vaginismus
coital pain	dyspareunia

function becomes inhibited.

Today's method of treating those hypophilias which are based on inhibition of the reversible type is the method of dual-team, couple therapy worked out by Masters and Johnson. It exemplifies the rule of sexology that treatment is of the partnership, not the individual. It also exemplifies the rule that prevention will prove better than cure, for it is very difficult to get effective and long-lasting results with, as yet, no guaranteed method of being predictably able to alter fantasies that interfere with proper and desired genital function.

In sexological practice, hyperphilias are rare, though not unknown. They also are connected with erotic arousal fantasies, though in a compulsive or addictive, rather than an inhibitive way.

Paraphilias, hypophilias and hyperphilias occasionally can be traced to disorders of the nervous system or the vascular system. Such cases are a reminder not only of the wisdom of the differential diagnosis, but also of the developmental fact that all function, as it develops, becomes built into the system as a whole. Eventually, the ideal will be not only that prevention is better than cure, but that there are techniques—neurological, vascular and other—of intervention to bring about cure when prevention has failed. In sexology that also is science fictional, as of the present.

The conceptive phase of human sexuality is the one on which most scientific energy has been expended to date. It is also the phase for which the most varied forms of somatic intervention are available. Under the title of Human Reproduction, it escapes the stigmatization lavished on that aspect of human sexuality for which there still is not even a decent scientific name, only the still vulgar term, fucking. What an indictment of us all in the last quarter of the 20th century, that there is not a decent scientific name for an aspect of our humanity that is as important to us all, to you and me, as is nutrition, respiration, circulation, and excretion—as food, air, blood and . . . There, I have hit another taboo!

Note

Originally presented at a symposium in celebration of the 50th anniversary of the University of Rochestesr Medical Center, April, 1976, and published in *Frontiers of Medicine* (G. M. Meade, ed.). New York, Plenum Press, 1977. [Bibliog. #2.215]

PART V
Sexology and Sexosophy:
Principles and Polemics

THIRTY-FIVE

Obstacles to Sex Research

Science and Value Change

Look back at history. Science has many times collided with personal values widespread in the culture of the era. Vesalius defied popular values about the sanctity of the human corpse in order to advance the science of anatomy.

Galileo broke with established religious values when he affirmed mathematical rationality and not divine revelation as the way to understand natural phenomena, and thereby established the foundation of all modern science.

The ruckus over Darwin's assault on religious values about the sanctity of man still has not completely faded and is familiar to all.

The rift between the prudish values of society and the open-minded values of the Freudian investigators is now well known.

Apart from its subject matter, however, the Freudian rift is like all other scientific breaks with established values. Primarily these scientific breaks are a declaration of the right of scientists to investigate phenomena and examine principles that people hitherto have considered too sacred, taboo, dangerous or immoral to tamper with.

Why should the public be perturbed? Basically they are perturbed because they see the thin edge of the wedge being driven into their customary values by the very approach of science. That which was avoided, concealed or reversed is brought into full view and minutely scrutinized.

The scientist himself no longer partakes of the old fear or respect which would keep him at arm's length from the phenomena of his study. His values have changed. What others consider sacred, taboo, dangerous or immoral, he considers neutral and safe to study. He has set an example for a change of values. He is in the vanguard of value change. Before long all society might follow suit.

Society might not only follow suit, but it might also go further still. For example, a scientist studies the extent of intercourse among high school students. In so doing he lifts the ban on public inquiry into this matter. He does not lift the ban on premarital coitus itself. Other people, however, may take this additional step. Again, a society that can become impartial about the scientific study of abortion is likely to be one that becomes impartial about its practice.

Change is a form of instability. Change begets change in a sort of chain reaction. Once the stability of a value system is broken, the resultant chain of events, until stability is re-established, is unpredictable. We are not far enough advanced as social scientists to be able to predict and control such complex happenings. It is all a gamble.

Now, the thing about gambling and taking risks is that some people have a great capacity for it. and some no capacity at all. Whole societies differ in their commitment to risk-taking, and a single society may differ in its different historical epochs.

At the present time, for example, our society is in a great mood to take a gamble on nuclear power and outer space, not knowing where the risks will lead, nor how they will boomerang back on to society itself. It is in no mood, however, to risk any genetic experimentation on human mutation and the breeding of pure-strain subspecies.

What would be the ultimate effect on society and its personal values of the breeding of a pure strain of sexually precocious human beings who would mature normally by the age of six? We don't know, and we probably won't have the chance to find out, unless, maybe, some dedicated enthusiast gets it into his head to lead a crusade in the cause of science.

In sexual research, the question is this: how prepared is the scientist to risk becoming a martyr in the cause of the advancement of knowledge? Whether he likes it or not, the scientist breaking new ground is something of a prophet who may be made a martyr. He proclaims that what he is doing ought to be permitted, and that to permit it is a good thing.

The student of sexual behavior like adultery, premarital coitus and abortion might as well face the music. The value system on which his work is premised is going to conflict with the value systems of many other people. He therefore has no alternative but to pay the price of being on the frontier of knowledge, a price which may vary from mild ostracism to public contempt and condemnation.

At the severest extreme for instance, the scientist who might do fieldwork research on abortion by setting up in collaboration with an abortionist would almost certainly get into legal hot water, in our culture at least.

The application of the fieldwork-participant method, which has been borrowed from anthropology, to the study of phenomena of sexual behavior has considerable merit. It diminishes the chances that data will be biased through the mistrust, evasiveness, deception or confabulation of the informant. Information is obtained at first hand instead of second hand, and from the actions of people, not only their verbal reports.

The hazard of the fieldwork-participant method is that the investigator may run foul of the law on a charge of approving, or at least of failing to disapprove, of values disagreeable to society.

An investigator may possibly get on the right side of the law by taking the precaution of informing the authorities of what he is doing. Participant investigators, doing undercover work for the law, do have the protection of the law, even while they are participating in illegal activities. Narcotic peddling is an example. But these men are agents, spying. They work in order to make an arrest and book charges against the offender.

It is still novel in our society for a person to be legally protected in order to obtain information on socially unsanctioned activities for the purposes of science and not of the courts. The poets and novelists, not the scientists, are the ones who participate in the disreputable and then come forth to publish a report on their experience.

In our society there is, however, the time-honored tradition of privileged communication and the Hippocratic oath. Thus, there is a strong precedent permitting fieldwork study of the forbidden, provided one remains an impartial observer with a minimum of personal participation other than observing.

A good example of first-class fieldwork research of the privileged communication type is that being done by a well-known sex-scientist, Evelyn Hooker, on the sociology of the homosexual community and the psychology of the individual homosexual.

In this research the scientist is working with members and friends of members of the Mattachine Society, many of whom could be eligible for encounters with the law. The scientist studies the very propensity that makes the subjects vulnerable, but breaks no taboos except to deal with a taboo subject—thereby risking the tongue-clackings of the Mrs. Grundies of our society.

Strategies

Sometimes controversy is provoked less by the conduct of research than by its publication. There are many experiments that upset people's susceptibilities that can be conducted discreetly in private. Publication is what would create a public furor. Kinsey ran into this problem with regard to brain-wave data during human copulation.

In such a situation, the scientist can once again become the prophet of a new public opinion, at the risk of being publicly martyred. Or, he may take the discreet way out by publishing obscurely through a foreign press.

History has usually favored the emergence of data from obscurity. Eventually the data have circulated back home and changed the climate of public opinion. After a time lag, such data become acceptable in the public forum, and related experiments are no longer condemned. There is a lot to be said for the judicious way of breaking new ground.

The sex scientist may follow another way in making a truce with antagonistic popular values. He may approach a touchy topic, carrying his investigation only to the limit of what is socially tolerable. This sort of thing is done quite widely today.

For example, it is acceptable to do a public opinion poll on attitudes to abortion or extramarital sex. The information so obtained is a sample of verbal behavior only. The statements released by each informant are those which he feels willing to have attributed to his name when they are circulated among even a confidential audience. Provided their limitations are recognized, such data are valuable. They are not, in themselves, an accurate prognosticator of actual behavior.

Go West, young man, go West! This advice against constriction and restraint at home can apply to the sex scientist. Abortion in Japan, premarital love in Sweden, homosexuality in Denmark, casual love in Polynesia, prostitution in Mexico—somewhere the sexual activities frowned on at home are tolerated and approved. Many scientific questions that are too hot to raise at home can, therefore, be answered by the expedient of moving one's laboratory to a cooler climate.

More than ever in this type of study, where moral values, attitudes and taboos may intrude, is there need to guard against the usual hazards of sampling, to make sure that the group being studied is a representative one. Sampling may be biased by the operation of some prior principle of selection. Studies of homosexuals in jail, or of abortion clients subsequently admitted to a hospital for example, give only a distorted picture of the whole population of homosexuals or people who resort to abortion.

Sampling may also be biased by the use of volunteers. They may turn out to be a typical bunch of crackpots with an exaggerated confessional or publicity need. The idea is to set a criterion for the kind of sample one wants and, among cases that conform to the criterion, to select on a random basis. Even then the danger of sampling bias may creep in in the form of a high refusal rate. Especially on touchy issues of sex, the refusal rate may be high, thereby introducing an undefined skewing of the sample.

What now about the personal values of the scientist?

The one thing that differentiates the scientist from nonscientists is his attitude toward the phenomenon of his research. In his value system, it is safe and desirable to study the phenomenon, no matter how abhorrent his proximity to the phenomenon may be to others. The syphilologist does not have a syphilis phobia. If he did, he would be unable to study the disease. Similarly, the abortion researcher does not go into a paroxysm of revulsion every time the occurrence of abortion is mentioned.

There is an important distinction to make between the scientist's approval of *studying* a phenomenon and his approval of the *occurrence* of that phenomenon.

The behavioral scientist is always tolerant of the subject's behavior, however distasteful or deviant it may be. Others may bypass judgment and apply the legalistic values of a prosecutor. The scientist accepts what is and studies it, applying the impartial values of the physician.

Yet, he may be trying to wipe out the occurrence of a phenomenon, to institute its universal occurrence, or to control its occurrence sometimes positively, sometimes negatively.

Thus, the syphilologist's approval of the study of syphilis and his pleasure at finding an adequate number of new cases for his sample does not signify his approval of the occurrence of the disease. In fact, in this particular case, he is interested in wiping out the disease.

The contrary holds true in, say, the occurrence of female orgasm: the scientist of this phenomenon is interested in making the experience accessible to all women.

Study of the fertility cycle is an example of a scientist's sitting astride the fence. Knowledge of fertility can be applied either to the promotion of fertility in childless marriages, or to its discouragement in overproductive marriages.

The scientist's values, long or short term, bear no constant relationship to another factor, namely his own personal experience or inexperience as a participant in the phenomenon of his study. The blind make good teachers of Braille, but so do the seeing. A physician who has practiced abortion may make as competent an investigator of abortion as one who hasn't, or he may be worse.

Similarly, a woman who has had an abortion is not incapacitated as a scientific investigator, nor is she necessarily made a better one because of her experience.

In brief, it is neither necessary nor unnecessary to be personally experienced as a participant in order to be a competent scientist of a particular aspect of human sexual behavior.

Experience or the lack of it, however, may be of utmost significance in motivation. There is no doubt that many people, on the basis of the psychologic mechanism of a reaction formation, have done significant research on problems that had their first urgency as personal problems.

What motivates a person to serve on the risky frontiers of science? Honestly speaking, this question cannot be answered at the present time. Yet it does appear that, when a new technique or a new insight comes to light, the search for new knowledge is sooner or later irresistible.

As in the past, some intrepid souls will come forward, as did Galileo and the rest, to challenge society and its personal values, when there is the promise of a new harvest from the tree of sexual knowledge.

Note

Originally published in *Sexology,* 28:548–553, 1962, as a revised version of a presentation to the Society for the Scientific Study of Sex, in December, 1960. [Bibliog. #4.4]

THIRTY-SIX

Sexology: Behavioral, Cultural, Hormonal, Neurological, Genetic, Etc.

Sexology as Science

The nineteenth century founders of modern sexual research did not find a name under which their science could be known and pursued today. Sexology is the natural contender, but that term is dismissed by many as having an aura of prurient commercialism. Any word with sex as its etymological stem is likely to be so branded in our sexually prurient society. We all run scared of being labeled sexologists—and not unrealistically so when it comes to applying for research funds. Perhaps, now, it is time to stand up and fight. A science does indeed need a name.

The early sex researchers staked out sex as the unit of their scientific claim on phenomenological, not causative grounds. Sexology should, by this criterion, have scientific status cognate with urology, gynecology, endocrinology, psychology, and so forth.

A science that is defined phenomenologically may turn to sciences below or adjacent to it in the hierarchial structure of knowledge in order to find explanatory principles for itself. It may also look upward and itself supply a source of basic explanatory principles for another science. Early in its career, sexology turned both ways.

For example, Krafft-Ebing drew on vaguely formulated concepts of pedigree genetics and of neuroanatomy to explain sexual psychopathology. Magnus Hirschfeld rather arbitrarily called on heredity and hormones to explain one postulated kind of homosexuality, and on environmental learning to explain the other. Havelock Ellis focused his attention more on sexology as a branch of psychology and was content to let psychology do whatever explaining it could in terms of biographical experience, perhaps with a touch of heredity and hormonal drive. Eugene Steinach turned primarily to the newly emerging science of endocrinology to explain, often in a statistically unsophisticated way, his experiments on sexual drive, its failure and rejuvenation, and its incongruities.

By contrast with reductivist theorists of the above type, Freud was a sexological constructivist. He formulated a conceptually rather simple drive theory, elaborated it with Oedipal theory, and then applied it to the explanation of psychopathology in his psychoanalytic doctrine. Freud expected that his drive or libido theory would one day be reducible to biochemistry, but he expounded it as a doctrine that belongs to the metaphysical rather than the corporeal body of man. In a more jocular and irreverant vein, I sometimes say that libido or drive

500

theory belongs to the astral body, and behavioral, neural, endocrine and genetic theory to the secular body. There is more than a joke here, however. There is a very disquieting disjunction between two theoretical persuasions in sexology, the reductivist and the constructivist.

Sexology cannot afford this disjunction, for a viable science needs to be able both to reduce and to construct. It needs to reduce some of its own phenomena so that they can be explained in terms of less complex phenomena. It needs also to construct concepts or hypotheses that can be used to explain more complex phenomena. To illustrate, some sexual phenomena need to be reduced to hormonal, neural, or genetic explanations; and some sexual concepts need to be used to explain the phenomena of psychopathology or of the social behavior of groups.

Without a coherent body of theory that gives it at least the promise of predictive power, sexology, or any science, will not be viable. It will, instead, fragment and be distributed among "foster sciences." Historically, there has already been a strong tendency in this direction, so that today sex research is farmed out to gynecology, urology, endocrinology, and psychiatry, in the clinical departments of medical schools; to ethology, social psychology, sociology and anthropology in the social sciences; and to neurophysiology, neuroendocrinology, behavior genetics, behavioral endocrinology and behavioral biology in the basic sciences and their recent offshoots.

In this process of farming out, not only sexology, but also sex as a personal experience is fragmented. Fertility and sterility are separated from love and copulation. Pregnancy and childbirth are treated as a disease instead of events in a complex interaction of paired eroticism. Contraception is a lesson in population growth, rather than a personal decision about a whole future way of parental life. Abortion is surgery rather than a psychic event and a persistent memory. Sex education is the physiology of reproduction, rather than love, affection, and the sexual partnership. Impotence is a disorder of the penis and not of love. Unsanctioned anomalies of sexual behavior are legal perversions more often than they are behavior disorders. Marriage is a sociological contract rather than a personal set of expectations. And so on.

It is, of course, perfectly legitimate to separate one kind of research from another—research into the endocrinology of sex, for example, from research into the sociology of sex. It is not, however, legitimate to leave them apart, separated as though unrelated. That is why an organized body of sexological theory is imperative—to show that what was separated for the sake of empirical convenience can be brought together again; and to prevent silly debates of the nature vs. nurture, soma vs. psyche type, which still plague sexual studies. Even if this organized body of theory should need frequent updating, it will nonetheless always serve to remind sex researchers of the need to coordinate their various hypotheses, findings and concepts.

Developmental Sexual Dimorphism

In my own dealings with sexological theory, I have been singularly impressed by the fact that, among the systems of the human body, the sexual system is unique in being dimorphic. Thus, any explanation of its development and functioning must also be an explanation of its differentiation as a dimorphic system. Embryonal sexologists have never had difficulty with this requirement, but hormonal sexologists laid a trap for the unwary when they named the hormones androgen and estrogen (male and female, respectively). These hormones are not sex specific, but sex shared, though in different quantities. Behavioral sexologists traditionally have not done well in their attempt to explain behavioral dimorphism, even when employing a bisexual drive theory.

My own experience in behavioral sexology, especially in human hermaphroditic studies, has taught me that effective theoretical coverage of dimorphism of differentiation in sex begins with chromosomal genetics. The sex chromosomes, XY in the male and XX in the female, carry the genetic code that tells the indifferent embryonic gonad whether to differentiate into male or female form, respectively. Thenceforth, the gonads, not the sex chromosomes, instruct the embryo how to differentiate sexually. It is quite possible that there are no further genetic instructions whatsoever pertaining to sexual function, though the issue must be left open, at least in special cases. In the 47, XXY (Klinefelter's) syndrome, for instance, it is possible that the presence of the supernumerary X chromosome in every cell of the body accounts for an end organ resistance to androgen at puberty, with resultant poor virilization and relative indifference to, and infrequency of, orgasmic experience and sexual pairing. The supernumerary X in all the cells of the nervous system may also account for the increased developmental risk of psychopathologic symptoms, among which sex behavioral pathology may be included.

The principle by which the embryonal gonad instructs the embryo to differentiate sexually is this: if the gonad stays silent, as it normally does if it is an ovary, or if the gonad is missing, then the sexual morphology differentiates as female. If the gonad is a testis, it releases an inhibitor substance, not yet clinically identified, which instructs the mullerian ducts not to develop into a uterus and fallopian tubes, but to vestigiate instead. The testis then proceeds to instruct the wolffian ducts to develop and form the male internal organs. It does so by releasing male sex hormone. This hormone also instructs the *anlagen* of the external organs to differentiate as male. The genital tubercle becomes a penis instead of a clitoris, wrapped by the skin that would otherwise be the clitoral hood and labia minora, and the labioscrotal folds fuse to become a scrotum instead of two separate labia majora.

The sudden expansion in recent years of research in animal neuroendocrinology has proved that androgen, the hormone released by the fetal testis, has an effect on the central nervous system. Administered at the critical developmental period, androgen can prevent a female rodent from ever having estrous cycles. She will be acyclic instead, like the male. It does so by its action on neurohumoral releaser cells in the hypothalamus which thenceforth are unable to instruct the pituitary gland (and through it the ovaries) to release its stimulator hormones in cycles.

Neuroendocrine findings offer strong presumptive evidence that fetal androgen may also affect brain cells, probably in the hypothalamus and nearby limbic system (the old cortex), which subsequently will regulate certain aspects of sexually dimorphic behavior. Human hermaphrodite studies, as summarized in Money and Ehrhardt (1972), suggest a parallel phenomenon in man. Thus it seems likely that fetal androgen can instruct the central nervous system to lower the threshold for vigorous, competitive energy expenditure in childhood, to lower the threshold for dominance assertion (but not aggression per se), and to elevate the threshold for rehearsal of parentalism in childhood play. Fetal androgen may possibly also lower the threshold for spontaneous pelvic thrusting movements in infancy, for wandering and territorial surveyal in childhood, and for postpubertal erotic response to the visual image, as contrasted with the erotic tactile stimulus.

The fetal testis, having completed its hormonal instructions, enters a long period of hormonal quiescence until the onset of puberty. The issuance of instructions regarding dimorphic differentiation then passes on to the external genitalia, and a completely new principle of instruction appears: the external genitalia direct their instruction to the cerebral cortex in other people. The route is primarily by way of the eyes, or indirectly by verbal report (how parents-to-be wait for the announcement from the place of delivery!). The baby eventually gets the visual instruction too, but with a proprioceptive one added.

The sexually dimorphic responses of other people are, like their native language, culturally prescribed. They are as potent in shaping a growing baby's sexually dimorphic behavior as are their utterances in shaping the baby's own speech. It is true that speech cannot be learned except by a human brain, but it is equally true that there must be a social input. The social input is equally important for sexual dimorphism of behavior (from which gender identity may be construed).

There are two models of sexually dimorphic behavior in the social environment of a growing child: the identification (same sex) model, and the complementation (other sex) model. The child codes both in the brain, the one to implement in action, the other to use as a guide in what to expect in reaction.

The two models are most expeditiously acquired if there is consistency between the proponents of each in the mutual delineation of boundaries of difference and overlap, and if there is consistency between them in what they mutually approve and disapprove (the contingencies of reinforcement) in the child's reactions.

So much of behavioral dimorphism remains to be differentiated postnatally that there is ample opportunity for impairment and error. Boys appear to be more vulnerable than girls (as they were in utero and will be again in pubertal differentiation). The determinants of error are not yet systematically understood or controllable. Some impairments will affect subsequent erotic behavior broadly, as in the paraphilias. Some will locally inhibit subsequent sex-organ performance. Some even will have a neural feedback influence on the hormonal system, postpubertally, and inhibit its function (as in behaviorallly influenced, reversible amenorrhea). Some may possibly even delay the timing of puberty.

After the long childhood period of social instruction in the dimorphic sexual differentiation of behavior (and of its coding in the brain), puberty begins. With the onset of puberty, the issuance of instructions regarding sexual dimorphism again becomes the province of the gonads. The hormonal rule is now changed, however. It is no longer a case of adding something to differentiate a male. Androgen differentiates the male, and estrogen plus progesterone the female. The pituitary's gonadotropic hormones are shared by both sexes. The pubertal hormones complete the differentiation of body morphology and activate reproduction. They lower the threshold for erotic behavior, androgen being important to both sexes in this respect.

In adulthood, the hormones continue to issue sexually dimorphic instructions with respect to menstruation, gestation and lactation in the female, and impregnation, in the male. These are the irreducible differences in sexual differentiation. They cannot be interchanged. Physique and body build, including even the morphology of the genitalia, can be interchanged by hormonal intervention, appropriately timed, as can neurohormonal dimorphism. Behavioral differentiation postnatally can be interchanged by social or cultural decree, but only within the limits imposed by these irreducible dimorphisms. That allows for extensive variety and experimentation in the dimorphism of sexual behavior, but complete and total reversal of dimorphic sexual differentation is not yet attainable in mammalian sexology. It can occur, however, in fish and amphibian sexology.

Hormonal instructions on sexual dimorphism continue to be issued until, with age, they become fainter. There is no new source of instructions in adulthood, unless the brain malfunctions and thereby allows the balance between the dimorphism of identification and complementation in sexual behavior to become disrupted. Such disruption may occur in the presence of a brain lesion, especially in the temporal lobe. Dimorphically incongruous behavior may then be released, possibly in association with epilepsy. In advanced old age, senile deterioration of the brain also may possibly release dimorphically incongruous sexual behavior.

Definition and Conclusion

Sexology is the science of sex, or more precisely, of the differentiation and dimorphism of sex. Its branches are genetic sexology; morphologic sexology; hormonal sexology; neurohormonal sexology; neural sexology; behavioral sexology; sociocultural sexology; conceptive and contraceptive sexology; gestational and parturitional sexology; and parental sexology.

The subdivisions of sexology according to the life cycle are: embryonal and fetal sexology; infanthood and childhood sexology; pubertal and adolescent sexology; adulthood sexology; and geriatric sexology.

Sexology has no formal and financial recognition as a science in the United States at the present time. Among the branches of sexology, the least developed are behavioral, sociocultural, and parental sexology. Their support and development would be of immeasurable benefit to the welfare of mankind.

Reference

J. Money and A. A. Ehrhardt, *Man and Woman, Boy and Girl: Differentiation and Dimorphism of Gender Identity from Conception to Maturity* (Johns Hopkins University Press, Baltimore, 1972).

Note

Address delivered, November 2, 1972, to the Fifteenth Annual Conference of the Society for the Scientific Study of Sex, Palm Springs, CA, on the occasion of receiving the Society's Research Award. Originally published in *The Journal of Sex Research,* 9:3-10, 1973. [Bibliog. #2.163]

THIRTY-SEVEN

The Development of Sexology as a Discipline

Abstract

The founding of the SSSS in 1957 was perhaps one portent of the sexual revolution of the sixties, which would break some of the power of the antisex forces. At the time, the Society had no competition, whereas now there are various splinter groups. It would be better had sexologists kept united in the common cause of founding a new academic discipline of sexology. Meantime, there is no department of sexology in any medical school or teaching hospital in the Western hemisphere. Sexology, because human beings are a sexually dimorphic species, deals basically with a partnership, not an individual. It has four branches: experimental and investigative; clinical and therapeutic; education and training; and standards and certification. The SSSS and JOSR can contribute to a more systematic and less laissez faire growth of sexology as an academic discipline.

Historical Context

Nineteen fifty seven: This date marks the foundation of the Society for the Scientific Study of Sex. It was one year short of the tenth anniversary of the year in which the Red Sea of sex research divided—1948, the publication year of the Kinsey Institute's first report, Sexual Behavior in the Human Male.

This was the McCarthy era in American politics—the era when the 20th century senator of the Inquisition, himself sexually suspect, was witch-hunting communists and sexual deviates in governmental and other prominent positions. It took some guts in the America of the 1950s to declare that one's professional purpose was in any way, shape, or form sexual.

When it was founded, the SSSS had no rival and no competition. In all the world, there was no other group of sexologists who had banded together to defy the all but universal taboo on the study of human sexuality in its recreational as compared with its purely procreational function. The International Journal of Sexology, published in Bombay, had folded with Volume 8, in 1955, and it had no successor.

Centers for sex research and treatment existed in only a handful of places. Magnus Hirschfeld's Institute in Berlin had been obliterated by Hitler in the early 1930s. After World War II, German sexology reemerged in the Sex Research Institute headed by the late Hans Giese at the University of Hamburg. Only in Prague, at the Sexuological Institute of Charles University, under the leadership of Joseph Hynie, did prewar sexology survive into the postwar era,

506

but without the strategy to become a worldwide rallying point for academic sexology.

In the United States, at the conclusion of World War II, the only center for sex research was Kinsey's Institute at the University of Indiana. Miraculously, it survived the assaults of the academic establishment on its 1948 "Sexual Behavior of the Human Male," and the consequent cancellation of research funds at the time, notably by the Rockefeller Foundation.

In 1957 when the group of sexologists who would form the SSSS gathered in the New York office of Harry Benjamin, M.D., they had no way of knowing whether they would, by history, be judged charismatic or criminal. Professionally, they were all engaged publicly in such matters sexual as were, in those days, politically, legally, and morally suspect: trial-tests of the contraceptive pill; overt advocacy of the positive value of recreational sex in or out of marriage; endorsement of hormonal and surgical sex reassignment of patients whose diagnosis of transexualism had formerly been medically unrecognized; explicit sex therapy for people in trouble with their sex lives as well as their love lives; and advocacy of the rights of women to legal abortion.

The founders of the SSSS were as much concerned with social issues as with science in sex. They named their society Scientific rather than Social. The duality is evident in the membership and in the articles that get into the *Journal of Sex Research*. The Journal continues to attract a relatively disproportionate number of social-issues manuscripts, at the expense of conventional scientific reports. Membership, especially in the Western Region of the Society, is chiefly attractive to practitioners of sex therapy.

At its inception, the SSSS had no organized competition, and the Journal, which first appeared in 1965, had no rival. Now there are both. As sexology has become less stigmatized, professionally and scientifically, the SSSS has proved to be less of a magnet than a centrifuge, as various splinter groups establish themselves and their journals which now include: Hormones and Behavior; Archives of Sexual Behavior; Journal of Sex and Marital Therapy; Journal of Homosexuality; Journal of Homosexual Counseling; Journal of Sex Education and Therapy; Sex Roles; and Psychoneuroendocrinology. In addition there are various other experimental journals in which animal sex research is preferentially published.

The SSSS today has a membership of 500, and an additional Journal subscribership of 800. The members are an eclectic group for whom it is difficult to define a true unity of purpose and effort, except that they belong on the frontier of sexology, rather than in the scientific establishment. The Journal serves the purpose of opening up novel and controversial issues, and presenting, as well as regular scientific reports, pilot studies, and case reports which may not otherwise see the light of day.

Sexology and Medicine

The Society and its Journal might have a more homogeneous constituency and purpose if there were, in the U.S., an organized acceptance of sexology as a specialty discipline. There is no such specialty. In fact, in the entire Western hemisphere, as in the rest of the world, there is not a single medical school and/or its teaching hospital that houses a department of sexology. The one academic department of sexology is Canadian, at the University of Quebec at Montreal, but it is not medical. The sexological system is the only one of the body's systems which does not have specialty status.

Sexology is difficult for medicine to accommodate, not only because of society's long-standing taboo on eroticism and sexuality, but also because the sexual system, being dimorphic, involves people in twos. Its function in health and disease is the function of a partnership, not an individual. The new couple method in sex therapy recognizes the partnership as a unit, whereas in general the strong tradition in medicine is to treat individually.

Actually, there are three approaches to therapy in modern medicine: treatment of the lab. reports, the organ system, and the patient as a whole person. To treat lab. results is quite an expeditious public health approach to an epidemic. In sexology, the approach might apply to a V.D. epidemic, even though it would do not justice to individual patients in need of more extensive help.

Treatment of an organ system, quasi-independently of the person it belongs to, is a standard procedure in today's biochemical era of therapy. This method as, for example, in the treatment of a uterus or a prostate, does justice to a patient only when the formula for an effective cure is known. Too often, it leaves the patient feeling too much like a veterinary specimen, unable to communicate.

Treatment of the person as a whole is the only method of treatment when the most that therapy can offer is essentially supportive, ameliorative, or rehabilitative. The approach may need to be extended, when the symptoms involve other people, to include a partner (as in couple therapy) or a family (as in sexual child abuse). In sexology, all the problems of erotic dysfunction are of the type that involve another person, either in practice or imagery. These problems do not, therefore, lend themselves to individual traditions of treatment typically found in today's clinics for gynecology, urology, endocrinology and psychiatry. They require the establishment of a new specialty service, that is to say sexology.

As a specialty discipline, sexology's territory will be delineated, on the basis of sexual dimorphism, in terms of the sexual-erotic interaction of partners. It will not be exclusively behavioral and psychological, nor exclusively somatic, but both. Sex is as much in the head and the mind as in the crotch. No sexological disorder can be treated as purely psychologic or purely somatic. The mind-body split simply cannot be applied to sexology.

The new sexology is evolving so as to have an experimental and investigative branch. Here the neuroendocrine principles of sexual function and behavior are being worked out. The greatest burst of new knowledge, based primarily on animal experiments, applies to prenatal hormonal effects on sexual pathways in the brain and, later in life, to the role of neurotransmitters and releaser hormones produced by brain cells in the hypothalamus. In human beings, the tie-in between neuroendocrinology and sexual imagery and behavior is still fragmentary. Its clinical application is to problems of fertility rather than of eroticism. For the most part, sexual behavior and imagery are studied independently of hormones, mostly in a social-science context, though sometimes in a clinical context. The weight of the taboo on the study of infantile and juvenile sexual behavior and imagery effectively prevents the developmental research which is imperative to the ultimate understanding of sexuality and its dysfunctions in adolescence and adulthood.

The clinical branch of the new sexology continues some of the older traditions of counseling and psychotherapy, including behavior modification, to which is added couple therapy. Adjunctive hormonal therapy is usually inappropriate. One new hormonal development is the use of antiandrogen plus counseling for sex offenders. Unorthodox sexual behavior is still, however, more likely to be adjudged criminal than medical, and to lead to the jail rather than the hospital.

A third branch of the new sexology is education in human sexuality. In a minority of American medical schools, there is still no course in human sexuality. Explicit sexual and erotic teaching materials are used in some undergraduate and graduate schools, but in high schools the taboo on them remains pretty much intact. Ultimately, effective sex education will become part of a program of preventive sexological medicine. The public at large still needs to be taught how to use sexology, like psychiatry, preventively, instead of at the end of the road, as an admission of defeat.

Practitioners of the new sexology, notably sex therapists and educators, are beginning to respond to the issue of certification and standards. The drift so far has been more toward the example set by psychoanalysis, namely that of certification by independent institutes rather than academic departments. The future of sexology will be more secure and less vulnerable to charlatanism if sexology develops within the universities. The places of training need to be certified, as well as the individuals trained; and there is a place for a national certification examination, on the model of other specialty board examinations in medicine.

The *SSSS* and *The Journal of Sex Research* have in their own way contributed substantially to the new sexology. It is time now to be less laissez faire and more systematic and rigorous in shaping the next phase of sexology's emergence as a part of medicine and science.

Note

Presidential address, delivered November 1, 1975, to the Seventeenth Annual Conference of the Society for the Scientific Study of Sex, New York, NY. Originally published in *the Journal of Sex Research*, 12:83-87, 1976. [Bibliog. #2.194]

THIRTY-EIGHT

Three Editorials from *Forum* Magazine and One from the *New York Times*

The Sexual Revolution: A Manifesto

Revolutions are not triggered by the theories and desires of social dissidents, as many people may believe, and the sexual revolution is no exception. It was triggered, above all, by the technology of contraception.

The date that stands as a milestone in history is 1876, the year of the Philadelphia Exposition. There, on the nation's centennial birthday, the first public display of the rubber condom took place. Although penis sheaths made of animal membranes had long been known, it was the invention in 1839 of the vulcanization process of making rubber that led to the first feasible and effective methods of birth control: the condom and the diaphragm.

However, vulcanized rubber condoms were clumsy to use, and the mores of the Victorian age did not allow easy availability of diaphragms to women. It was not until the invention of the latex rubber process in the late 1920's, which made possible very thin condoms, that the contraceptive revolution began in earnest. That was just half a century ago—not long enough for American society to catch up with all the ramifications of this revolution.

One contribution of the contraceptive revolution to the sexual revolution stands out above all others: it allows people of all ages, whether monogamous, married, multi-partnered, or unmarried, to separate recreational sex from procreational sex. Before the advent of contraception, only those who were sterile, or too young or too old to procreate could take part in recreational sex. All others had to fear the possibility of pregnancy every time they copulated.

Following the rules of logic, the invention of contraception should have quickly revolutionized the sex lives of all people not ready to assume parenthood. Officially, however, contraception was first euphemized as family planning—a means of allowing married couples to space out the births of their children and to predict family size. This attitude, of course, has little to do with recreational sex and true sexual freedom.

As long as men held the authority, and the use of contraceptive devices remained under their control, it was more or less inevitable that there would be restrictions on their use by women, for men have always been reluctant to grant women equality in sexual matters.

Thus, it took some time before women in general, single as well as married, assimilated the full impact of the contraceptive revolution, namely, that it permitted them, too, to have sex with a partner without an automatic commitment to parenthood.

The contraceptive revolution accelerated as the Pill was perfected in the 1950's, and the IUD perfected soon after that. These methods—along with the diaphragm—have given women control over their own bodies. Thus, it was in the 1960's that the sexual revolution gained its greatest momentum.

The revolution that has occurred in sexual attitudes as well as sexual actions has not been easily won. During the time of the Inquisition, and until the end of the seventeenth century, thousands of women were burned as witches for having falsely confessed, under torture, to the crime of having dreamed that they were seduced by a demon or Satan himself and had copulated with him. During this period in history, more than at any other time, people were obsessed with the idea that the erotic imagination was evil and must be exorcised.

In the middle of the eighteenth century, under the leadership of Simon-André Tissot, a Swiss physician, a new theory of demonic possession emerged, in which masturbation—believed to be degenerative behavior which would result in insanity and debilitation of the body—replaced erotic dreaming as the origin of all evil. It required the full force of scientific evidence and theory in the twentieth century to dispel this myth.

Alfred Kinsey and his associates struck a heavy blow for sexual freedom when they published, in 1948 and 1953 respectively, *Sexual Behavior in the Human Male* and *Sexual Behavior in the Human Female,* and demonstrated just how great a discrepancy there was between official sexual dogma and the reality of what people said they thought and did about sex.

Kinsey did more than ask people to talk about their sexual histories. He took some physiological measurements during orgasm, and even recorded some sexual activities on film. But the censorship laws, as well as interstate restrictions on the dissemination of sexual materials, based on the fanatical efforts of the nineteenth-century anti-sex crusader Anthony Comstock, made it impossible for Kinsey to release this material to the public.

Taking up where Kinsey left off in the 1950's, Dr. William Masters and Virginia Johnson made very extensive studies of the physiology of orgasm, which they published in 1966 as *Human Sexual Response.* The publication of their book made a great impression on the general public, and also helped to establish in the medical world their right, and the right of all sexologists, to study the technique and physiology of human sexuality.

Masters' and Johnson's second book, *Human Sexual Inadequacy,* published in 1970, helped to advance the sexual revolution even further. In this book, they showed that sexual problems such as impotence and frigidity could be successfully treated with direct, short-term therapy using the dual-team approach, thus saving the time and expense of the older, more indirect, psychoanalytical approach.

This new doctrine coincided with the beginnings of a major change in psychiatric thinking—the move away from the traditional psychoanalytical approach toward behavior modification. Since it is not necessary to be an M.D. to practice behavior modification, this opened the field of sex therapy to a broader range of professional practitioners.

As the field of sex therapy expanded, both therapists and patients began to realize the existence of a desire for knowledge about erotic fantasy and imagery, particularly women's sexual fantasies, an almost totally restricted field of knowledge.

The women's liberation movement and the gay liberation movement (as well as the consciousness-raising efforts of people involved in sadomasochism and bondage) have played a powerful role in the exploration and understanding of the sexual fantasies and imagery of women and gays. Naturally, the emergence of these fantasies in the public arena has allowed all people—men and women, straights and gays—to learn more about their own, and other people's, sexuality.

However, it was not sexologists or sex therapists who first perceived this interest in sexual imagery and fantasy as a significant part of the sexual revolution. Instead, as is often the case, it was artists and entertainers who saw it, and with them the commercial entrepreneurs who maintain them in the public eye.

However, this eroticism has not really been accepted by society on its own terms. Instead, it has been labeled pornography and smut, and has become the heir to erotic dreaming and masturbation as the alleged scourge of our society. In the name of decency, the maintenance of the taboo against eroticism (and sex in general) has been an integral part of our society, and total enforcement of "decency" has resulted in the eradication or suppression of erotic entertainment.

Even when the well-planned research sponsored in the U.S. by the Commission on Obscenity and Pornography showed in 1970 that erotic imagery in pictures, movies, and literature does not injure either the individual or society, politicians were afraid to open up the last frontier of freedom—erotic freedom.

The U.S. Supreme Court has performed no better. Instead, in a series of decisions, it has endeavored to hold the line against the sexual revolution.

These decisions involve the denial of the right of a man, in the state of Washington, to teach school if his erotic imagery is predominantly homosexual; the denial of the right of a poor teenage girl to obtain a federally funded abortion if her heterosexual imagery leads her to have sex while not being prepared for pregnancy, and the denial of the right of the public to enjoy sexual imagery by purchasing and viewing sexually entertaining books and films.

What has happened is that, as the sexual revolution has advanced, reaction has set in. More and more traumatized by the threat of change, ultra-conservative and reactionary people have mobilized against that change. And they have the weight of organized authority on their side.

By contrast, the sexual revolution is a piecemeal affair. Its forces are uncoordinated, each element involved in its own battles. What is needed is a coordinated movement, an administrative structure, a joint manifesto, and an assertive, militant, political and educational strategy.

If these four conditions are fulfilled, we may be able to keep the sexual revolution moving. For in a democracy, sexual freedom is as important as any other freedom. Of course, it is subject to the same constraints as any other freedom, for freedom is not synonymous with license.

America has not been able to free itself entirely from the heritage of the Inquisition and the sexual mores of Western culture. Our sexuality has always been subverted by tyrannous restraints—restraints on birth control, on abortion, on sex education, on recreational sex, on sexual entertainment, on homosexuality, on women's sexual equality. There are also restraints on sexological research, therapy, and teaching, and attempts to discredit the practitioners of sexology.

We in America do not live in a sexual democracy, but in a sexual tyranny. Politically that is very dangerous, as all tyranny is dangerous. Dictators, including Hitler and Stalin, have always used sexual tyranny as a means to total tyranny. After people have bowed under the weight of sexual tyranny, they often bow under the weight of total tyranny, mistaking their martyrdom for righteousness.

Already, there are signs of a backlash against the sexual revolution. However, although the older generation of sexual revolutionaries can be easily defeated (they constitute a minority without a unified voice) their children will not be so easily defeated, for they have been brought up in an atmosphere of sexual freedom which they consider their birthright.

In any case, people do not abandon new cultural artifacts easily. Therefore, we will not abandon our contraceptive devices, and the contraceptive revolution will continue to flourish. No one knows which direction the sexual revolution will take, for that is subject to various sociological events (economic events, for example) that cannot be prophesied.

However, the politics of sexual democracy ought not to be left to chance. Political democracy has always been a delicate plant, in danger of being cut down by tyranny, and American democracy is no exception. Thus, by mobilizing their forces against the sexual revolution, unscrupulous politicians could pave the way for the totalitarianism of a police state.

The citizens of a democracy must always be on guard against the encroachments of tyranny. That is why the sexual revolution, with its ultimate goal of sexual democracy, is very important and must be defended.

At this moment in our history sexual freedom is the last great frontier of human freedoms. Let us keep it open, for this frontier is our birthright, natural and divine.

The Best of *Forum;*
Introduction: Sexual Democracy, American Birthright!

Sexual democracy, American birthright! This is *Best of Forum's* slogan for the 80's. But it is more than a slogan. It is a battle cry summoning the readers of

Forum to become a guerrilla force organized and equipped to destroy the tyranny of sexual dictatorship wherever it shows us its Medusa head. Because this
Medusa is everywhere, a group of *Forum*-reading Canadians in 1978 formed, in
Toronto, the Center of Human Freedom and Sexuality to act as a guardian of
sexual democratic rights and civil liberties. It is not too late for the movement to
take root in the U.S., but there is no time for dallying. Sexual democracy is not
a tree that grows untended. To survive, it needs constant attention and support
against the virulent and unremitting destruction caused by sexual dictatorship.

We have never had full democratic sexual freedom in America, and we
are not used to organizing ourselves to defend and extend as much of it as we
have. Our society has barely begun to become a sexual democracy, but at least
a beginning has been made. Many Americans now take for granted the democratic sexual right to birth control and to being able to separate sex as recreation from sex as procreation. The church, however, in many instances dictates otherwise.

There was a time, not too remote in our history, when the church was a
tyrant of sex, dictating a suppression of everything sexual except procreation.
Today the sexual dictatorship of the church has been partly secularized and is
supplemented by the sexual dictatorship of lawmakers, law enforcement officers,
and the courts. Most Americans have grown up under the influence of this
partly ecclesiastical and partly secular sexual dictatorship. In consequence they
do not ingenuously accept sexual democracy as a birthright.

Readers of *Best of Forum,* for example, become accustomed to the uncensored and honest frankness they find in each issue of *Forum.* Yet they are
also aware that this very frankness is anathema to those who formerly imposed
sexual tyranny on them in their youth. Thus, for them, the sexually frank and
the sexually illicit are one and the same! Caught in this double bind, a reader is
like St. Peter when the cock crowed thrice—he denies or hides the evidence
should he ever be accused of, let us say, contributing to the delinquency of a
minor by allowing *Forum*'s explicit sexual writings to be available.

What the reader should do is actively defend his right to sexual democratic
freedom at all costs. To be effective, he cannot act alone. That is why the
readership of *Forum* needs to become a powerful, organized pressure group
that not only accepts sexual democracy but demands it from those who otherwise dictate sexual tyranny.

The pendulum of history often swings from civil liberty to civil tyranny
for, as soon as the growth of liberty becomes clearly evident, the forces of
reaction lash back to restore the status quo. The vengeance of the sexual
backlash gained momentum during the 70's and it has not yet spent itself. Its
tyranny is evident in the campaigns of the Anita Bryants of religion and psychiatry against gay rights and, in my very own university, against transexuals'
rights; of the right-to-lifers against abortion; of the antifeminists against ERA;
of the antisex-education zealots against knowledge of coitus and contraception
for teenagers; and of the foes of pornography against erotica in the media.

The issue of pornography illustrates the malignant effectiveness of tyranny insofar as those most active in sexual democracy for women, namely feminists themselves, are now tyrants wrongfully attacking all explicit erotica (pornography) by confusing it with that very small segment of such material which portrays the pathology of brutal sadism and lust murderism.

Against these forces of darkness, *sexual democracy* means:

1. greater enlightenment regarding sexual censorship and what is and is not harmful in sexual publications;

2. a complete overhaul of ideas and attitudes regarding children's sexual health and rights;

3. upgrading and equalization of the rights of both sexes;

4. revision of the penal code for sex offenders, differentiating the socially harmless from the assaultive and dangerous;

5. greatly increased flexibilty and tolerance regarding sexual lifestyles;

6. new honesty about nonerotic nudity;

7. vastly increased funding of sexual research leading to new knowledge applicable to fertility, contraception, population size, pair-bonding, parenting, and to the sexual health and happiness of humankind everywhere.

These are constituents of *sexual democracy*.

These are an American birthright. Apply your war paint! Man your battle stations! Make the 80's sexually joyful for yourselves and for us all.

Sex, Taboo and the Media

> How fair, how pleasant you are!
> O Love, daughter of delights.
> Your stature resembles the palm,
> Your breasts the clusters.
> I dream I'll climb the palm,
> I'll grasp its branches.
> Let your breasts be like grape clusters,
> The scent of your vulva like apples
> Your palate like the best wine
> Flowing (for my love) smoothly,
> Stirring sleepers' lips.
>
> I belong to my beloved,
> and for me is his desire.
>
> Song of Solomon 7:6–10

A taboo, by its very nature, is able to survive fire, earthquake, flood, war, political upheaval, revolution, scientific exposé and educated intelligence. In our society, the sexual taboo, the woolly mammoth of all taboos, is embedded not only in our daily habits and customs, but also in our religious doctrines and, ominous above all, in our laws. Break the taboo and you may be put in jail. You will be ostracized, and you may lose your job, your wealth and even your family.

A taboo masquerades as a principle of righteousness. In fact, it is an insidious strategy for social control. Perhaps some prehistoric tyranny of ruler priests made the brilliant discovery that they could rule their population if they banned certain activities normal to the species and punished all expressions of them, beginning with the young.

It is normal for children, and for the young of all primates, to engage in sexual rehearsal play as a prerequisite to sexual health in adulthood. When prohibited and punished, as they are in our taboo-ridden culture, all expressions of sexual rehearsal play make a child feel either guilty and ashamed or defiantly disobedient and subject to more punishment.

The price of obedience is to become a convert who believes in the taboo and puts it into practice. Indeed, most children are converted because, if they rebel, they will have no one to help and support them. When they become parents themselves, they impose the taboo on their own children as vigorously as it was forced on them. Some of these people actually grow up to be self-righteous and fanatical guardians of the sexual taboo.

For the majority of adults, however, the sexual taboo is honored as much in the breach as in the observance. Many of us lead double lives. We have our cake and eat it too. But for the majority, scandal is the formula for breaching the taboo while observing it at the same time.

Scandal goes hand in hand with newsmongering. It is the public disclosure of the hidden story of someone else's lapse from grace. The revelation may present all the details, even including illustrations, of how, when, where, why and with whom it happened. The telling of the story is socially sanctioned—if and only if the tone of the telling is condemnatory.

Scandal is the formula par excellence with which the majority of the media breaches the sexual taboo. The formula enables the media to report salacious topics with tongue-clucking sanctimony and an implication of moral superiority—but to tell the forbidden details and titillate the readership nonetheless.

This is precisely how journalists dealt with syphilis at the turn of the century. They preyed on famous vaudeville and theater actors, listening for the vocal changes and looking for the motor incoordination that heralded the third, degenerative stage of syphilis. Then they sniggered about their malady in print. They do the same today in reporting the sex lives of celebrities—particularly if they are unorthodox.

For the most part, reporters, editors and producers in the media have no training in sexological science, medicine, law or education. Professionally, they have exactly the same taboo-ridden sexual concepts and prejudices as their public. The scandalizing of sex is the negation of sex. It precludes the simple and explicit presentation of positive approval and joy—such stories are routinely censored as obscene or pornographic.

Science also has become obligingly subservient to the insatiable power of taboos—so much so that scientists have in recent years invented the bastard science of sexual victimology in order to get governmental or private research grants. Today, sexual research is funded only when it defines sex as a crime, focuses on the alleged victim and excludes the alleged offender, whose fate is under the jurisdiction of the law, not of sexual science and medicine. The offender is very often incarcerated, as epileptics once used to be.

There is no research funding for sex as a positive experience, for falling in love and pair-bonding, for lovesickness or for the sexual rehearsal play of childhood. I cannot conceive of any researchers submitting a grant application to study juvenile love affairs, or juvenile lust and intercourse!

Yet without a proper knowledge of the healthy development of sexuality in childhood, there can be no rational assurance whatsoever of sexual health in adulthood.

The alternative is to muddle along, hoping that everything will somehow change for the better. But the only certainty is that the sexual taboo will give way.

The clock of change is already ticking. It was set off by the discovery of successful contraception, a discovery that affects every minute of our waking existence because it shapes our reproductive patterns. The consequences of this contraceptive revolution are as profound and far-reaching in human affairs as were the consequences of the discovery of how to make fire.

The fire-making revolution applied not only to domestic cooking and heating, agricultural and hunting burn-offs, and fighting, but also to the divine flame of religious worship on altars of burnt offerings.

The contraceptive revolution, by contrast, has not yet been applied to or incorporated into religious worship. Rather, religion is still in the throes of ideological adjustment to the new era of contraception and the freedom and sexual reformation that it has sparked.

Change threatens those whose security it endangers. The sexual reformation is mightly opposed today by those who would prefer, if only they could, to turn back the clock of history. They fanatically embrace the sexual taboo.

This zealotry has no ear for reason and compromise. That is why the nation needs a sexually reformed religion, organized to challenge the negations of the anti-sexual zealots of the ultra-conservative New Right.

The new church of the sexual reformation would have an ideology, a positive sexosophy based on life and the joy of love-bonding. It would be King Solomon's Song of Songs amplified and broadcast to the world.

Why should the new institution of positive sexosophy be a church? As a legal institution, a church is tax exempt and has the constitutional privilege and protection accorded to religion! Moreover, a religion is a repository of belief, and is founded on faith. People need to be able to believe in the positive benefits of sexuality. Their credo needs a voice and preachers who can, from the pulpit, the radio and the television tube, spread the message to the infidels and convert them to a renewal of joyful life.

Perhaps the sexual taboo may be forced to yield up some of its abominable power. And then the media can deal with sexuality in a more honest and emancipated way, without fear of scandalizing the people.

Recreational and Procreational Sex

The need for a new ethic of recreational sex is not a luxury or an option. It is an imperative from which there is no escape. Our old ethic is, like Venice, sinking imperceptibly into the sea. We have succeeded neither in shoring up the old customs and morality of sexual relationships nor in restructuring them to meet the new tide of history.

The new tide is driven partly by the force of contemporary contraceptive methods, and partly by changes in life span that make recreational sex without procreation all the more desirable. The age of the onset of puberty has been lowering by four months every ten years, from late to early teens. Life expectancy, since a century ago, has increased by thirty years, from age 40-45 to 70-75. Men and women both, therefore, may plan many years of recreational sex together during which they are either too young or too old to embark on parenthood.

Still another force propels the new tide of history: the world's population excess. To have everyone breeding at maximum fertility rate would bring personal and social disaster. Abstinence is not a practicable ideal for the majority. The only practicality is sex without procreation.

The established generation of adults has pretty much abdicated its responsibility toward youth. Ethically, parents look backward rather than forward. Youth, meanwhile, appears to be developing a new code of betrothal—a relationship of recreational sex that is not promiscuous but that also is not a permanent commitment to procreation.

Legal marriage and breeding come later, perhaps after several unsuccessful betrothal relationships have been terminated. There is a good possibility that this new ethic will greatly lower the need for terminating procreational sex by divorce. The age of the new ethic of recreational sex coincides with the age of technology, which for the first time in human history makes it possible to minimize sex-coded roles: With prepared baby foods the father can take care of an infant until his wife returns, and with labor-saving machinery a mother can do even the heavy work of providing food, shelter and clothing.

The undesirability of too long a period of procreational sex, and the increase in life expectancy, have made it imperative for a woman to have some form of extradomestic career for about thirty years of her adult life. By the same token, a man has time enough to spend part of his life at home rearing his children, though most men do not yet see this as an asset but a liability.

The imperative sex differences are that men impregnate, and that women menstruate, gestate and lactate. A reversal of these functions is a science-fiction possibility—just as sex reversal in some species of fish is a normal part of the life cycle—though not in the immediately foreseeable future.

Meantime, all other sex-coded roles of work, play, mores and the law are optional and potentially reversible, and are equally appropriate for both sexes. Historically, their sex coding is arbitrary, and not programed in the genes, the hormones or the brain.

Change in the ethics of recreational sex and in the morality of sex-coded roles are the basis of the sexual revolution. Historically, change in sexual customs has always been part of a larger tide of change that includes heresy (that later becomes accepted dogma) and expansion of intellectual freedom and scientific knowledge; the pendulum has swung between freedom and authoritarianism. The age of the Inquisition was the blackest epoch of antisex, antiheresy and antiscience. Today, while we are still emerging from the age of Victorian compromise into an epoch of greater freedom, there is grave danger of retrogression.

The forces of antiscience are powerful, as are the forces of religious authoritarianism, whether the religion be orthodox, neomystic or Marxist. The forces of antisex cry in moral outrage when confronted with the evidence of paraphilic sexual disabilities, and blame the new freedom. In fact they should blame the excess of inhibition and punishment regarding sex during the childhood of those whose sexuality is now disabled.

The antisexual, antiheretical and antiscientific forces make it extremely difficult to get institutional endorsement and financial support of sex research. We have all heard the caterwauls of politicians objecting to the expenditure of public money on sex research. Yet, we need new research knowledge to guide us in formulating a new code of sexual ethics to meet the changes wrought by the new tide of history.

The alternative to drifting on the tide, laissez-faire, is to plan. We may learn a lesson from societies that have recently changed to the metric system. They prepared the way for change in a vigorous policy of public education. Then finally the change was made by legislative decree, and everyone obeyed. To achieve consensus, once a new code has been devised, sudden change is best.

Notes

The Sexual Revolution: A Manifesto, originally published in *Forum*, 7(6):62–64, 1978. [Bibliog. #2.233]

Introduction, originally published in *The Best of Forum*, Winter 1980, pp. 4–5. [Bibliog. #4.70]

Sex, Taboo, and the Media, originally published in *Forum*, 12(1):41–43, 1982. [Bibliog. #4.92]

Recreational and Procreational Sex, originally published on the Op-Ed page of the *New York Times*, Saturday, September 13, 1975, p. C23. [Bibliog. #5.15]

THIRTY-NINE

Childhood: The Last Frontier in Sex Research

Forbidden Research

You don't know how difficult it is to do postpubertal—let alone prepubertal—sex research until you try to finance it. Then you crash, head-on, into the major taboo of our society, the sex taboo, which is diligently guarded by politicians, bureaucrats, and others who guard public and private funds.

Consider what happened before a 1976 conference on the ethics of sex research and sex therapy held under the auspices of Masters and Johnson. The organizers were advised to delete the term *sex* from the title of their application for Public Health Service supporting funds. Imagine the expurgated title: "Ethics of S . . . Research and S . . . Therapy," as prim as if the unmentionable word were F . . .

S . . research is equated with f . . . research by professional and lay people alike, especially in the sexology of childhood. In consequence, childhood sexuality remains a research frontier, unopened to empirical and operational study. Any attempt to cross the frontier is subject to condemnation, as if juvenile sexology constituted a branch of pornography, which, in turn, is stigmatized as illicit and immoral. The social mechanisms for maintaining the taboo on juvenile sex research include the withholding of funds, academic ostracism and the mouthing of falsely pious platitudes about the "informed consent" of infants and children as subjects of research. (For their protection, participants in clinical investigative treatment must now sign a consent form after receiving a complete explanation of what will be done, and what the risks are. Children, it is claimed, have no legal rights, and therefore no capacity to give their informed consent.)

The hidden assumption behind the common attitude toward juvenile sex research is that childhood is an age of sexual innocence that would be tarnished by research. Innocent children must be protected from the depravity of sexologists. Paradoxically, another hidden assumption is that because children are conceived in iniquity and born in original sin, they are programed for sexual depravity unless supervised and disciplined. In consequence, juvenile sex research encourages juvenile sexual depravity.

What proponents of the doctrine of original sin define as sexual depravity in childhood is, in fact, nothing more than the sexual rehearsal play that is typical in the development of the young of many, if not all, species of primates. Not only is early sexual rehearsal play typical in the behavioral development of most primate species, it is a prerequisite to the proper maturation of adult sexual behavior.

520

Sexual Rehearsal Play

The evidence in support of this proposition has been well established in rhesus monkeys. In late infancy and early childhood, these animals engage in presenting and mounting play. Initially, they mount the head end and the sides, as well as the tail end. Gradually they acquire directional orientation. The males become accustomed to mounting and the females to presenting. When the males first accustom themselves to mounting the female's rear, they stand with their feet on the floor. Later, they achieve adult positioning with their feet clasping the legs of the female above the ankle (Plate 1).

When infant monkeys are reared in social isolation without playmates and without even a mother in place of playmates, they are deprived of all social and sexual rehearsal play. Then, after puberty, they are unable to establish a sexual partnership. Even with a gentle and experienced partner, the deprived animal— male or female—is unable to get properly positioned for copulation. They do not breed. If pregnancy is experimentally induced, the female becomes an abusing mother—so abusive, in fact, that she almost certainly will kill her baby. Atypical and bizarre sexual behavior associated with excessive isolation in captivity has been recorded also in a higher primate, the chimpanzee. But infantile deprivation in chimpanzees has not yet been systematically documented, as it has been in rhesus monkeys.

Human children, like the young of other primates, also engage in sexual rehearsal play. In our culture, the natural history of sexual rehearsal play cannot be ascertained, because free sexual expression among children is prohibited. In some children the prohibition takes effect successfully, and sexual play is suppressed. In others, the prohibition simply sends sexual play underground where it may never become known to adults. Thus, we know only about sexual play, such as infantile masturbation, which occurs before the prohibition takes effect, or play which is intruded upon by adults and, typically, subject to further prohibition (Plate 2).

Beyond our own culture, we can glimpse at what may be the natural way in which children's sexual rehearsal play evolves. The Aboriginal inhabitants of Arnhem Land on the Australian north coast, for example, traditionally have no taboo against infantile sexuality, and, despite Westernization, some of the old traditions survive. Once in a while in nursery school at nap-time a boy may press up against a girl, his body making pelvic thrusting movements, an innocuous rhythmic contentment resembling in significance the thumb-sucking of other children nearby.

Aboriginal children a year or two older, aged five or six, may play at more explicit coital positioning when going to sleep outdoors around the campfire. Adults often laugh their approval, as if to say: "Isn't it cute? They will know how to do it right when they grow up." It is not clear whether these children would invent such positioning in play if they had no model to copy or whether they mimic the play of older children. They may see adolescents and adults copulating, but that is not likely, since Aboriginal adults typically copulate in private, usually in the dark.

Rehearsal of pelvic thrusting and coital positioning is not the beginning of sexuality in childhood. In fact, the first phase of sexual rehearsal may begin even before birth with erections in boys. Certainly erections occur neonatally and throughout infancy and childhood. Even if erections are not observed during waking hours, they can be seen to occur from birth onwards during REM sleep (when rapid eye movements indicate that the sleeper is dreaming). The corresponding phenomenon in girls has not been fully identified and documented.

The first postnatal phase of sexual rehearsal is sensuous rather than sexual and it is not play so much as part of living—the haptic sensuousness of skin contact in clinging, cuddling and hugging. If children are delivered by natural childbirth methods, skin contact begins at birth when the baby emerges from the vagina and lies on the mother's belly. In the first few hours after delivery the pairbond between mother and infant is established, partly through the sense of sight, but chiefly through the haptic, or tactual, sense. This bonding is not only of great importance to the well-being of mother and child; it is a rehearsal, so to speak, of the pair-bonding of romantic love, which usually happens for the first time in adolescence or young adulthood.

Sensuous pair-bonding in infancy is essential for human behavioral development. It continues during breast-feeding, lessens gradually during weaning, is maintained during childhood, and has a great resurgence as an erotic pair-bond at or after puberty. The infant's first pair-bond is necessarily with the mother, but a parallel bond is established between infant and father, beginning even at delivery if the father is present.

When Freud formulated his theory of infantile sexuality, he overlooked the haptic phase, possibly because it is initially contemporaneous with what he termed the oral phase. Freud's second, or anal phase, is not exclusively sensuous. It also coincides with the onset of sphincter control and is a programed phase of learning in which a connection is established between the stimulus to eliminate and the response of finding a place to eliminate.

The genital phase proposed by Freud is the beginning of authentic sexuality in that the child experiences the sensuousness of the sex organs. In Europe until the eighteenth century, parents and guardians soothed fretful children by masturbating the genitals. In the aftermath of the Inquisition, however, masturbation came to be viewed as the cause of insanity and other symptoms of degeneracy, and adults who played with children's genitals were punished as child molesters.

In modern terms, Freud's oedipal phase of late infancy and early childhood does not relate only to genital and erotic sexual rehearsal but also to differentiation of gender identity and role as masculine, feminine, or in some cases, ambivalent. The two principles involved are identification and complementation. Identification is *with* people of the same sex—chiefly parents. Complementation is *to* people of the opposite sex—also chiefly parents. At kindergarten age it is

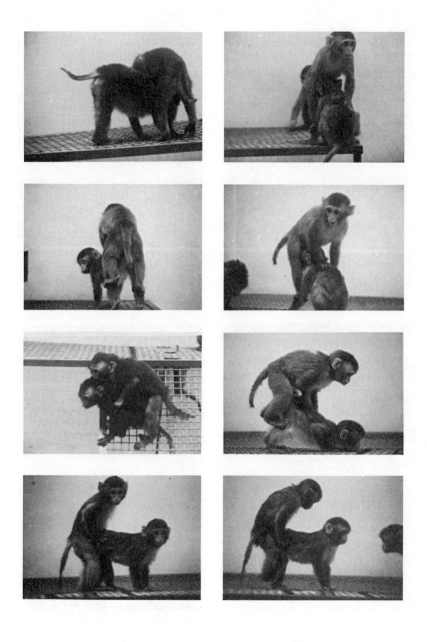

PLATE 1. Normal juvenile sexual rehearsal play in rhesus monkeys as manifested between three months and a year of age. Sequence reads from left to right and down. (Photos courtesy of David Goldfoot, Ph.D.)

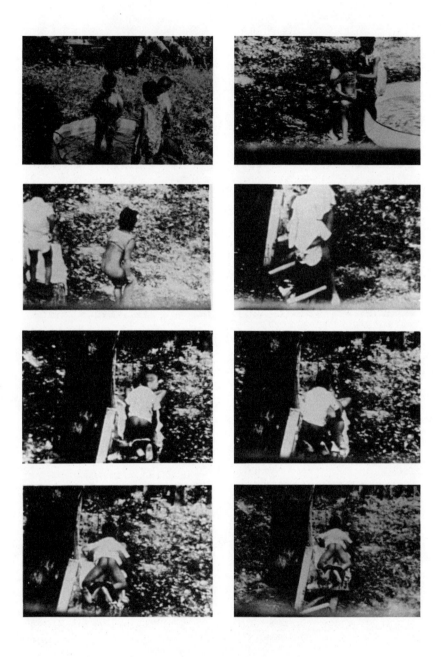

PLATE 2. Normal juvenile sexual rehearsal play in children five or six years of age. Sequence reads from left to right and down. (Telephoto lens, photographer anonymous, 1960.)

common to observe daughters flirting with their fathers, and sons with their mothers, in a way that clearly rehearses the flirtation of what, in adolescence and adulthood, will be known as the proceptive phase. Proception is a new term for erotic invitation, solicitation, or courtship which postpubertally leads up to the phase of acception (copulation), which then may or may not be followed by the phase of conception. Prior to puberty, flirtation in infancy may become frankly erotic, but actual erotic rehearsal during this phase is more likely to be enacted with peers.

Such rehearsal ensures that the behavioral sex differences that are bona fide sexual and erotic will be amalgamated with those differences which are sex-coded by tradition and are actually optional rather than imperative. If rehearsal of the bona fide sex differences—those that ultimately will be associated with impregnation in the male, and menstruation, gestation and lactation in the female—is thwarted, there is a risk that disordered or anomalous erotic, sexual, and psychosexual function will evolve. Such disorders or anomalies come into full bloom when the hormones of puberty lower the threshold for their expression.

As far as sexual rehearsal play is concerned, the middle years of childhood are not latency years as Freud believed. On the contrary, in cultures where sexual play is not forbidden, children express their sexuality from time to time, but not obsessively or excessively. During this phase, children may establish romantic pair bonds or love affairs in play rehearsal, but there is not enough evidence for a firm statement to be made about such behavior.

At puberty, sexual rehearsal play gradually relinquishes its rehearsal function and emerges as the finished performance. The hormones of puberty are the chief agent of this change. Apart from producing obvious changes in the body, these hormones also lower the barrier or threshold to the expression of sexuality in imagery and dreams, and in practice. Puberty does not determine what will be expressed. Rather, it releases that which has already been determined by rehearsals during infancy and childhood.

Nature's ideal developmental program of sexual rehearsal play in childhood is not known; nor do we know all the noxious influences that can misdirect it. Noxious influences on sexuality need not themselves be explicitly sexual. The death of a parent, sibling, or other close relative, for example, may adversely affect a child's psychosexual development. By contrast, a childhood sexual experience, such as being the partner of a relative, or of an older person, need not necessarily affect the child adversely. If violence or trauma are involved, however, the probability of an adverse effect is exponentially increased.

What may be important in some cases is not the event itself, but the context in which it is experienced. If a child intrudes on copulating parents—the so-called primal scene—the effect may be adverse if, as is common in our middle class society, the parents have no formula ("playing the mommy-daddy game," for example) for coping with the interruption. In scores of other societies, however, children sleep in the same room with their parents and inevitably see coitus. They know about copulation from as far back as they can remember— even if convention dictates that they not talk about it.

Research Strategies

Although there is no firm knowledge of what constitutes a natural program of sexual rehearsal, nor what effect various experiences may have on sexual development, it is almost certain that human beings, like the other primates, require a period of early sexual rehearsal play in order to ensure the maturation and manifestation of functional mating behavior during puberty and later. It could well be that the dysfunctional mating behavior that is prevalent among us as adults comes as an unplanned, unbargained-for result of the imposition of the taboo on sex play in childhood.

Whether this hypothesis is true or false cannot be decided by armchair speculation or doctrinal moralizing. It can be decided only by evidence—the hard-science evidence of well-planned, systematic, and long-term observational research.

It would not be technically difficult to test whether harsh, negative attitudes toward childhood sexuality produce sexual abnormality or inadequacy at puberty, and in adolescence and adulthood.

One could follow two groups of children, one group with a closed-minded, punitive sexual upbringing, and the other raised in an open-minded unpunitive sexual atmosphere. By keeping complete and systematic records, year by year, until puberty and adolescence, one would learn how many children in each group became sexually and psychosexually normal, and how many abnormal. There are already some parents in our society who are open-minded about their children's sexual upbringing, as well as many who are not. It would be possible to do this study at any university or medical school in the country.

An even more attractive research possibility would be to compare two or more different cultures in a cross-sectional rather than longitudinal experiment. One would select each culture on the basis of preliminary evidence that it was either open-minded, or closed-minded with respect to childhood sexuality. Then, one would collect further evidence on the sexual rearing of children in each society. One would also collect evidence on how well or how poorly the adults in these societies were getting along in their sex lives—frequency of marital problems, sexual dysfunction, sex offenses, so-called perversions, and other psychosexual anomalies.

There is a dearth of even preliminary evidence of this type, for cultural anthropologists, by and large, have been as prudish as most other scientific and medical people and have not thoroughly recorded sexual matters. In addition, cultural anthropologists are not trained in sexology. No university in the U.S. has a department of sexology. In fact, in all of the Western Hemisphere, only the University of Quebec, in Montreal, Canada, has a department of sexology. And that department is not yet affiliated with a medical school or hospital.

Clearly, information on childhood sex is lacking. Parents do not have sexologically sound facts and good theory to guide them in child-rearing. All they have is the folk belief that children's sex play, if discovered, should be severely disciplined, that children should be made to feel guilt and shame, and that the sensuous pleasure found in the sex organs is sinful. Whether they accept or reject this belief, parents must do so as an act of faith, not of reason.

Further research into childhood sexuality could provide the much needed information on which to base reasoned decisions. Why then, does society stand in the way of childhood sex research?

No final and complete answer can be given to this question. It essentially asks why our society has a strong sexual taboo. Not only is that taboo of great antiquity, it is also only one manifestation of a total social order. Perhaps, far back in history, our forebears' ruler-priests invented the sex taboo as a principle of child rearing. Inculcation of a taboo ensures the presence of guilt, anxiety and shame, which can be used as a lever to control all sorts of behavior.

Whatever the origin of the sex taboo, one major rationale for maintaining it has today begun to disappear, and that is the prevention of premarital pregnancy. With the invention of the crude rubber condom last century, and the improvement of birth control in this century, the sex play of children and the continuation of that play in actual sex among adolescents need not pose the danger of pregnancy.

The strength of the taboo on sex is evident in that birth control technology alone has not eliminated it. Society's ability to separate recreational and procreational sex is still a source of cultural and moral indigestion.

The sex taboo resists extinction. Punitive treatment of childhood sexuality is the norm. And it is practiced in ignorance. Parents do not know whether punishing sexual rehearsal play may make their children sexual paragons or cripples in adulthood. They do not know whether treating sexual play with dignity and respect will benefit their children, allowing them to lead more fulfilling sexual lives as adults. They need to know, and research into childhood sexuality can help provide the answers—provided, that is, that society, the Congress, and the private foundations will change their timid policy and allocate funds for research into sexuality and its development at all ages, childhood included.

Note

Originally published in *The Sciences,* 16(6):12ff. November/December, 1976. *The Sciences* is the official publication of The New York Academy of Sciences. [Bibliog. #2.191]

FORTY

Service and Science in Pediatric Psychology

Know Your Syndromes

A young colleague, allocating his budget for professional memberships, asked me why my rating of the Society of Pediatric Psychology was only lukewarm. His question required me to formulate my philosophy regarding pediatric psychology.

I had joined the Society at the time of its inception in 1970. It promised me an escape from scholarly isolation that dated back to 1951. In that year I had qualified as a pediatric psychologist by reason of joining the fledgling pediatric endocrine clinic in the Department of Pediatrics at Johns Hopkins. The first of its kind in the world, it had been founded in 1946 by Lawson Wilkins. The pediatric psychoendocrine unit that I established was also the first of its kind. Hence the sense of scholarly isolation. There were no other psychologists with a specialty interest in clinical psychoendocrinology; and, indeed, no other psychologists who identified themselves as pediatric psychologists. Child psychologists identified themselves as clinical psychologists. In children's hospitals and clinics, they were affiliated with child psychiatry, or child guidance units. I became officially designated not as a clinical psychologist, but as a medical psychologist assigned to pediatrics. De facto, I was a pediatric psychologist. My specialty was clinical psychoendocrinology in childhood and adolescence, with longterm followup into adulthood.

In order to be a participating member in a specialty clinic, it is imperative to assimilate a specialist's knowledge of the syndromes (some named as diseases, disorders, defects, or conditions) specific to that clinic—their etiology, their diagnosis, and their prognosis relative to the available methods of intervention, psychological intervention included. In 1951, the endocrine syndromes of childhood and adolescence were, for the most part, a psychological terra incognita. Therefore, from the outset of my career as a pediatric psychologist, I formulated the axiom: Know your syndromes. Self-applied, this axiom required first that I learn what was known about the hormonal etiology, diagnosis, treatment and prognosis of the endocrine syndromes of childhood and adolescence. It required also a knowledge of the chromosomal or genetic basis of some syndromes, as applicable. More to the point, this axiom imposed on me the responsibility of seeking new knowledge to fill in the voids that existed concerning the psychologic sequelae, both primary and secondary, of hormonal dysfunctions—deficits, excesses, or other anomalies. The converse also applied, namely to seek new knowledge concerning the induction or potentiation of hormonal disorder secondary to environmental determinants, some of which might be construed as psychological (as in the syndrome of child-abuse dwarfism).

In brief, the task that was set out before me was to build a psychology of syndromes in the speciality of pediatric endocrinology. To know the psychology of a syndrome greatly expedites the psychological case management in each individual case. It permits phenomena that are syndrome derived to be distinguished from those that have to be attributed to other sources; and it also safeguards against oversights and omissions in the case workup.

Turner's syndrome provides a good illustration. As often happens, academic planning is the issue. The psychologist who knows the syndrome, knows even before he sees the patient that specific praxic and mathematical disability is a common characteristic in girls with Turner's syndrome, whereas verbal ability is not impaired. Thus, he completes his evaluation more expeditiously and makes recommendations more efficaciously than does his counterpart who lacks such knowledge. For the Turner patient in teenage, the knowledgeable psychologist is also far more effective in counseling, if he knows that psychosexual infantilism in the syndrome is chronologically determined in synchrony with clinical delay in the induction of puberty with estrogen replacement therapy. The purpose of this delay is to allow more time for increased growth in height to help offset the statural dwarfism that is another characteristic of the syndrome. Puberty does not occur spontaneously, owing to embryological agenesis or dysgenesis of the gonads. Once puberty is induced with estrogen, bone growth is rapidly brought to a close with consequent cessation of growth in height. However, there is for each individual an optimal age beyond which the onset of puberty should not be postponed. The basic defect in Turner's syndrome is chromosomal. The typical karyotype is 45,X, there being neither a second X nor a Y chromosome.

Basic and Applied Science

In the history of pediatric psychology, the construction of a psychology of syndromes has been, for the most part, haphazard. What is now needed is a systematic and coordinated effort on the part of the profession as a whole. The goal is to build a research effort in each subspecialty of pediatrics that would lead, eventually, to a comprehensive textbook of the psychology of pediatric syndromes. In many syndromes, the psychology of the syndrome will be not syndrome specific, but shared by other syndromes of either acute or chronic suffering. By contrast, in other syndromes, the psychology of the syndrome will be directly derived from syndrome-specific genetic, metabolic, hormonal, or nervous-system anomalies and impairments.

A pediatric psychology that is able to differentiate psychologic symptoms of a syndrome that are a direct expression of the pathology of the syndrome from those that are general sequelae of being in the role of a sick person will be looked upon as genuinely scientific. It will be a science in its own right, characterized chronologically by being developmental, theoretically by having etiological explanations, and phenomenologically by having its own subject matter. It will be a science for pediatric psychologists to be proud of.

At the present time pediatric psychologists cannot, in all honesty, be truly proud of their science, for it is named not for the pediatric determinants and uniqueness of its theory, but for the age group on whom it is practiced, and for the location in which it is practiced. On the chronological criterion, it is an applied science on the same spectrum as neonatal, ephebiatric, young adult, adult, menopausal, and geriatric psychology. On the locational criterion, pediatric psychology is yet again an applied science, but on a different spectrum. This spectrum encompasses, for example, ecclesiastical, military, astronautical, penal, industrial, academic, and other varieties of applied psychology that are named for the arena in which they are applied.

The defining characteristic of any applied science is that it applies theory borrowed from one or more basic science. Applied science is to basic science as engineering technology is to mathematics and physics. Pediatric psychology as an applied science borrows its theory, if not indiscriminately, then eclectically from Skinner's behaviorism (behavior modification), psychogenics and modified Freudianism, and from a rather diffuse neuroscience entity known as organicity.

When applied scientists form a professional society and meet together on a regular basis, their major interest is in advances in technique, and in the preservation of their monopoly through legislated licensing or certification. The Society of Pediatric Psychology is not typical in this respect, for its members engage in political lobbying, if at all, through their respective state psychological associations, and through the national American Psychological Association. With politicking excluded, one would expect, therefore, that pediatric psychologists would associate professionally by reason of a common interest in the basic science of pediatric psychology. This science would have its counterparts in other branches of psychology, each with its own theoretical principles, as for example, the cognitive, sexological, hormonal, neurochemical, ethological, cytogenetic and other branches.

The theoretical principles that pediatric psychology might claim as its own are those that can be researched and formulated as the principles belonging to the psychology of the syndromes of pediatrics. These principles may overlap with those of the psychology of the syndromes of other age groups. Their uniqueness is that they are additive to the principles of syndromes that have their onset prenatally, and are attached to the principles of syndromes that extend into adolescence and beyond. They are, in other words, developmental. Their discovery and formulation will give pediatric psychologists a sense of scientific mission, a validation by other scientists, and an experience of the excitement of scientific scholarship which presently is poised on the threshold of expansive new growth. For the newcomer to a career in pediatric psychology, that prospect of new scientific growth is intellectually more invigorating than the prospect of burnout from the delivery of scientifically dubious services. It changes the temperature of pediatric psychology from lukewarm and weak, to hot and strong.

Note

Originally published in *Newsletter of the Society of Pediatric Psychology,* pp. 3-5, Oct., 1984. [Bibliog. #4.102]

FORTY-ONE

Progress of Knowledge and Revision of the Theory of Infantile Sexuality

Change and Dogma

It is not at all rare in the history of science, as in religion as well, that a theory is perpetuated as dogma because it is the hallmarked property of an Establishment. It is then not unlike a self-fulfilling prophecy, insofar as it predicts the explanation of given phenomena and then claims validity when they occur. There is not much that one can do to prevent an Establishment from using a theory in this way. Like the phlogiston theory, it will die, if at all, from the displacement of the old Establishment by the new, which has no place for it. In science, the displacement of the old Establishment is usually effected as the result of the introduction of new methods, investigative and applied, which dictate new theories and command a larger following.

Dr. Chodoff does very well to ask the psychoanalytic Establishment to reconsider the theory of infantile sexuality. He will probably meet with little immediate success, since any change will trigger off a revision of the entire body of psychoanalytic doctrine. This is too much to ask all at once, with no consolidated body of opposing doctrine available as a substitute. Nonetheless, the handwriting is already on the wall. Change is inevitable.

New Experimental Knowledge

This inevitability of change is dictated, as is usually the case, by the accumulation of new knowledge, especially that derived from newly discovered techniques and methods of obtaining knowledge pertinent to sexual theory. This new knowledge pertains, for example, to the new genetics of chromosome counting, behavior genetics, and the relationship of psychosexual development to the sex chromosomes in certain clinical populations. There is new knowledge also of hormones administered to the pregnant mother that will reverse the sex of the external organs of the offspring—androgen will produce a genetic and ovarian female with a penis and empty scrotum, and cyproterone, an antiandrogen, will produce a genetic and testicular male with perfectly simulant female external genitals.

Perhaps even more startling is the new knowledge, from the lower mammalian species, of hormonal substances as neural organizers in the fetal hypothalamus. These early organizers are capable of regulating subsequent cycling of pituitary function and the correspondingly appropriate sexual behavior. There is

530

also new knowledge that radioactive labeled hormone can be traced to the sexual centers of the hypothalamus that absorb it, even into the very cells. In the world of behavioral experimentation, it is equally startling to follow the macaque monkey studies of Harlow and his group at Wisconsin and to learn of the extraordinary importance of clinging and the haptic sense, during a critical period of infancy, to the subsequent psychosexual normalcy of monkeys. The same experiments show the extraordinary effects of childhood play, including sexual play, on subsequent psychosexual function; for play deprivation induces subsequent inability to copulate and breed. Taken together, these various new additions to knowledge show that there are more variables to be accounted for in the process of psychosexual development than are presently recognized in psychoanalytic theory of infantile sexuality.

Hermaphroditism

It is not simply a matter of new variables to be accounted for, however. My own work with human hermaphrodites, especially those of identical genetic, gonadal, hormonal and morphologic status whose assigned sex differed, has forced me to the realization that there is a very basic conceptual deficit in the logic of psychoanalytic sexual theory. This deficit lies concealed in the very name of the theory, for it is a theory of psychosexual development exclusively and not of psychosexual differentiation as well. It should also be a theory of psychosexual differentiation. As contrasted with, for example, the respiratory system, development in sex from the embryo onward is always differentiation into male or female as well as development per se.

Masculinity is Something Added

Psychoanalytic theory, like the Book of Genesis, more or less derives the feminine from the masculine. Primacy is attributed to the masculine trend in development. By contrast, there has been a convergence of evidence from divergent sources in recent years showing that nature's first disposition would appear to be to differentiate a female. Males are more delicate and vulnerable, as witness the greater loss of male conceptuses and of males after birth. Nature compensates with a ratio of 106 male to 100 female births. The general developmental rule seems to be that, to obtain a male, something must be added. Thus, it is the addition of the male sex hormone that accounts for the embryonic differentiation of male morphology, particularly externally: if the embryo is castrated before the critical embryonic period of sex-organ differentiation, genetic males have the sexual morphology of females. It is the male sex hormone, likewise, that accounts for the masculinization of neurohumoral centers in the hypothalamus in estrous species, as a consequence of which cyclic functioning of the pituitary to produce the sexual cycle will not occur. It is quite possibly the presence of male hormone at a critical, early developmental period that makes human males more erotically responsive to visual and narrative stimuli, whereas females are more dependent on touch stimulation.

In adulthood, the presence and strength of sexual drive and erotic initiative in males—though not the capacity for erotic imagery—is androgen dependent. Estrogen, as used in the treatment of prostatic cancer, is functionally castrating. Androgen given to women as in the treatment of breast cancer adds, in many cases, a new intensity of sexual urge that a woman may resent and find embarrassing.

Psychosexual status is dependent not only on prenatal antecedents and hormone levels, however. Psychosexual differentiation in hermaphrodites of the same diagnostic status at birth, but different sex assignment and subsequent rearing, demonstrates that psychosexual status is also heavily dependent (as is one's native language) on what happens after birth—especially on what happens in social interaction within the family and community. Here, once again, nature's greater difficulty at differentiating a male is further exemplified, for it is in males that the psychosexual aberrations occur with greater frequency than in females. Some such aberrations are exclusively found in men. Apparently because the differentiating task is more complex, there are more opportunities for casualties along the way.

Bisexual Theory

There are some males in whom masculine psychosexual differentiation is complete. No feminine vestiges remain in evidence. By contrast, a few males signally fail to differentiate psychosexually as males. In them, feminine traits, instead of being vestigial, are very much in evidence. A third group are those whose psychosexual differentiation is ambiguous. They remain epicene, bisexual and ambivalent. In converse, much the same may be said about females, in that some of them become bisexual and some strongly masculinized, though a relatively larger proportion differentiate as feminine. The general rule here is not that all members of the species grow up bisexual, but that they are bipotential at the outset and differentiate to become, as a general rule, unipotential. Whatever the outcome, masculine, feminine or ambivalent, it becomes fixed. The paradigm here is probably that of the internal reproductive structures, where development of the wolffian organs is reciprocated by vestigiation of the müllerian and vice versa, except in rare cases of male or true hermaphroditism where both remain side by side. Freudian bisexual and Oedipal theory needs revising in the light of these considerations.

Components of Psychosexual Identity

Possible though it is to generalize as if psychosexual differentiation were a unitary process and psychosexual identity a single entity, it is necessary also to pay attention to the component elements. Elucidation of the nature of these component elements is a matter of continuing discovery, subject to continuing revision. Five that have emerged from my own investigations are energy expenditure and energy level, which is generally greater in boys than girls; maternalism, which is greater in the play and activities of girls than boys; perceptual stimulation of erotic genitopelvic arousal, which, after the pubertal age, is more haptic and less visual or narrative in girls than boys; erotic imagery as it relates to the body image and the sexual dimorphism of body morphology; and social insignia of sex as exemplified in cosmetic and clothing preference, gestural habits and movements, and chosen pastime and vocational interests that are sex stereotyped.

Breast and Pregnancy Envy

The second of these components is worthy of special attention in view of its traditional psychoanalytic neglect in the theory of childhood sexuality. Breast and pregnancy envy in boys deserves at least as much attention as penis envy and castration anxiety in girls. Moreover, the developmental—and evolutionary—relationship of oral and anal functioning to sex has less to do with copulation than parturition and infant grooming. To give birth, mammals must use the mouth in proximity to the vagina and must eat the afterbirth. In childcare they lick the young. Even a species as high as the chimpanzee cleans the baby of feces by licking them away. It is in these biological sources that one most sensibly looks for the relationship between the head and the rear parts in sex, whether as rehearsed fragmentarily in infantile development or coordinated with orgasm in the sexual proclivities of adults. In any consideration of oral and anal theory, it goes without saying that the functional development of the oral and anal systems applies to food intake and elimination as well as or more than to sex and libido.

Oral and Anal Imprinting

Regarding food, one developmental function is the discrimination of dietary from non-dietary foods. This discrimination is the cultural elaboration of the biological imperative to avoid poisoning by ingesting unselected, instead of traditional, habit-determined foodstuffs. This learning of food preferences, often manifested in food binges and food fads in the behavior of young children, may be looked upon as a human variant of what ethologists refer to as imprinting. The concept of imprinting may also be called upon in connection with the development of toilet training. In many mammalian species, voluntary control of the sphincters of elimination is accomplished simultaneously with imprint-learning of where to go to eliminate—which is the basis of being able both to housebreak a kitten to use a box of sand or a spread-out newspaper and to teach a child to use a commode or toilet. These considerations of imprinting need to be incorporated into the total body of childhood psychosexual theory.

Conclusion

Dr. Chodoff is to be congratulated for calling professional attention to the need for a revision of psychoanalytic theory of infantile sexuality. I would suggest an international convention for the purpose of working out a revision that will bring Freudian theory up to date, consistent with today's experimental and clinical findings, and versatile in the production of new hypotheses to test.

Note

Originally published in *International Journal of Psychiatry*, 4:50-53, 1967. [Bibliog. #3.14]

FORTY-TWO

Issues and Attitudes in Research and Treatment of Variant Forms of Human Sexual Behavior

Truth and Ethics

It was formerly part of the faith of scientists that they were seekers of pure truth, insulated from the moral and political concerns of how the findings of their pure truth might be applied or misapplied. Ethics was the specialty of philosophers and theologians. Hiroshima destroyed all that. Scientists have been rudely awakened to a sense of moral responsibility for the principles they are discovering and the technology to which they are applying them.

In medicine a quarter of a century ago, ethics was pretty much a fossilized discipline, embedded in the Hippocratic oath. The good patient, like the good child, was to be seen and not heard. His records were inaccessible to him, and his prescriptions, more than likely, were written in incomprehensible, abbreviated Latin. No more! Today the ethics of informed consent is the new "in" thing.

The practice of medicine is affected by informed consent insofar as a patient has increased ease of access to his record. It is the conduct of medical research, however, that is most affected by the new ethics of informed consent. In some instances the very existence and continuance of clinical investigation among human beings is threatened.

Research Design

In clinical investigative design, the randomly selected group is a major casualty of the new concern with the ethics of informed consent. It is now absolutely impossible to get a genuinely random sample of human beings for any type of medical study, whether it be blood chemistry or sexuality. Informed consent implies the right of either refusal or cooperation. Cooperation is voluntary. Thus, under the new rules of informed consent, volunteer bias is universal in both treatment and control groups.

Occasionally one will be able to obtain a sample for investigative study that constitutes a complete census of a diagnostic group. An alternative in research design is to resort to the method of matched comparison or contrast groups. To illustrate, a group of 47, XXY men might be matched and compared with a group of 47, XYY men. Each group constitutes an experiment of nature and is homogeneous relative to the criterion by which it is identified. The composition of each group is equally subject to volunteer bias. Other possible biases, such as

535

the secondary effects of being hospitalized or being followed in a clinic, are shared by both groups. That is to say, between groups, the uncontrolled variables are either sufficiently constant or sufficiently random as to permit consistent differences to show up. In the example noted, the independent variable is the chromosomal status. The dependent variable—the one being studied—may be fertility, serum testosterone level, IQ, behavioral pathology, and so on.

To circumvent volunteer bias, one may also have recourse to that research design in which volunteers act as their own controls in a before-and-after investigative strategy.

Ideological Constraint

The constraint imposed on human clinical investigation by the volunteer bias of informed consent may be irksome, but it is imperative in order to protect human beings from being treated amorally as experimental animals. Another form of constraint is far more insidious and dangerous. It masquerades as ethical, whereas in actuality it is ideological. It abrogates, by edict, the right of some human beings to have informed consent and the right of investigators to conduct their clinical studies. It also restricts the topics of clinical investigation. Its prime victims, at present, are children and prisoners; and its most vetoed topics are sex research and fetal research. This ideological form of constraint operates by way of legal threat, legal action, suing for malpractice, disapproving research protocols, and promulgating decrees and regulations pertaining to funding and the withdrawal of funds for research. On occasion it operates by way of terrorism.

The paradox and tragedy of this ideological constraint on human clinical investigation is that its proponents believe themselves to be protecting the welfare of research subjects. In fact, they have allowed the protective pendulum to swing too far. They are now depriving subjects, especially prisoners and children, of their right of informed consent; and they are depriving themselves and all mankind of the right to the benefits of clinical research.

Case Example: XYY Syndrome

Recently there was a much-publicized attack on the Harvard study of the incidence of anomalies of chromosomal karyotype in the newborn.[1] Though the study was endorsed by the Harvard faculty, its principal investigator eventually discontinued it because his wife and children were subjected to continual harassment and intimidation.[2]

The attack appears to have been instigated by a militant political-action group, with support from a legally oriented civil-liberties group. Both groups may have been seeking public exposure quite apart from their social philosophy of protecting the public against science. They focused their attack only on the ascertainment of the 47,XYY anomaly. They used the rationale of the self-fulfilling prophecy, namely, that parents who knew they had an XYY baby would rear him to become a violent criminal, since the media had publicized the extra Y chromosome as the crime chromosome. No matter that the media were wrong!

There is already evidence to contradict the sensationalization of the supernumerary Y—the evidence that there are XYY citizens who do not get into trouble with the law. There is also evidence that the parents of XYY babies are profoundly grateful for whatever counseling they receive in rearing the XYY child, which is, by and large, an exceptionally difficult task. XYY boys are at risk for a high degree of impulsiveness. Their response to punishment is impulsive and destructive. They do far better on a program of incentive training than on punishment training.

According to the evidence available, it is an asset rather than a liability for a baby with a cytogenetic anomaly to have parents who know about it.[3] From now on the chances are that American children will be deprived of this asset, for their chromosomal status will either be unascertained or undisclosed—which is as foolish as suppressing a diagnosis of meningitis in the false belief that knowledge of the diagnosis itself will cause death.

Case Example: Therapy for Sex Offenders

Nonviolent sex offenders—exhibitionists, for example—who are arrested and found guilty frequently get inordinately severe and lengthy sentences. Studies begun in 1966 show that sex offenders may gain in self-regulation of sexual behavior if given a period of treatment with antiandrogen, preferably accompanied by counseling.[4,5] In Germany the newly discovered antiandrogen cyproterone acetate was used. Its use is still prohibited in the United States by the Federal Drug Administration; medroxyprogesterone acetate (Depo-Provera) is used instead. The first trials with Depo-Provera were conducted at Johns Hopkins in an era prior to the requirement of approval by a clinical investigations committee.

By 1972 it was necessary to have committee approval, which was given with the proviso that no prisoners or men under arrest be treated. The committee was responding to the implications of federal policy regarding the rights of informed consent. In effect, it was saying that by being under arrest or in jail, a man forfeits his right to informed consent, for he is likely to sign anything that promises a lighter sentence or an earlier parole. That is a specious, if not a vindictive, argument, for being in jail is a fact of life for a prisoner just as being in a hospital is for a patient. The facts of our lives shape all of our judgments, including those of informed consent.

Being arrested or in jail is a trauma that allows the sex offender to seek treatment. Ordinarily, sex offenders do not feel any more hurt or disabled because of their sex lives than do nonoffenders. They know their behavior is socially stigmatized and punishable, but the threat of punishment is not traumatic enough to induce them to seek treatment. Thus, to fail to provide treatment at the time of arrest or imprisonment is, in most cases, to fail forever.

The precedent for resolving the foregoing dilemma was established by a sex offender serving concurrent life sentences for rape and attempted rape. Recently he took his case to federal court and obtained an agreement from the prison authorities that they would make him available for treatment if he was accepted into the Johns Hopkins antiandrogen program. Then he received from the same judge a ruling that his consent to treatment was indeed informed consent: A physician and a psychologist informed him in the courtroom of the pros and cons of treatment. He has since been treated on a weekly basis in jail.

Power of Decision-Making

The foregoing illustrations exemplify an erosion of the power of medical people to make their own decisions. The law has long imposed certain constraints on doctors, for example, regarding abortion and euthanasia. But here we have two dangerous precedents. In one case a research decision was made not by experts, with all the data at their fingertips, but by militant dilettantes. In the other case, a therapeutic decision was taken out of the hands of experts who had researched the new form of therapy and was made by a judge who took a courtroom course on the treatment of sex offenders with antiandrogen. It goes without saying that a lone judge is no more and no less error-free than a lone doctor. One does not guarantee the rights of prisoners by handing over the guardianship of those rights to a judge instead of a doctor. It is a jury that is needed, and preferably a jury of one's expertly informed peers.

There is no ready explanation for why medical people are being robbed of, and are giving up, their rights of informed decision-making. Yes, it does reflect the antiscientism of our era, and antiscience may itself represent a backlash against the immense influence of scientific research on our daily existence. Despite the problems still unresolved, medicine has a life-and-death power undreamed of at the onset of this century.

Wherever power lies, there also lies someone to usurp it. Medical personnel and other people engaged in sexological research and therapy do not seem very alert in this respect. Those who should be natural allies snipe at one another in rivalry. The enemy rejoices. Meanwhile, our combined forces are not yet strong enough to have given rise to a single department of sexology in an American medical school.

Moral Standards

The current debate on the ethics of informed consent is a reminder that there are no absolute moral standards of right and wrong—only a series of approximations as new data, new events, new artifacts, and new people require the updating of old standards.

Intellectual obedience, studious self-discipline, and ethical conformity are prerequisites to beating the competition in order to enter and be successful in medicine and the allied professions. There are notable exceptions, but, as a group, medical professionals are more likely to endorse the ethical status quo than to question it. Once in a while a paroxysmal change occurs: Witness recent upheavals in the definition of mental illness and normality and in the reclassification of homosexuality as an erotic alternative rather than a pathology.

Such changes have major implications for priorities in research and therapy. For example, an exhibitionist is an inconsequential person in a nudist camp or a society unperturbed by nudity, whereas in hospitals and courtrooms such behavior is always regarded as pathological. Similarly, during and prior to the eighteenth century in Europe, adults who fondled infants' genitals were pacifying them, whereas today they would be jailed for pedophilia or incest, or both.

It is quite possible that medical attention today is too much focused on research and therapy of individual sexual and erotic pathology, as defined by today's criteria. We might well spend more time in medical anthropology. We might then discover that, like our relatives and neighbors, we are all overzealous in applying the sexual prejudices and taboos specific to our heritage. Without them, we may be able to make our heritage preventative; that is, the children of future generations might grow up free from the complaints to which we today so assiduously address ourselves.

Professional Nonjudgmentalism

Variant forms and expressions of human sexuality are among those human conditions and syndromes that absolutely demand a professionally nonjudgmental attitude on the part of the person who investigates or treats them. Neither you nor I would like to be morally chastened by a physician to whom we took a case of VD for treatment. If that happened, we would probably seek treatment from someone else.

Judgmentalism belongs to the law, but not to medicine. Since Hippocrates society has accorded to the physician the responsibility shared with the attorney and the priest, of privileged communication. It is a responsibility of utmost importance to the patient, for the physician is often the only person in society to whom a patient may turn for help with problems to which all other people react with moral condemnation. For problems of sexual conduct, the therapist's nonjudgmental impartiality in the doctor-patient relationship is as essential to therapeutic success as it is in, say, temporal lobe epileptic behavior, suicidal behavior or self-injurious behavior.

Nonjudgmentalism toward the patient as the person manifesting a syndrome is not synonymous with absence of judgment regarding the prognosis and treatment. Nor is the nonjudgmentalism toward the patient synonymous with lack of judgment regarding one's own personal conduct and morality. Nonjudgmentalism toward the patient is professional nonjudgmentalism. It is as essential to one's medical professionalism as is technical competence. I make this point because I have found that medical students, when I lecture them on human sexuality, have difficulty differentiating the principle of professional nonjudgmentalism from the principle of personal moral responsibility. Sex therapists and investigators may have the same difficulty.

It is easier to be professionally nonjudgmental with respect to etiology and diagnosis than with prognosis, and least easy with respect to treatment. The doctor must make a decision regarding the disposition or treatment of a case, and in so doing must have recourse to his own judgment as to what to do. It is not easy to be nonjudgmental when dealing with what society judges as the immoral, illegal, and bizarre manifestations of human sexuality.

Ethics of Tolerance and the Intolerable

Among those variant forms of human sexuality that constitute the paraphilias, some are harmless and others are harmful to the partner or the self. Harmless forms are often defined as crimes in today's law. Even so, they do not pose as great an ethical challenge to the therapist or the researcher as do the harmful paraphilias that constitute crimes with victims, such as lust murder, brutal rape, sadomasochist homicide or suicide, and erotic self-strangulation. In my own practice and teaching, I draw an ethical dividing-line between harmless and harmful paraphilias on the basis not simply of the criterion of partner consent—for one can encounter cases such as that of a masochist who consents to, and indeed stage-manages, his own murder. Harmful sexual practices are those that invade the personal inviolacy of one or both partners and bring about severe and injurious personal abuse, up to and including death. Like child abuse, these are intolerable practices that demand some degree of obligative, nonelective intervention and help with a view to bringing about change.

Ethics and Homosexuality

Many, if not most physicians, both clinical and investigative, are deeply enough imbued with our culture's sexual traditions that they are unable to accept as ethical the idea of treating a heterosexual person so as to bring about a homosexual response, even briefly and reversibly. There are cultures, however, in which homosexuality as one component of a tradition of developmental bisexuality is the ideological norm.[6] In such a culture, young males experience only homosexual erotic activities in the early years of their maturity, formally changing to heterosexuality after negotiating a bride-price and getting married in young adulthood. They are subsequently able to resume homosexual activity when working away from home, but such episodes are transient and do not impair the sexual relationship of marriage.

There is no absolute criterion by which to evaluate a bisexual cultural tradition as either superior or inferior to a monosexual one. The very existence and cultural viability of a bisexual society does, however, require that we in our society do not set up exclusive heterosexuality as an absolute norm. An exclusively heterosexual society is neither superior nor inferior to a bisexual one. Thus, it is purely rhetorical to ask whether or not heterosexual persons could be so treated as to become homosexual for a time. Nonetheless, the rhetorical question is a valuable exercise in both logic and ethics, for its obverse and precise counterpart is the question of whether homosexuals should be treated to become heterosexual (or bisexual) and whether such treatment should be enforced by edict.

Until the advent of modern sexology in the nineteenth century, homosexuality was classified in Western Christian culture as belonging with heresy and treason; there was no better way to dispose of a political enemy than to accuse him of homosexuality, for he was then eligible to be accused of heresy and treason as well. The sanctions and punishments were ruthless. In the Victorian era, some of the old ruthlessness remained and was even enforced legislatively while it was simultaneously being replaced by the new view of science and medicine—the same new view that had earlier removed the mentally ill from dungeons (where they were punished for having allowed themselves to be devil-possessed) and placed them in asylums or hospitals, ostensibly for treatment. Homosexuals became reclassified as sick people, their sickness being that they did not conform to the ideological norm. They were to be pitied instead of punished, and offered whatever treatment was in fashion for their supposed cure.

It goes without saying that medicine has throughout its history taken on more conditions than it can cure, more indeed than it can even ameliorate. In addition, medicine has also been indiscriminate as to what it defines as a condition needing cure; it has had no systematic philosophy, set of principles, or criteria as to what constitutes health or disease. The very etymology of the latter term tells the story: dis-ease. Traditionally, it has pretty much been left up to the patient to decide whether he or she was suffering or at ease, that is, in need of a cure or to be left to his or her own devices.

Germ theory in the nineteenth century changed all that, for it brought to medicine the first genuine theory of etiology and the first genuine possibility not only of cure but also of prevention. The theory of prevention became the basis of public health, notably with respect to preventing the spread of contagion. Prevention raised a new ethical issue: the right of society to enforce treatment on unwilling patients who were not yet diseased and who did not appreciate the risk of becoming diseased with sufficient urgency to accept preventive treatment.

The ethics of prevention, or the right to enforce treatment, is still a matter of unsettled debate and controversy; witness the controversies over fluoridization of water and over population growth, both of which arouse intense religious and political passions.

As a result of controversy over individual rights and the ethics of prevention, special subgroups within the population at large have become increasingly attentive to their ethical rights with respect to enforced treatment and with respect to being classified as diseased and in need of treatment. The issue is especially sensitive in the case of those conditions or diseases for which the etiology is still so imperfectly understood that there is no guaranteed method of either prevention or cure.

Sexuality is one of these conditions. Theory as to the origins and development of a person's sexuality—whether it be bisexual, heterosexual, or homosexual—still has virtually zero predictive power regarding either prevention or cure. Inchoately at first, homosexual people have in the last two decades formulated a revision of the concept of whether they should be considered diseased or simply representatives of an unorthodox, atypical variant form of sexuality that could exist unobtrusively and unthreateningly in society, in much the same way as left-handedness and redheadedness exist amongst a majority who are different.

Homosexual men and women formulated this new view of themselves as they organized into a liberation movement contemporaneous with the women's liberation movement, in the era of widespread social change regarding acceptance of sexuality that goes under the name of the sexual revolution. Militant homosexual activists made direct attacks on the medical profession, especially its psychiatric representatives, and helped to bring about, despite a rear-guard defensive action, the declassification of homosexuality as a disease in America.

The ethical issue here is not denial of psychiatry or counseling to any men or women whose homosexual responses distress them. Rather, the issue is stigmatization—labeling people as in need of treatment when they consider that they can function satisfactorily. The result of the stigmatization process itself is impairment of a person's abilities. Historically, the wheel has turned from sin to sickness to social acceptability. That does not mean that research into the origins of sexuality will cease. It does mean that researchers will come to realize that their true interest lies in the origins of sexuality in general, not just homosexuality in particular. Eventually, when enough is known predictively to permit effective prevention and cure, in the authentic sense of cure, it will be time to engage in ethical debate as to whether our society, with its own special history and culture, will be improved or impoverished by providing a place for homosexuals and bisexuals as well as heterosexuals. Without the homosexuals who have contributed to the growth of Western civilization, its science, its art, and its literature, we would be sadly deprived; but there is, as of the present, no implementable research design for deciding the verdict one way or the other.

Ethics and Sex Reassignment of Transexuals

In the mid-1960s, I had a personal part to play in the history of the ethics of sex reassignment when the procedure for the rehabilitation of transexuals first became accepted in the United States. I shall tell the story autobiographically.

In the early 1950s and early 1960s, I became acquainted with cases of sex reassignment in hermaphroditism, and also with some cases of reassignment of nonhermaphroditic transexuals whose surgery had been performed overseas. Following surgery at the well-known clinic in Casablanca, two patients of Harry Benjamin in New York came to Baltimore in order to be examined surgically by the gynecologist Howard W. Jones, Jr., and psychologically by me. Jones and I had worked together for years on cases of hermaphroditism. We had also shared cases of nonhermaphroditic transexuals, many of whom in those days had self-diagnosed themselves as hermaphroditic in an attempt to justify the necessity of reassignment surgery.

Convinced by the evidence that sex reassignment, in appropriate cases, could be rehabilitative, Jones and I were confronted with the ethical and legal issues involved in legitimizing this controversial procedure.

Jones held the opinion that some decisions in medicine, ethical as well as empirical, are the responsibility of the specialists involved. Only they are fully informed of all the facts of the case. Only they have the full range of information on which to base a decision.

Some years earlier, I had heard the same philosophy expressed by Lawson Wilkins, the founder of pediatric endocrinology and a specialist in neonatal and juvenile hermaphroditism. He was dismayed that a local judge of his acquaintance refused to cosponsor a seminar on legal and medical issues in the sex assignment and treatment of hermaphroditic babies, focusing especially on the legal status of therapeutic castration, which is necessary in some cases. Wilkins' verdict was that his past decisions involving castration might, on a technicality, have gotten him jailed but that, had he waited on the law to make a decision for him, he would have made no progress in the treatment and rehabilitation of hermaphroditic children.

Here was an instance of medicine's needing to lead the law rather than calling on the law for a decision that it was, through lack of precedent, powerless to give. The law would function later, should the physician's action be contested. In the meantime, the doctor had to put himself and his career on the line, so to speak, ready to face the consequences even if they were negative. In no other way could change be brought about.

The situation was the same with respect to sex-reassignment surgery for transexuals. Approval of the first case of male-to-female reassignment surgery was, in the last analysis, made by Howard Jones and me. Administrative approval was subsequently institutionalized. A year later public approval was institutionalized in the wake of a press release strategically timed and designed to circumvent gossip and to inform and educate the public. The press release on

November 21, 1966, was successful in mobilizing public support and stilling criticism.[7]

The lesson from transexualism is that professionals must sometimes assume the burden and responsibility of the ethics of a decision for which no custom or precedent exists. They must then assume the further responsibility of educating their colleagues and the general public about the rationale for and outcome of their decision. Left to chance, the professional and public response may too easily become negative. A positive strategy positively influences public opinion and policy in favor of the ethics of the new decision.

In the case of transexualism, the public attitude toward a variant form of sexuality became more open-minded. Prospectively, that change in public attitude was as important to me in planning (and risking) the first transexual operation at Johns Hopkins as was the improvement in well-being of the individual patient.

Today, as compared with 1965, I am not sure that transexual surgery could be introduced for the first time at Johns Hopkins. Here is yet another example of how, under the pressure and encroachment of bureaucratic regulations regarding ethics of informed consent, medical researchers and physicians have all too readily surrendered their own rights of informed consent with respect to innovative and investigative procedures and treatments. It is time to call a halt.

Clinical Research Plus Service

For me it has been an imperative that, when human beings are the subjects, clinical investigation must be combined with clinical service. The service may be as simple as reporting on and interpreting findings or as complex as providing a continuous referral-and-treatment program, which is of particular importance in longitudinal study, for example, of anomalies of gender-identity differentiation.

Provision of service builds in a guarantee that any untoward side effects, somatic or psychological, will not be missed and will be subject to remediation. It thus meets one of the needs of informed consent, namely, that concerned with possible risks. Moreover, it helps build a positive reciprocal relationship between investigator and subject (doctor and patient) and guards against attrition of patients during follow-up.

Provision of service extends beyond the specifics of a particular piece of research. It deals with the well-being of the subject in toto. In other words, one treats not only the lab results, nor the single organ system, but the person as an entirety. This means, in some instances, extension from the person to his or her relationship with a sexual partner, or a child or parent. Herein lies a potential advantage for research: In the case of an exhibitionist, sadist, or other paraphiliac, for example, a subtle degree of collusion exists between the sex offender and his partner. Contact with the partner is necessary if all the facts are to be known and if attempted treatment is to be effective. For example, an abused and martyred wife in collusion with her sadistically paraphilic husband, together with the therapist, can take steps to prevent her brutal injury and his imprisonment as a consequence. Thus, by working with both partners, one can circumvent ethical problems that might otherwise arise, for one is able to discharge one's ethical responsibilities jointly to each member of the partnership without betraying confidentiality.

References

1. Culliton, B. J. Patients' rights: Harvard is site of battle over X and Y chromosomes. *Science* 186:715-717, 1974.

2. Culliton, B. J. XYY: Harvard researcher under fire stops newborn screening. *Science* 188:1284-1285, 1975.

3. Franzke, A. Telling parents about XYY sons. *New England Journal of Medicine* 293:100-101, 1975.

4. Laschet, U. Antiandrogen in the treatment of sex offenders. Mode of action and therapeutic outcome. In J. Zubin and J. Money (eds.), *Contemporary Sexual Behavior: Critical Issues in the 1970's.* Baltimore: Johns Hopkins University Press, 1973.

5. Money, J., Wiedeking, C., Walker, P., Migeon, C., Meyer, W., and Borgaonkar, D. 47,XYY and 46,XY males with antisocial and/or sex-offending behavior. Antiandrogen therapy plus counseling. *Psychoneuroendocrinology* 1:165-178, 1975.

6. Money, J., and Ehrhardt, A. A. *Man and Woman, Boy and Girl: The Differentiation and Dimorphism of Gender Identity from Conception to Maturity.* Baltimore: Johns Hopkins University Press, 1972.

7. Money, J., and Schwartz, F. Public opinion and social issues in transsexualism: A case study in medical sociology. In R. Green and J. Money (eds.), *Transsexualism and Sex Reassignment.* Baltimore: Johns Hopkins University Press, 1969. Chap. 17.

Note

Originally published in *Ethical Issues in Sex Therapy and Research* (W. H. Masters, V. E. Johnson and R. C. Kolodny, eds.). Boston, Little, Brown, 1977. [Bibliog. #2.218]

FORTY-THREE

Sexual Dictatorship, Dissidence, and Democracy

Wrong Deeds and Wrong Ideas

It is not illegal to publish pictures or stories of actual murders, nor to depict murders on stage, in films or in television dramas, nor to narrate explicit murder scenes in books or magazine stories. A person must specifically substantiate a murder threat or actually commit the act before being arrested, accused and tried for murder. The law deals primarily with deeds and misdeeds and only secondarily with the mental state that engendered them. In fact, the law does not have good criteria for dealing with such mental states as knowing right from wrong, irresistible impulse, and planned intention versus fortuitous or provoked response. The law also lacks good criteria for dealing with treason and heresy, in both of which not deeds but ideology goes on trial.

Treason applies to the secular authority or political system, and heresy to the ecclesiastical authority or theological system. The two terms are not much used with contemporary reference, but what they stand for is by no means extinct in the running of society.

Today the Iron Curtain synonym for treason is Capitalism. In the west the synonym for treason is Communism, even though it carries much less force than it did in the United States in the days of Senator Joe McCarthy in the 1950s. Treason means to contravene the authority of the governing power by endorsing an opposing ideology, especially that of an enemy power.

The synonym for heresy in today's pluralistic and ecumenical theology is sex. In the church, heresy pertains to masturbation, contraception, abortion, legal prostitution, homosexuality, children's sexuality, women priests and married clergy.

Secularization of Sexual Heresy

In contemporary democratic states, the church's ecclesiastical authority to enforce doctrinal obedience and punish sexual heresy is limited by the secular authority of the judiciary. However, where ecclesiastical authority fails, secular authority succeeds. The law steps into the shoes vacated by the church and, wearing them, pursues with inquisitorial zeal the eradication of sexual heresy. The charges are the same and the indictment does not change. The only alteration is the secularization of the prosecuting authority. Defying redefinition, sexual heresy has survived the transfer of antiheretical authority and power of enforcement from church to state.

546

One's first impulse is to marvel that this astonishing sociological phenomenon could, indeed, have occurred. Pragmatically, it is not so astonishing, however, insofar as legal heresy hunters receive only their authority from the state, not their personal faith as to what moral sexosophy is dogma and what is heresy. Their faith is a direct legacy from the church transmitted through the common law, the statutes of the states and, above all, folk adherence, in the rearing of children, to sexual doctrine and taboo which is still the official teaching of the church.

Sociologically, there is an additional explanation of how the definition of sexual heresy has survived the transfer of antiheretical authority and power of enforcement from church to state. To an unknown degree, the church utilizes the methods of espionage as employed internationally by nation states and terrorists groups, and domestically by guerrilla movements and crime syndicates. That is to say, the church brings covert pressure to bear on its own members employed in positions of secular power, or educates its students to become superior candidates for appointment to positions of secular power. In Customs, for example, or Justice, or the Post Office, a high ranking official who understands the will of the church is able to assign priorities about what to investigate, what to seize, and what to prosecute.

So it is that the secular authority performs the inquisitional function of suppressing sexual heresy, and of dictating and censoring what the people should and should not know or do sexually. When a secular authority dictates, it becomes a dictatorship. We live today in a sexual dictatorship that restricts not only what people may do sexually, but also what they may read, see, hear, or otherwise have existing in their minds. Any deviation qualifies as secular heresy.

Legal Definition of Sexual Heresy

In a democracy, it is actually an embarrassment to the judiciary to have to arbitrate on what is sexually the secular equivalent of heresy and what is not. To do so infringes on the right of freedom of conscience and freedom of speech, and comes dangerously close to abrogating the principle of separation of church and state. In what follows, I use the United States as my example, simply because I know its system best. Unless you come from Denmark, you may substitute the name of your own country and you will not, by and large, be wrong. In the United States, the Supreme Court has for the most part evaded the basic constitutional issue of whether the federal judiciary may justifiably address itself to defining and regulating secular heresy with respect to sex. Instead, it has acted on a principle of decentralization that identifies sexual heresy as a local phenomenon, locally defined and locally regulated. Abortion, for example, is now a heresy, though only for poor people who have no money to pay for it, since local or regional authorities have the right to disqualify the use of public funds to pay for it. Likewise, the demand of civil rights for homosexuals must be argued locally, for the Supreme Court has, to date, declined to accept appeals from lower courts. The heresy of explicit erotica, otherwise known as obscenity and pornography, also clearly illustrates the Supreme Court's policy of sexual decentralization, as is evident in what follows.

According to what is now known as the Miller decision, the Supreme Court of the United States in 1973 updated its criteria of the obscene or pornographic in sex. The judge is the average man or woman in the role of member of the jury. The standard is that of the contemporary community, with no regional limits stated. The material to be decided upon is to be evaluated as a whole.

To qualify as obscene or pornographic, material should: 1) appeal to the prurient interest; 2) depict or describe sexual conduct in a patently offensive way; 3) lack serious literary, artistic, political, or scientific merit.

Etymologically, prurient means itching, and also to have longing for something. In contemporary usage, when the connotation of the longing is sexual, it is immoral or indecent. *Webster's Dictionary* defines prurient not as amative, romantic, or erotic, but as lustful, lewd, or lascivious. Here the law is blatantly tautological, for it connotes as indecent that which has prurient appeal, and prurience has the connotation of indecent appeal. To escape this logical trap, the courts have extended the definition of prurient to mean shameful and morbid appeal. This escape is illusory for average people. For example, heterosexual jury members do not consider the kind of sex that appeals to them to be shameful and morbid, but normal and healthy. Average people are heterosexual. Therefore heterosexual intercourse cannot be judged shameful and morbid, and hence as having prurient appeal. Paradoxically, it is erotic material which does not appeal to them, and perhaps even disgusts them, that average people are likely to classify as shameful and morbid. To whose prurient interest, then, does such material appeal? The only formula that the courts have devised to answer this question is to define a shameful and morbid appeal in terms of the presumptive target audience or readership to whom a given type of material is addressed. Homosexuals, for example, are defined as having a shameful and morbid interest in homosexual erotic materials. Homosexuality is thus, in effect, given the status of secular heresy, and so is any other form of sexual expression that does not conform to the ideology officially espoused, though not necessarily privately practised, by the members of the average jury.

Once erotic material has been declared shameful and morbid because of the special group, the heretics to whom it appeals, it is a foregone conclusion that, applying contemporary community standards, it will also be declared patently offensive to the average person.

In Hitler's Germany, Jews, dwarfs, and homosexuals were declared patently offensive to the average person, applying Hitler's contemporary community standards, and the average German condoned the extermination of millions of them. In an earlier century, at the height of the Inquisition, the average person had condoned the extermination of entire villages for the heresy of witchcraft. The average person all too often is wrong—just plain wrong!

Material that is adjudged shameful, morbid and patently offensive surely, it would seem, must lack serious literary, artistic, political, or scientific value. But such is not the case. All materials have scientific value for the scientists into whose speciality they fall. Thus, all sexual materials are of scientific value to the science of sexology. Likewise, their literary, artistic, or political value cannot be measured against absolute standards, for there are none. These values, like scientific value, are relative to the appraiser. Like beauty which resides in the eye of the beholder, and like color-blindness which is in the eye of the viewer, and not in the view, all values are intensely subjective and privately engendered. Values may be highly idiosyncratic or unusual, without being debased.

Jury Definition of Obscenity

There is no way in which the Supreme Court's attempt to define obscenity and pornography can be salvaged. It is flawed irreparably by the transcendental fallacy of defining good and bad not in terms of deeds performed, or their outcome, but in terms of mental states that have no exact definition and no dimensions by which to be measured—arousal of prurient interest, a feeling of offensiveness, and a judgment of literary, artistic, political, or scientific merit.

Normally a jury is required to weigh evidence as to whether an act was or was not committed, and under what circumstances. Not so in a pornography trial. There, in no more than a few days, and without preliminary study and preparation, a jury is imploded with information from expert witnesses that a graduate student would spend an entire semester digesting. Then, without a public-opinion poll as a guide to community standards, the jury must believe that its own subjective reactions are typical of the community at large.

What in fact the jury does do in defining obscenity and pornography is what all people do: it judges erotica material as obscene or pornographic if to read, hear, or see it breaks a taboo or prohibition formerly intensively inculcated, especially in childhood, and so creates a feeling of being sneaky and of doing something wrong. This judgment is made irrespective of the content of the tabooed and prohibitive material. The fact that the prohibition was insistently inculcated early in life is what counts. The sexual taboo in our society has great antiquity and is enormously powerful, pervasive, and broad in the scope of what it prohibits. It allows only a narrow range of human sexual expression that is doctrinally correct. All the rest is heresy. A jury usually has no difficulty, therefore, in bringing in a guilty verdict. With few exceptions, its verdict in effect brands all erotic material as heresy.

Sexual and Political Dissidence: Parallelism

The modern political name of heresy is dissidence. Dissident writings, graphics, or speeches may be defined as those which promulgate ideas which, taken as a whole, are adjudged by the average person applying contemporary community standards to have shameful and morbid appeal, to be patently offensive, and to lack serious literary, artistic, political and scientific merit. You perceive, of course, that this definition is identical with the definition of obscenity and pornography in the Supreme Court of the United States. It demonstrates an extraordinary parallelism between the United States and Russia, regarding ideological nonconformity, of which, I suspect, neither country is aware. The sexual dissident in the United States is the counterpart of the political dissident in Russia. Both are kept under police surveillance, and are subject to police harassment and entrapment. Both are arrested and brought to trial at enormous expense to the taxpayer. Both are subject to sanity tests and both may be sentenced to custody in either a psychiatric institution or a prison. Both are professionally dispossessed and cannot return to their former occupations. Both have their families economically ruined and morally traumatized. Both are defined as "Prisoners of Conscience" by Amnesty International insofar as, in 1977, the International Council of Amnesty International resolved that Prisoners of Conscience include persons detained or imprisoned because of sexual orientation or behavior, provided that those persons have not infringed the human rights of any other person. The reference to sexual orientation is in particular to homosexuality.

A further similarity between both types of dissident is that the materials they produce and publish do not disappear. They achieve subversive fame and circulate on an underground or black market. In some instances, especially regarding sexual materials, the black market may produce great wealth, and with it corrupt political power for the bootleggers of the crime syndicate which exploits it. Thus does society's persecution of the dissident boomerang disastrously upon itself, insofar as black-marketing inflates prices, and encourages blackmail, extortion, murder, and corruption of politicians and law enforcement officers. It also robs from the public purse billions of dollars in untaxable blackmarket revenue. In the United States, the history of Prohibition taught us that lesson with respect to alcohol, but we are poor students who fail to learn the lessons of history.

Harmfulness versus Wrongfulness

The prohibition of dissidence is often defended with arguments that amount to a belief in the social contagion of sinfulness. Monkey see, monkey do! This is the maxim of how wrong is perpetuated, always at the expense of righteousness. Belief in the social contagion of sinful sex is the residual survival of its inquisitional predecessor, belief in demonic possession. As a belief, and despite a total absence of empirical support, the contagiousness myth has exhibited extraordinary survival and power. The most likely reason is that any explanation is better than none when people are afraid—and they are afraid of difference, especially in those who differ sexually from themselves. Intolerance and persecution of nonconformity or difference, irrespective of its origin, is widespread in the animal kingdom. Both are overinclusive rather than individually discriminative. The harmless suffer with the harmful.

Harmfulness is a covert component of the idea of wrongfulness that people attribute to sexual nonconformity. Here again overinclusiveness characterizes the way people think. Society overreacts and labels too much as harmful, without checking the facts. Nonetheless, harmfulness cannot be dismissed altogether. Quite to the contrary! The concept of harm can be used to establish the dividing line between what society should and should not tolerate in the way of individual sexual nonconformity. Lust murder, for example, is out. So are violent rape, violent sadism, and forced pedophilia.

Sexual Harmfulness Defined

Harmful sexuality can be defined as nonconsensual, imposed, or enforced. It infringes upon the personal inviolacy of the partner. Spelled out in operational terms, an infringement of personal inviolacy means that the partner is unable to enter into a consensual relationship because the terms of the contract are not fully specified. The beginning does not predicate the end.

The principle of noninfringement of personal inviolacy is, like any statute or law, a broad generalization that needs to be applied and tested, case by case, in order to establish examples and precedents. Some cases are unambiguous, and the violator will always be subjected to detention or therapy, if therapy is available as, for example, combined antiandrogen-plus-counseling therapy for crimes of violent sex. Lust murder is an example, insofar as the victim does not predicate his or her death as the culmination of the sexual encounter. Violent sexual assault and mutilation are comparable. Logically, an exception may be argued in the case of a masochist who stage manages his own mutilation and death at the hands of a sadistic lust murderer who himself stage manages the uncertainty of whether he will be caught, or not. Such a case represents a rare and extreme type of reciprocal sadomasochism. Perfectly reciprocal matching of a couple in a pact of mutilation, suicide or murder of one or both partners is statistically difficult to achieve, and so it seldom challenges society. So long as the couple maintain total privacy, society is none the wiser. Society is alerted only when privacy is not maintained, either because the relationship is not perfectly reciprocal and one of the partners complains, or because a third party becomes discovered as a witness or accessory who fails to complain. If a hypothetical third party should make a movie of consensual sadomasochistic mutilation, suicide, or murder, then paradoxically, according to today's laws, it would qualify as illegal, not because it depicted mutilation and killing, but because it depicted exposed genitalia in action.

Paraphilic Themes

All of today's erotic movies that qualify as obscene and illegal earn that qualification because they depict the exposed genitals being used erotically. Normal heterosexual intercourse in a movie is condemned as obscene, but with less vehemence than if the movie also depicts a paraphilic theme, of which lust murder or mutilation are examples. In terminology that is now becoming obsolete, a paraphilia used to be known as a perversion or deviation, and in the vernacular, as bizarre or kinky sex. For many people, paraphilic imagery seems not only weird but also so repulsive that they want to get rid of it. They define it as socially dangerous and believe that it spreads by social contagion. As a test case, consider urophilia, a paraphilia which dictates that a person, almost invariably a man, will be able to get erotically aroused and be able to perform sexually to orgasm, only if his partner urinates on him and in his mouth. To its critics, this ritual seems filthy and disease-infecting, as well as repugnant. Repugnance and infection are not, however, the same thing. In actual fact, in healthy beings, urine is a sterile fluid. Many animals keep their babies clean by licking up their excreta. In Kenya, among the Masai, a major source of nourishment is a mixture of the milk, blood and urine of cows. In India, a former prime minister, Morarji R. Desai, drank some of his own urine each morning for medicinal purposes. Exposure to this information about ingestion of urine is powerless to turn those so exposed into urine drinkers, even if they read or hear it hundreds of times. Likewise, hundreds upon hundreds of exposures to urophilic narratives, pictures or movies will not convert a single person into being a urophiliac. None of the paraphilias is transmitted by social infection. Each paraphilia appeals only to a person who already has that same paraphilia. All the paraphilias have their origin in early childhood development, before puberty. A paraphilia is a developmental dissidence, and the prime suspect in the etiology of all paraphilias is excessive restriction of normal infantile and childhood sexual rehearsal play, plus excessive punishment for being caught at it. Restriction and punishment produce a sexual dissidence, which is then subject to more restriction and further punishment. The formula is repeated on the next generation, and so our ancient heritage of sexual taboo perpetuates itself with incredible tenacity.

Dictatorship versus Sexual Democracy

A taboo by its very nature always restricts something, like eating or sex, that human beings ordinarily do. The great taboos that human beings have devised for themselves pertain to eating, conversing, sex, elimination and disposal of the dead. They tend to be distributed regionally, and their origins are lost in pre-recorded history. They all have religious or sacred significance. The sexual taboo is not unique to the Judeo-Christian tradition, but was incorporated into it.

A taboo is inculcated into the members of a society in early childhood, according to the principle of avoidance or punishment learning. Infringement brings retribution, and establishes shame and guilt, which enables the taboo to maintain itself throughout life and to be transmitted to the next generation. Parents use shame and guilt to demand conformity from their children. Clerics do the same with their congregations, as do rulers with their subjects, and politicians with their voters.

Most politicians endorse the sexual taboo in our society. For example, when the Report of the National Commission on Obscenity and Pornography came before the U.S. Senate in 1970, the vote was 60-5 to reject it on the basis of a forewarning that it was not sufficiently condemnatory of explicit erotica.

Inchoately, politicians like parents realize their advantage in being able to manipulate the lever of guilt and shame in order to obtain conformity. A political or religious crusade to clean up smut is a Pied Piper's tune that sends voters flocking to the polls, eager to approve of anything the Piper dictates. Thus legislatures, like clerics, are loath to remove the last great barrier to full democratic freedom, the barrier against sexual democracy.

Democratic freedom is not, of course, equivalent to license. It does not mean anything goes. It means that sexual freedom is your birthright and mine, so long as it does not cross the dividing line of infringing on the personal inviolacy of the partner. Across that dividing line, the violator may in some cases be tolerated as an eccentric. In other cases he may be offered whatever medicine has to offer by way of its expanding therapeutics and rehabilitation. In only rare cases will the violation be so dangerous and the violator so unresponsive to nonincarcerative treatment that prolonged detention will be the only resort.

Today's politicians, attorneys, law-enforcement officials, news reporters, health professionals and researchers all in their various ways take advantage of sexual dictatorship and the suppression of sexual democracy. They thereby gain various combinations of notoriety, power, profit, and career advancement, unendangered by retaliation or reprisal. The public, if it does not overtly condone, apathetically bows under the yoke of the system; it lacks the factual knowledge with which to protest. Sexologists either have this knowledge, or else the skills with which to obtain it. With them rests the responsibility of transmitting this knowledge first to their fellow educators and clinical professionals, then to the news media, the law, the policy makers in politics, and the church, until finally it filters down to people everywhere.

To protest the status quo is to become a dissident oneself, victimized by the immense power of the social machinery of taboo maintenance. Some sexologists will find the status of protester too demanding. Some will scale sexology's Mt. Everest.

Note

Originally presented at a conference on Human Freedom and Sexuality, October, 1978, in Toronto; and incorporated, in part, into the opening address to the Third International Congress of Medical Sexology, Rome, October 25-28, 1978. This address was published untitled, in a report of the Congress in the *British Journal of Sexual Medicine,* 6(48):27ff., 1979; in translation, also untitled, into Dutch in the periodical, *Sekstant,* 2:25-27, 1979; and, under the title of "Ideas and Ethics of Psychosexual Determinism," in the proceedings of the Congress, *Medical Psychology* (R. Forleo and W. Pasini, eds.), Littleton, MA, PSG Publishing Company. The Italian translation of the proceedings was published by Feltrinelli, Milan, 1981. The version of the paper here reproduced was originally published in *The International Journal of Medicine and Law,* 1:11-20, 1979 (discontinued after Vol. I); and as a chapter in *Love and Love Sickness* (J. Money, Baltimore, Johns Hopkins University Press, 1980). [Bibliog. #2.237]

FORTY-FOUR

The Genealogical Descent of Sexual Psychoneuroendocrinology from Sex and Health Theory: The Eighteenth to the Twentieth Centuries

Abstract

In the aftermath of the Inquisition, secular health theory became separate from sacred health theory. Both assimilated vital spirits or sympathies as explanatory concepts. Sympathies were progressively transformed into internal secretions and the hormones of endocrinology. The sexual genealogy of psychoneuroendocrinology traces back to the sexual transplantation experiments of John Hunter (1728-93). Sexology, the science, has the same genealogy, whereas sexosophy, the philosophy, does not. In sexosophy, the theory that vital spirits or sympathies lost by masturbation caused debility or degeneracy became, along with health-food and exercise theories, popular in 19th-century health doctrine. Graham crackers and Kellogg's corn flakes were by-products of the diet/abstinence doctrine. With police power under the Comstock Law (1873), 19th-century sexosophy negated sexuality so effectively that human sexual psychoneuroendocrine research remains muffled and deprived of funds to this day.

Experimental Transplants

The genealogy of contemporary endocrine and psychoendocrine science began with sex and the gonads when, at some far-distant and unrecorded time, the effect of castration on domesticated animals and enslaved eunuchs was discovered. The first endocrine experiments also were sexual and involved the gonads. They were performed by John Hunter (1728-93), the renowned English anatomist and surgeon (Jørgensen, 1971).

Hunter devised the technique of surgical transplantation and demonstrated that the spur from the leg of a hen chick could be transplanted onto a cock chick's leg. There it would mature and attain the adult size of a cock's spur. Conversely, an immature cock's spur transplanted to a hen chick would attain only the smaller female size.

Hunter succeeded also in transplanting the cock testis into the abdominal cavity of the hen. Three of his anatomical specimens preserved in London's Hunterian Museum still testify to the success of his experiments. It is fortunate that they have survived, for Hunter did not report his experiments except in brief references and notes.

He may have considered his findings too incomplete to report, for he subsequently wrote that he had 'formerly transplanted the testicles of a cock into the
abdomen of a hen, and they had sometimes taken root there, but not frequently,
and then had never come to perfection'. Alternatively, he may have refrained
from reporting to avoid publicity and the possible accusation of witchcraft.
Fallout from the gruesome centuries of the Inquisition had still to be reckoned
with (the last witch was burned in Scotland in 1728)—and crowing hens and
sexually denatured beasts and men were signs of witchcraft.

Vital Spirits and Sympathies

The end of the Inquisition brought with it the end of demon possession as an
omnibus explanation of misfortunes, defeats, illnesses, plagues and other assorted woes of humankind. In matters of health, this marked a theoretical
watershed. On one side of the divide would flow the new secular stream of
scientific explanations of health and disease, and on the other, the traditional
sacred stream of theological explanations of health and disease.

The new secular heritage of Renaissance science became incorporated into
medical explanations of the 18th century. The four humors of Galenic medicine
gave way to vapors, vital spirits and sympathies. It was by way of sympathies
that intercommunication was postulated to take place between the various
organs of the body. Sympathies would eventually prove to be the conceptual
forebears of, *inter alia,* today's hormones and neurohormones.

Sympathies also would eventually give their name to the sympathetic nervous system. The life-regulating function of the nervous system was a prominent
principle in the physiology of William Cullen (1712-90) in Edinburgh, and of his
pupil, Benjamin Rush (1745-1813) in Philadelphia. Rush was influenced also by
two French physicians, Xavier Bichat (1771-1802) and his colleague, François
Broussais (1772-1832), who survived him. They postulated two nervous systems,
one that regulated the external life within the world, and one the internal life
within the self. They were, respectively, the animal (now known as the central)
nervous system (named after Erasistratus's 3rd-century B.C. teaching of Aris-
totle's animal spirit of the brain, vs. the vital spirit of the heart), and the organic
or vegetative (now known as the autonomic) nervous system. The former
functioned in conjunction with the special senses, and the latter with the internal
organs. For Broussais, the relationship of the gut to the 'great sympathetic nerve'
was the equivalent of that of the spinal cord to the animal nervous system.

The organic nervous system would, in the 20th century, become linked up
with sympathies, renamed first internal secretions and then hormones, from the
endocrine glands. However, the transmutation of sympathies into hormones was
slow.

Internal Secretions

Hunter's transplantation findings had no scientific progeny until 1849 when Arnold A. Berthold (1803-61) in Göttingen replicated them, and also showed that a testis implant in a capon would restore its precastration characteristics as a cock. Berthold concluded that something from the testis had affected the blood (Jørgensen, 1971). Berthold's experiments, like those of Hunter before him, proved difficult to replicate—no doubt because of the immune rejection phenomenon, which hindered the progress of endocrine science until a technique could be devised for preparing a glandular extract.

The first successful glandular extract was made not from the testis, but from the thyroid gland. G. R. Murray (1865-1939) reported the first use of an injection of thyroid extract for the treatment of hypothyroidism in 1891—with dramatic success. The concept of an internal secretion (Claude Bernard, 1813-78) was now empirically related to an internally secreting gland.

With thyroid extract Murray had succeeded with what Brown-Séquard (1817-94) had attempted with testicular extract. Before the Société de Biologie in Paris, in 1889, Brown-Séquard announced that, at the age of 72, he had been reinvigorated and rejuvenated by a series of six subcutaneous injections of a *liquid orchidique* over the course of two weeks (Olmsted, 1946). The liquid was an aqueous extract obtained from dog or guinea pig sperm, testis and testicular-vein blood. Despite his own attempt to guard against autosuggestion, he almost certainly was a victim of it. Later laboratory knowledge would prove that his aqueous extract was inert.

Despite the discredit that ultimately overtook Brown-Séquard's claim, the publicity gave great impetus to the concept of an internal secretion produced by the testis, and ensured that the idea would be pursued until the secretion was discovered.

Hormones

In the meantime, the concept of an internal secretion as a chemical messenger released into the bloodstream from glandular cells was formulated not with respect to the gonads, but to the duodenum. W. M. Bayliss (1860-1924) and E. H. Starling (1866-1927) in 1904 were responsible for naming this type of secretion a hormone. They called the hormone they had been working with secretin, a polypeptide released from the duodenal lining to govern the release of pancreatic juice and bile.

The successor of Brown-Séquard in the pursuit of what would eventually become known as male hormone, androgen, or testosterone, was Eugen Steinach, a teacher of Harry Benjamin (1885-   ) who is still living, aged 101. In 1910, Steinach took up again the implantation technique of Hunter and Berthold and, in so doing, also did the first modern experiment in sexual psychoendocrinology. He castrated neonatal male guinea pigs and then transplanted into them heterotypical gonadal tissue, thus achieving 'an intentional reversal of sex . . . with pronounced female sex characteristics and feminine psyche'. The quote is translated from the title of one of his reports (Benjamin, 1944; 1945).

Testicular implants were immunologically unsatisfactory for reinvigoration and rejuvenation of the aged. On the basis of experimental vasoligation of aging animals, Steinach developed the hypothesis, and in 1920 published his findings to the effect, that the vasoligated testis undergoes tubular degeneration with compensatory interstitial-cell hypertrophy and a consequent increase in hormonal output and rejuvenation.

Steinach's rejuvenation theory was both acclaimed and ridiculed. Many older people, some of them wealthy and famous, underwent the 'Steinach operation'. Among them was Freud (1856-1939) who confided to Benjamin (1945) that he thought its effect had been beneficial, perhaps even on his cancer of the jaw.

Even while being ridiculed, the claim of rejuvenation through vasoligation did help to weaken the stringency of the Victorian sexual taboo, by generating public discussion of sex. Covertly, it set the stage for further public endorsement and support of sex and sex-hormonal research.

After 1920, Steinach's focus on research became less on surgical and physiological endocrinology and more on hormonal biochemistry. He was responsible for Progynon, the first commercially marketed estrogenic extract. In the 1920s, the search for the hormones that regulated the female cycle went on apace in several different centers—the modern age of laboratory endocrinology had begun. Estrogen and progesterone were named, along with testosterone, and were isolated in purified form. Next, their chemical formulas were determined. By 1934, A. F. Butenandt (1903-   ) had worked out the formula for testosterone, and the modern era of sex-hormone therapy began.

Hormones and Behavior

In the 1930s, some psychology texts began to suggest the possibility that the secretions of the ductless, or endocrine, glands would one day prove to be a key to the understanding of instinctual drives and behavior. This homage to hormones was perfunctory, however. Psychology was not a respectable science in those days. Nor was psychiatry, which was just on the verge of its Freudian era. The relationship of endocrinology and psychology was something of a standoff— or at least of mutual indifference.

A psychoendocrine rapprochement began to appear in the 1950s. Geoffrey W. Harris (1913-71) moved endocrinology toward psychology and behavior. Speaking for myself (John Money, 1921-   ), I moved psychology and behavior toward endocrinology. Harris began exploring the site of neurohormonal action in the brain, notably in the region of the hypothalamus, with respect to its effect not only on pituitary secretions, but also on the release of sexual behavior. In the development of psychoneuroendocrinology, it was once again the sexual system that was in the forefront—not only in Harris's animal experimental research, but in human clinical studies also.

My approach to sexual psychoendocrinology had been human and clinical. It began in pediatric endocrinology* in a psychohormonal research unit for the longitudinal study of behavioral and psychological development of children with a history of endocrine disorder. One early, long-range study was of a sexual disorder, the congenital form of virilizing adrenal hyperplasia that in fetal life in girls induces female hermaphroditism. This syndrome became hormonally treatable for the first time in 1950, after the discovery and synthesis of the glucocorticoids. Thus, over the long term, it became feasible to investigate the effect of prenatal, as well as postnatal, hormonalization on behavior related to gender status (Money & Lewis, 1966; Money, 1974).

Sexology and Sexosophy

The sex-dimorphic names given to the sex steroids when they were first isolated in the 1920s has had far-reaching consequences for the development of psychoneuroendocrine theory. It has proved all but irresistible to attribute to male hormones the power to cause male behavior, and to female hormones the power to cause female behavior, whereas, in fact, men and women share both sets of hormones. It is their ratio that differentiates men and women, not their absolute presence or absence. This relativity, though not explicitly denied in principle, is often not applied in research practice, for the stereotype of an absolute male/female dimorphism, behavior included, is so grounded in the stereotypes of folk wisdom that it is simply taken for granted. This obedience of the stereotype is obedience also to the principles of social sexosophy, not to the principles of scientific sexology.

Sexology is the science of sex, and modern scientific sexual endocrinology is one of its major divisions. Sexosophy is the doctrine of sex pertaining to the dogmas, beliefs, values and laws regarding sex in personal or group life. Psychoneuroendocrinology does have a sexosophy, implicitly if not explicitly, and it is still deeply rooted in the more general sexosophy extant in society at large. This general sexosophy has its own history—the history of the sacred side of the watershed, opposite that on which John Hunter was an early exponent of secular sexology, the science.

---

*The psychohormonal unit originated in the Pediatric Endocrine Clinic, the first of its type anywhere, which had been established on a full-time basis by Lawson Wilkins, M.D., in 1946.

The Sin of Onan

In the Inquisitional sexosophy of demon possession, it was the sinfulness of the witch possessed that made her responsible for having cohabited with the devil or one of his demons—or, more accurately, for having done so in a dream falsely confessed under torture. The sin of the witch was the sin of sexual imagination. In the theology of the era, it caused disease, suffering and death. In the theology of the 18th century, their causes also would be sexual, namely, the sin of onanism. This new theory was an improvement over demonic possession, insofar as one could be admonished or coerced to cease masturbating, whereas for demon possession the only cure was by being burned to death at the stake.

Though the sin named for Onan (Genesis 38:9) was actually coitus interruptus, onanism became a synonym for spilling the seed instead of using it for procreation. 'Self-pollution' began *Onania,* an anonymous tract published in London early in the 1700s, 'is that unnatural Practice, by which Persons of either Sex, may defile their own Bodies, without the Assistance of others, whilst yielding to filthy Imaginations, they endeavour to imitate and procure to themselves that Sensation, which God has order'd to attend the carnal Commerce of the two Sexes, for the Continuance of our Species'.

Onania; or the Heinous Sin of Self-Pollution, and All its Frightful Consequences, in both Sexes, Considered. With Spiritual and Physical Advice to those, who have already injur'd themselves by the Abominable Practice was published in Boston in 1724 as a reprinting of the tenth London edition. In style it was a sermon, expounding an absolute dogma and proving it with written testimonials and confessions of the corruptions of the heinous sin.

There was no limit to the list of the corruptions of the body attributed to onanism. Palsies, distempers, consumptions, gleets, fluxes, ulcers, fits, madness, childlessness—all the syndromes of the day were included, even death itself. The common denominator was debility, brought on by the loss of semen. It could affect offspring. They were born sickly and ailing, and died or became a dishonor to the human race.

The equation of conservation of semen with conservation of strength has great antiquity as a folk belief, and it is still widely disseminated in ethnic Asia and Africa. It appears in the writings of Hippocrates, and in the texts of ancient Ayurvedic medicine still in use in India. In *Onania,* a new refinement appeared: in the testicular tubules, 'the Blood is made into Seed, which is further elaborated and purify'd in the Epidydimides . . . the oftner the Vesiculae Seminales are emptied, the more work is made for the Testicles, and consequently the greater Consumption of the finest and most Balsamick part of the blood'.

Degeneracy Theory

Debility theory was more or less tangential in *Onania.* In the 1750s, it became transformed into the more systematic theory of degeneracy *(dégénérescence)* by the Swiss physician, Simon André Tissot (1728-97). After several French editions, Tissot's *Treatise on the Diseases Produced by Onanism* was published in English in New York in 1832.

In the tradition of his day, Tissot relied on citing authority rather than empirical evidence. Thus he quoted 'one of the greatest men of his age' (unidentified) on the power of semen retained in the seminal vesicles: '. . . it excites the sexual desires of the animal; but the greatest part, the most volatile, the most odorous, that which has the most power, is resumed by the blood, and produces on entering it, remarkable changes, the hairs and the beard; it alters the voice and the manners, for age does not produce these changes in animals; they are caused by the semen alone, as they never occur in eunuchs'.

To be logically systematic, Tissot needed to fit women into onanistic degeneracy theory. He wrote:

> The symptoms which supervene in females, are explained like those in men. The secretion which they lose, being less valuable and less matured than the semen of the male, its loss does not enfeeble so promptly, but when they indulge in it to excess, as their nervous system is naturally weaker and more disposed to spasms, the symptoms are more violent. Sudden excesses produce symptoms similar to those of the young man mentioned above, and we have seen a case of this kind. In 1746, a prostitute, twenty-three years of age, had connected in a single night with six Spanish dragoons near Montpelier. The next morning she was brought into the city in a dying state; she expired in the evening bathed in uterine hemorrhage which flowed in a constant stream. (p. 45.)

To be systematic, Tissot found reasons why seminal loss in masturbation was more pernicious than in coition. He attributed to Sanctorius (1561-1636) the idea that when the seminal vesicles were not semen-filled, imagination and habit could more easily excite masturbation and thereby not only deprive nature of what was necessary for her healthful operations in coition, but also, as imagination always does, enfeeble all the faculties of the mind, and particularly the memory. His most irrefutable argument, however, relied upon the *torrens invisibles:*

> The exhalant vessels of the skin exhale at every instant an extremely thin fluid . . . at the same time another kind of vessels admit a part of the fluids which surround the body and carry them into the other vessels. These are the *torrens invisibles,* which leave our bodies and enter them again . . . These observations explain how the young woman with whom David slept, gave him strength . . . A person perspires more during coition than at any other time. This perspiration is perhaps more active and more volatile than at any other time: it is a real loss, and occurs whenever emissions of semen take place, from whatever cause, since it depends on the agitation attending it. In coition it is reciprocal, and the one inspires, what the other expires. This exchange has been verified by certain observations. In masturbation there is a loss without this reciprocal benefit. (pp. 50-1.)

Despite the virtues of coition, long periods of abstinence were strongly recommended as a health measure in marriage. The ancient theological doctrine of sex for procreation, not for passion, was now medically endorsed.

Intemperance and Debility

In conformity with the medical conventions of his time, Tissot offered proof of his assertions in anecdotal case examples and by citing authorities. His American translator, in an appendix to the American edition of 1832, cited a leading figure in American medicine, Benjamin Rush (aforementioned), as offering scholarly justification of his having presented Tissot's sexual degeneracy theory of disease in translation:

> This appetite, which was implanted in our natures for the purpose of propagating our species, when excessive, becomes a disease of both the body and the mind, . . . [Rush had written]. When restrained, it produces tremors, a flushing of the face, sighing, nocturnal pollutions, hysteria, a hypochondriasis, and in women the furor uterinus. When indulged in an undue or a promiscuous intercourse with the female sex, or in onanism, it produces seminal weakness, impotence, dysury, tabes dorsalis, pulmonary consumption, dyspepsia, dimness of sight, vertigo, epilepsy, hypochondriasis, loss of memory, manalgia, fatuity and death. (p. 109.)

In formulating his own theory of disease, Rush was influenced by his predecessors, Tissot included, as well as by his contemporaries, Bichat and Broussais (see above). He formulated a substitute for the doctrine of bloodletting, according to which George Washington had been bled to death at the age of 67 in 1799. Rush taught that there was only one disease, namely, different forms of morbid excitement induced by irritants acting upon a previous debility. Debility increased susceptibility to morbid excitement or erethism. Debility itself could be indirect and induced by overstimulation or direct and induced by understimulation (Nissenbaum, 1980).

There were three great intemperances, each with its own prior history in medical doctrine, that produced debility: intemperance in eating and drinking; intemperance in bodily fitness and insufficient exercise; and intemperance in sex. Alcohol and tobacco use in any amount was, by definition, intemperate. The corresponding three great principles of health pertained to proper diet, proper exercise and proper sex.

Commercialization

As a product of medical scholarship, degeneracy theory achieved its most sophisticated expression as formulated by Rush. It survived chiefly in its practical applications until, in 1876-7, it was rendered out of date by the discoveries of

Louis Pasteur (1822-95) and Robert Koch (1843-1910) that established the germ theory of disease. Thereafter, it survived only as a popularized and commercialized medical doctrine.

Its first popularizer was Sylvester Graham (1794-1851), a preacher and health reform zealot who began his public career in 1830, as a lecturer for the Pennsylvania Temperance Society. Ralph Waldo Emerson (1803-82), as quoted by Nissenbaum (1980), dubbed him the prophet of bran bread and pumpkins, because of his fanatical vegetarianism and obsession with the virtues of home-grown, home-milled, home-baked wholewheat bread as an all-purpose health food. (Graham's name has been handed down to posterity as the eponym for Graham flour and Graham crackers). His dietary regimen, especially avoidance of meat and 'high-seasoned food' was, however, integral to his doctrines of exercise and sexual abstinence. He claimed that it promoted physical and mental vigor and remedied morbid concupiscence and prurience of the imagination (Graham, 1834).

Historically, Kellogg's corn flakes were a second-generation descendant of Graham flour. The first generation was a health-food product, Granula, marketed early in the 1860s by James Caleb Jackson (1814-95), proprietor of a health institute, Our Home on the Hillside, in Dansville, in rural upstate New York. Granula was a baked brown flour and water wafer, broken up and rebaked. It was the original cold breakfast cereal, served in warm milk, not very tasty, and not a commercial success.

In 1878, a rival product, Granula, that later was changed to Granola*, was marketed by John Harvey Kellogg (1852-1943), medical director of the Battle Creek Sanitarium, run by the then new Seventh Day Adventist sect. Kellogg had been trained in the Grahamite tradition and was a zealous adherent of Graham's dietary, fitness and sexual doctrines. Jackson took Kellogg to court for infringement of patent rights and won. Kellogg went on experimenting in the nutrition laboratory attached to the kitchen of his Sanitarium, and came up with corn flakes. By 1898 he manufactured them on a small scale as a health food, in the Grahamite tradition, as an adjunct to abstinence and chastity. In 1906 his younger brother, Will Keith Kellogg, took over the firm, sweetened corn flakes with sugar, and made a fortune.

Antisexualism

In the years following 1840, the year of Graham's retirement, the tide of antisexual books on advice for young men, women, husbands and wives became a veritable publication flood. Kellogg spent his honeymoon in 1879 writing *Plain Facts for Old and Young: Embracing the Natural History and Hygiene of Organic Life*. It went through many editions and revisions and, in expanded

---

*In the 1960s the term Granola was revived as the name of a health-food cereal product which continues to be commercially popular.

form, was reissued in the early 1900s as far away as India and Australia. For sheer professional arrogance and anachronistic disregard of scientific medical knowledge even in its later editions, it is unsurpassed in medical nonsense (see Appendix). It luridly described all the diseases caused by masturbation, including consumption—with the effect that families hid their afflictions rather than disclose the sin of masturbation by seeking treatment.

The antisexualism of which Kellogg was so prestigious an exponent had immense police power to suppress dissent under the federal Comstock Law of 1873. Anthony Comstock (1884-1915), its originator, was a Y.M.C.A. crusader against vice and obscenity. He became the chief postal inspector and censor of sexual materials, including information on contraception, sent in the U.S. mail.

Beyond Antisexualism

The death knell of Victorian antisexualism was sounded in Philadelphia in 1876, at the nation's Centennial Exposition, but its significance was unrecognized at the time. There the public saw a rubber condom, on display for the first time ever, which was made possible by the technology of vulcanizing rubber. Though slow and tentative in its first fifty years, the birth control era had begun. It had immense repercussions for women's rights and for a reshaping of the traditions of the sexual and breeding relationship. It also opened the door for the entry of sexual medicine, beginning with sexual endocrinology, into medical science of the 20th century.

The phenomenon of cultural lag is plentifully in evidence, however. Victorian sexosophy still exerts its effect on sexual psychoneuroendocrinology. The neuroendocrine part of this conjoined discipline is now scientifically respectable, whereas the psycho-behavioral part is not, at least in human investigation. The latter is poorly funded. It is still stigmatizable as obscene and degenerate. To be too closely associated with it depletes, if not one's vital spirits, then one's professional status.

It is time for a change, though its occurrence may be contingent on the formulation of a new theory, one that does not split mind and behavior from body and biomedical science. This split presently divides psychoneuroendocrine scientists into those who deal with the erotosexual from those who deal with the reproductosexual. It denies them a unitary universe of discourse in which to work, each using a common scientific language and syntax and together advancing clinical and laboratory sexual psychoendocrinology as an undivided science.

Acknowledgment

Supported by U.S.P.H.S. Grants HD 00325 and HD 07111.

References

Anon. (1724) *Onania; or, the Heinous Sin of Self-Pollution, and All its Frightful Consequences, in both Sexes, Considered. With Spiritual and Physical Advice to those, who have already injur'd themselves by this Abominable Practice.* John Phillips, Boston, Mass. Facsimile reprint in *The Secret Vice Exposed!* Arno Press, New York (1974).

Benjamin, H. (1944) Eugen Steinach—a tribute. *Proc. Rudolph Virchow Med. Soc.* 3, 88-92.

Benjamin, H. (1945) Eugen Steinach, 1861-1944; A life of research. *Scient. Mon.* 61, 427-442.

Graham, S. (1834) *A Lecture to Young Men.* Cory, Providence. Facsimile reprint. Arno Press, New York (1974).

Jørgensen, C. B. (1971) *John Hunter, A. A. Berthold, and the Origins of Endocrinology.* Odense University Press, Odense, Denmark.

Kellogg, J. H. (1888) *Plain Facts for Old and Young: Natural History and Hygiene of Organic Life.* I. F. Segner, Burlington, Iowa. Facsimile reprint. Arno Press, New York (1974).

Kellogg, J. H. (1908) *Ladies Guide in Health and Disease: Girlhood, Maidenhood, Wifehood, Motherhood.* Signs of the Times, Warburton (Australia), London, Cape Town and Calcutta.

Money, J. & Lewis, V. (1960) IQ, genetics, and accelerated growth: Adrenogenital syndrome. *Bull. Johns Hopkins Hosp.* 118, 365-373.

Money, J. (1974) Prenatal hormones and postnatal socialization in gender identity differentiation. In *Nebraska Symposium on Motivation, 1973,* J. K. Cole and R. Dienstbier (eds.), University of Nebraska Press, Lincoln.

Murray, G. R. (1891) Note on the treatment of myxoedema by hypodermic injection of an extract of the thyroid gland of a sheep. *Br. Med. J.* 2, 796-797.

Nissenbaum, S. (1980) *Sex, Diet, and Debility in Jacksonian America: Sylvester Graham and Health Reform.* Greenwood Press, Westport, Conn.

Olmsted, J. M. D. (1946) *Charles-Édouard Brown-Séquard: A Nineteenth Century Neurologist and Endocrinologist.* Johns Hopkins Press, Baltimore, Maryland.

Tissot, S. A. (1832) *Treatise on the Diseases Produced by Onanism.* Collins & Hannay, New York. Facsimile reprint in *The Secret Vice Exposed!* Arno Press, New York (1974).

Appendix: Kellogg on Masturbation

The following excerpts from the 1888 revised edition of Kellogg's *Plain Facts for Old and Young* illustrate his antimasturbation doctrine:

Influence of Stimulants—The use of stimulants of any kind is a fruitful cause of the vice. Tea and coffee have led thousands to perdition in this way. The influence of tobacco is so strongly shown in this direction that it is doubtful if there can be found a boy who has attained the age of puberty, and has acquired the habit of using tobacco, who is not addicted to this vile practice. Candies, spices, cinnamon, cloves, peppermint, and all strong essences powerfully excite the genital organs, and lead to the same result.

It should be further added that there is evidence that a powerful predisposition to this vice is transmitted to the children of those who have themselves been guilty of it. [pp. 244-5]

The Race Ruined by Boys—The human race is growing weaker year by year. The boys of to-day would be no match in physical strength for the hale, sturdy youths of a century ago, their great-grandparents. An immense amount of skillful training enables now and then one to accomplish some wonderful feat of walking, rowing, or swimming; but we hear very little of remarkable feats of labor accomplished by our modern boys. Even the country boys of to-day cannot endure the hard work which their fathers did at the same age; and we doubt not that this growing physical weakness is one of the reasons why so large a share of the boys whose fathers are farmers, and who have been reared on farms, are unwilling to follow the occupation of their fathers for a livelihood. They are too weakly to do the work required by an agricultural life, even by the aid of the numerous labor-saving inventions of the age.

What is it that is undermining the health of the race, and sapping the constitutions of our American men? No doubt much may be attributed to the unnatural refinements of civilization in several directions, but there can be no doubt that vice is the most active cause of all. Secret sin and its kindred vices ruin more constitutions every year than hard work, severe study, hunger, cold, privation, and disease combined. [pp. 345-6]

Suspicious Signs—The following symptoms, occurring in the mental and physical character and habits of a child or young person, may well give rise to grave suspicions of evil, and should cause parents or guardians to be on the alert to root it out if possible. [There follows thirty-nine paragraphs of text, of which only the subheadings are reproduced here.]

General debility; early symptoms of consumption; premature and defective development; sudden change in disposition; lassitude; an unnatural dullness and vacantness of the eyes; sleeplessness; failure of mental capacity; fickleness, untrustworthiness; love of solitude; bashfulness; unnatural boldness; mock piety; easily frightened; confusion of ideas; aversion to the other sex, or its opposite, wantonness; round shoulders; weak backs, pains in the limbs, and stiffness of the joints; paralysis; gait; bad positions in bed; lack of development of the breasts; capricious appetite; extreme fondness for unnatural, hurtful, and irritating foods; eating clay, slate-pencils, plaster, and chalk; disgust for simple food; the use of tobacco; unnatural paleness; acne, or pimples; biting the finger nails; sunken eyes, with red edges, soreness and dark rings; habitually moist, cold hands; palpitation of the heart; hysteria; chlorosis, or green sickness; epileptic fits; wetting the bed; unchastity of speech. [pp. 249-59]

(For girls, two other suspicious signs appeared in *The Ladies Guide* (1908): "Ulceration about the roots of the nails, especially affecting one or both of the first two fingers of the hand, usually the right hand, is an evidence of the habit which depends upon the one just mentioned, the irritation of the finger being occasioned by the acrid vaginal discharge.

"Biting the finger-nails is a habit, which, when very marked, may be regarded with some degree of suspicion. The irritation of the fingers which gives rise to the habit, grows out of the irritable condition of the nails described in the preceding paragraph.") [p. 152]

Kellogg continues in *Plain Facts:*

Cure of the Habit— . . . Through the courtesy of Dr. Archibald, Superintendent of the Iowa Asylum for Feeble-Minded Children we have become acquainted with a method of treatment of this disorder which is applicable in refractory cases, and we have employed it with entire satisfaction. It consists in the application of one or more silver sutures in such a way as to prevent erection. The prepuce, or foreskin, is drawn forward over the glans, and the needle to which the wire is attached is passed through from one side to the other. After drawing the wire through, the ends are twisted together, and cut off close. It is now impossible for an erection to occur, and the slight irritation thus produced acts as a most powerful means of overcoming the disposition to resort to the practice.

In females, the author has found the application of pure carbolic acid to the clitoris an excellent means of allaying the abnormal excitement, and preventing the recurrence of the practice in those whose will-power has become so weakened that the patient is unable to exercise entire self-control. [pp. 295-6]

Note

Originally published in *Psychoneuroendocrinology*, 8:391-400, 1983. [Bibliog. #2.270]

FORTY-FIVE

Sexosophy and Sexology, Philosophy and Science: Two Halves, One Whole

Abstract

In today's world, truth is no longer the exclusive criterion by which science is judged. It must also pass a moral and aesthetic test. Biomedical and social science research using human subjects must conform to the standards of an unnamed body of information utilized by an institutional ethics review board. For the new science of sexology, the new name for this body of information is sexosophy. Sexosophy comprises the philosophy, principles, and knowledge that people have about their own personally experienced erotosexuality and that of other people, singly and collectively. It includes values, personal and shared, and it encompasses culturally transmitted value systems. Its subdivisions are historical, regional, ethnic, religious, and developmental or life-span. The customs and traditions of a culture's sexosophy are idiographically learned and grafted into their phylogenetic roots. The organ of conjunction is the human brain. Taboo is a pivotal principle around which all else sexosophical revolves. The sexual taboo is of great antiquity and widespread across the globe. It relates to the ancient concept of the bride as a chattel of the male lineage. It has led to a contemporary polarization of the madonna and the whore, the paterfamilias and the playboy, and of love above the belt and lust below the belt. Three subdivisions of the sexual taboo pertain to restrictions imposed on relationships according to the criteria of age-discrepancy, degree of familiarity or intimacy, and male/female discrepancy, respectively. The age-avoidancy taboo restricts communication between people discordant for age. It greatly hinders sex education and is disastrous for research into child sexology. The intimacy-avoidancy taboo makes a person disclosing intimate erotosexual self-data vulnerable to blackmail or vengeance, and so hinders research. The allosex-avoidancy taboo imposes segregation of males and females and limits the amount of their shared erotosexual information and experience. Its restrictions on research can be circumvented if male and female sexologists work conjointly. Longitudinal sexological research needs institutional support and funding, for without developmental foundations in fetal life and childhood, sexology will be an incomplete and inadequate science. Organized sexology should not wait for another lone Kinsey to defy the establishment, but should itself take on the founding, funding, and political defense of the sexology of childhood.

Truth, Aesthetics, Ethics

Science and technology, the pure and the applied, are a familiar juxtaposition in the idiom of physics and chemistry, the so-called hard sciences. Pure science is basic. Its metaphysical foundation is truth, and truth is exclusively the criterion by which its value is, and traditionally has been judged. Applied science, technology, is utilitarian. Its metaphysical foundation is power, economic and political power, by which criterion alone its value is and traditionally has been judged.

Until very recently, scientific truth and technological power paid no homage to aesthetics and ethics, two other great categories of metaphysical value-judgment. As recently as in the youth of my own career, it was the boast and the vanity of pure science that its singleminded dedication to truth needed no other justification. All that has changed now. The champions of ecology and the environment are as much the adversaries of pure science as they are of technology. They command pure science to put its entire house in order, and to pay attention not only to its technological applications, but also to its ethical and aesthetical implications. Ethics boards are now arbiters of all biomedical and social science research employing human subjects, their fluids, or their tissues.

Sexosophy Defined

There is no single term for the body of ethical and aesthetic knowledge that belongs to each science. Scientists have, therefore, been obliged to borrow conceptions of their own ethics and aesthetics from theologians and moralists. In this respect, science in general may have something to learn from, in particular, sexology, one of its infant progeny. Sexology was borne of moral philosophy and theology so recently that it is still, to paraphrase William Wordsworth, trailing clouds of glory whence it came. These clouds of genesis need a name, and that name should properly be sexosophy.[5] Sexosophy comprises the philosophy and the moral principles of the male/female relationship. Sexology is the science of that relationship.

Sexology is defined as that body of knowledge that comprises the science of sex, or, more precisely, of the differentiation and dimorphism of sex and of the erotosexual pairbonding of partners. Its primary data are behavioral-psychological and somatic, and its primary organs are the genitalia, the skin, and the brain. The scientific subdivisions of sexology are: genetic, morphologic, hormonal, neurohormonal, neuroanatomical, neurochemical, pharmacologic, behavioral, sociocultural, conceptive-contraceptive, gestational-parturitional, and parental sexology. The life-cycle subdivisions of sexology are: embryonal-fetal, infantile, child, pubertal, adolescent, adult, and geriatric sexology.[5]

Sexosophy is defined as that body of knowledge that comprises the philosophy, principles and knowledge that people have about their own personally experienced erotosexuality and that of other people, singly and collectively. It includes values, personal and shared, and it encompasses culturally transmitted value systems. Its subdivisions are historical, regional, ethnic, religious, and developmental or life-span.[5]

Every system of sexosophy can be analyzed according to rules of pairbonding and reproduction that pertain to: age, same or different; physique, juvenile, adolescent or adult; sex, same or different; kinship, related or not by genealogy, clan, or race; caste/class, same or different; number, unity or plurality of partnerships; overlap, single or multiple partnerships sequentially or concurrently; span, casual or constant partnerships; organs, genital or nongenital; privacy, public or concealed behavior; fertility, promoted or curtailed with contraceptive devices, surgery or abortion; accessory erotic artifacts (sex toys), permitted or prohibited; public disclosure, partnerships overt or covert; training, explicit and illustrated instruction accepted or rejected; and outcome, recreation or procreation.[6]

The conceptual distinction between the two bodies of knowledge, one sexosophical and the other sexological, let alone between the two terms by which they are named, is not yet established in professional usage. The confusion of the two may well be, at least in part, a legacy of Hitler's denunciation and extermination of European sexological institutions and libraries as pornographic and obscene. In English, sexology became an under-the-counter term, opprobrious and lewd. For science it was respectably paraphrased as sexual behavior (Kinsey), sexual response and inadequacy (Masters and Johnson) and human sexuality (Calderone). Human sexuality has become something of a catchword, combining sexological science and sexosophical doctrine, defined by those who use it only diffusely and by assumption.

History, ethnic tradition and religion mold the sexosophy of a people or region. Sexology, the science, to be comprehensively complete, must have no limit on the number of sexosophical variations it can accommodate. Sexology, however, extends far beyond comparative sexosophy. Sexology is not limited to being only a social science. Hermeneutically, it does not exist as ideation, imagery, and behavior only, independently of its other components—genetic, hormonal, morphological, vascular, neural, neurotransmitter, neuroendocrine, pharmacologic, et cetera. Its determinants are multivariate. They are also sequential in their effects, thus creating a complexity that defies simple cause-effect analysis, and requires complex computer programs of statistical analysis that have not yet been devised.

The data of sexology are generated as much between the ears as between the groins—mind-sex and body-sex. The brain is the organ where both conjunct, where erotosexual ideation, imagery, and behavior form a union with physiology. The penis and the vulva are very long organs! They quite literally reach up to the brain. There, at the centrum, messages are sent to, and received from the periphery, via the spinal cord; and there the genitalia, the organs of copulation, have their governance. It is there, in the brain that ontogeny and phylogeny meet; there that the social customs and traditions of sexosophy are assimilated and fused with one's species' heritage. In the brain sociopsychophysiomatic and/or somatophysiopsychosocial are one!

Sexosophy and Taboo

The definitive textbook of the sexosophy of Western culture, when it is written, must accede that the sex taboo is a pivotal principle around which all else sexosophical revolves.

Among the peoples of earth, the manifestations of taboo are five-fold. Each applies to one of the fundamental functions of being: talking, eating, eliminating, reproducing, and disposing of the dead. The chief among these is reproducing: the sex taboo covers more of the earth than all four others combined.

A taboo is an arbitrary restriction or set of restrictions on something that human primates, if not subjected to that restriction, would ordinarily develop to do. Subhuman primates and other mammals prohibit and punish certain types of behavior in their young; but human beings alone have institutionalized prohibition and punishment into taboo.

The prehistoric origin of taboo is lost along with those who created it, but the dynamic of its effectiveness persists. This is a three-phase dynamic of authoritarian power: denunciating, making guilty, and controlling allegiance. Taboo is transmitted from one group to another—from the missionary to the heathen, for example, or more typically from the older generation to the younger. Some recipients of taboo's denunciations and restrictions may be rebelliously defiant. The majority, if noncompliant, suffer guilt and shame, which eventually ensures complete compliance and allegiance. A lever of domination is thus installed. It is transferable. It can, for example, be transferred from parent to teacher, preacher, cult leader or political leader. Eventually, compliancy becomes so complete that it makes of the person a new recruit enlisted in the service of taboo enforcement. By the same principle, the abused becomes the abuser.

The sexosophy of our Western culture is at odds with itself regarding the sexual taboo in infancy and childhood. On the one hand it declares childhood to be the age of innocence which must be guarded from contamination from the serpent that brought about the downfall of Adam and Eve. On the other hand, it declares that Adam's sin, and Eve's, cause all of today's children to be born in original sin and to have a disposition to transgress. They must be watched for signs of transgression, namely, species typical erotosexual rehearsal play, i.e. play that involves the genitals, sexual positioning, and erotic stimulation. This kind of play is typical in primates. It is essential to healthy erotosexual development. Its prohibition, prevention, and punishment in children amounts to what is, indeed, a form of child abuse.

The Janus Face of Love and Lust

A taboo is always Janus-faced. It must permit some manifestation of the behavior it simultaneously restricts. Otherwise, both the form and the substance of the taboo would become extinct. To illustrate, an absolutely complete sexual taboo would leave no progeny to practice the taboo.

The Janus-face of our sexual taboo has a very long history of association with the abuse of the female as a chattel of the male lineage—first the lineage of her father, and then the lineage of the male to whom she became assigned in marriage.[7] The marriage was a contract to unite wealth and power in the two lineages, as well as to copulate and produce progeny.[3] For both the husband and the wife, copulation was a reproductive obligation, to be performed perfunctorily, if not with passion. If perfunctory for the wife, then she had no alternative but to tolerate it. If perfunctory for the husband, however, then the system provided him with other possible options, one being concubinage (etymology: with + to lie down). His concubine would be a lover whose lineage made her ineligible for marriage, but whose support he could provide in his household. Instead of a concubine, if he lived where polygamy prevailed, a secondary wife or wives would be an option. Insofar as polygyny disregards the sex ratio, when it is widespread the counterpart of the private harem is the public harem, the whorehouse, which may offer also another option for the perfunctory husband.

Aphoristically, the difference between the perfunctory relationship and its various options is epitomized as the difference between, in the female, the madonna and the whore, in the male, the paterfamilias and the playboy, and in both, the saint and the sinner. It is also the difference between the impassive nondescript service of conjugal insemination, and the impassioned orgasmic ecstasy and lust of romantic love.

In the early Christian centuries, the church expanded the scope of the sexual taboo by outlawing passionate love from the conjugal bed.[2] To inseminate was an injunction, but to enjoy copulating was a sin. By the end of the 11th century, love and passion began to reassert themselves in public, circumventing the taboo, in love lyrics first sung by the troubadours of southern France.[9] The courtly love of which they sang, however, was the love of a knight or noble for a fair lady who, in marriage to another, would be forever held inaccessible. The troubadours romantically idealized a love forlorn that would never be contaminated by carnal passion. Andreas Capellanus,[4] the chronicler of courtly love at the end of the twelfth century, deferring to the dictates of the church, taught that, if two lovers should perchance be eligible to marry, then their love ought not continue lest it provoke in them the sin of carnal passion.

The legacy of the troubadours still shapes today's sexosophy.[1] Love, lyricism, and romance exist above the belt. Lust, bawdry, and carnality exist below the belt. Love above the belt is refined, spiritual, virtuous, sensuous, chaste, loyal, committed, jealously possessive and, to use today's jargon, a meaningful relationship. Lust below the belt is uncouth, physical, wanton, sensual, libertine, opportunistic, irresponsible, expediently casual, and an exploitative relationship. The very words here listed disclose that our sexosophy of lust is negative, and of love, positive, whereas there is in the actuality of people's lives a mixture of negative and positive in both. This is an important issue in sex therapy which tends to be biased against lust and to exaggerate too much the positive in love, to the neglect of its debit side.

One side effect of the love/lust polarization is terminological. There is a paucity of operationally defined and precisely unambiguous terms with which to give scientific precision to the sexological analysis of a complete erotosexual episode, so that every component, from beginning to end, has a name. Nor indeed is there a term for the entire episode itself. Making love is used both for romance and as a euphemism for genital union. Foreplay might include oral copulation, but if either cunnilingus or fellatio climax in orgasm, then surely sucking and being sucked is something more than foreplay. Intercourse, coitus, copulation, and the earthy word, fuck, are all used to specify genital union, but do not etymologically exclude any of the other components of what people say and do along with conjoining their sex organs.

Lust without love is compatible with reproduction of the species, but love without lust is not. Thanks to the legacy of the troubadours, the contract of marriage in Western culture today is not solely the product of an arrangement to join two lineages, but predominantly the product of the attraction and pair-bondedness of a love affair between two people. The criteria of the status of having fallen-in-love or having been love-smitten, newly named the state of limerence,[8] are not standardized. Young people supply their own criteria based on subjective idiosyncracy added to what they are taught by today's troubadours, who, in a marvel of historical continuity, are rock-and-roll and other popular singers. Their songs constitute a prime educational source of the sexosophy of love and lust in the youth culture of our time.

Love and lust have not yet defied the rigors of the sexual taboo to become wholly reunited in any system of sexosophy, popular or academic. One popular and partly religious approach connotes coitus as sacred and beautiful, provided it is reserved for the sacrament of marriage.

The Contraceptive Age

The experience of limerence or being fallen-in-love is essentially as lusty as it is lovely. In every generation of poets, there have been some who tell us that! But it is not what they tell us that will enable us to change and unify love and lust. Rather, it is the revision of the status quo of sexosophy that was engineered by the discovery of contraceptive devices approximately a century ago. The first public display of a condom was in 1876 at the International Centennial Exposition in Philadelphia. It was a product of the newly discovered process of vulcanizing rubber. Another fifty years elapsed before the contraceptive age got truly under way, with the invention of the latex rubber condom.

Contraception, need it be said, permits the separation of recreational from procreational sex for all fertile couples regardless of age, marital status, monogamy, or whatever. Youth need no longer denounce lust as lewd and obscene—though paradoxically to be saved for the sanctity of marriage! Lust below the belt need no longer invariably be correlated with a sexosophy of parenthood and childcare. It is now as feasible to have a moral sexosophy of love/lust—love in combination with lust—without a marital contract for procreation, as it is to unite love and lust in marriage with procreation. This new sexosophy of youth is already evident in the restoration of the custom of betrothal and living together as sexual partners before being married. This custom belonged to the pre-Christian sexosophy of Europe. It survived until the 20th century only in the Scandinavian north and in Iceland.

Age-Avoidancy

The sexosophy of being betrothed but not married as sexual partners is a taboo topic in today's sex education of children and teen-agers. It is not solely the topic of betrothal and living together that is taboo, however, but also the very practice of sex education. Sex education violates that subsection of the sexual taboo that specifies avoidancy of communication on sexual topics between people discordant for age. This is the age-avoidance taboo. It applies especially to communication between adults and juveniles or adolescents. Youth itself learns the age-avoidancy taboo so well that children of twelve may censor the information that they might share with others younger than themselves.

The age-avoidancy taboo affects communication between parents and their own children. Some families have become emancipated. Among those who have not are numbered many who are opposed to sex education at school, where the age-avoidancy taboo would be broken. They claim that sex education belongs in the home, which is where they have power to veto and can ensure that sexual information does not cross the age barrier, but is censored instead. In some schools that give sex education, age-avoidancy is deferred to insofar as teachers are forbidden to trasmit to their students information on selected topics like coitus, orgasm, and erotic imagery.

Age-avoidancy applies not only to exchange of information, but also to erotosexual participation. Among children who are age-discrepant, the sanctions against erotosexual rehearsal play are more punitive for those who are older, especially if they are postpubertal. Among adults, age-discrepant sexual partnerships are legal, but when one partner is much older the age-avoidance taboo is applied in the attenuated form of leering, smirking, and jesting.

Intimacy-Avoidancy

Age-avoidancy overlaps with intimacy-avoidancy in the sexosophy of taboo with which we live. The more personally intimate the information, the less likely that it crosses the age-barrier. Thus eggs, sperms and fertilization are more acceptable in a sex education curriculum than are genital love-play, body sensuousness, and ability to climax.

Intimate personal disclosure of erotosexual ideation, imagery, or practice is dangerous. As recently as three centuries ago, the church burned people at the stake for confabulating, under torture, erotic dreams they had not had. Today, intimate disclosure makes a person vulnerable to blackmail or vengeance. That is ensured by the very existence of the taboo against intimacy. In the State of Maryland, or in the District of Columbia, the Capital of the United States, for example, anyone can be blackmailed or brought to face charges for the practice of oral sex, for it is illegal no matter who the partner.

The mass media, especially television, are scrupulously attentive to the intimacy-avoidance taboo. Society is thus deprived of an immense public-health resource for the improvement of its own erotosexual health.

Even in an erotosexually emancipated family, disclosure of intimacy is subject to constraint in our society—the constraint of not personally demonstrating coitus, for example. Since our sexosophy dictates coital privacy for parents, the children of those parents who might disobey this dictate have the burden either of keeping the information secret or, if they disclose it, even though inadvertently, of having sanctions imposed on themselves and their parents.

The taboo against intimacy invades even the most intimate of relationships. Lovers and spouses, for example, may withhold intimate information, either negative or positive, about their own personal erotosexual sensuousness, and even more about their idiosyncratic erotosexual imagery and fantasy. The rationale for the treatment of couples in sex therapy is that breaking the taboo on intimacy is a two-way street.

Allosex-Avoidancy

The taboo-prescribed avoidancies of age and intimacy in our society's sexosophy are two of a trio of overlapping avoidancy relationships. The third is the allosex-avoidancy. It prescribes, relative to age or intimacy, what must be avoided in the presence of the other sex, and must not, or need not be avoided in the presence of one's own. Allosex-avoidancy applies in particular to exposure of the body, and to vocabulary and topics of conversation.

Avoidancy of nudity varies according to extent and organs of the body exposed; age of the exposed individual and the observers; degree of intimacy or familiarity between those involved; and the sex of the exposed and of the observers. The taboo on nudity has been relaxing in recent years, but it is still only among the elite of the nudist movement in Western culture that one finds both sexes of all ages and all degrees of acquaintanceship playing and socializing together totally nude. Exposure of the body under these circumstances is not, per se, erotosexual, just as exposure, per se, of the woman's face is not erotosexual in a society where no woman's face is veiled.

Avoidance of erotosexual words and conversation in mixed company once was simply an extension of widespread segregation of the sexes in education, play, work, politics and religion. In addition, females were, and to a large extent still are excluded from certain erotosexual rites and ceremonials of the "men's house." Growing up, males had their segregated circle jerks, dirty books, dirty stories, burlesque shows, freak shows at the fair, stag movies, bachelor parties, and in some cases group visits to the whorehouse. Since boyhood, they had learned their own explicit sexual vocabulary, stigmatized as crude, vulgar, and impolite (and to a large extent, in English, derived from Anglo-Saxon rather than Latin). It gave them a common denominator of words with which to compare their common denominator of erotosexual learning.

Girls had no corresponding common denominator of erotosexual terms, except, perhaps the terminology of menses as the curse, keeping a boy in his place or getting pregnant, and waiting for the right one to come along. For the female growing up, the counterpart of the segregated "men's house" was the slumber party, soap opera, true romance magazine, girl-talk about cute boys, and maybe a bridal or baby shower. That was the common denominator of their erotosexual learning.

To further ensure that developing girls and boys had no mutual common denominator of shared erotosexual experience on which to converse, classes or lectures in sex education were usually sex segregated. Sex education at home, if it existed was from mother to daughter, and father to son.

The allosex-avoidancy taboo has been relaxing in recent years. Nonetheless, to an unknown degree it still maintains and reinforces the stereotypes of male and female erotosexualism by preventing mutual and widespread exchange of ideas and information. Bantering and ribaldry, institutionalized as the joking relationship, is one way of breaching the taboo, but it is only a beginning. Many books written in the last quarter century have attempted to explain men and women erotosexually to one another, and to liberate them. Nonetheless, the allosex-avoidancy taboo dies hard. It gets reinforced from most unlikely places, for example, from militant feminists, as part of their current all-out attack on men by pejoratively classifying all visuoerotic arousal not as erotica (even pictures of themselves!) but as pornography. The power of the sexosophy of our time is, indeed, deeply pervasive! It even redefines reluctance as being raped.

Sexological Research and Taboo

Sexosophy, through its taboos, has always held the power to police sexology, the science, and to dictate not only the terms of what it may and may not do, but the charter of its very existence. There is an analogy in the relationship between anatomy and taboo. In the 16th century, Vesalius in defiance of religious doctrine on the resurrection of the dead, broke the taboo on defiling the human corpse by dissecting it. Today, the taboo is not defunct, but lives on, in refusals to permit autopsies and, reinforced by an alliance with the sexual taboo on abortion, in its application to the fetal corpse.

Of the three taboo-prescribed avoidancy relationships, allosex-avoidancy is the least troublesome for sexological research today, since sexologists are both women and men. They can, therefore, work together, each augmenting what the other cannot do alone, whether their research be on men, women, or couples. This principle of research collaboration applies not only to male/female collaboration. It extends also to those who are different in age level, language spoken, ethnicity, and erotosexual lifestyle.

The intimacy-avoidancy taboo imperils sexological research. It restricts the availability of research subjects, introduces volunteer bias, and limits the range of information that an individual provides. It makes some knowledge dangerous to possess. For example, detailed disclosures of exhibitionism, voyeurism, incest, pedophilia, rape, lust murderism, or any other paraphilia legally-classified as a sex offense, given by research volunteers without a police record, might be reported or subpoenaed and misused. Failure to report, might lead to legal charges being brought against the researcher, even on the initiative of his own work associates. Intimate and confidential information, especially of the case history type, quite often must be withheld from publication or even professional discussion at meetings, because of the risk of a malpractice claim, even though a signed release had been obtained.

Sexology is already being siren-sung into service under the dictatorship of the intimacy-avoidance taboo. The siren sings of large grants and easy funding for those who collaborate with the criminal justice system in the new and bastard science of victimology. Victimology equates sex with wrongdoing. It studies only what it condemns: abortion, pornography, assault, rape, incest, molesting. It deprives itself of half of its legitimate subject-matter. The raptophiliac—the true rapist—for example, gets handed over to the criminal justice system, and only the victim of rape gets the victimologist's attention. The same happens to the pedophile whose relationship with the younger partner is defined as abuse or molestation, never as love or affection. The scientific challenge, namely to understand more about the phenomenon of prepubertal or early nonabusive pairbond with an older person, is lost.

Imposition of the intimacy-avoidancy taboo in some instances of sex-offending is absolute. It dictates that the offender, once convicted, becomes the property of a penal system from which sexological research is absolutely excluded. The offender must die, perhaps condemned to execution, with the secrets of the etiology of his paraphilic syndrome, and its prognosis and prevention, scientifically unexplored and undisclosed. Society is, of course, the ultimate loser, burdened by the continuing weight of its own ignorance to prevent the recurrence of the sex-offending paraphilias in the next generation.

Lest you consider me unduly alarmist, consider this: early in 1981, the legislature of the State of California enacted a statute whereby every girl or woman who had had unmarried sexual intercourse before her eighteenth birthday was classified as a sexual victim. Her physician or any other professional to whom she disclosed the fact that she had had intercourse became a law breaker, unless he/she reported the so-called victim to the police or to the child abuse authorities. It is true that, under pressure from the California Medical Association, the statute was later declared unconstitutional. Nonetheless, it serves as a warning of the continuing power of the age-avoidance taboo in preventing younger women patients from telling older professionals that they had copulated without being the victims of copulation. All health care professionals, sexologists included, had themselves fallen victim to their own victimology.

Taboo-prescribed age-avoidance outweighs the other two avoidancy relationships in the magnitude of its adverse consequences for sexological research. In fact, it is a research disaster, because it eliminates developmental sexology as a science. It eliminates the possibility of institutional support for either unfunded or funded research into the uncensored, unsuppressed erotosexual manifestations of normal childhood; and it eliminates also the possibility of grant support. The sexology of human adulthood cannot exist independently of its developmental underpinnings in the sexology of the fetus, the infant, the child, and the adolescent. Whatever can be learned from animal models, including the higher primates, will not substitute for additional longitudinal study of human erotosexual development, and the variables that affect the development from the day of conception onward. There will be no other way in which to discriminate between the determinants of male and female erotosexualism that are prenatal or postnatal, juvenile or postpubertal, normal or pathological, fixed or modifiable, species specific or biographically specific, phylographic or idiographic. In other words, there will be no complete science of sexology in the absence of longitudinal research and a sexology of childhood.

There may already be some unknown and undisclosed Vesalius of the sexology of childhood, protected from the glare of publicity. It is unlikely. What then of the future? Sexologists around the world and here at this World Congress have, as one option, to pass the proverbial buck, and to wait for a lone Vesalius to take on the sexosophy of the establishment, as Kinsey did. The other option is that we ourselves accept the responsibility of founding, funding, and politically defending the scientific sexology of childhood. Do we have the resolve? If we do, we will rewrite sexosophy. Then the theme of this Congress, Applied Sexosophy, will truly have been applied to the reconciliation of sexosophy and sexology as the two halves of one whole.

References

1. Boswell, J. (1980): *Christianity, Social Tolerance, and Homosexuality*. University of Chicago Press, Chicago, IL.
2. Bullough, V. L. (1976): *Sexual Variance in Society and History*. Wiley, New York, NY.
3. Ladurie, E. L. R. (1978): *Montaillou: The Promised Land of Error*. Braziller, New York, NY.
4. Locke, F. W., Editor (1957): *Andreas Capellanus: The Art of Courtly Love*. Frederick Ungar, New York, NY.
5. Money, J. (1980): *Love and Love Sickness: The Science of Sex, Gender Difference and Pair-bonding*. Johns Hopkins University Press, Baltimore, MD.

6. Money, J. and Ehrhardt, A. A. (1971): *Man and Woman, Boy and Girl: The Differentiation and Dimorphism of Gender Identity from Conception to Maturity.* Johns Hopkins University Press, Baltimore, MD.

7. Murstein, B. L. (1974): *Love, Sex, and Marriage Through the Ages.* Springer, New York, NY.

8. Tennov, D. (1979): *Love and Limerence: The Experience of Being in Love.* Stein and Day, New York, NY.

9. Valency, M. (1961): *In Praise of Love: An Introduction to the Love Poetry of the Renaissance,* Macmillan, New York, NY.

Note

Originally presented as the opening lecture of the 5th World Congress of Sexology, Jerusalem, June 21-26, 1981 and published with selected papers of the congress in *Sexology, Sexual Biology, Behavior and Therapy* (Z. Hoch and H. I. Lief, eds.). Amsterdam-Oxford-Princeton, Excerpta Medica, 1982. [Bibliog. #2.261]

FORTY-SIX

Sexual Reformation and Counterreformation in Law and Medicine

Abstract

Though the birth-control revolution originated a century ago, its current momentum dates from the invention of the latex condom in the late 1920s. It has a daily impact on our lives comparable with that of the fire-making revolution. Whereas the sacred flame has long since become incorporated into religious worship, contraception has, under the pervasive force of the ancient sexual taboo, so far been denied positive religious status. Contraception is changing the customs of pairbonding and family formation, as in the contemporary revival of betrothal in which love and lust unite in a test of compatibility for parenthood. The tide of history imposes on us all the imperative of a new ethic of the male/female relationship, a veritable Sexual Reformation, which is met within powerful segments of the religious establishment by Sexual Counterreformation. The Sexual Reformation needs a legally constituted church of its own. Otherwise the Sexual Counterreformation may succeed in establishing a sexual and military dictatorship, exploiting overpopulation of the people of poverty by depriving them of the rights of contraception and abortion. Sexual Reformation will have an effect on developmental sexual health in childhood through adulthood; on both women's and men's liberation and emancipation; and on the increase of knowledge through expansion of sexological research. Its effect will reach both Law and Medicine.

Birth-Control Revolution

Fire-making and birth-control, their respective discoveries spanning untold millennia of human history, are intellectual monuments that share in common the revolution that they wrought in our daily lives.

The fire-making revolution changed dark into light, cold into warm, raw into cooked, trees into horticultural ash, assailants into fleeing victims and inert fuels into working energy. The birth-control revolution is barely a century old. It changed conception from chance to prediction. It allowed recreational sex to be distinct from procreational sex during the years of adult fertility; and it permitted family size and chronology to be fixed ahead of time.

The fire-making revolution had not only utilitarian applications, but also religious ones. The sacred flame burned on altars of sacrifice and worship as candles still, today, burn in sanctuaries and votive places. The birth-control revolution is too recent in onset to have been accorded not only utilitarian but also religious application. There is no contraceptive equivalent of the sacred flame. People do not yet, in any of the major religions of the world, offer public prayers or votive offerings in thanks for a completed family and a continued sex life, safe from further pregnancies—though they readily do so, in supplication for a wanted pregnancy they fail to conceive.

Sexual Taboo in Christian Ideology

Established religions, being old and venerable institutions, cling to their old and venerable ideologies and policies. They update them only after a prolonged period in which the proponents of change are persecuted as heretics.

In Christendom today, ecclesiastical doctrine regarding sexual matters is indeed old and venerable, for it incorporates and perpetuates the sexual taboo, the ancient origin of which undoubtedly predates the Bible. Christian sexual doctrine owes less to the Bible itself, however, than to the 5th century ideologies of St. Jerome and, especially, St. Augustine.[3] Both ideologies vigorously repudiated sexuality—Jerome's the sexuality of women, and Augustine's the sexuality of the genitals. Augustine gave special distinction to concupiscence or lust that excites the genitals as the very wellspring of sin. In marriage, to have sexual intercourse for its carnal pleasure, instead of for its procreative expediency, was a sin requiring forgiveness. The penitentials of the 6th century, the earliest that have survived, specified the penances incurred for experiencing orgasm, including the orgasm of the nocturnal emission, in ways that excluded the possibility of procreation.[2]

Though copulation of the infertile was not blacklisted, nor that of those few who lived long enough to survive the menopause, recreational sex and procreational sex were for the most part absolutely irreconcilable.[1] Procreational sex itself, outside of marriage, was a sin. Within marriage, sexual continence was required for 40 days before and 40 after the celebration of both Christmas and Easter. For the remainder of the year, intercourse was proscribed on Mondays, Wednesdays, and Fridays.

Mediterranean Marital System

The church's doctrine of legitimizing copulation only as a procreational insemination service devoid of passion, and only for married couples, has its antecedents in the marital system of ancient Rome. The Roman system itself had antecedents of even greater antiquity in the Eastern Mediterranean. According to this ancient system, the system of arranged marriage, the families negotiated a match between two young people as an alliance of lands, wealth and power; and of class, religious and ethnic status. With the price of a son-in-law represented by the girl's dowry, her father gave to him his daughter's hand in marriage, and with it the legal authority of owning her and the offspring with which he inseminated her. It was essential that she be a virgin and that she preserve the chastity of her womb for her husband's insemination alone. In effect, she was his womb, and its copulatory obligation was to be inseminated, without the accompaniment of erotic arousal and passion.

This was the system not only of the virgin bride, but also of the double standard. For copulatory passion, the man was variously entitled to a private harem, to slave girls, concubines, or mistresses; or to a harlot from the public harem, the brothel; or to dalliance with a widow, or a girl of lower social station—a servant or peasant girl who may, herself, by reason of having been born out of wedlock, be stigmatized as unmarriageable.[6]

Nordic Marital System

The marital system of pre-Roman and pre-Christian Europe eventually became confined to the Arctic borders of Scandinavia and Iceland where alone it survived intact, as a legitimate institution, into the 20th century. This is the Nordic system, the system of betrothal and the love match of erotic equality between the sexes. According to this system, it was traditional for young romance to bloom in spring and summer when the climate was warm enough for households no longer to need to sleep in the kitchen, kept from freezing to death by a great log fire. Then the daughters and hired girls of a farming or fishing family moved their sleeping quarters to the loft of a small storage building called the girls' house or, in Finnish, the night-foot house, where local boys came, taking a walk on their night-feet, to serenade them. Instead of opening the trap-door to invite the boys into their loft, the girls would throw a rope ladder from the window for them to climb up. If a boy and a girl became love-smitten, the others would arrange for them subsequently to be left alone overnight. Then, according to customary ritual, the boy would progress from sleeping fully clothed above the covers, to under the covers, and then undressed under the covers. It was appropriate for them to announce to their families that they were betrothed, and ready to celebrate the announcement with guests at a great party. They expected, of course, to have a baby. If they proved their fertility, they were permitted to be married, otherwise not. In Sweden, it was as late as the 18th century that marriage in a church became legally required, in the place of betrothal marriage. In America, the betrothal system was known in 18th century New England as bundling. With later waves of peasant European immigrants it was preserved in the somewhat debased form that today is known simply as unwed motherhood or teenaged illegitimacy.

Love and Lust

Rivalry between the two systems of marriage, the betrothed love-affair, and the arranged expediency is epitomized in the life of St. Augustine. As a young man, he lived for 15 years and had a son in a betrothed relationship of which his mother disapproved. He broke up the relationship. "And this was a blow," he wrote in his *Confessions,* "which crushed my heart to bleeding, because I loved her dearly." His well known prayer, as he struggled with "lust and wantonness," was: "Give me chastity and continence, but, no, not yet." While waiting for a marriage to be arranged, he had another love affair. Then, undergoing a religious conversion he renounced "nature's appetites," and took the God of the Christian religion as the true goal of love.[3]

So well did the Christian ascetic marital ideology displace the betrothal ideology of pairbonded love, that the concept of a relationship based on falling in love lost its place in recorded European history until, in the 13th century, the troubadours of Provence began singing of it once again. The troubadours were diffusing a romantic tradition, dating back probably to Hellenistic Greece and Persia and rediscovered perhaps in Arabic verse and songs of Moorish Spain, and also in the Hebrew language of the Sephardic Jews of Spain.

Romantic love as sung by troubadours and their successors was the love of gallant knights courting their ladies fair. It was love unattainable, and predestined to be forever unrequited, for the fair lady would already have been either given or promised to another in an arranged marriage. Ardor fulfilled would have entailed punishment and even death for the sins of adultery or fornication. Nonetheless, it was better to die of lovesickness and of ardor unfulfilled, than never to have known the ecstasy of having been in love's toils.

Andreas Capellanus, from the court of Eleanor of Aquitaine, in his *De arte honeste amandi* (*The Art of Courtly Love*[7]) written in the late eleven hundreds, questioned whether two lovers, if permitted to marry, could continue to be in love. The answer was no, for they would be unable to restrain themselves from the carnal sin of passion while having intercourse. Eight centuries later, this split between love and lust still today has not been reconciled.

Of course, there are some contemporary couples who, obedient to the system, reconcile love and lust by having no passion in either the courtship or the marriage. By contrast, there are other couples who outwit the system and reconcile passionate love in the courtship with passionate lust in the marital bed. Countless other couples, however, are victims of the irreconcilability of love and lust in their marital relationship, and of its pathological spin-off in their private lives, and the lives of their family unit. Expanding exponentially, the number of pathologically affected families sooner or later reaches a critical point, and society itself is confronted with the crisis of an institution, the family, that fails to function. We are, indeed, in such a crisis with respect to the nuclear family in our own society today. In large segments of the population, across all social classes, the nuclear family simply does not maintain itself.

Young adults of today are aware, albeit in a less than explicit way, that the families of their youth all too often did not sustain the optimal well-being of either themselves or their parents. They know that the rewards of being in love, as promised by today's electronic troubadours, the lyricists and singers of rock-and-roll, do not necessarily materialize in the sexual life of marriage. They take for granted that the contraceptive revolution is upon them, and that the ethic of the nuclear family no longer, therefore, monopolizes the ethics of the male/female relationship. Without cognizance of their debt to history, and without a formal declaration, they are endorsing again the betrothal system. They enter into couple relationships as "live-ins." They live together not to test their fertility, as in the old system of betrothal; but because, in the age of contraception, they can test their compatibility as sexual partners before committing themselves to parenthood.

Amerafrican Marital System

In the United States, there is another great tradition of procreation and child-care, the Amerafrican system that had its origins in slavery. American slaves had no legal right to marry, for they had no legal rights at all. Slave girls were permitted, encouraged, or required to breed young, and with partners either white or black (but a white female's pregnancy by a black male was, by definition, evidence of rape). The young slave parent had no rights of parent-hood, including childcare. The rearing of infants and young chidren was the work of the yard slaves, the infirm and elderly, of grandparental age. This skipped-generation system of child-rearing is still widely distributed in both the rural and urban culture of poverty.

One change is that food, shelter, and clothing, formerly provided at the discretion of the plantation manager, may now be provided by a welfare check and food stamps. More accurately, it is underprovided, for the system is still geared to exploit poverty for cheap labor. If made economically viable, the three-generation family of the Amerafrican system would have positive solutions for problems that the nuclear family so far has not solved. It does not require prolonged postponement of childbearing until the late twenties or thirties. It provides youth with the opportunity of a betrothal relationship in which love and lust coexist. It provides for the young mother the logistics of combining parenthood with an extradomestic, professional career. It allows for the commitment to permanent living together in wedlock and family care to be delayed until the maturity of mid-life. It gives to the elderly the self-respect of having an important family position—a position not to be taken lightly, since life expectancy has increased from 45 to 75 years, more or less, in this present century.

Contemporary Betrothal

One aspect of contemporary betrothal that is still undecided is the etiquette and protocol with which "live-ins" (there is no formal noun with which to name them) will be recognized in society, and in the family of origin. Some few parents, emancipated by reason of contraception from the unwanted burden of illegitimate grandparenthood, make peace with their teenagers and allow the boyfriend/girlfriend couple to sleep together in their own bed at home. In the Amerafrican system, however, though the pregnancy is accommodated in the home, the coitus that brought it into being is not. It is considered disrespectful for the young couple to let it be known when or where they copulate, particularly if it is in the boy's mother's home.

Young people denied betrothal status at home must catch as catch can until, living elsewhere and managing their own resources, they can live-in together. Officially and bureaucratically, their status is tolerated rather than respected. Yet, because there is no etiquette for integrating "live-ins" into the formalities of social mixing, it is within the informality of their own age group they are most at ease, socially, as a couple. Sooner rather than later, there will be needed a formal etiquette for the institution of betrothal; and some symbolic way of informing society at large to accord a couple betrothal status.

Doomsayers who equate betrothal with immorality misrepresent it as promiscuous or casual. Not so! Betrothed people are pairbonded. To become pairbonded and in love, or limerent (to use the new term) is as inalienable a feature of us human beings as is genital lust and copulation.

Casual or promiscuous sex is not a substitute for pairbondedness. For some people, however, it has the intrinsic merit of variety with which to augment a permanent relationship. It has always been that way. The prevalence figures may change in the age of conception, and the age of relatively effective control of sexually transmitted disease. There may be more open relationships in which both partners have multiple other partners, while maintaining their primary allegiance. But the bugaboo of equating erotic or sexual emancipation with promiscuity is both moral fiction, and science fiction.

Prophets of doom notwithstanding, betrothal whether in the Nordic tradition, or the skipped-generation Amerafrican tradition, is not immoral. It has its own intrinsic morality, and it is a morality in which love and lust may coexist, undivided. It is a morality that, if it fulfills its early promise, will reconstitute the institution of the family and protect children from the traumatic hazards of the breakup of the nuclear family.

In the famous American melting pot, it is our historical destiny to be now in the process, whether we like it or not, of melding together the Nordic-betrothal and the Amerafrican skipped-generation systems of family formation with the Mediterranean-arranged system. This is one of the great dimensions of change in our era. It constitutes, in effect, if not a Revolution, then a Reformation in our sexual morality.

Sexual Counterreformation

Like all change, this Reformation, this dimension of change is anathema to those whose ideological or material security it threatens. Their response to reformation is to mount a counterreformation. That precisely is what the guardians of the new right are presently engaged in. Their policies add up to what is essentially a Sexual Counterreformation in defense of the Mediterranean sytem of the virgin bride, the arranged or family-approved marriage in which copulation is only a procreational insemination service, and in defense of the double standard by which the husband is an absolute patriarchal dictator. To implement this defense of erotic asceticism and misanthropy, the counterreformationists' policies actively negate educational instruction regarding technique and positioning in coitus; regarding erotic response and orgasm; and regarding also contraception; abortion; masturbation; and homosexuality. The counterreformationist policy excludes also erotic illustrations and entertainment, all of which are condemned by being labeled obscene, pornographic, and antifeminist. Counterreformationists have legislated a policy of federally funding centers to promote virginity. They have proposed a policy of the death sentence for all homosexuals. They define any degree of sexual coercion or imposition as rape, even in marriage. They divert funds from pure sexological research to the application of untested theories for the policing and punishment of rape and sexual child abuse. The sex-negative is funded. The sex-positive is not.

Sexual and Military Dictatorship

The publicly declared counterreformationist policies conceal an undeclared hidden agenda, namely sexual dictatorship and the probability of military dictatorship.

Population expansion is an inevitable consequence of negating contraception and illegalizing abortion. In the actualities of the everyday world, this population expansion will take place disproportionately among the people of poverty. Those with enough wealth will, more readily than the poor, have access to information on contraceptives and abortion, and on how to procure them.

Counterreformationist leaders and the politicians and jurists who represent them may in some cases be unscrupulous or duplicitous, but they are not mental retardates with no reasoning power. One is obliged to infer, therefore, that they know what they are doing, and that it is part of their master plan to enforce the breeding of the poor, so as to disproportionately enlarge this segment of the population. Then there would ensue the risky possibility of an uprising of the poor, in riot, terrorism, and revolution that would bring about the very extermination of the counterreformationist leaders and their supporters. Self-genocide can exist even in a master plan, witness the 1978 history of Jonestown, but it is a rare type of morbidity. It is more likely to be written into the master plan that the overpopulous poor will be exploited, either economically or militarily or both. For that to be effective, it would be necessary for a democracy to transform itself into a military dictatorship with complete control over its citizens. Under a dictator, the population would be militarized, dissidents would be persecuted in a new form of the Inquisition, and offensive warfare would be feasible.

The lesson of history is that enforced population increase has indeed been decreed under military dictatorships, and that sexual reformation has been outlawed in favor of taboo-ridden sexual austerity. Applied to ourselves, the possibility of change to a military dictatorship is nightmarish, but not too farfetched. It is a dimension of change that could overtake us, and with it the victory of the Sexual Counterreformation.

A Church of Sexual Reformation

The Sexual Counterreformation has a secure, centralized and well-financed base of operations in ultraconservative and fundamentalist religion. The Sexual Reformation has an insecure, decentralized and insufficiently financed base of operations, and its constituency is both secular and religious. It would exercise more authority and power if it were to organize itself legally as a religion—the new Church of Sexual Reformation—complete with theology, as well as with the constitutional privileges, including tax-exempt status, accorded to religion in the United States. As an organized religion, Sexual Reformation could project the message of love-positive sexual philosophy, or sexosophy[10] to radio and television congregations, as well as to local pulpit congregations. Should it ever be formed, a Church of Sexual Reformation would create a new, and hitherto unexpected dimension of positive change in family, sexuality, and social roles. This change would, like a stone in a pond, spread its beneficent ripples widely, affecting, for example, our understanding of the developmental sexuality of childhood, the liberation of both sexes, and the uncensored advancement of sexual knowledge through research.

Sexual Reformation and Childhood

Sexual Reformation has, as yet, barely scraped the surface of the developmental sexuality and eroticism of childhood. Habituated to the mythology of innocence and the latency period, we justify what is, in effect, criminal neglect of our children's erotosexual health and welfare—the only aspect of their development that we deliberately neglect. At the same time, habituated to the contradictory mythology of original sin, we lay in wait for any manifestation of the normal sexuality of childhood sexual rehearsal play, and, in response, subject our children to the discipline of what is, in effect, criminal child abuse.

There are some very telling monkey experiments from the Wisconsin primate center[4, 5] that prove the importance of sexual rehearsal play in infancy and childhood. Infant monkeys reared in isolation and totally deprived of play with their age mates grew up to be entirely unable to perform sexually as adults. If their species had depended on them to breed, it would have become extinct. Even so little as one half hour of play a day was sufficient to swing the pendulum, but only for one out of each three monkeys, and even for them the birthrate was abnormal and low.

In another monkey experiment, the prevention of male/female heterosexual rehearsal play, but not the play of all-female, or all-male groups increased the prevalence of same-sex coupling later in life.

The question must be asked: Are we human beings guilty of too heavily imposing the sexual taboo on our children, so as to lay the foundations of genital dysfunction, couple incompatibility, and anomalous or "kinky" sexual rituals in maturity? The verdict is a resounding yes. There are societies on earth with no history of the sexual taboo to which we ourselves are heir, and their citizens are not afflicted with sexual "hangups" in adulthood to the extent that we are.[12]

Sexual Reformation and Liberation

The Sexual Reformation, if applied to childhood, would have an especially beneficial effect on girls who, under the negations of the sexual taboo, have been robbed of their erotosexual birthright even more than have boys. One especially regrettable consequence is that antisexualism and, even more, antieroticism has crept into their adult lives. It has also crept, misguidedly, into some of the policies of the women's liberation movement, alienating potential supporters. For example, it is a mistake to define all visual erotica as pornography,[11] and to define all pornography as the victimization of women, as in bondage and discipline, sadism, or lust murder. Whereas only some women are dependent on their eyes to become erotically turned on in the ordinary, heterosexual way, almost all men are. It is a mistake for those who are erotically indifferent to the visual image, to judge sons, husbands and lovers by themselves. If they are responsive to picture books and movies of an erotic nature, it does not signify that they respond to women only as sexual objects. They fall in love, too.[8]

It is a mistake, also, to jump onto the kiddy-porn bandwagon, and to equate all manifestations of juvenile sexuality with victimization or child abuse. One needs to be more discriminating, so as not to conspire in robbing children, developmentally, of their sexual and erotic birthright.

It is likewise a mistake to equate all insistent or even coercive sexual advances with victimization and rape, while neglecting the possibility, in the alleged victim, of a combination of seduction followed by phobia of genital contact. Genuine rape is a special syndrome, raptophilia, one of the paraphilias[9, 14] and it almost always involves an unsuspecting stranger. Mistakes of the aforesaid type narrow and retard the dimensions of change by which women's liberation, an imperative of our future, becomes effected. A widened and accelerated dimensions of change must be a mutual liberation of men and women together.

Sexological Research

The Sexual Reformation will, if successful, exert its influence beyond everyday applications to men's and women's roles[8] to basic sexological research. At the present time, it is virtually impossible to get funding for affirmative sexological research. A blatantly conspicuous lack is research into laying the foundations of adult sexual and erotic health in the development of childhood.

Sex-research money today is predominantly for research that is sexologically negative—for sex as a behavioral disease scheduled to be eradicated, or law-breaking scheduled to be punished. In deference to this sexual negation, the new, bastard science of victimology has come into existence. In sexual victimology, the role of the victim is to be diagnosed and authenticated, even at the cost of being further traumatized, and then to be rehabilitated with methods of treatment that have not yet been scientifically validated. The role of the offender is to be proved guilty and punished, usually imprisoned. Research into the cause or etiology of the condition or syndrome that led to the offense and that produced the victim is, with rare exceptions, disregarded.

Victimologists might do well to learn a lesson from the social eugenics movement of the 19th and early 20th century. Pfäfflin[13] traced this movement in the early history of sexology. Many of the founders of sexology jumped on the bandwagon of eugenic purity and advocated castration of the unfit. Many of them lived to see the day when Hitler used their own theory against them, not to castrate, but to exterminate them because they were racially unfit to be members of his eugenic nation.

Today's victimologists whose work is to pass judgment on others are not immune to being themselves judged. The very bureaucracy they have built requires only a change of political wind to adopt a new vogue and criterion of abuse. Then, victimologists could become victims of their own bureaucracy.

Victimology is an applied science that lacks the principles of a pure science which it applies. This lack stems in large part from the failure of any university or medical school in either the New World or the Old to establish a full department of sexology or sexual medicine. Divisions, clinics or programs in human sexuality exist in some institutions, but they have neither the prestige and power accorded to a full department, nor the full range of subspecialties housed therein. There are a handful of organizations for sex research associated with universities in North America and Europe, but their budgets are inadequate to encompass all the subspecialties, from neuroscience to ethnology, that should be encompassed. A fully endowed university department or institute for sex research could advance the momentum of discovery applicable to new dimensions of change. It could provide the facts needed for effective evaluation of the policies and principles, pro and con, revolutionary and counterrevolutionary, as applied to the human sexual condition in both law and medicine.

References

1. Boswell, J. (1980). *Christianity, social tolerance, and homosexuality: Gay people in Western Europe from the beginning of the Christian era to the fourteenth century.* University of Chicago Press, Chicago.
2. Bullough, V. L. (1976). *Sexual variance in society and history.* Wiley, New York.
3. Gaden, J. R. (1981). The church and sexuality—on not getting it together. *St. Mark's Review* (Canberra, Australia), June 1981, pp. 13-33.
4. Goldfoot, D. A. (1977). Sociosexual behaviors of nonhuman primates during development and maturity: social and hormonal relationships. In: Schrier, AM (ed.). *Behavioral primatology: Advances in research and theory, vol 1.* Erlbaum, Hillsdale, NJ.
5. Goldfoot, D. A., Whalen, K. (1978). Development of gender role behaviors in heterosexual and isosexual groups of infant rhesus monkeys. In: Chivers, D. J., Herbert J. (eds.). *Recent advances in primatology, vol 1: Behaviour.* Academic Press, London, New York.
6. LeRoy, Ladurie E. (1978). *Montaillou, the promised land of error.* Braziller, New York.
7. Locke, F. W. (1957). *Andreas Capellanus: the art of courtly love.* Ungar, New York.
8. Money, J. (1980). *Love and love sickness: the science of sex, gender difference and pairbonding,* Johns Hopkins University Press, Baltimore.
9. Money, J. (1981). Paraphilias: phyletic origins of erotosexual dysfunction. *Int J. Mental Health* 10:75-109.
10. Money, J. (1982). Sexosophy and sexology, philosophy and science: Two halves, one whole. In: Hoch, Z., Lief, H. I. (eds.). *Sexology, sexual biology, behavior and therapy.* Excerpta Medica, Amsterdam, Oxford, Princeton.
11. Money, J., Athanasiou, R. (1973). Pornography: Review and bibliographic annotations. *Am J Obstet Gynecol* 115:130-146.
12. Money, J., Cawte, J. E., Bianchi, G. N., Nurcombe, B. (1977). Sex training and traditions in Arnhem Land. In: Money, J., Musaph, H. (eds.). *Handbook of sexology.* Excerpta Medica, Amsterdam, New York.
13. Pfäfflin, F. (1986). The connections between eugenics, sterilization, and mass murder in Germany 1933-1945. *Medicine and Law,* 5:1-10.
14. Money, J. (1984). Paraphilias: phenomonology and classification. *Am J Psychotherapy* 38:164-179.

Note

Derived from an address presented at the Sesquicentennial Conference, "Dimensions of Change," convened at New York University, October, 1981, by the late Werner Brandt, Professor of Physics. Originally published in *Medicine and Law,* 4:479-488, 1985. [Bibliog. #2.293]

FORTY-SEVEN

The Conceptual Neutering of Gender and the Criminalization of Sex

Abstract

Thirty years ago the term gender was borrowed from philology for use in sexological psychology in a paper on hermaphroditism (Money, 1955). As originally defined, gender role consists of both introspective and the extraspective manifestations of the concept. In general usage, the introspective manifestations soon became separately known as gender identity. The acronym, G-I/R, being singular, restores the unity of the concept. Without this unity, gender role has become a socially transmitted acquisition, divorced from the biology of sex and the brain. Sex and gender have been partitioned between body and mind, respectively. The desexualization of gender is in accord with the Zeitgeist of contemporary sexual politics together with victimology and an expanding criminalization of sex. The funding of sexological research is being diverted to victimology, which is, de facto, a branch of law enforcement. Victimologists—and sexological professionals among them—are vulnerable to a backlash of being themselves criminalized. This happens as a result of false accusations of various types of malpractice, including sexual abuse of clients, especially children. Under Hitler, there was an historical parallel when the destruction of sexology was effected by the application of the theory of social eugenics and racial purity which sexologists had endorsed. They were among the first of Hitler's victims.

History of Gender and Hermaphroditism

Today the term *gender* in idiomatic English and in translation, applies to human beings in such expressions as gender role, gender identity, and gender gap. Thirty years ago, however, these expressions did not exist in any language. The standard dictionaries of the time defined gender as having only a grammatical usage, namely to refer to the sex of nouns, pronouns, and adjectives, or their suffixes. Only colloquially and rarely was it used to refer to the sex of human beings. The expansion and present popularity of the concept of gender as a human attribute dates to 1955 and to a paper, the first of a series on hermaphroditism, published in the *Bulletin of the Johns Hopkins Hospital* (Money, 1955).

I recall regularly burning the midnight oil at that time, struggling to formulate a concise conceptualization of the data I had on my desk. I had reviewed 60 years of medical literature on cases of hermaphroditism (Money, 1952). I had also interviewed and tested, first-hand, 60 hermaphroditic children and adults distributed in 10 clinical categories (Money, 1955).

I needed a terminology that would permit me to write about their sexual and procreative lives as male or female, despite the handicap of having been born with a birth defect of the sex organs and despite the relative success or failure of attempted surgical repair of the defect. I also needed terminology that would permit me to write about the lives of these same patients as male or female, despite the degree of endocrinological success or failure in regulating hormonal masculinization or feminization of the body appropriately at puberty.

This same terminology that I needed would also permit me to write about the lives of hermaphroditic patients in terms of their adherence to traditional social coding and stereotyping of activities and interests as belonging to either males or females, respectively. These activities and interests are recreational, educational, vocational, and legal. They pertain to manners and morals, grooming and personal adornment and clothing style as well.

The terminology that I needed precluded the word *sex* as a unified entity, insofar as the birth-defective sex organs of hermaphroditism preclude using these organs as the criterion of all of the variables of a hermaphrodite's sex. The morphology of the external genitalia of a hermaphrodite, even if it is not ambiguous but the morphology of a normal penis or a normal vulva, is not a preordained indicator of the other variables of sex. Indeed, it was from the phenomenology of hermaphroditism that I had already devised the differentiation and classification of the variables of sex that are not inevitably correlated with one another, namely: chromosomal or genetic sex; gonadal sex; prenatal hormonal sex; internal morphologic sex; external morphologic sex; and pubertal hormonal sex. In addition, there was the sex of assignment, and the sex of rearing.

In the different syndromes of hermaphroditism, it is possible for one or more of these variables of sex to be discordant with the others. I wanted to be able to investigate each variable independently as a possible determining influence in the hermaphroditic person's existence in society as a boy or girl, man or woman. For this social variable, I might have used the term *social sex,* but that term carries too strong a connotation of adherence to a social code of behavior as a male or a female in public, independently of the intimate social use of the sex organs in private with a participating partner—or a series of partners.

Among psychologists, there had developed an academic application of the term *sex role* to refer to a person's social role as a male or female. Dimorphism of the anatomy of the genitalia was taken for granted as the criterion of male and female, though the social use of the genitalia in private as a component of sex role was prudishly evaded. There could be no defense of such prudishness in the case of birth-defective sex organs. Quite the contrary! In these cases, the role of the genitalia in male or female relationships cannot be taken for granted. It must be specified. It is, indeed, literally the sex role—the genital and erotic sex role. Its masculine or feminine completeness is a function of the original nature of the birth defect and of the degree of success achieved by surgical intervention.

I could not use the term sex role to mean the genitoerotic sex role, since it already had been preempted by social scientists to mean the nongenitoerotic, social sex role. I might have made do with complex expressions like "social sex exclusive of genital sex," or "social sex inclusive of erotic imagery as male or female." To avoid this pedantry, I decided not to further overburden the word *sex,* which already must do service as a civil status as well as an activity in bed. Instead, I borrowed *gender* from its sequestered place in grammar and philology, and used it in the term *gender role.*

Gender Role and Gender Identity

I was mindful of the dramatist's meaning of *role* as a part played by an actor, and also of the fact that a great actor may enter into a role so completely that he does not leave it in the theatre with his costume after each performance. For as long as the play runs he may inhabit the role in much the same way as, in everyday life, a person lives his role as a scholar, parent, worker, employer, politician, and so forth. In this latter sociological sense, a role is not simply a social script to be changed with everyday's change of clothing. It becomes in the brain an enduring template or mental map that is personalized for its owner to live by.

An individual is not only the bearer of his/her gender role but is also its exemplar, through whom it is transmitted socially as a model for others, especially those of the new generation, to assimilate. In this respect, gender role is like native language. In 1955, when I first used the term gender role in print, I defined it as having, like two sides of the same coin, a dual significance, namely, of being not only a personal attribute of the self, but also a social expression communicable to others in word and deed. This definition reads thus: "The term gender role is used to signify all those things that a person says or does to disclose himself or herself as having the status of boy or man, girl or woman, respectively. It includes, but is not restricted to, sexuality in the sense of eroticism" (Money, 1955, p. 254).

In the years after 1955, the term gender role entered first the professional, and then the vernacular language fairly rapidly, not only in English but in translation as well. Obviously, it filled a linguistic void and satisfied a conceptual need of many people—not, however, the same conceptual need for which I framed the definition, above. People adopted the term and gave it their own definition.

The first change was to separate the two sides of the same coin, and to name one side gender role, and the other side *gender identity.* Gender role became assigned to sociology as a socially prescribed mode of conduct which might, or might not be faithfully adhered to in an individual's development.

Gender identity, to the best of my knowledge, was first proposed by Evelyn

Hooker. I recall its appearance in an exchange of correspondence I had with her in reference to her homosexual studies. Gender identity became assigned to clinical psychology as a psychodynamic state of being, along with other attributes of identification current in psychoanalytic doctrine. Gender identification posed a problem for psychoanalytic theory that Robert Stoller (1964) solved by proposing the concept of *core gender identity* which, he said, is "produced by the infant-parents relationship, by the child's perception of its external genitalia, and by a biologic force that springs from the biologic variables of sex" (Stoller, 1968, pp. 29-30). Core gender identity formation antedates the classical Oedipal period of masculine and feminine development of the psyche, as represented in psychoanalysis.

Sex and Gender

The second change imposed on the original meaning of gender role was brought about by the partitioning of sex and gender. This change was heralded in the title of Stoller's book, *Sex and Gender* (1968). Its outcome was to restore the metaphysical partitioning of body and mind. Sex was ceded to biology. Gender was ceded to psychology and social science. The ancient regime was restored!

On the sex side of the partition, sex has retained its subdivisions into chromosomal or genetic sex, gonadal sex (prenatal and pubertal), and morphological sex (internal and external). For the biologically devout, these variables, acting either alone or as a combinatory vital force, preordain the entirety of masculinity or femininity of development in childhood through adulthood. For some of these devout it is enough to karyotype the chromosomes of a newborn hermaphrodite in order to decide the sex of assignment, regardless of the anatomy of the genitals. For others, the dogma is a laboratory diagnosis, as in the currently popular instance of 5-alpha reductase deficiency, when it exists, as the exclusive criterion for assigning a hermaphroditic baby as a male.

On the gender side of the partition, gender has retained its separation into gender identity and gender role. The definition of gender identity has been constricted to the simple self-declaration, "I am a boy," or "I am a girl"—or man, or woman (Stoller, 1964). This self-declaration might be either concordant or discordant with the anatomy of the genitalia. The discordancy that exists in the case of transexualism is so complete that, in technical jargon, gender identity is sometimes used as an attribute of only the discordant cases. One effect of this usage has been that some theoreticians of homosexuality have been entrapped into attributing a male gender identity to all homosexuals, provided they do not repudiate their self-declared status as male. The qualifier is then added that the homosexual, despite a male identity, has a male object choice or sexual preference. This nomenclature is totally illogical in cases of gynemimetic homosexuals, or drag queens, who impersonate women in variable degrees on a full-time basis. It is more straight-forward to attribute to homosexuals a gender identity that is homoerotic, and in its nonerotic components may or may not conform to the masculine stereotype.

Whereas the definition of gender role has not been constricted so severely as that of gender identity, it has been metamorphosed by having been divorced from biology and from the genital and erotic meaning of sex. Many textbooks of human sexuality and chapters in psychology texts now introduce the definition of gender by defining sex as a biological entity—and as what one is born with. Gender is a social entity, which one acquires after birth, and gender role is the social casting or ordainment of gender. This is the strategy by which gender role has been neutered. It has become devoid of any connection with biology and reproduction. It is defined instead as the product of social history, with male and female roles having been more or less arbitrarily assigned on the basis of male superiority and female inferiority. By today's definition gender role has thus become the intellectual property of social science and sexual politics—especially the sexual politics of the women's movement and, to a lesser degree, of the gay liberation movement. Vested interest groups within social science and sexual politics put up a spirited defense of their intellectual property. The opposition claims biology as the exclusive determinant of all gender differences. They maintain an equally one-sided defense of their a priori claim by ceding gender role to the social relativists, and defining gender identity as the entity that is biologically determined—though in a global and amorphous way. Thus, in applying biological determinism to hermaphroditism, they assert that hermaphroditic children may switch their gender identity at puberty, when in fact the correct statement should be that, after an ambiguous childhood, their official status in society is changed.

Nature/Nurture and Critical Period

The zealots of social determinism and of biological determinism are the darlings of the media. The majority of journalists and producers apply the ancient adversarial principle of the law to the search for truth, and ignore the more recent principle of science, which is the principle of consensus. A good fight makes for readership and audience appeal. Consequently, media people have not shifted from the nineteenth-century anachronism of juxtaposing nature and nurture, heredity and environment, constitutional and acquired, or biological and social.

The media thus endorse for nonspecialists the failure of most specialists to adopt an integrated psychobiological or sociobiological way of thinking about gender difference. This integration requires a paradigm shift away from the two-term juxtaposition of nature/nurture to a three-term integration of nature/critical-period/nurture. The three-term paradigm has long been known in embryology—far longer than in behavioral science. It means that nature and nurture interact at a critical period of development, that the outcome of this interaction is governed by its timing, and that the outcome, whether normal or abnormal, will be henceforth indelible.

In the dogma of social determinism, the emancipation of gender role from biology is also prerequisite to its emancipation from its genital and erotic component. This emancipation defers to the ancient and pervasive taboo on genital and erotic sex in our society by circumventing it. Gender is not a dirty three-letter, or four-letter, word. It is a clean, six-letter one.

Gender role, as defined in social science and sexual politics, is a clean term. The double entendre of the term, *sex gap,* if it were ever used, would be an absolute embarrassment to the politics of the gender gap. As a term, *gender gap* has none of the genital, erotic, and breeding stigma that sex gap would have. It refers only to those present differences between men and women that pertain to play, manners, fashion, schooling, career, and legal rights.

End-of-the-century society obviously needs the cleansed term, gender, to replace the soiled term, sex, in its political feuding for equal rights between men and women. Since the body politic is far larger than the body of sexological scientists, it is inevitable that politics will be able to preempt the term gender for its own usage.

Nonetheless, following the example of the dictionary, sexological science could also lay claim to its own scientific meaning. That, however, seems highly unlikely, so long as sexology, psychology, and sociology continue their present anarchic inability to agree. Unlike other sciences that convene an international assembly for the purpose of generating agreement on defintion of terms, policies, and procedures, sexology has been unable to do so with respect to gender research, pure and applied.

G-I/R

My own bridging of the chasm between the social and the biological definitions of gender is based on not separating gender role as a social phenomenon from gender identity as a biological one. Instead, the two are like obverse sides of the same coin. They constitute a unity. To prevent the subdivision of the unity of gender identity and role, I have adopted the practice of using an acronym for Gender-Identity/Role—G-I/R. Being singular, G-I/R enforces the union of identity and role. The defintion of G-I/R (Money, 1980, p. 215) is as follows:

> *Gender-Identity/Role (G-I/R):* Gender identity is the private experience of gender role, and gender role is public manifestation of gender identity. Gender identity is the sameness, unity, and persistence of one's individuality as male, female, or ambivalent, in greater or lesser degree, especially as it is experienced in self-awareness and behavior. Gender role is everything that a person says and does to indicate to others or to the self the degree that one is either male or female, or ambivalent. G-I/R includes but is not restricted to sexual arousal and response.

Developmentally, G-I/R is formed as a product of multivariate components. Not only are they multivariate, but also sequential in the chronology of their influence on the differentiation of G-I/R.

The concept of the multivariate, sequential differentiation of G-I/R has been widely disseminated. Nonetheless, the application of the concept has lagged far behind the rival concepts of the exclusivity of either biological (organic) determinism, or the social determinism of acquired learning.

Perhaps it is futile to fight the tide of dissension. That, however, could prove to be an abdication of scientific responsibility. It would deepen the chasm between the behavioral phenomenology of gender difference, and the neuroscience of its representation in the brain. In the ultimate analysis, gender differences reside in the brain, regardless of how they got there, whether as a consequence of prenatal or neonatal hormonal programing, postnatal social programing, pubertal hormonal programing, adult unfolding of prior programing, or geriatric deterioration of the programing from earlier years. The task confronting sexological science is to differentiate the input of these various programs—not excluding the program of social learning, of course. Let it never be forgotten, however, that learning itself is represented in the brain. There is, indeed, a brain biology of learning, irrespective of our ignorance of it at the present time.

Advancement in knowledge of how, when, and where G-I/R is represented in the functioning of the brain will undoubtedly bring about an advancement in the application of that knowledge in a more rational approach to the prevention of G-I/R syndromes, and to the treatment of those that do occur. A rational consensus among experts is absolutely prerequisite to the ability of patients and, in the case of neonatal hermaphrodites, for example, the ability of the parents to give their informed consent to the program of case management. Without a legitimate basis for fully informed consent, it becomes increasingly popular in a litigious society for patients, or their parents, to find a malpractice attorney. He, in turn, can easily find an expert from within a divided profession, who will testify on his side of the adversary system in the courtroom.

Victimology and the Criminalization of Sex

The inability of experts to agree has another ominous spin-off which I have headlined in the title of this paper as the "neutering of gender." The sociological definition of gender role as an acquired product of social learning would apply quite well if human beings were robotic dolls with nothing but smooth plastic between their legs. Their sex would reside exclusively above the belt, with the anatomy below the belt being a neutered zone. Then breeding would presumably take place by cloning, or parthenogenesis. Human beings, however, are not monecious, but diecious. They reproduce not by parthenogenic cloning, but by male-female mating below the belt. The connection between what takes place in the diecious anatomy below the belt, and what takes place in the mating brain above the belt, is mediated as the imagery of erotic arousal.

Erotic imagery and its relationship in perception or fantasy to erotic arousal and erotic performance is the Achilles heel in the social dogma of gender-role determination. In one school of social dogma, erotic imagery is totally ignored. In another, pioneered by militant women against pornography, all erotic imagery, not only that of sadomasochistic violence or rape, is equated with pornography; all pornography is, by their own definition, equated with the subjugation of women as men's sex objects and the victims of their power and violence. Among extremists, all sexual intercourse is either enforced rape or enforced exploitation of the female by the male—the husband included, in many jurisdictions of the United States.

The neutering of gender is part of a tidal wave of antisexualism that spreads its octopus tentacles into the politics of what could become a new and dictatorial era of antisexualism. America is, by reason of its historical roots in the antisexualism of Puritanism, vulnerable in this respect. It is vulnerable also because it presently has a media image of itself as having become sexually too permissive. In actual fact, America is not sexually too permissive. What the media misconstrues as sexual permissiveness is erotic permissiveness. Moreover, it pertains chiefly to eroticism above the belt, as exemplified in the titillation and innuendo of sexual advertising and entertainment, in both of which official policy is to avoid explicit mention of the genitalia.

In the funding of research the de facto policy of both the government and the private philanthropies is not to fund explicit investigations of genital sexuality, nor of falling in love. Funds that should be released through scientific channels for sex research are, by and large, released through criminal-justice channels instead, and they are tagged primarily for the practice of the newly minted specialty of victimology.

Victimologists are professionals trained mostly in psychology or social work, occasionally in medicine, and only rarely in sexology. They counsel victims, often on an improvisational basis, and also prepare them as witnesses. Currently, victimology addresses itself mostly to wife abuse, child abuse, rape, child molestation (pedophilia), incest, and, to some extent pornography.

Victimologists who specialize in child abuse, pedophilia, and incest, if they serve the recipient, or victim, are obliged by law to report the initiator as the perpetrator of a crime. Thus, in addition to their professional role as health-care providers, they become paralegal agents of law enforcement. Their paralegal status creates an ethical dilemma, since it is in conflict with the ethics of informed consent and confidentiality in the delivery of health care.

This ethical dilemma becomes apparent in, for example, a case in which an adolescent or adult is prevented from seeking help as a participant in a pedophilic relationship, since disclosure of the relationship would be self-incriminating, and would lead to arrest. For the same reason it is impossible for participants in pedophilia to volunteer as research subjects.

In the United States it is now possible to qualify as a pedophilic criminal if, after reaching the age of eighteen, you take nude pictures of your boyfriend or girlfriend who has not reached the age of eighteen, even if by only one day. On May 21st, 1984, the President signed Public Law 98-292, the Child Protection Act of 1984. In effect, this law requires that all Americans have the sexual status of being children until their eighteenth birthday. It specifies as a crime the depiction of anyone under the age of eighteen with the genitals exposed, or in simulated or nonsimulated sexual acts, not only if it is distributed for commercial purposes, but also as a gift or exchange. Obscenity is not a legally required criterion. Strictly applied, the law makes it a crime for young parents to send to their baby's grandparents a nude picture of the baby, genitals exposed, in the bathtub. It also makes it a crime for sexologists studying the sexuoerotic development of childhood to make a pictorial record of children's normal, healthy sexual rehearsal play.

The criminalization of sex is nothing new in Christendom. It has a long history in both canonical and secular law. What is new is the criminalization of sex on an expanding basis as the price paid for the desexualization of gender. Gender equality is equality in everything except the sexual and the erotic. The myth that women are sexually inert and anerotic is thus maintained. Simultaneously, a new myth is being created—the fiction that all sexual intercourse is an act of violence by which men dominate and degrade women and children.

As this new myth takes root in state legislatures and courtrooms, sexologists either admiringly endorse its growth, or else stand idly by, fiddling while Rome burns. They are naively unaware that the contemporary criminalization of sex makes them extremely vulnerable to being charged as sex criminals themselves. Before his/her eighteenth birthday, any child wily in the ways of juvenile crime can falsely accuse a sexologist—or, indeed, any victimologist—with child molestation, and thus ruin a professional career on the basis of guilt by accusation. By the same token, children can also retaliate against their parents by laying a false charge of incest before the child abuse authorities.

Earlier in the present century, European sexologists, also fiddling while Rome burned, endorsed the then popular social-eugenics theory of racial purity and the elimination of the unfit by castration to prevent their breeding (Pfäfflin, 1986). With the knowledge of hindsight, they would have foreseen sexology consumed by its own theory when Hitler decided that sexologists, homosexuals, and Jews were among the racially impure.

It is time for today's sexologists not to wait for the knowledge of hindsight, but to have the foresight to take political action now against the sinister implications of the new wave of the criminalization of sex and the conceptual neutering of gender.

References

Money, J. (1952). *Hermaphroditism: An Inquiry into the Nature of a Human Paradox*. Doctoral Dissertation, Harvard University Library. (University Microfilms Library Services, Xerox Corporation, Ann Arbor, Michigan 48106, 1967).
Money, J. (1955). Hermaphroditism, gender and precocity in hyperadrenocorticism: Psychologic findings. *Bulletin of The Johns Hopkins Hospital*, 96:253-264.
Money, J. (1980). *Love and Love Sickness: The Science of Sex, Gender Difference, and Pair-bonding*. Johns Hopkins University Press, Baltimore.
Pfäfflin, F. (1986). The connections between eugenics, sterilization and mass murder in Germany 1933-1945. *Medicine and Law*, 5:1-10.
Stoller, R. J. (1964). A contribution to the study of gender identity. *The International Journal of Psycho-analysis*, 45:220-226.
Stoller, R. J. (1968). *Sex and Gender: On the Development of Masculinity and Femininity*. Science House, New York.

Note

Presented, September 20, 1984, as an invited lecture at the Tenth Annual Meeting of the International Academy of Sex Research, Cambridge, England; and published in the *Archives of Sexual Behavior*, 14:279-290, 1985. [Bibliog. #2.295]

FORTY-EIGHT

Forensic and Family Psychiatry in Abuse Dwarfism: Munchausen's Syndrome by Proxy, Atonement, and Addiction to Abuse

Abstract

The syndrome of abuse dwarfism is characterized by gross impairment of statural and intellectual growth and social maturation while the abused child remains in the domicile of abuse. The parents collude as child abusers, and are medical imposters regarding the symptoms of abuse. The syndrome as a whole is appropriately named Munchausen's syndrome by proxy. Though the mother typically initiates abuse, she cannot give a rational explanation for doing so. In her own history there is a sin that is expiated or atoned for symbolically by the sacrifice of the child—explainable in terms of the theory of opponent-process learning. In the two cases presented, the sin was the mother's own birth out of wedlock, in one case as a sequel to incest. The child's addiction to abuse is a challenge to the program of rehabilitation. With respect to parents at risk, the data of this study are relevant to the prevention of a predisposition toward, or the actual implementation of child abuse, though a program of prevention needs still to be formulated. The sexological relevance of this study is that the data demonstrate that the effects of sexual abuse may be transmitted to the next generation and manifested as child abuse which is not necessarily sexual in content.

Concepts and Purpose

This article is one in a series of the psychoendocrine syndrome of abuse dwarfism.[1-11] Also known as psychosocial dwarfism, this syndrome is characterized by extreme failure of growth in stature, intellect, and sociobehavioral status. All three components of growth failure persist and eventually become irreversible, unless the child is rescued from the abusive environment, usually the parental home, where he/she has been the victim of multiple practices of child abuse and neglect. The earlier the rescue, the greater the amount of physical, mental, and social catch-up growth that can be achieved.

Parents who abuse their children so contravene our society's idealization of the sanctity of the family that the evidence of abuse is either euphemized as discipline or, if that fiction cannot be maintained, prosecuted as a crime. Though the reality of child abuse is acknowledged in traditional children's literature, the

601

responsibility is laid on witches and wicked stepmothers. Actual parents are exonerated. A century ago, when society first admitted that children have a right not to be abused by their parents,[12] actual parents were exonerated if they were respectable native-born Americans. The blame for child abuse was laid on illiterate immigrants, drunkards, prostitutes, and mental defectives. Today it is known that parental child abuse is not a prerogative of the disadvantaged or disabled. Well-educated, nondrinking, pious parents of the middle class and privileged elite of society may also be child abusers.

After a century of neglect, when child abuse was rediscovered under the name of the battered child syndrome,[13] it became a sexist vogue to exonerate mothers. Along with their children, they were considered victims of the brutality of their child-abusing husbands. Now, however, it is known that the mother herself may be the instigator of child abuse. Her husband acquiesces in what is, in effect, a folie à deux—a conspiracy or collusion to abuse.[7, 8] This is a phenomenon that still awaits an adequate scientific explanation. It is not clear whether any husband (or wife) could be enlisted as a collusional partner in child abuse; or whether, before they are married, there is a particular collusion-prone matching of the personalities of the two parents. Once their collusion in abuse gets under way, siblings of the victim are also locked into it. Even the agents of society may acquiesce, or be indifferent.

The phenomenon of the instigator as well as the colluder in child abuse also awaits an adequate scientific explanation. Extreme child abuse is too complexly systematic and bizarre to be written off as a simple deficiency of parenting, or ignorance of child care. Moreover, typically abuse is meted out not to all children in a family, but to one victim, with a second child being possibly a stand-in. Thus, child abuse cannot be attributed to a syndrome of psychopathology characterized by generalized neglect, or by indiscriminate violence and rage attacks. Rather, it is a syndrome of persecution and torture, unremittingly applied to a selected victim.

This syndrome is not yet recognized in the official nosology. As a psychopathological entity, it gets lost under the larger, and chiefly legal rubric of child abuse. It resembles Munchausen's syndrome, in that it involves medical impostoring: The history of child abuse is not disclosed if the child is ever brought to a physician or a clinic. Confabulatory explanations for abusively inflicted or induced symptoms are given instead. In Munchausen's syndrome, symptoms are self-inflicted. When they are inflicted on the child, one has, therefore, to speak of Munchausen's syndrome by proxy.[7, 14]

The purpose of the present report is to illustrate, in two cases of abuse dwarfism, the existence of Munchausen's syndrome by proxy, and the concepts therein of sacrifice and atonement. The child is sacrificed as a surrogate to atone for the transgressions of one or more of its forebears. The two cases illustrate also that the victim becomes addicted to abuse, and so becomes a participant in the collusion of the abusers.

Sample and Procedure

From among 50 cases of abuse dwarfism seen in the Johns Hopkins Psychohormonal Unit, these two cases, one male and one female, were selected because they were abused very severely for a longer period of time, until age 16 and 8 respectively, than any other case. In both cases, because the parents were prosecuted, information from witnesses in court supplemented information obtained in the clinic. The patients themselves have been maintained in follow-up, the boy for 15 years, and the girl for 8 years, and so have been able to provide details of their own story. Interviews with both patients, and in each case with one relative familiar with the period of abuse and rescue, were recorded and transcribed verbatim. While in prison, the girl's parents consented to be interiewed, but it was not possible to contact the boy's parents.

From the patients' consolidated psychoendocrine histories, information was indexed, organized, abstracted and tabulated in accordance with the subheadings that follow.

Medical Impostoring

In each of the two cases, the history and evidence of child abuse was irrefutable. The history of abuse was confirmed in the courtroom on the basis of evidence produced by police and social welfare officials, and by family and community members. The evidence of bodily abuse was confirmed by physical and laboratory examinations conducted in hospitals to which the children were taken at the time of rescue.

In each case, the most dramatic evidence of abuse pertained to the post-rescue acceleration in growth rate, which is typical and, indeed, pathognomonic of abuse dwarfism. Thus, whereas the boy's chronological age at the time of rescue was 16, his height was that of an 8-year-old, and his bone age, 11. Mental age (IQ 59) and social developmental age were correspondingly retarded, as was the onset of puberty. In the year following rescue, statural growth accelerated, with a phenomenal gain of 13 inches in three years. The onset of puberty was similarly rapid, whereas catch-up intellectual growth and social maturation were both protracted.

In the case of the girl, her chronological age at the time of rescue was 8:10. Her height was that of a baby of 2 years, and her bone age was 3 years. In the year following rescue, there was a gain in height of 10.5 inches. Catch-up mental and social growth was, as expected, less rapid. The IQ at the time of rescue was 43. The onset of puberty was at the age of 11:9.

In neither case had the parents responded in the normal way to their child's extreme growth failure, namely, by taking the child to a pediatrician or a pediatrics clinic. The boy's mother threatened relatives with a butcher knife if they questioned her treatment of him. She developed the fiction that she was his benefactor by not putting him away in an institution, claiming that he was so retarded as to be like an animal—witness his crawling on all fours while the other children ate, waiting for them to throw scraps of food to him. She did not disclose that she forbade him to be fed in any other way, and deprived him of food and water which he had to obtain by subterfuge—drinking out of the toilet bowl, for example, and eating from the garbage can.

In the case of the girl, when a neighbor made inquiries about a rumor that a child was kept locked in a closet, the mother assured him that this child was no longer in the home, but had been put away in an institution. Thenceforth, if ever she left the house with her parents, she was required to lie on the floor behind the front seat of the car, so that no one would see her. At home she was kept locked in the closet. Only a few family members knew of her failure to grow. Her sister, two years older, would sneak food to her. Once when a cheese wrapper was found in the closet, the sister herself was subjected to being locked in a similar closet for a month, and similarly deprived of food, water, toilet facilities, clothing, and space to lie down to sleep.

The boy also had the fate of being locked in a closet and deprived of food, water, and amenities. His siblings were, under threats of reprisals, unable to disclose his ordeal, or to engineer his rescue. Once a week, he was tied to a newel post, and they were forced to beat him with a broomstick, or else be beaten with it themselves.

In the hospital, in both cases, the physical examination revealed old scars and burn marks that confirmed the testimony of relatives regarding injuries inflicted by beating and burning. There was visible as well as radiographic evidence that the girl's left leg had been broken and allowed to heal untreated. It was crooked and an inch shorter than the right leg. Radiography showed that the boy's right arm had been fractured in two places, and not set; and also that he had suffered skull fractures. In both cases the fractures had been inflicted. The girl's mother explained the deformity of the left leg as the result of a car accident, but did not explain the failure to seek medical attention. The boy's parents avoided the hospital after he was rescued, and so were not obliged to confabulate explanations for his injuries.

In both cases, the parents succeeded as medical impostors, who produced symptoms in their children without being discovered. Their impostures succeeded partly through threats and reprisals that coerced juvenile siblings and other potential informants into colluding with them. In addition, the parents succeeded as impostors by keeping the abused child away from medical attention. They succeeded also because the agents of society, by their indifference, became agents of collusion.

In each child's history, there was an occasion when the relatives alerted the police to child abuse. When police officers came to the girl's home, the father excused himself for long enough to remove the child from the locked closet and put her in bed beside her sister. The officers saw her in bed and departed, leaving her for two more years of abuse.

In the boy's case, the police officers removed the nails with which his closet door was sealed, photographed him seated in his own excrement, and did not prosecute. He was abused for two more years. His relatives then appealed to the school authorities to investigate his total lack of schooling. After several attempts, truant officers finally succeeded in taking him away for a day of evaluation. The story of abuse was professionally recorded and, along with the test results, filed. No further action was taken, so that the boy was locked away and abused for two more years, until he was rescued at age 16.

In both cases, when rescue was finally effected, the exposure of the parents' abuse was so convincing that their imposture of normality was no longer persuasive. Their alibis simply would not hold up. They were prosecuted and penalized.

Transgression and Atonement

Publicly exposed as impostors who in private have been torturing and persecuting a child, abusive parents have no defense, other than the self-righteous imposture of parental morality with which to mitigate their guilt. They are without defense, because they do not have a genuine explanation of the genesis of themselves as child abusers.

Morally naked and on view in public, they have no alternative with which to counteract the philosophy of their accusers, namely, that they acted on the basis of free will and voluntarily chose to be evil. They do not have an image of child abusing as a syndrome of disease, and of themselves as victims of it.

With some justification, they are haughty and indignant at the prospect of being labeled with a psychiatric diagnosis, for the nomenclature itself has no satisfactory etiology for child abuse. Indeed, up to a point, harsh discipline and the infliction of bodily injury and pain on children at home and school is condoned as normal and healthy, not as pathological and abusive.[15] Without discipline and punishment, it is said, there is disobedience and no character building. Moreover, there is religious sanction against sparing the rod and spoiling the child. Punishment is a penalty for sin and wrongdoing. Penance and sacrifice expiate sin. They are an atonement. Atonement is a powerful institute that permeates all our social life.

Parents who abuse their child are, in effect, sacrificing their child. Whether they know it or not, they have assimilated the example of Abraham of old whose abusive knife got perilously close to sacrificing Isaac. It is the vengeance of a wrathful God that demands the sacrifice of one's own son. A wrath of such magnitude implies a sin of comparable magnitude.

Today's child-abusing parents do, indeed, in some cases sacrifice their children. Literally, they kill them. If, before that, the parents bring the child to a hospital, it is not to prevent it from dying, but to prolong its life as a living sacrifice. To send the child back home is to guarantee its continued abuse and, possibly, its ultimate death.

This is the apogee of child abuse. Even when the sacrificial child survives, however, professionals and others are mystified as to the reason for the sacrifice. So also are the parents themselves. The sin that is being atoned for in the sacrifice of the child is either unspeakable, unspoken of, or logically disconnected from the child's suffering.

In the two cases of this report, it was the mother who was heir to a sin so great that it could not be atoned for, except by sacrifice. In the case of the boy, the woman who engineered his abuse was actually his stepmother. His birth mother and her paramour, his father of conception, had died in an auto crash when he was a baby. He was three years old when his deceased mother's husband, his legal father, remarried. The new wife had had four children of her own. The oldest had been born out of wedlock when the mother was a teenager. The next three were children of her first marriage. These three, but not the oldest daughter, were given up for adoption after the marriage failed. At the time the mother was clinically diagnosed as depressed, but she did not pursue treatment.

In middle teenage, this woman's personality had reputedly undergone a rapid change. From a well-behaved religious girl, she became a rebellious delinquent. The change followed hospitalization for third degree burns suffered when her robe caught on fire, apparently accidently. While she was in the hospital, her grandmother, devoutly religious, prepared her for the possibility of final absolution, by disclosing to her the secret of her birth. Her father was not the same man as the father of her siblings, she being their half-sister. She herself had been born out of wedlock. Her grandmother's husband, the man she knew as grandfather, was actually her father. Knowing this incest secret traumatized and reshaped her life. When she remarried, the three-year-old boy in the household who, like herself, had been conceived out of wedlock, became the sacrificial lamb, destined to atone for her own original sin. Intellectually, she herself did not make this connection. Nor, apparently, did her husband who colluded in the sacrificial abuse of the child. He may have been trapped into collusion, because family life was too complex for him to manage as a single parent and wage earner.

In the other case, that of the girl, the mother's sin was, according to what she had been told, that she had been conceived by an unknown father. Her mother had been stigmatized as promiscuous. Before she was born, her mother promised to give her to a tavern companion, a woman with a childless marriage. This woman and her husband raised the child from birth. As a 16-year-old, the child escaped what she considered an intolerable home life by marrying a serviceman. They had two children. While he was overseas, she had a brief affair and became pregnant again. By age three months, the baby was so grossly neglected, along with two older sisters, that all three were taken from their mother and placed in foster care. Upon the husband's return, the family was reunited, out of state. The marriage ended in divorce. The mother married another serviceman who had recently returned from Southeast Asia. The new stepfather collaborated with his wife in the continued abuse of her youngest daughter. Later, he naively attributed the error of his ways to an excessive devotion to military discipline. However, he may also have had no escape from a trap in which collusion in the abuse of the youngest child was a trade-off for a pedophilic relationship with the oldest one. The mother herself did not explicitly relate her abuse of her youngest daughter to either her own or the child's out-of-wedlock birth; but she was pathologically explicit in saying that she had rejected her abused daughter since her birth and had long wanted to "give her up." Thus, she partially replicated with her daughter what her birth mother had done to her. She recalled never having seen her birth mother until she was fully grown and in her twenties.

Addiction to Abuse

One of the self-justifications used by abusing parents is that their child instigates abuse. More fully explained, this claim may signify a failure of parent-child bonding, even from birth onward. Subsequently, it may signify also that the abused has become addicted to abuse: The response to abuse is to stimulate more of it. The neurochemistry of this addiction may well be linked to the neurosecretion of brain endorphin which has a morphine-like effect. There is as yet, no direct evidence in support of this proposition.

The indirect evidence is from the clinic, namely that children with the syndrome of abuse dwarfism exhibit signs of pain agnosia while they live under conditions of abuse.[10] Rescued and in the hospital, they regain an aversive response to pain in about two weeks. During the same period of time, they regain also normal levels of pituitary growth hormone secretion which, in the domicile of abuse and growth failure, is at a near-zero level.

In the two cases of this report, the children's addiction to abuse became evident soon after they had been rescued and were living for a period in a children's recovery center, and for a period with a foster family. It is typical in the syndrome of abuse dwarfism that, following rescue from the home of abuse, the child goes through a phase of noisy hyperactivity. This phase persists for several months, and possibly for as long as two years. It is marked by disputatiousness and noncompliance which exasperates other people and provokes their retaliation. At first glance, it may seem that the naughtiness and disobedience of this early postrescue phase is no different than that encountered in children without the same history of severe abuse. A closer search, however, reveals a difference.

Thus, in the case of the girl, her foster mother told of how the child had asked why she hadn't been paddled as her foster sister had been. "I guess she thought I didn't love her, if I didn't paddle her, the way her mother used to beat her," the foster mother conjectured. This foster mother was unable to cope with the challenge of rehabilitating an abused child, and requested that the girl be placed elsewhere. The new placement was in a home for the retarded, not an ideal placement for a family-deprived child, since it replicated the deprivation of close parent-child bonding to which the child had so long been subjected.

In the case of the boy, the first foster parents encountered a similar problem. They also were unable to meet the challenge of rehabilitating him in their home, as they had hoped to be able to do. His next placement was in the children's recovery center. There he was said to provoke fights with other children. Though he yearned to be accepted by his relatives, they neglected him. On one occasion he became upset and protested that people were mean to him. He said he wanted to die. After an emergency session with his therapist, he went to sleep. The next morning he continued with wanting to die. He went to a storage room to get some personal belongings, but instead wrapped around his neck a belt and a wire coat hanger. They were removed by two staff members who found him. Next day, considered to be a suicide risk, he was put in an unfurnished room. There he swung from overhead pipes, and banged his head against the wall.

The staff considered the aforesaid behavior as psychotic and had the boy transferred to a state mental hospital. With the knowledge of hindsight, another interpretation is possible, namely, that the boy was homesick for the only family life that he knew, in which the only child-to-parent bond familiar to him was that of victim to victimizer. This is the kind of bonding that has recently become known as the Stockholm syndrome, named from the case of a woman held captive in a bank robbery in Stockholm. She became so captivated by the terrorist who held her in captivity that she remained faithful to him throughout his prison term, at the cost of abandoning her erstwhile fiancé.

In the present case, the boy was eventually located in a church-sponsored institution for the chronically mentally retarded, not an ideal environment to foster intellectual and social catch-up growth in the syndrome of abuse dwarfism. With the passage of years, he was able to live away from the institution, but only with the help of a disability pension. He continued to attract abusive attacks on himself by at times tangling with members of an organized street gang, and at other times antagonizing the police with minor misdemeanors childishly unsuited to his adult age. He needed a protector and did, in fact, have several people who took on that role. His most recent protectors are a police officer and his wife. With their assistance, he seems finally to have outgrown, at age 32, his former addiction to abuse.

Discussion

In the foregoing, the section on *impostoring* raises the issue of whether deception and evasion on the part of child-abusing parents should be regarded as evil or illness. Historically, when our society has been intolerant of behavior, the initial response has been to set up sanctions against it as sinful or criminal. Its cause has been attributed to the voluntary pursuit of wickedness. Society's energy and money have been directed toward the establishment of right or wrong, innocence or guilt. By fiat, without proof, the doctrine of prevention is equated with the doctrine of punishment and the death sentence.

It is a recent phenomenon of the last two centuries that some manifestations of socially condemned behavior have been reclassified as syndromes of illness. Society's money and energy have then been directed toward diagnosis, prognosis, and treatment. The doctrine of prevention is equated with the doctrine of etiology or cause. Indeed, the reclassification of criminality as pathology may be contingent on the discovery of its etiology and, thus, of the possibility of its cure or prevention.

In the present instance, it is without question that parental child abuse is as much a social evil as is cholera, or radiation from nuclear waste. The question is whether child abuse should be classified as a crime and the parents prosecuted, as were both sets of parents herein reported, or whether it should be reclassified as a disease.

In this paper, it is classified as a disease, and given the name of Munchausen's syndrome by proxy. The rationale for this strategy is that, by possessing a name as a syndrome instead of as a moral pejorative, the source of the syndrome, and its eradication as a social ill will be sought biomedically.

The section of this paper on *atonement,* achieved by offering up one's offspring as a sacrifice, shows how pervasively the paradigms of our religious culture may be assimilated and practiced. Whereas this theme of atonement by sacrifice has some etiological significance, it provided only a necessary, but not sufficient cause for the syndrome of abuse. What still is needed is an explanation of how forbidden and repugnant behavior becomes endorsed and practiced. For so complete a reversal of negative into positive, Solomon[16] formulated and tested the theory of opponent-process learning. Opponent-process is seen in action when, for example, the initial panic and terror of a novice practicing a daredevil sport gives way to the exhilaration and ecstasy of the aficionado. This conversion is undoubtedly accompanied by a corresponding change in the neurochemistries of the learning brain. Deciphering them will require further advances in neuroscience.

A special instance of the opponent-process principle is the principle of identification with the aggressor. This principle is used in brainwashing of political prisoners, and in the training of recruits in terrorism and torture. The same principle is at work in the Stockholm syndrome above mentioned; and in the martyrdom of *addiction to abuse,* the topic of the third section of this paper.

Becoming addicted to abuse is the human equivalent of, among horses, becoming broken-in to harness. In former times, the same principle applied to the breaking-in of slaves. Among children who have had sufficiently severe and prolonged abuse, as in the present two cases, the outcome is not rage, rebellion, and revenge. On the contrary, it is appeasement, appealing to be nurtured, and yearning to be worthy of good parents.

This outcome of abuse interferes with the development of autonomy and adult independence. In the syndrome of abuse dwarfism, it represents an impairment of social maturation that is the counterpart of impaired intellectual growth and statural growth. The longer the period of abuse, the more severe these impairments, and the less the final achievement in catch-up growth in stature, intellect, and social maturity, as a sequel to rescue.

Appendix: Endocrine and Behavioral Nature of the Syndrome of Abuse Dwarfism

The syndrome of abuse dwarfism is characterized by a domicile-specific impairment of statural growth and of growth hormone secretion.[17] Along with various other pathological features of the syndrome, both impairments occur as sequelae of child abuse.[1] All impairments are reversible upon change of domicile, away from abuse, into an environment of rescue. Taxonomically, the syndrome today is usually known as abuse dwarfism[1] or psychosocial dwarfism.[18] However, the syndrome has had various diagnostic labels: environmental failure to thrive;[19] deprivation dwarfism;[20] and maternal deprivation and emotional deprivation.[21, 22]

Three primary impairments in the syndrome are deficits in physique age, mental age, and social age relative to chronological age. Physique age includes height age, identified as dwarfed when the height is below the third percentile for chronological age. Physique age includes also the age of onset of puberty which is delayed if abuse is sufficiently prolonged. Intellectual development is retarded so that the M.A. (mental age) and IQ are defective.[2, 3] Social maturation also is retarded so that social age, including academic achievement age and psychosexual age, is deficient.

There are three known hormonal impairments in the syndrome. Growth hormone impairment is associated with statural growth impairment resulting in a physique age discrepant with chronological age. Impaired gonadotropin (LH and FSH) secretion is associated with delayed puberty. Impaired response of ACTH (adrenocorticotropic hormone) reserve as tested by metyrapone stimulation is partial—total impairment would be lethal.

The pathognomonic characteristic of the environment of growth failure is child abuse. Recovery from abuse takes place after rescue. An initial hospitalization for a short period of time, approximately two weeks, allows for the resumption, of growth hormone secretion, and leads to the onset of catch-up statural growth, both of which are essential to establish the diagnosis of abuse dwarfism.

After continued rescue, intellectual catch-up growth has been measured by an increase of as much as 84 IQ points.[3] The rate of intellectual catch-up growth is positively correlated with the rate of catch-up statural growth.[2]

Another developmental deficit that is reversible upon rescue from abuse pertains to unusual social behavior. Eating may be from a garbage can, for example, and drinking from a toilet bowl; or there may be binges of polydipsia and polyphagia, possibly followed by vomiting. There can also be a history of such reversible behavior symptoms as enuresis, encopresis, social aloofness or inertia, crying spasms, insomnia, eccentric sleeping and waking schedules,[11] and pain agnosia and self-injury,[10] all occurring only in the growth-retarding environment of abuse.

References

1. Money, J.: The syndrome of abuse dwarfism (psychosocial dwarfism or reversible hyposomatotropinism): Behavioral data and case report. *American J Dis Child* 131:508-513, 1977.

2. Money, J., Annecillo, C., Kelley, J. F.: Abuse-dwarfism syndrome: After rescue, statural and intellectual catchup growth correlate. *J Clin Child Psychol* 12:279-283, 1983.

3. Money, J., Annecillo, C., Kelley, J. F.: Growth of intelligence: failure and catchup associated respectively with abuse and rescue in the syndrome of abuse dwarfism. *Psychoneuroendocrinol* 8:309-319, 1983.

4. Money, J., Annecillo, C., Werlwas, J.: Hormonal and behavioral reversals in hyposomatotropic dwarfism. In E. J. Sachar (ed.), *Hormones, behavior, and psychopathology.* New York, Raven, 1976.

5. Money, J., Needleman, A.: Child abuse in the syndrome of reversible hyposomatotrophic dwarfism (psychosocial dwarfism). *Pediat Psychol* 1:20-23, 1976.

6. Money, J., Needleman, A.: Impaired mother-infant pair bonding in the syndrome of abuse dwarfism: Possible prenatal, perinatal, and neonatal antecedents. In G. J. Williams, J. Money (eds.), *Traumatic abuse and neglect of children at home.* Baltimore, Johns Hopkins University Press, 1980.

7. Money, J., Werlwas, J.: Folie à deux in the parents of psychosocial dwarfs: Two cases. *Bul Amer Acad Psychiat Law* 4:351-362, 1976.

8. Money, J., Werlwas, J.: Paraphilic sexuality and child abuse: The parents. *J Sex Marital Ther* 8:57-64, 1982.

9. Money, J., Wolff, G.: Late puberty, retarded growth and reversible hyposomatotropinism (psychosocial dwarfism). *Adolescence* 9:121-134, 1974.

10. Money, J., Wolff, G., Annecillo, C.: Pain agnosia and self-injury in the syndrome of reversible somatotropin deficiency (psychosocial dwarfism). *J Autism Childhood Schiz* 2:127-139, 1972.

11. Wolff, G., Money, J.: Relationship between sleep and growth in patients with reversible somatotropin deficiency (psychosocial dwarfism). *Psycholog Med* 3:18-27, 1973.

12. Williams, G. J.: Cruelty and kindness to children: Documentary of a century, 1874-1974. In G. J. Williams, J. Money (eds.), *Traumatic abuse and neglect of children at home.* Baltimore, Johns Hopkins University Press, 1980.

13. Kempe, C. H., Silverman, F. N., Steele, B. F., Droegemueller, W., Silver, H. K.: The battered child syndrome. *JAMA* 181:17-24, 1962.

14. Meadow, R.: Munchausen syndrome by proxy: The hinterland of child abuse. In G. J. Williams, J. Money (eds.), *Traumatic abuse and neglect of children at home.* Baltimore, Johns Hopkins University Press, 1980.

15. Hyman, I. A.: Corporal punishment in the schools: America's officially sanctioned brand of child abuse. In G. J. Williams, J. Money (eds.), *Traumatic abuse and neglect of children at home.* Baltimore, Johns Hopkins University Press, 1980.

16. Solomon, R. L.: The opponent-process theory of acquired motivation. *Amer Psychol* 35:691-712, 1980.

17. Patton, R. G., Gardner, L. I.: Deprivation dwarfism (psychosocial deprivation): Disordered family environment as cause of so-called idiopathic hypopituitarism. In L. I. Gardner (ed.), *Endocrine and genetic diseases of childhood,* 2nd ed. Philadelphia, Saunders, 1975, pp. 85-98.

18. Reinhart, J. B., Drash, A. L.: Psychosocial dwarfism: Environmentally induced recovery. *Psychosom Med* 31:165-171, 1969.

19. Barbero, G. J., Shaheen, E.: Environmental failure to thrive: A clinical view. *J Pediat* 71:639-644, 1967.

20. Silver, H. K., Finkelstein, M.: Deprivation dwarfism. *J Pediat* 70:317-324, 1967.

21. Powell, G. F., Brasel, J. A., Blizzard, R. M.: Emotional deprivation and growth retardation simulating idiopathic hypopituitarism. I. Clinical evaluation of the syndrome. *N E J Med* 276:1271-1278, 1967.

22. Powell, G. F., Brasel, J. A. Raiti, S., Blizzard, R. M.: Emotional deprivation and growth retardation simulating idiopathic hypopituitarism. II. Endocrinologic evaluation of the syndrome. *N E J Med* 276:1279-1283, 1967.

Note

Originally published in the *Journal of Sex and Marital Therapy,* 11:30–40, 1985, with C. Annecillo and J. Werlwas Hutchison as coauthors. [Bibliog. #2.296]

Author's Comment: Religious Sexosophy

The syndrome of abuse dwarfism is of great theoretical significance because it dramatically demonstrates how events in the social environment affect the functioning of the neuroendocrine system and the growth of the body, as well as the growth of intelligence and the maturation of behavior in childhood. The syndrome is additionally significant because it also demonstrates, as is evident in this paper, that events in the social environment may have a two generational effect. In the two cases reported in this paper, the mother atoned for the illegitimacy of her own origin through the protracted sacrifice of her child.

Here then is a hitherto unrecognized psychopathological phenomenon, namely the insidious and unsuspected alliance of two tenets of our cultural heritage in sexosophy and religion, namely, the sinfulness of sex and the expiation of sin through sacrifice. How, and in whom, this alliance is able to become established and perpetuated in the brain and behavior is still, scientifically, a mystery. The fact that such an alliance can take place, however, may open up a new approach to religious counseling and psychotherapy. The religious sexosophy of our society is more pervasive than we fully comprehend.

Bibliography

Author's Explanatory Note: This bibliography of publications from the Psycho-hormonal Research Unit has a history of having been compiled annually. In 1974, the years from 1948 through 1974 were consolidated, with separate categories and numberings for books, scientific papers, reviews and book chapters, et cetera. The second consolidation covers the years 1975–1979. From 1980 to the present, there is a separate supplement annually. However, the numbering within each category of publication is continuous, not annual. All books are listed continuously from 1952 through 1986. On coauthored scientific papers, the name of the senior author is not invariably listed first, but sometimes last. The responsibility of the senior author, as director of the Psychohormonal Research Unit, was to design, supervise, write, and edit each paper.

Part One: 1952–1986

BOOKS

1.1 Money, J. *Hermaphroditism: An Inquiry into the Nature of a Human Paradox.* Doctoral Dissertation, Harvard University Library, 1952. University Microfilms Library Services, Xerox Corporation, Ann Arbor, Michigan 48106, 1967.

1.2 Money, J. *The Psychologic Study of Man.* Springfield, Ill., Charles C Thomas, 1957.

1.3 Money, J. (ed.), *Reading Disability: Progress and Research Needs in Dyslexia.* Baltimore, Johns Hopkins Press, 1962.

1.4 Money, J. (ed.), *Sex Research: New Developments.* New York, Holt, Rinehart and Winston, 1965.

1.5 Money, J., Alexander, D. and Walker, H. T., Jr. *A Standardized Road-Map Test of Direction Sense.* Baltimore, Johns Hopkins Press, 1965.

1.6 Money, J. (ed.). *The Disabled Reader: Education of the Dyslexic Child.* Baltimore, Johns Hopkins Press, 1966.

1.7 Money, J. (sub-ed.). Section VI, Biologic Age, Cerebral Function and Psychologic Growth. In *Human Growth: Body Composition, Cell Growth, Energy and Intelligence* (D. B. Cheek, ed.). Philadelphia, Lea and Febiger, 1968.

1.8 Money, J. *Sex Errors of the Body: Dilemmas, Education and Counseling.* Baltimore, Johns Hopkins Press, 1968.

1.9 Green, R. and Money, J. (eds.). *Transsexualism and Sex Reassignment.* Baltimore, Johns Hopkins Press, 1969.

1.10 Money, J. (ed.). *Sexual Behavior—Readings V: Introduction to Psychiatry and the Behavioral Sciences.* Baltimore, Dept. of Psychiatry and Behavioral Sciences, The Johns Hopkins University School of Medicine, 1970.

1.11 Money, J. and Ehrhardt, A. A. *Man and Woman, Boy and Girl: The Differentiation and Dimorphism of Gender Identity from Conception to Maturity.* Baltimore, Johns Hopkins University Press, 1972.

1.12 Zubin, J. and Money, J. (eds.). *Contemporary Sexual Behavior: Critical Issues in the 1970s.* Baltimore, Johns Hopkins University Press, 1973.

1.13 Money, J. and Tucker, P. *Sexual Signatures.* Boston, Little, Brown, 1975.

1.14   Schaie, W. K., Anderson, E., McClearn, G., and Money, J. (eds.). *Developmental Human Behavior Genetics*. Lexington, Mass., D. C. Heath, 1975.

1.15   Money, J. and Musaph, H. (eds.). *Handbook of Sexology*. Amsterdam/New York, Excerpta Medica, 1977.

1.16   Money, J. and Musaph, H. (eds.). *History and Ideology, Vol. I, Handbook of Sexology.* New York, Elsevier/North-Holland, 1978 (Paperback).

1.17   Money, J. and Musaph, H. (eds.). *Genetics, Hormones and Behavior, Vol. II, Handbook of Sexology.* New York, Elsevier/North-Holland, 1978 (Paperback).

1.18   Money, J. and Musaph, H. (eds.). *Procreation and Parenthood, Vol. III, Handbook of Sexology.* New York, Elsevier/North-Holland, 1978 (Paperback).

1.19   Money, J. and Musaph, H. (eds.). *Selected Personal and Social Issues, Vol. IV, Handbook of Sexology.* New York, Elsevier/North-Holland, 1978 (Paperback).

1.20   Money, J. and Musaph, H. (eds.). *Selected Syndromes and Therapy, Vol. V, Handbook of Sexology.* New York, Elsevier/North-Holland, 1978 (Paperback).

1.21   Money, J. *Love and Love Sickness: The Science of Sex, Gender Difference, and Pairbonding.* Baltimore, Johns Hopkins University Press, 1980.

1.22   Williams, G. and Money, J. (eds.). *Traumatic Abuse and Neglect of Children at Home.* Baltimore, Johns Hopkins University Press, 1980.

1.23   Wolman, B. B. and Money, J. (eds.). *Handbook of Human Sexuality.* Englewood Cliffs, N.J., Prentice-Hall, 1980.

1.24   Williams, G. and Money, J. (eds.). *Traumatic Abuse and Neglect of Children at Home. Abridged Edition.* Baltimore, Johns Hopkins University Press, 1982 (Paperback).

1.25   Money, J. *The Destroying Angel: Sex, Fitness, and Food in the Legacy of Degeneracy Theory, Graham Crackers, Kellogg's Corn Flakes, and American Health History.* Buffalo, Prometheus Books, 1985.

1.26   Money, J. *Lovemaps: Clinical Concepts of Sexual/Erotic Health and Pathology, Paraphilia, and Gender Transposition in Childhood, Adolescence, and Maturity.* New York, Irvington Publishers, 1986.

Part Two: 1948-1974

SCIENTIFIC PAPERS

1948

2.1   Money, J. Delusion, belief and fact. *Psychiatry,* 11:33-38, 1948.

1949

2.2   Money, J. Unanimity in the social sciences with reference to epistemology, ontology and scientific method. *Psychiatry,* 12:211-221, 1949.

1951

2.3   Money, J. Observations concerning the clinical method of research, ego theory and psychopathology. *Psychiatry,* 14:55-66, 1951.

1954

2.4   Money, J. An examination of the concept of psychodynamics. *Psychiatry,* 17:325-330, 1954.

1955

2.5   Hampson, J. G. Hermaphroditic genital appearance, rearing and eroticism in hyperadrenocorticism. *Bulletin of The Johns Hopkins Hospital,* 96:265-273, 1955.

2.6   Hampson, J. G. and Money, J. Idiopathic sexual precocity in the female. *Psychosomatic Medicine,* 17:16-35, 1955.

2.7   Hampson, J. L., Hampson, J. G. and Money, J. The syndrome of gonadal agenesis (ovarian agenesis) and male chromosomal pattern in girls and women: Psychologic studies. *Bulletin of The Johns Hopkins Hospital,* 97:207-226, 1955.

2.8   Money, J. Hermaphroditism, gender and precocity in hyperadrenocorticism: Psychologic findings. *Bulletin of The Johns Hopkins Hospital,* 96:253-264, 1955.

2.9   Money, J. Linguistic resources and psychodynamic theory. *British Journal of Medical Psychology,* 28:264-266, 1955.

2.10 Money, J. and Hampson, J. G. Idiopathic sexual precocity in the male. *Psychosomatic Medicine,* 17:1-15, 1955.

2.11 Money, J., Hampson, J. G. and Hampson, J. L. An examination of some basic sexual concepts: The evidence of human hermaphroditism. *Bulletin of The Johns Hopkins Hospital,* 97:301-319, 1955.

2.12 Money, J., Hampson, J. G. and Hampson, J. L. Hermaphroditism: Recommendations concerning assignment of sex, change of sex, and psychologic management. *Bulletin of The Johns Hopkins Hospital,* 97:284-300, 1955.

1956

2.13 Money, J. Mind-body dualism and the unity of body-mind. *Behavioral Science,* 1:212-217, 1956.

2.14 Money, J. Psychologic studies in hypothyroidism, and recommendations for case management. *Archives of Neurology and Psychiatry,* 76:296-309, 1956.

2.15 Money, J., Hampson, J. G. and Hampson, J. L. Sexual incongruities and psychopathology: The evidence of human hermaphroditism. *Bulletin of The Johns Hopkins Hospital,* 98:43-57, 1956.

1957

2.16 Money, J. Case illustration: Hermaphroditism, sex reassignment. From Chapter 9 in *The Psychologic Study of Man.* Springfield, Ill., Charles C Thomas, 1957.

2.17 Money, J., Hampson, J. G. and Hampson, J. L. Imprinting and the establishment of gender role. *Archives of Neurology and Psychiatry, 77:33-336, 1957.*

1960

2.18 Green, R. and Money, J. Incongruous gender role: Nongenital manifestations in pre-pubertal boys. *Journal of Nervous and Mental Disease,* 130:160-167, 1960.

2.19 Money, J. Components of eroticism in man: Cognitional rehearsals. In *Recent Advances in Biological Psychiatry* (J. Wortis, ed.). New York, Grune and Stratton, 1960.

2.20 Money, J. Phantom orgasm in the dreams of paraplegic men and women. *Archives of General Psychiatry,* 3:373-382, 1960.

1961

2.21 Green, R. and Money, J. Effeminancy in prepubertal boys: Summary of eleven cases and recommendations for case management. *Pediatrics,* 27:286-291, 1961.

2.22 Money, J. Components of eroticism in man. I: The hormones in relation to sexual morphology and sexual desire. *Journal of Nervous and Mental Disease,* 132:239-248, 1961.

2.23 Money, J. Components of eroticism in man. II: The orgasm and genital somesthesia. *Journal of Nervous and Mental Disease.* 132:289-297, 1961.

1962

2.24 Green, R. and Money, J. Binocular rivalry of gender-significant pictures in a stereoscope. *Journal of Psychiatric Research,* 2:19-27, 1962.

2.25 Shaffer, J. W. A specific cognitive deficit observed in gonadal aplasia (Turner's syndrome). *Journal of Clinical Psychology,* 18:403-406, 1962.

1963

2.26   Money, J. Cytogenetics and psychosexual incongruities, with a note on space-form blindness. *American Journal of Psychiatry,* 119:820-827, 1963.
2.27   Money, J. Problems of sexual development. Endocrinologic and psychologic aspects. *New York State Journal of Medicine,* 63:2348-2354, 1963.
2.28   Money, J. and Hirsch, S. R. Chromosome anomalies, mental deficiency and schizophrenia: A study of triple X and triple-X/Y chromosomes in five patients and their families. *Archives of General Psychiatry,* 8:242-251, 1963.
2.29   Shaffer, J. W. Masculinity-femininity and other personality traits in gonadal aplasia (Turner's syndrome). In *Advances in Sex Research* (H. G. Beigel, ed.). New York, Hoeber, 1963.

1964

2.30   Alexander, D., Walker, H. T., Jr. and Money, J. Studies in direction sense. I. Turner's syndrome. *Archives of General Psychiatry,* 10:337-339, 1964.
2.31   Everett, H. C. Sneezing in response to light. *Neurology,* 14:483-490, 1965.
2.32   Money, J. Two cytogenetic syndromes: Psychologic comparisons. I. Intelligence and specific-factor quotients. *Journal of Psychiatric Research,* 2:223-231, 1964.
2.33   Money, J. and Lewis, V. Longitudinal study of IQ in treated congenital hypothyroidism. In the Ciba Foundation Study Group No. 18, *Brain-Thyroid Relationships* (M. P. Cameron and M. O'Connor, eds.). London, J. & A. Churchill, 1964.
2.34   Money, J. and Pollitt, E. Cytogenetic and psychosexual ambiguity: Klinefelter's syndrome and transvestism compared. *Archives of General Psychiatry,* 11:589-595, 1964.
2.35   Pollitt, E., Hirsch, S. and Money, J. Priapism, impotence and human figure drawings. *Journal of Nervous and Mental Disease,* 139:161-168, 1964.
2.36   Pollitt, E. and Money, J. Studies in the psychology of dwarfism: I. Intelligence quotient and school achievement. *Journal of Pediatrics* 64:415-421, 1964.

1965

2.37   Alexander, D. and Money, J. Reading ability, object constancy and Turner's syndrome. *Perceptual and Motor Skills,* 20:981-984, 1965.
2.38   Money, J. Biographical sketch, Lawson Wilkins, M.D. In *The Diagnosis and Treatment of Endocrine Disorders in Childhood and Adolescence,* 3rd ed. (L. Wilkins). Springfield, Illinois, Charles C Thomas, 1965.
2.39   Money, J. Negro Illegitimacy: An antebellum legacy in obstetrical sociology. *Pacific Medicine and Surgery,* 73:350-352, 1965.
2.40   Money, J. Psychological aspects of reading disability. *Transactions of the Pennsylvania Academy of Ophthalmology and Otolaryngology,* 18:16-24, 1965.
2.41   Money, J. Psychologic evaluation of the child with intersex problems. *Pediatrics,* 36:51-55, 1965.
2.42   Money, J. Psychology of intersexes. *Urologia Internationalis,* 19:185-189, 1965.
2.43   Money, J. The Sex instinct and human eroticism. *Journal of Sex Research,* 1:3-16, 1965.
2.44   Money, J. and Granoff, D. IQ and the somatic stigmata of Turner's syndrome. *American Journal of Mental Deficiency,* 70:69-77, 1965.
2.45   Money, J. and Hirsch, S. R. After priapism: Orgasm retained, erection lost. *Journal of Urology,* 94:152-157, 1965.
2.46   Money, J., Walker, H. T., Jr. and Alexander, D. Development of direction sense and three syndromes of impairment. *The Slow Learning Child: The Australian Journal on the Education of Backward Children,* 11:145-155, 1965.

1966

2.47   Alexander, D., Ehrhardt, A. A. and Money, J. Defective figure drawing, geometric and human, in Turner's syndrome. *Journal of Nervous and Mental Disease,* 142:161-167, 1966.

2.48 Alexander, D. and Money, J. Turner's syndrome and Gerstmann's syndrome: Neuropsychologic comparisons. *Neuropsychologia,* 4:265-273, 1966.
2.49 Drash, P. W. Case 5: Arrested literacy. In *The Disabled Reader: Education of the Dyslexic Child* (J. Money, ed.). Baltimore, Johns Hopkins Press, 1966.
2.50 Drash, P. W. and Money, J. Motor impairment and hyperthyroidism in children: Report of two cases. *Developmental Medicine and Child Neurology,* 8:741-745, 1966.
2.51 Green, R. and Money, J. Stage-acting, role-taking and effeminate impersonation during boyhood. *Archives of General Psychiatry,* 15:535-538, 1966.
2.52 Money, J. On learning and not learning to read. In *The Disabled Reader: Education of the Dyslexic Child* (J. Money, ed.). Baltimore, Johns Hopkins Press, 1966.
2.53 Money, J. Case 1: Space-form deficit. *Ibid.*
2.54 Money, J. Case 2: Directional sense rotation and poor finger localization. *Ibid.*
2.55 Money, J. Case 3: Conceptual idiosyncracy. *Ibid.*
2.56 Money, J. Case 4: Phonetic-graphemic matching defect. *Ibid.*
2.57 Money, J. and Alexander, D. Turner's Syndrome: Further demonstration of the presence of specific cognitional deficiencies. *Journal of Medical Genetics,* 3:47-48, 1966.
2.58 Money, J. and Ehrhardt, A. A. Preservation of IQ in hypoparathyroidism of childhood. *American Journal of Mental Deficiency,* 71:237-243, 1966.
2.59 Money, J. and Lewis, V. IQ, genetics and accelerated growth: Adrenogenital syndrome. *Bulletin of The Johns Hopkins Hospital,* 118:365-373, 1966.
2.60 Money, J. and Pollitt, E. Studies in the psychology of dwarfism: II. Personality maturation and response to growth hormone treatment. *Journal of Pediatrics,* 68:381-390, 1966.
2.61 Money, J. and Wang, C. Human figure drawing: I. Sex of first choice in gender-identity anomalies, Klinefelter's syndrome and precocious puberty. *Journal of Nervous and Mental Disease,* 143:157-162, 1966.
2.62 Money, J., Weinberg, R. S. and Lewis, V. Intelligence quotient and school performance in twenty-two children with a history of thyrotoxicosis. *Bulletin of The Johns Hopkins Hospital,* 118:275-281, 1966.

1967

2.63 Alexander, D. and Money, J. Reading disability and the problem of direction sense. *The Reading Teacher,* 20:404-409, 1967.
2.64 Ehrhardt, A. A. and Money, J. Hypercalcemia: A family study of psychologic functioning. *Johns Hopkins Medical Journal,* 121:14-20, 1967.
2.65 Ehrhardt, A. A. and Money, J. Progestin-induced hermaphroditism: IQ and psychosexual identity in a study of ten girls. *Journal of Sex Research,* 3:83-100, 1967.
2.66 Money, J. Adolescent psychohormonal development. *Southwestern Medicine,* 48:182-186, 1967.
2.67 Money, J. Breasts in intersexuality and transexualism: II. Body image and gender identity. *Journal of the American Medical Women's Association,* 22:869-875, 1967.
2.68 Money, J. Dwarfism: Questions and answers in counseling. *Rehabilitation Literature,* 28:134-138, 1967.
2.69 Money, J. Cytogenetic and other aspects of transvestism and transsexualism. *Journal of Sex Research,* 3:141-143, 1967.
2.70 Money, J. Learning disability and the principles of reading. *The Slow Learning Child: The Australian Journal of the Education of Backward Children,* 14:69-87, 1967.
2.71 Money, J. Sexual problems of the chronically ill. In *Sexual Problems: Diagnosis and Treatment in Medical Practice* (C. W. Wahl, ed.). New York, Free Press, 1967.
2.72 Money, J. The genetics of homosexuality. *New Zealand Medical Journal,* 66:745-748, 1967 (Published by title only).
2.73 Money, J. The laws of constancy; and learning to read. In *Selected Conference Papers: International Approach to Learning Disabilities of Children and Youth* (Third Annual International Conference, March 1966). Tulsa, Oklahoma 74105: The Association for Children with Learning Disabilities, Inc., 3739 South Delaware Place; 1967, pp. 80-97.
2.74 Money, J. Panel discussion: Implications for research. *Ibid.* 262-265.
2.75 Money, J. and Alexander, D. Eroticism and sexual function in developmental anorchia and hyporchia with pubertal failure. *Journal of Sex Research,* 3:31-47, 1967.

2.76   Money, J., Drash, P. W. and Lewis, V. Dwarfism and hypopituitarism: Statural retardation without mental retardation. *American Journal of Mental Deficiency,* 72:122-126, 1967.

2.77   Money, J. and Epstein, R. Verbal aptitude in eonism and prepubertal effeminacy—a feminine trait. *Transactions of the New York Academy of Sciences,* 29:448-454, 1967.

2.78   Money, J. and Hosta, G. M. Laughing seizures with sexual precocity: Report of two cases. *Johns Hopkins Medical Journal,* 120:326-336, 1967.

2.79   Money, J., Lewis, V. G., Ehrhardt, A. A. and Drash, P. W. IQ impairment and elevation in endocrine and related cytogenetic disorders. Chapter 3 in *Psychopathology of Mental Development* (J. Zubin, ed.). New York, Grune and Stratton, 1967.

2.80   Money, J. and Meredith, T. Elevated verbal IQ and idiopathic precocious sexual maturation. *Pediatric Research,* 1:59-65, 1967.

2.81   Money, J. and Neill, J. Precocious puberty, IQ and school acceleration. *Clinical Pediatrics,* 6:277-380, 1967.

2.82   Money, J. and Raiti, S. Breasts in intersexuality and transexualism: I. Mammary growth. *Journal of the American Medical Women's Association,* 22:865-869, 1967.

2.83   Money, J. and Wang, C. Human figure drawing: II. Quality comparisons in gender-identity anomalies, Klinefelter's syndrome and precocious puberty. *Journal of Nervous and Mental Disease,* 144:55-58, 1967.

2.84   Money, J. and Yankowitz, R. The sympathetic-inhibiting effects of the drug Ismelin on human male eroticism, with a note on Mellaril. *Journal of Sex Research,* 3:69-82, 1967.

2.85   Pollitt, E. and Granoff, D. Mental and motor development of Peruvian children treated for severe malnutrition. *Inter-American Journal of Psychology,* 1:93-102, 1967.

1968

2.86   Borgaonkar, D. S., Murdoch, J. L., McKusick, V. A., Borkowf, S. P., Money, J. and Robinson, B. W. The YY syndrome. *Lancet,* 2:461-462, 1968.

2.87   Drash, P. W., Greenberg, N. and Money, J. Intelligence and personality in four syndromes of dwarfism. Chapter 39 in *Human Growth: Body Composition, Cell Growth, Energy and Intelligence* (D. B. Cheek, ed.). Philadelphia, Lea and Febiger, 1968.

2.88   Drash, P. W. and Money, J. Statural and intellectual growth in congenital heart disease, in growth hormone deficiency, and in sibling controls. Chapter 42 in *Human Growth: Body Composition, Cell Growth, Energy and Intelligence* (D. B. Cheek, ed.). Philadelphia, Lea and Febiger, 1968.

2.89   Ehrhardt, A. A., Epstein, R. and Money, J. Fetal androgens and female gender identity in the early-treated adrenogenital syndrome. *Johns Hopkins Medical Journal,* 122:160-167, 1968.

2.90   Ehrhardt, A. A., Evers, K. and Money, J. Influence of androgen and some aspects of sexuality dimorphic behavior in women with the late-treated adrenogenital syndrome. *Johns Hopkins Medical Journal* 123:115-122, 1968.

2.91   Eldridge, R., Berlin, C. I., Money, J. and McKusick, V. A. Cochlear deafness, myopia and intellectual impairment in an Amish family. *Archives of Otolaryngology,* 88:49-54, 1968.

2.92   Lewis, V. G., Money, J. and Epstein, R. Concordance of verbal and nonverbal ability in the adrenogenital syndrome. *Johns Hopkins Medical Journal,* 122:192-195, 1968.

2.93   Money, J. Cognitive deficits in Turner's syndrome. Chapter 4 in *Progress in Human Behavior Genetics* (S. G. Vandenberg, ed.). Baltimore, Johns Hopkins Press, 1968.

2.94   Money, J. Discussion on hormonal inhibition of libido in male sex offenders. In *Endocrinology and Human Behavior* (R. P. Michael, ed.). London, Oxford University Press, 1968.

2.95   Money, J. Influence of hormones on psychosexual differentiation. *Medical Aspects of Human Sexuality,* 2(11):32-42, November, 1968.

2.96   Money, J. Intellect, brain and biologic age: Introduction. Chapter 37 in *Human Growth: Body Composition, Cell Growth, Energy and Intelligence* (D. B. Cheek, ed.). Philadelphia, Lea and Febiger, 1968.

2.97   Money, J. Psychologic approach to psychosexual misidentity with elective mutism: Sex reassignment in two cases of hyperadrenocortical hermaphroditism. *Clinical Pediatrics,* 7:331-339, 1968.

2.98   Money, J. and Bobrow, N. A. Birth defect of the skull and face without brain or learning disorder: A psychological and pedagogical report. *Journal of Learning Disabilities,* 1:289-298, 1968.
2.99   Money, J. and Brennan, J. G. Sexual dimorphism in the psychology of female transsexuals. *Journal of Nervous and Mental Disease,* 147:487-499, 1968.
2.100   Money, J., Cohen, S., Lewis, V. G. and Drash, P. W. Human figure drawings as index of body image in dwarfism. Chapter 40 in *Human Growth: Body Composition, Cell Growth, Energy and Intelligence* (D. B. Cheek, ed.). Philadelphia, Lea and Febiger, 1968.
2.101   Money, J. and Drash, P. W. Juvenile thyrotoxicosis: Behavioral and somatic symptoms and antecedents leading to referral and diagnosis. *Journal of Special Education,* 2:83-91, 1968.
2.102   Money, J. and Ehrhardt, A. A. Correlation of mental functioning and calcium regulation in a rare case of pseudohypoparathyroidism. *Johns Hopkins Medical Journal,* 123:276-282, 1968.
2.103   Money, J. and Ehrhardt, A. A. Prenatal hormonal exposure: Possible effects on behaviour in man. Chapter 3 in *Endocrinology and Human Behaviour* (R. P. Michael, ed.). London, Oxford University Press, 1968.
2.104   Money, J., Ehrhardt, A. A. and Masica, D. Fetal feminization induced by androgen insensitivity in the testicular feminizing syndrome: Effect on marriage and maternalism. *Johns Hopkins Medical Journal,* 123:105-114, 1968.
2.105   Money, J. and Hosta, G. M. Negro folklore of male pregnancy. *Journal of Sex Research,* 4:34-50, 1968.
2.106   Money, J. and Primrose, C. Sexual dimorphism and dissociation in the psychology of male transsexuals. *Journal of Nervous and Mental Disease,* 147:472-486, 1968.

1969

2.107   Ehrhardt, A. A. *Zur Wirkung fötaler Hormone auf Intelligenz und geschlechtsspezifisches Verhalten.* (Tr.: The effect of fetal hormones on intelligence and sex-related behavior). Dissertation zur Erlangung des Doktorgrades der Philosophischen Fakultät der Universität Düsseldorf, 1969.
2.108   Masica, D. N., Money, J., Ehrhardt, A. A. and Lewis, V. G. IQ, fetal sex hormones and cognitive patterns: Studies in the testicular feminizing syndrome of androgen insensitivity. *Johns Hopkins Medical Journal,* 124:34-43, 1969.
2.109   Money, J. Fatherhood behavior and gender identity. *Medical Aspects of Human Sexuality,* 3, 9:67-80, September, 1969.
2.110   Money, J. Sex reassignment as related to hermaphroditism and transsexualism. Chapter 5 in *Transsexualism and Sex Reassignment* (R. Green and J. Money, eds.). Baltimore, Johns Hopkins Press, 1969.
2.111   Money, J. and Alexander, D. Psychosexual development and absence of homosexuality in males with precocious puberty: Review of 18 cases. *Journal of Nervous and Mental Disease,* 148:111-123, 1969.
2.112   Money, J. and Brennan, J. G. Achievement versus failure: Intelligence, education and career in seven female transexuals. *Journal of Learning Disabilities,* 2:76-81, 1969.
2.113   Money, J., Potter R. and Stoll, C. S. Sex reannouncement in hereditary sex deformity: Psychology and sociology of habilitation. *Social Science and Medicine,* 3:207-216, 1969.
2.114   Money, J. and Schwartz, F. Public opinion and social issues in transsexualism: A case study in medical sociology. Chapter 17 in *Transsexualism and Sex Reassignment.* (R. Green and J. Money, eds.). Baltimore, Johns Hopkins Press, 1969.

1970

2.115   Ehrhardt, A. A., Greenberg, N. and Money, J. Female gender identity and the absence of fetal gonadal hormones: Turner's syndrome. *Johns Hopkins Medical Journal,* 126:237-248, 1970.
2.116   Jones, H. W., Jr., Verkauf, B. S., Lewis, V. G. and Money, J. The relevance of surgical, psychologic and endocrinologic factors to the long-term end result of patients with congenital adrenal hyperplasia. A study of eighty-nine patients. *International Journal of Gynaecology and Obstetrics,* 8:398-401, 1970.

2.117 Lewis, V. G., Ehrhardt, A. A. and Money, J. Genital operations in girls with the adreno-genital syndrome: Subsequent psychologic development. *Obstetrics and Gynecology*, 36:11-15, 1970.

2.118 Money, J. Behavior genetics: Principles and examples from the XO, XXY and XYY syndromes, *Seminars in Psychiatry*, 5:11-29, 1970.

2.119 Money, J. Hormonal and genetic extremes at puberty. In *Psychopathology of Adolescence* (J. Zubin and A. F. Freedman, eds.). New York, Grune & Stratton, 1970.

2.120 Money, J. Matched pairs of hermaphrodites: Behavioral biology of sexual differentiation from chromosomes to gender identity. *Engineering and Science* (California Institute of Technology) *Special issue: Biological Bases of Human Behavior*, 33:34-39, 1970.

2.121 Money, J. Pituitary-adrenal and related syndromes of childhood: Effects on IQ and learning. In *Pituitary, Adrenal and the Brain* (Progress in Brain Research, Vol. 32, D. DeWeid and J. A. W. M. Weijnemen, eds.). Amsterdam, Elsevier Publishing Company, 1970.

2.122 Money, J. Sexual dimorphism and homosexual gender identity. *Psychological Bulletin*, 74:425-440, 1970.

2.123 Money, J. The positive and constructive approach to pornography in general sex education, in the home and in sexological counseling. In *Technical Report of the Commission on Obscenity and Pornography*. V:339-353. Washington, Government Printing Office, 1970.

2.124 Money, J. Use of an androgen-depleting hormone in the treatment of male sex offenders. *Journal of Sex Research*, 6:165-172, 1970.

2.125 Money, J. and Brennan, J. G. Heterosexual vs. homosexual attitudes: Male partners' perception of the feminine image of male transexuals. *Journal of Sex Research*, 6:193-209, 1970.

2.126 Money, J., Cawte, J. E., Bianchi, G. N. and Nurcombe, B. Sex training and traditions in Arnhem Land. *British Journal of Medical Psychology*, 43:383-399, 1970.

2.127 Money, J. and Ehrhardt, A. A. Transsexuelle nach Geschlechtswechsel: Partnerbeziehung, Beruf, Straffaelligkeit, psychiatrische Behandlung und subjektive Bewertung des Geschlechwechsels. (Trans.: Transexuals after sex reassignment: Marriage, employment, police records, psychotherapy, and subjective satisfaction.). In *Tendenzen der Sexualforschung* [*Beitraege zur Sexualforschung*, 49:70-87] (G. Schmidt, V. Sigusch and E. Schorsch, eds.). Stuttgart, Ferdinand Enke, 1970.

2.128 Money, J., Gaskin, R. and Hull, H. Impulse, aggression and sexuality in the XYY syndrome. *St. John's Law Review*, 44:220-235, 1970.

2.129 Money, J. and Gaskin, R. Sex reassignment. *International Journal of Psychiatry*, 9:249-282, 1970-1971.

2.130 Money, J. and Mittenthal, S. Lack of personality pathology in Turner's syndrome: Relation to cytogenetics, hormones and physique. *Behavior Genetics*, 1:43-56, 1970.

2.131 Nurcombe, B., Bianchi, G. N., Money, J. and Cawte, J. E. A hunger for stimuli: The psychosocial background of petrol inhalation. *British Journal of Medical Psychology*, 43:367-374, 1970.

1971

2.132 Bobrow, N. A., Money, J. and Lewis, V. G. Delayed puberty, eroticism, and sense of smell: A psychological study of hypogonadotropinism, osmatic and anosmatic (Kallmann's syndrome). *Archives of Sexual Behavior*, 1:329-344, 1971).

2.133 Ehrhardt, A. A. Der Eigfluss von fötalen Hormonen auf Intelligenz und geschlechts-spezifisches Verhalten. (The effect of fetal hormones on intelligence and sex-related behavior). In *Praxis der Klinischen Psychologie*, Band II (E. Duhn, ed.). Goettingen, Verlag für Psychologie, Dr. C. F. Hogrefe, 1971.

2.134 Masica, D. N., Ehrhardt, A. A. and Money, J. Fetal feminization and female gender identity in the testicular feminizing syndrome of androgen insensitivity. *Archives of Sexual Behavior*, 1:131-142, 1971.

2.135 Money, J. Differentiation of gender identity and gender role. *Psychiatric Annals*, 1:33-43, 1971.

2.136 Money, J. Pornography in the home. In *Sex in Childhood* (Third Annual Seminar). Tulsa, Oklahoma, Children's Medical Center, 1971.

2.137 Money, J. Prefatory remarks on the outcome of sex-reassignment in 24 cases of transexualism. *Archives of Sexual Behavior,* 1:163-165, 1971.
2.138 Money, J. Prenatal hormones and intelligence: A possible relationship. *Impact of Science on Society,* 21:285-290, 1971.
2.139 Money, J. Psychologic findings associated with the XO, XXY and XYY anomalies. *Southern Medical Journal,* 64: Supplement No. 1, 59-64, 1971.
2.140 Money, J. Sexually dimorphic behavior, fetal hormones and human hermaphroditic syndromes, with a note on XYY. In the *Neuroendocrinology of Human Reproduction: Biological and Clinical Perspectives.* (H. C. Mack and A. I. Sherman, eds.). Springfield, Ill., Charles C Thomas, 1971.
2.141 Money, J. Sexually dimorphic behavior, normal and abnormal. In *Enviromental Influences on Genetic Expression: Biological and Behavioral Aspects of Sexual Differentation* (N. Kretchmer and D. N. Walcher, eds.). Washington, D. C., U.S. Government Printing Office, 1971.
2.142 Money, J. The Aboriginal Australians of Arnhem Land and psychosexual differentiation in childhood. In *Sex In Childhood* (Third Annual Seminar). Tulsa, Oklahoma, Children's Medical Center, 1971.
2.143 Money, J. and Block, D. Speech, sexuality and the temporal lobe: An analysis of spontaneous speech of thirteen male transexuals. *Journal of Sex Research,* 7:35-41, 1971.
2.144 Money, J., Bobrow, N. A. and Clarke, F. C. Autism and autoimmune disease: A family study. *Journal of Autism and Childhood Schizophrenia,* 1:146-160, 1971.
2.145 Money, J. and Ehrhardt, A. A. Fetal hormones and the brain: Effect on sexual dimorphism of behavior—A review. *Archives of Sexual Behavior,* 1:241-262, 1971.
2.146 Money, J. and Walker, P. Psychosexual development, maternalism, nonpromiscuity and body image in 15 females with precocious puberty. *Archives of Sexual Behavior,* 1:45-60, 1971.

1972

2.147 Cohen, S., Money, J. and Uhlenhuth, E. A computer study of selected features of self-and-other drawings by 385 children. *Journal of Learning Disabilities,* 5:145-155, 1972.
2.148 Ehrhardt, A. A. and Money, J. Prenatal hormones and human behavior. *Illinois Medical Journal,* 141:386-389, 1972.
2.149 Jones, H. W., Jr., Money, J. and Meyer, J. K. An appraisal of the role of the gynecologist in the treatment of male transsexualism. In *The Year Book of Obstetrics and Gynecology 1972* (J. P. Greenhill, ed.). Chicago, Year Book Medical Publishers, 1972.
2.150 Money, J. Clinical aspects of prenatal steroidal action on sexually dimorphic behavior. In *Steroid Hormones and Brain Function* (C. H. Sawyer and R. A. Gorski, eds.). Berkeley, University of California Press, 1972.
2.151 Money, J. Determinants of human sexual identity and behavior. In *Progress in Family and Group Therapy* (C. J. Sager and H. A. Kaplan, eds.). New York, Brunner/Mazel, 1972.
2.152 Money, J. Identification and complementation in the differentiation of gender identity. *Danish Medical Journal,* 19:265-268, 1972.
2.153 Money, J. Phyletic and idiosyncratic determinants of gender identity. *Danish Medical Journal,* 19:259-264, 1972.
2.154 Money, J. Pubertal hormones and homosexuality, bisexuality, and heterosexuality. In *National Institute of Mental Health Task Force on Homosexuality: Final Report and Background Papers* (J. M. Livingood, ed.). Washington, D.C., U.S. Government Printing Office, 1972.
2.155 Money, J. Strategy, ethics, behavior modification and homosexuality: An editorial comment. *Archives of Sexual Behavior,* 2:79-81, 1972.
2.156 Money, J. and Ehrhardt, A. A. Gender-dimorphic behavior and fetal sex hormones. In *Recent Progress in Hormone Research* (E. B. Astwood, ed.), 28:735-763. New York, Academic Press, 1972.
2.157 Money, J., Wolff, G. and Annecillo, C. Pain agnosia and self-injury in the syndrome of reversible somatotropin deficiency (Psychosocial dwarfism). *Journal of Autism and Childhood Schizophrenia,* 2:127-139, 1972.
2.158 Walker, P. and Money, J. Prenatal androgenization of females. *Hormones* 3:119-128, 1972.

1973

2.159 Lewis, V. G., Bobrow, N. A. and Money, J. Psychologic study of boys with retarded statural and osseous growth, and normal age of pubertal onset. *Adolescence,* 8:445-454, 1973.

2.160 Money, J. Effects of prenatal androgenization and deandrogenization on behavior in human beings. In *Frontiers in Neuroendrocrinology* (W. F. Ganong and L. Martini, eds.). Vol. III. New York, Oxford University Press, 1973.

2.161 Money, J. Gender role, gender identity, core gender identity: Usage and definition of terms. *Journal of the American Academy of Psychoanalysis,* 1:397-403, 1973.

2.162 Money, J. Pornography in the home: A topic in medical education. In *Contemporary Sexual Behavior* (J. Zubin and J. Money, eds.). Baltimore, Johns Hopkins University Press, 1973.

2.163 Money, J. Sexology: Behavioral, cultural, hormonal, neurological, genetic, etc. *Journal of Sex Research,* 9:3-10, 1973.

2.164 Money, J. Some thoughts on sexual taboos and the rights of the retarded. In *Human Sexuality and the Mentally Retarded* (F. de la Cruz and G. LaVeck, eds.). New York, Brunner/Mazel, 1973.

2.165 Money, J. Turner's syndrome and parietal lobe functions. *Cortex,* 9:387-393. 1973.

2.166 Money, J. and Athanasiou, R. Pornography: Review and bibliographic annotations. *American Journal of Obstetrics and Gynecology,* 115:130-146, 1973.

2.167 Money, J. and Wolff, G. Sex reassignment: male to female to male. *Archives of Sexual Behavior,* 2:245-250, 1973.

2.168 Wolff, G. and Money, J. Relationship between sleep and growth in patients with psychosocial dwarfism. *Psychological Medicine,* 3:18-27, 1973.

1974

2.169 Money, J. Long-term psychologic follow-up of intersexed patients. *Clinics in Plastic Surgery,* 1:271-274, 1974.

2.170 Money, J. Prenatal hormones and postnatal socialization in gender identity differentiation. *Nebraska Symposium on Motivation,* 21:221-295, 1974.

2.171 Money, J. Psychologic consideration of sex assignment in intersexuality. *Clinics in Plastic Surgery,* 1:215-222, 1974.

2.172 Money, J. Two names, two wardrobes, two personalities. *Journal of Homosexuality,* 1:65-70, 1974.

2.173 Money, J., Annecillo, C., Van Orman, B. and Borgaonkar, D. S. Cytogenetics, hormones and behavior disability: Comparison of XYY and XXY syndromes. *Clinical Genetics,* 6:370-382, 1974.

2.174 Money, J. and Clopper, R., Jr. Psychosocial and psychosexual aspects of errors of pubertal onset and development. *Human Biology,* 46:173-181, 1974.

2.175 Money, J. and Nurcombe, B. Ability and cultural heritage: The Bender and Draw-A-Person tests in Aboriginal Australia. *Journal of Learning Disabilities,* 7:297-303, 1974.

2.176 Money, J. and Ogunro, C. Behavioral sexology: Ten cases of genetic male intersexuality with impaired prenatal and pubertal androgenization. *Archives of Sexual Behavior,* 3:181-205, 1974.

2.177 Money, J. and Wolff, G. Late puberty, retarded growth and reversible hyposomatotropinism (Psychosocial dwarfism). *Adolescence,* 9:121-134, 1974.

REVIEWS, ENCYCLOPEDIA AND TEXT BOOK CHAPTERS

1957

3.1   Hampson, J. L. and Money, J. The child with disorders of physical growth. In *Management of the Handicapped Child* (H. Michal-Smith, ed.). New York, Grune and Stratton, 1957.

1961

3.2 Hampson, J. L. and Hampson, J. G. The ontogenesis of sexual behavior in man. In *Sex and Internal Secretions,* 3rd ed. (W. C. Young, ed.). Baltimore, Williams and Wilkins, 1961.

3.3 Money, J. The sex hormones and other variables in human eroticism. In *Sex and Internal Secretions,* 3rd ed. (W. C. Young, ed.). Baltimore, Williams and Wilkins, 1961.

3.4 Money, J. Hermaphroditism. In *Encyclopedia of Sexual Behavior* (A. Ellis and A. Abarbanel, eds.). New York, Hawthorn Books, 1961.

1962

3.5 Money, J. Dyslexia, a postconference review. In *Reading Disability: Progress and Research Needs in Dyslexia* (J. Money, ed.). Baltimore, Johns Hopkins Press, 1962.

1963

3.6 Money, J. Developmental differentiation of femininity and masculinity compared. In *Man and Civilization: The Potential of Woman* (S. M. Farber and R. H. L. Wilson, eds.). New York, McGraw-Hill, 1963.

3.7 Money, J. Factors in the genesis of homosexuality. In *Determinants of Human Sexual Behavior* (G. Winokur, ed.). Springfield, Ill., Charles C Thomas, 1963.

3.8 Money, J. Psychosexual development in man. In *Encyclopedia of Mental Health* (A. Deutch, ed.). New York, Franklin Watts, 1963.

1964

3.9 Money, J. Reading disorder. In *Current Pediatric Therapy* (S. S. Gellis and B. M. Kagan, eds.). Philadelphia, W. B. Saunders, 1964.

1965

3.10 Money, J. Influence of hormones on sexual behavior. In *Annual Review of Medicine* (A. C. Degraff, ed.), 16:67-82. Palo Alto, Annual Reviews, Inc., 1965.

3.11 Money, J. Psychosexual differentiation. In *Sex Research: New Developments* (J. Money, ed.). New York, Holt, Rinehart and Winston, 1965.

1966

3.12 Money, J. Specific disability for reading (reading dysphoitesis). Chapter 15 in *The Pediatrician's Ophthalmology* (S. Liebman and S. Gellis, eds.). St. Louis, C. V. Mosby, 1966.

3.13 Money, J. The sex chromatin and psychosexual differentiation. Chapter 24 in *The Sex Chromatin* (K. L. Moore, ed.). Philadelphia, W. B. Saunders, 1966.

1967

3.14 Money, J. Progress of knowledge and revision of the theory of infantile sexuality. A response to a critique of Freud's psychosexual theory of infantilism. *International Journal of Psychiatry,* 4:50-54, 1967.

3.15 Money, J. Reading disorders in children. Chapter 14A in *Brennemann-Kelley Practice of Pediatrics,* Vol. IV. New York, Harper & Row, 1967.

1968

3.16 Money, J. Hermaphroditism and pseudohermaphroditism. In *Textbook of Gynecologic Endocrinology.* (J. J. Gold, ed.). New York, Harper & Row, 1968.

3.17   Money, J. Sexual behavior: Deviation: Psychological aspects. In *The International Encyclopedia of the Social Sciences,* Vol. 14 (D. L. Sills, ed.). New York, Crowell, Collier, Macmillan and Free Press, 1968.
3.18   Money, J. Intellectual and academic growth. Chapter 168 in *The Biologic Basis of Pediatric Practice,* Vol. II (R. E. Cooke and S. Levin, eds.). New York, McGraw-Hill, 1968.
3.19   Money, J. Psychologic disorders associated with genital defects. Chapter 112, *Ibid.*

1969

3.20   Drash, P. W. Psychologic counseling: Dwarfism. In *Endocrine and Genetic Diseases of Childhood* (L. I. Gardner, ed.). Philadelphia, W. B. Saunders, 1969, pp. 1014-1022.
3.21   Money, J. Developmental dyslexia. Chapter 19 in *Handbook of Clinical Neurology, Vol. 4: Disorders of Speech, Perception and Symbolic Behaviour* (P. J. Vinken and G. W. Bruyn, eds.). Amsterdam, North-Holland Publishing Co., 1969.
3.22   Money, J. Intellectual functioning in childhood endocrinopathies and related cytogenetic disorders. In *Endocrine and Genetic Diseases of Childhood* (L. I. Gardner, ed.). Philadelphia, W. B. Saunders, 1969, pp. 1004-1014. [2nd ed., 1975.]
3.23   Money, J. Psychologic counseling: Hermaphroditism. *Ibid.,* pp. 539-544. [2nd ed., 1975.]
3.24   Money, J. Sex errors of the body. In *The Individual, Society and Sex: Background Readings for Sex Educators* (C. B. Broderick, ed.). Baltimore, Johns Hopkins Press, 1969, pp. 285-317.

1970

3.25   Money, J. Paraphilias: Phyletic origins. In *Introduction to Psychiatry and the Behavioral Sciences—Readings V: Sexual Behavior.* Baltimore, Dept. Psychiatry and Behavioral Sciences, The Johns Hopkins University School of Medicine, 1970.
3.26   Money, J. Sex education: Infancy through maturity, kindergarten through college—A bibliography. *Professional Psychology,* 1:499-503, 1970.

1971

3.27   Money, J. Pornography and medical education. In *Macy Conference on Family Planning, Demography, and Human Sexuality in Medical Education* (V. W. Lippard, ed.). New York: Josiah Macy, Jr. Foundation, 1971.

1972

3.28   Money, J. Sex reassignment therapy in gender identity disorders. In *Treatment of the Sex Offender* (H. L. P. Resnik and M. C. Wolfgang, eds.). Boston, Little, Brown, 1972.

1974

3.29   Money, J. Intersexual and transexual behavior and syndromes. In *American Handbook of Psychiatry,* Vol. III, 2nd Edition, revised (S. Arieti and E. B. Brady, eds.). New York, Basic Books, 1974.
3.30   Money, J. Sex education. In *Advances in Human Growth Hormone Research,* (S. Raiti, ed.). Washington, D.C., U.S. Government Printing Office, 1974.

BRIEF COMMUNICATIONS, ABSTRACTS, TEACHING NOTES

1956

4.1   Hampson, J. G., Money, J. and Hampson, J. L. Teaching clinic. Hermaphroditism: Reccommendations concerning case management. *Journal of Clinical Endocrinology and Metabolism*, 16:547-556, 1956.

1961

4.2 Green, R. and Money, J. Tomboys and Sissies. *Sexology*, 28:304-307, 1961.
4.3 Money, J. Too early puberty. *Sexology*, 28:154-157 and 250-253, 1961.

1962

4.4 Money, J. Obstacles to sex research. *Sexology*, 28:548-553, 1962.

1963

4.5 Pollitt, E. Urge for sex change. *Sexology*, 29:737-739, 1963.

1964

4.6 Green, R. and Money, J. Prepubertal morphologically normal boys demonstrating signs of cross-gender identity: A five-year follow-up. *American Journal of Orthopsychiatry*, 34:365-366, 1964. (Abstract)
4.7 Money, J. "Female Penis": The role and function of the clitoris. *Sexology*, 30:367-369, 1964.

1966

4.8 Money, J. The strange case of the pregnant hermaphrodite. *Sexology*, 33:7-9, 1966.
4.9 Money, J. Judging teenage mores. *Journal of Sex Research* 2:41-42, 1966.
4.10 Money, J. Priapism: Continuous erection. *Sexology*, 32:849-851, 1966.
4.11 Money, J., Alexander, D. and Ehrhardt, A. A. Visual-constructional deficit in Turner's syndrome. *Journal of Pediatrics*, 69:126-127, 1966.

1967

4.12 Ehrhardt, A. A. and Money, J. Did pregnancy drugs turn girls into tomboys? *Sexology*, 33:814-816, 1967.
4.13 Money, J. Letter to Clark P. Polak, on homosexuality and psychopathology. In: Brief of the Homosexual Law Reform Society of America. Amicus Curiae, in the *Supreme Court of the United States*, October term, 1966, No. 440, Clive Michael Boutilier v. The Immigration and Naturalization Service. pp. 68-70.

1968

4.14 Money, J. Discussant. Gender identity and a biological force. *The Psychoanalytic Forum*, 2:327-329, 1968.
4.15 Primrose, C. and Money, J. Do "sex-change" men want to be mothers? *Sexology*, 34:634-636, 1968.

1969

4.16 Money, J. Answers to questions: Earlier maturation. *Medical Aspects of Human Sexuality*, 3(12):77, December, 1969.

1970

4.17 Money, J. Answers to questions: Clitoral size and erotic sensation. *Medical Aspects of*

Human Sexuality, 4(3):95, March, 1970.

4.18   Money, J. Critique of Dr. Zuger's manuscript. *Psychosomatic Medicine,* 32:463-465, 1970.

4.19   Money, J. Sexual identity and pathology. *Playboy Magazine,* 17:209-210, 1970.

4.20   Money, J. Viewpoints: What are the effects on children of overhearing sounds of love-making from the parents' bedroom? *Medical Aspects of Human Sexuality,* 4(9):16, September, 1970.

1971

4.21   Money, J. Panel discussion: Hormones and human sexual behavior. In *The Neuroendocrinology of Human Reproduction: Biological and Clinical Perspectives* (H. C. Mack and A. I. Sherman, eds.). Springfield, Ill., Charles C Thomas, 1971.

4.22   Money, J. Refractory period after orgasm in the male. *Sexual Behavior,* 1:15, 1971.

4.23   Money, J. Special sex education and cultural anthropology, with reference to mental deficiency, physical deformity and urban ghettos. *Journal of Special Education,* 5:369-372, 1971.

4.24   Money, J. Transexualism and the philosophy of healing. *Journal of the American Society of Psychosomatic Dentistry and Medicine,* 18:25-26, 1971.

4.25   Money, J. Viewpoints: Why are some orgasms better than others? *Medical Aspects of Human Sexuality,* 5(3):17, March, 1971.

4.26   Money, J. Viewpoints: What are your feelings toward sex-change surgery? *Medical Aspects of Human Sexuality,* 5(6):135, June, 1971.

4.27   Money, J., Kinsey, B. A., Proctor, J. T. and Spitz, R. First panel discussion. In *Sex in Childhood* (Third Annual Seminar). Tulsa, Oklahoma, Children's Medical Center, 1971.

1972

4.28   Money, J. Comments on papers by Johannes Nielsen and Alice Theilgaard. *Danish Medical Journal,* 19:282-285, 1972.

4.29   Money, J. Development of sexual identification. *Acta Paediatrica Scandinavica,* 61:246-247, 1972.

4.30   Money, J. Is there a relationship between homosexuality and creativity? *Sexual Behavior,* 2:49, 1972.

4.31   Money, J. Mann und Frau—Einheit der Gegensätze. Geschlechtsrolle durch Unweltein-flüsse stärker als von genetisher Anlage geprägt. (Tr.: Man and woman: Unity of opposites. Gender role is more strongly influenced by the environment than by genetic anlage.) *Sexualmedizin,* 2, 73-77, 1972.

1973

4.32   Money, J. A rejoinder to Edward Sagarin's review. *Journal of Sex Research,* 9:276-280, 1973.

4.33   Money, J. Answers to questions: Aren't the fetishists, transvestites, sado-masochists, and similar deviants psychotic? *Medical aspects of Human Sexuality,* 7(11):206, November, 1973.

4.34   Money, J. The birth-control age. *The Chronicle of Higher Education,* 8(8):20, November 12th, 1973.

4.35   Money, J. Unisex, ambisex, bisex? The liberation of both sexes. *The Johns Hopkins Magazine,* 24:4-5, 1973.

4.36   Money, J. Viewpoints: Castration for rapists? *Medical Aspects of Human Sexuality,* 7(2):17-20, February, 1973.

1974

4.37   Money, J. Answers to questions: Do women lose interest in sex if they are continually frustrated by husbands' poor technique or premature ejaculation? Do they still engage in coitus hoping "this time it will be better," or is it the nature of the sex drive not to be extinguished no matter what? *Medical Aspects of Human Sexuality,* 8(6):39-40, June, 1974.

4.38 Money, J. Differentiation of gender identity (Abstract). In *Proceedings of the "Congrès International de Sexologie Médicale,"* Paris, July, 1974.

4.39 Money, J. Discussion: Delayed sexual maturation, with special emphasis on the occurrence of the syndrome in the male. In *The Control of the Onset of Puberty* (M. M. Grumbach, G. D. Grave, F. E. Mayer, eds.) New York, John Wiley & Sons, 1974.

4.40 Money, J. Round table on transexualism: Summary of remarks. In *The Proceedings of the "Congrès International de Sexologie Médicale,"* Paris, July, 1974.

4.41 Money, J. SAM Panel: Exogene sexual hormone für infarkt—rehabilitanden. Nach plasma-testosteron abwägen: Endogene produktion (Tr.: Exogenous sexual hormone for post-coronary rehabilitation—Evaluate exogenous plasma testosterone level.) *Sexualmedizin*, 11:598-599, 1974.

4.42 Money, J. Why males are more easily aroused. *Medical Aspects of Human Sexuality*, 8(12):8-9, December 1974.

4.43 Money, J. and Mazur, T. Follow your nose to love. *Sexology*, 40:32-34, 1974.

EDITORIALS AND LETTERS TO THE EDITOR

1960

5.1 Money, J., Hampson, J. L. and Hampson, J. G. Correspondence—"Hermaphroditism". *Canadian Psychiatric Association Journal*, 5:131-133, 1960.

1963

5.2 Money, J. Letter to the Editor. *Psychosomatic Medicine*, 25:88, 1963.

1966

5.3 Money, J. Which sex doth prevail? *Journal of the American Medical Association* (Editorial), 196:447, 1966.

5.4 Money, J. The theatre and the homosexual. *Journal of the American Medical Association* (Editorial), 198:1027-1028, 1966.

1967

5.5 Money, J. Letter to the Editor. Wrongly assigned sex. *British Medical Journal*, 1:50, 1967.

1969

5.6 Money, J. Physical, mental and critical period. *Journal of Learning Disabilities* (Editorial), 2:144-145, 1969.

5.7 Money, J. XYY, the law and forensic moral philosophy. *Journal of Nervous and Mental Disease* (Editorial), 149:309-311, 1969.

1971

5.8 Money, J. Correspondence—Review of "Transsexuals" by James P. Driscoll (*Transaction*, 8(5 & 6):28, 1971) *Transaction*, 8(12):12, 1971.

1973

5.9 Money, J. A rejection from *Science*. *The Sciences*, 13(3):3, April 1973.

5.10 Walker, P. A. Letter to the editor. Transexualism. *Medical Journal of Australia*, 2:790, 1973.

1974

5.11   Money, J. Behavioral aspects of chromosomal disorders. *Southern Medical Journal,* 67:509-510, 1974.
5.12   Money, J. Letter to the editor. Bisexual intensity. *Time,* p. 8, June 24, 1974.
5.13   Money, J. Letter to the editor. *American Journal of Psychotherapy,* 28:319, 1974.

BOOK REVIEWS

1955

6.1   Money, J. *Manual of Psychological Medicine for Practitioners and Students,* second edition, by A. F. Tregold and R. F. Tregold. (Baltimore, Williams and Wilkins 1953). *American Journal of Psychiatry,* 12:158-160, 1955.

1956

6.2   Money, J. *Sexual Behavior in American Society: An Appraisal of the First Two Kinsey Reports,* by J. Himelhoch and S. Fleis Fava, eds. (New York, W. W. Norton, 1955). *Contemporary Psychology,* 1:232-234, 1956.

1957

6.3   Money, J. *The Abnormal Personality,* second edition, by Robert W. White. (New York, Ronald Press, 1956). *American Journal of Psychiatry,* 113:862-863, 1957.

1959

6.4   Money, J. *Existence: A New Dimension in Psychology and Psychiatry,* by Rollo May, Earnest Angel and Henri F. Ellenberger, eds. (New York, Basic Books, 1958). *American Sociological Review,* 24:138, 1959.

1964

6.5   Money, J. *Homosexuality. A Psychoanalytic Study of Male Homosexuals,* by I. Bieber and other members of the Society of Medical Psychoanalysis. (New York, Basic Books, 1962). *Journal of Nervous and Mental Disease,* 138:197-200, 1964.

1965

6.6   Money, J. *Problems of Dynamic Neurology.* L. Halpern, ed. (New York, Grune and Stratton, 1963). *Bulletin of the Orton Society,* 15:69, 1965.

1966

6.7   Money, J. *Sex and Behavior.* Frank Beach, ed. (New York, Wiley, 1965). *American Scientist,* 54:86A, 1966.

1967

6.8   Money, J. *Christine Jorgensen. A Personal Autobiography.* (New York, Paul S. Eriksson, Inc, 1967). *Baltimore Sunday Sun,* 9-17-67.

1969

6.9 Money, J. *The Hidden World of Sex Offenders* by Tony Parker (New York, Bobbs-Merrill, 1969). *Baltimore Sunday Sun,* 5-25-69.

1970

6.10 Ehrhardt, A. A. *A Psychiatric-Psychological Study of 50 Severely Hypogonadal Male Patients, Including 34 with Klinefelter's Syndrome; 47,XXY* by J. Nielsen, A. Sørensen, A. Theilgaard, A. Frøland, and S. G. Johnsen (Copenhagen, Munksgaard, 1969). *American Journal of Human Genetics,* 22:599-600, 1970.

6.11 Money, J. *Sex and Gender: On the Development of Masculinity and Femininity* by R. J. Stoller (New York, Science House, 1968). *Contemporary Psychology,* 15:226-227, 1970.

6.12 Money, J. and Lewis, V. G. *The Young Handicapped Child: Educational Guidance for the Young Cerebral Palsied, Deaf, Blind, and Autistic Child* by A. H. Bowley and L. I. Gardner (Baltimore, Williams and Wilkins, 1969). *American Journal of Disease in Childhood,* 119:380, 1970.

1971

6.13 Lewis, V. G. and Money, J. *From Conception to Birth: The Drama of Life's Beginnings* by R. Rugh and L. B. Shettles, with R. N. Einhorn; drawings by R. Van Dyke (New York, Harper and Row, 1971). *Archives of Sexual Behavior,* 1:276-277, 1971.

6.14 Money, J. *A Psychiatric-Psychological Study of 50 Severely Hypogonadal Male Patients, Including 34 with Klinefelter's Syndrome, 47,XXY* by J. Nielsen, A. Sørensen, A. Theilgaard, A. Frøland, and S. G. Johnsen (Copenhagen, Munksgaard, 1969). *Social Biology,* 18:92, 1971.

6.15 Money, J. *The Intersexual Disorders* by C. J. Dewhurst and R. R. Gordon (London, Balliere, Tindall and Cassell, 1969; Baltimore, Williams and Wilkins). *Journal of Nervous and Mental Disease,* 152:216-218, 1971.

1972

6.16 Money, J. *Sexuality and Homosexuality: A New View* by A. Karlen (New York, W. W. Norton, 1971). *Contemporary Psychology,* 17:355, 1972.

6.17 Money, J. *Klinefelter's Syndrome and the XYY Syndrome, A Genetical Endocrinological and Psychiatric-Psychological Study of 33 Severely Hypogonadal Male Patients and 2 Patients with Karotype 47,XYY* by J. Nielson (Copenhagen, Munksgaard, 1969). *Cytogenetics,* 11:67-68, 1972.

1973

6.18 Money, J. *Gender Differences: Their Ontogeny and Significance* by C. Ounsted and D. C. Taylor, eds. (Baltimore, Williams and Wilkins, 1972). *New England Journal of Medicine,* 288:1137-1138, 1973.

6.19 Money, J. *Males and Females* by Corinne Hutt, (Baltimore, Penguin Education, 1972). *Contemporary Psychology,* 18:603-604, 1973.

6.20 Money, J. *Splitting: A Case of Female Masculinity* by R. J. Stoller (New York, Quadrangle/The New York Times Book Co., 1973). *New England Journal of Medicine,* 289:700-701, 1973.

6.21 Money, J. and Athanasiou, R. *The Nature and Evolution of Female Sexuality* by Mary Jane Sherfey (New York, Random House, 1972). *Contemporary Psychology,* 18:593-594, 1973.

1974

6.22 Money, J. *Clinical Sexuality: A Manual for the Physician and the Professions,* 3rd ed., by John F. Oliven (Philadelphia, Lippincott, 1974). *New England Journal of Medicine,* 291:25, 1974.

6.23   Money, J. *Male and Female Homosexuality: A Comprehensive Investigation* by M. T. Saghir and E. Robbins. (Baltimore, Williams and Wilkins, 1973). *New England Journal of Medicine,* 290:114, 1974.

6.24   Money, J. *Pornography and Sexual Deviance* by M. J. Goldstein and H. S. Kant, with J. J. Hartman. (Los Angeles, University of California Press, 1973). *Medical World News,* April 12, p. 74, 1974.

6.25   Money, J. *Two Births* by J. Brown, E. Lesser, S. Mines and E. Buryn (New York, Random House/Bookworks, 1972). *Archives of Sexual Behavior,* 3:178-179, 1974.

6.26   Money, J. *Beyond Monogamy: Recent Studies of Sexual Attitudes in Marriage* by J. R. Smith and L. G. Smith, eds. (Baltimore, Johns Hopkins University Press, 1974). *The Johns Hopkins Magazine,* 25:5-6, 1974.

6.27   Money, J. and Early, J. *Being Different: The Autobiography of Jane Fry* by Thomas Bogdan (New York, John Wiley and Sons, 1973) and *Sex Change: The Achievement of Gender Identity Among Feminine Transsexuals* by Thomas Kando (Springfield, Ill., Charles C Thomas, 1973). *American Journal of Psychiatry,* 4:1974.

6.28   Money, J. and Higham, E. *The Inevitability of Patriarchy* by S. Goldberg (New York, William Morrow and Co., 1973). *American Journal of Diseases of Children,* 128:262-264, 1974.

6.29   Money, J. and Schwartz, M. F. *Gender Differences: Their Ontogeny and Significance* by C. Ounsted and D. C. Taylor, eds. (Baltimore, Williams and Wilkins, 1972). *Archives of Sexual Behavior,* 3:598-599, 1974.

6.30   Money, J. and Schwartz, M. F. *Father, Child, and Sex Role* by R. Biller (Lexington, D. C. Heath). *SIECUS Report,* 3(1):8-9, September, 1974.

6.31   Money, J. Walker, P. A. and Higham, E. *The Female Orgasm: Psychology, Physiology, Fantasy* by Seymour Fisher (New York, Basic Books, 1973). *Contemporary Psychology,* 19:399-400, 1974.

6.32   Walker, P. A. and Money, J. "The male transvestite" (audio cassette tape), 1974. Personal Counseling Services, Inc., Box 56, Tappan, New York 10983. *SIECUS Report,* 3(1):13, September, 1974.

REPUBLICATIONS AND TRANSLATIONS

1954

7.1   Money, J. Observations concerning the clinical method of research, ego theory and psychopathology. (Synopsis) *Annual Survey of Psychoanalysis,* II (J. Frosch, ed.). New York, International Universities Press, 1954, pp. 49-50 and 111-116. [Repub. #2.3]

1956

7.2   Hampson, J. G. Hermaphroditic genital appearance, rearing and eroticism in hyperadrenocorticism: Psychologic findings. In *Adrenal Function in Infants and Children: A Symposium* (L. I. Gardner, ed.). New York, Grune and Stratton, 1956. [Repub. #2.5]

7.3   Money, J. Hermaphroditism, gender and precocity in hyperadrenocorticism: Psychologic findings. In *Adrenal Function in Infants and Children: A Symposium* (L. I. Gardner, ed.). New York, Grune and Stratton, 1956. [Repub. #2.8]

1966

7.4   Money, J. Reading disorder. In *Current Pediatric Theory* (S. S. Gellis and B. M. Kagan, eds.). Philadelphia, W. B. Saunders, 1966. [Repub. #3.9]

1967

7.5   Money, J. Components of eroticism in man: I. The hormones in relation to sexual morphology and sexual desire. In *Hormones and Behavior* (R. E. Whalen, ed.). Princeton, Van Nostrand, 1967. [Repub. #2.22]

1968

7.6   Money, J., Hampson, J. G., and Hampson, J. L. Imprinting and the establishment of gender role. In *Human Adaptation and Its Failures* (L. Phillips, ed.). New York, Academic Press, 1968. [Repub. #2.17]

7.7   Money, J., Hampson, J. G. and Hampson, J. L. An examination of some basic sexual concepts: The evidence of human hermaphroditism. Chapter 6 in *Theory and Practice in Family Psychiatry* (J. G. Howells, ed.). London, Oliver and Boyd, 1968. [Repub. #2.11]

1969

7.8   Money, J. Cytogenetics and psychosexual incongruities, with a note on space-form blindness. In *Behavioral Genetics: Method and Research* (M. Manosevitz, G. Lindzey and D. D. Thiessen, eds.). New York, Appleton-Century-Crofts, 1969. [Repub. #2.26]

7.9   Money, J. and Brennan, J. G. Sexual dimorphism in the psychology of female transsexuals. Chapter 7 in *Transsexualism and Sex Reassignment* (R. Green and J. Money, eds.). Baltimore, Johns Hopkins Press, 1969. [Repub. #2.99]

7.10 Money, J. and Primrose, C. Sexual dimorphism in the psychology of male transsexuals. Chapter 6 in *Transsexualism and Sex Reassignment* (R. Green and J. Money, eds.). Baltimore, Johns Hopkins Press, 1969. [Repub. #2.106]

7.11 Money, J. Developmental differentiation of femininity and masculinity compared. Chapter 12 in *Issues in Child Psychology* (D. Rogers, ed.). Belmont, California, Brooks/Cole, 1969. [Repub. #3.6]

7.12 Money, J. *Koerperlich-sexuelle Fehlentwicklunger.* (Tr.: Sex Errors of the Body: Dilemmas, Education and Counseling.). Hamburg, Rowholt, 1969. [Repub. #1.8]

7.13 Money, J. Hampson, J. G. and Hampson, J. L. An examination of some basic sexual concepts: The evidence of human hermaphroditism. Condensed in *Panorama of Psychology* (N. H. Pronko, ed.). Belmont, California, Brooks/Cole, 1969. [Repub. #2.11]

1970

7.14 Money, J. Two cytogenetic syndromes: Psychologic comparisons. 1: Intelligence and specific-factor quotients. Retitled as: Genetic abnormality and intelligence. In *The Ecology of Human Intelligence* (L. Hudson, ed.). Baltmore, Penguin Books, 1970. [Repub. #2.32]

7.15 Money, J. Phantom orgasm in paraplegics. *Medical Aspects of Human Sexuality,* 4(1):90-97, January, 1970. [Repub. #2.20]

7.16 Money, J. XYY, the law and forensic moral philosophy. *Acta Psiquiátrica y Psicológica de América Latina* (Editorial), 16:74-76, 1970. [Repub. #5.7]

1971

7.17 Money, J. Hermaphroditism. In *Sex and Today's Society. Encyclopedia of Sexual Behavior* (Vol. 5, Ace Paperback #441-20654-095) (A. Ellis and A. Abarbanel, eds.). New York, Ace Publishing Co. (1120 Avenue of the Americas, New York, 10036), undated. [Repub. #3.4]

7.18 Money, J. et al. Sex training and traditions in Arnhem Land. *Transcultural Psychiatric Research Review,* 8:139-140, October, 1971. [Repub. #2.126, Abridged]

7.19 Money, J. Sexual dimorphism and homosexual gender identity. Abridged in: *Mental Health Digest,* 3:23-32, 1971. [Repub. #2.122]

7.20 Money, J. and Bobrow, M. A. Birth defect of the skull and face without brain or learning disorder: A psychological and pedagogical report. In *Educational Perspectives in Learning Disabilities* (D. Hammill and N. Bartel, eds.). New York, John Wiley and Sons, 1971. [Repub. #2.98]

1972

7.21 Ehrhardt, A. A., Epstein, R. and Money, J. Fetal androgens and female gender identity in the early treated adrenogenital syndrome. In *Readings in the Development of Behavior* (V. H. Denenberg, ed.). Stamford, Connecticut, Sinauer Associates, 1972. [Repub. #2.89]

7.22   Ehrhardt, A. A. and Money, J. Progestin-induced hermaphroditism: IQ and psychosexual identity in a study of ten girls. In *Readings in the Development of Behavior* (V. H. Denenberg, ed.). Stamford, Connecticut, Sinauer Associates, 1972. [Repub. #2.65]

7.23   Money, J. *A Psychiatric-Psychological Study of 50 Severely Hypogonadal Male Patients, Including 34 with Klinefelter's Syndrome, 47,XXY* by J. Nielsen, A. Sørensen, A. Theilgaard, A. Frøland, and S. G. Johnsen (Copenhagen, Munksgaard, 1969). *Cytogenetics,* 11:66-67, 1972. [Repub. #6.14]

7.24   Money, J. Psychosexual differentiation. In *A First Reader in Physiological Psychology* (J. F. Lubar, ed.). New York, Harper and Row, 1972. [Repub. #3.11]

7.25   Money, J. Sex reassignment therapy in gender identity disorders. In *Sexual Behaviors: Social, Clinical, and Legal Aspects* (H. L. P. Resnik and M. E. Wolfgang, eds.). Boston, Little, Brown, 1972. [Repub. #3.28]

7.26   Money, J. Sexual dimorphism and homosexual gender identity. In *National Institute of Mental Health Task Force on Homosexuality: Final Report and Background Papers* (John M. Livingood, ed.). Washington, D.C., U.S. Government Printing Office, 1972. [Repub. #2.122]

7.27   Money, J. Sexual dimorphism and homosexual gender identity. In *Readings on the Psychology of Women* (J. Bardwick, ed.). New York, Harper and Row, 1972. [Repub. #2.122]

7.28   Money, J. The therapeutic use of androgen-depleting hormone. In *Sexual Behaviors: Social, Clinical, and Legal Aspects* (H. L. P. Resnik and M. E. Wolfgang, eds.). Boston, Little, Brown, 1972. [Repub. #2.214]

7.29   Money, J. The therapeutic use of androgen-depleting hormone. In *Treatment of the Sex Offender* (H. L. P. Resnik and M. E. Wolfgang, eds.). Boston, Little, Brown, 1972. [Repub. #2.214]

1973

7.30   Jones, H. W., Jr., Money, J. and Meyer, J. K. An appraisal of the role of the gynecologist in the treatment of male transexualism. *Current Medical Dialogue,* 40:379-385, 1973. [Repub. #2.149]

7.31   Money, J. Hermaphroditism and pseudohermaphroditism. Retitled as: Intersexual problems. *Clinical Obstetrics and Gynecology,* 16:169-191, 1973. [Repub. #3.16]

7.32   Money, J. Krankheit setzt Grenzen [Tr. #2.71: Sexual problems of the chronically ill]. In *Sexualmedizin,* 5:246-248, May, 1973.

7.33   Money, J. The birth control age. Retitled as: Living in the age of birth control. In *Mankato Free Press,* Mankato, Minn., December 8th, 1973. [Repub. #4.34]

7.34   Money, J. Cawte, J. E., Bianchi, G. N. and Nurcombe, B. Sex training and traditions in Arnhem Land. In *The Psychology of Aboriginal Australians: A Book of Readings* (G. E. Kearney, P. R. de Lacey and G. R. Davidson, eds.). Crows Nest, N.S.W., Australia, John Wiley and Sons, 1973. [Repub. #2.126]

7.35   Money, J. and Ehrhardt, A. A. Prenatal hormonal exposure: Possible effects on behavior in man. In *Early Human Development* (S. J. Hutt and C. Hutt, eds.). London, Oxford University Press, 1973. [Repub. #2.103]

7.36   Nurcombe, B. Bianchi, G., Money, J. and Cawte, J. A hunger for stimuli: The psychosocial background of petrol inhalation. In *The Psychology of Aboriginal Australians: A Book of Readings* (G. E. Kearney, P. R. de Lacey and G. R. Davidson, eds.). Crows Nest, N.S.W., Australia, John Wiley and Sons, 1973. [Repub. #2.131]

1974

7.37   Money, J. Components of eroticism in man: The hormones in relation to sexual morphology and sexual desire. In *Hormones and Sexual Behavior* (S. Carter, ed.). Stroudsburg, Pa., Dowden, Hutchinson and Ross, Inc., 1974. [Repub. #2.22]

7.38   Money, J. Sexual Dimorphism and homosexual gender identity. In *Sex Research: Selected Readings* (N. Wagner, ed.). New York, Behavioral Publications, 1974. [Repub. #2.122]

7.39   Money, J. and Ehrhardt, A. A. *Man and Woman, Boy and Girl: Differentiation and Dimorphism of Gender Identity from Conception to Maturity.* New York, Mentor, New America Library, 1974. [Paperback.] [Repub. #1.11]

7.40   Money, J. and Mazur, T. Liebe geht durch die Nose Sexuelle Stimulation durch vaginale Pheromones (Tr. #4.43: Love is in the nose. Sexual stimulation via vaginal pheromones). *Sexualmedizin,* 6:304, 1974.

7.41   Money, J., Wolff, G. and Annecillo, C. Pain agnosia and self-injury in the syndrome of reversible somatotropin deficiency (psychosocial dwarfism). In *Annual Progress in Child Psychiatry and Child Development* (Vol. 6, S. Chess and A. Thomas, eds.). New York, Brunner/Mazel, 1974. [Repub. #2.157]

7.42   Money, J./Ehrhardt, A. A. *Männlich, Weiblich: Die Entstehung der Geschlechtsunterschiede.* (Tr. #1.11: Man and Woman, Boy and Girl: The Differentiation and Dimorphism of Gender Identity from Conception to Maturity). Hamburg, Rowholt, 1975.

MULTIPLE AND REVISED EDITIONS

1967

8.1   Money, J. Hermaphroditism. In *The Encyclopedia of Sexual Behavior,* 2nd edition revised (A. Ellis and A. Abarbanel, eds.). New York, Hawthorn Books, 1967.

1969

8.2   Money, J. and Brennan, J. G. Sexual dimorphism in the psychology of female transexuals. In, Vol. 147, #5, Journal of Nervous and Mental Disease (1968), reissued as *The Psychodynamics of Change of Sex Through Surgery.* Baltimore, Williams and Wilkins, 1969.

8.3   Money, J. and Primrose, C. Sexual dimorphism and dissociation in the psychology of male transexuals. In, Vol. 147, #5, Journal of Nervous and Mental Disease (1968), reissued as *The Psychodynamics of Change of Sex Through Surgery.* Baltimore, Williams and Wilkins, 1969.

FILMS AND TAPES

1972

9.1   Money, J. Interview on film. *Insights.* 16mm, sound/color, 20 min., 1972. EDCOA Productions, Inc., 520 South Dean Street, Englewood, New Jersey 07631.

9.2   Money, J. Interview on film. *"Our Birth Film." Prepared Childbirth: The Human Drama of a Woman and Man in the Delivery Room.* 16mm, sound/color, 26 minutes, 1974. Milner-Fenwick, Inc., Baltimore, Maryland.

1974

9.3   Money, J. Tape recorded report, "Professional autobiography." Privately published, 1974. (No copies available.)

Part Three: 1975-1979

SCIENTIFIC PAPERS

1975

2.178 Money, J. Ablatio penis: Normal male infant sex-reassigned as a girl. *Archives of Sexual Behavior,* 4:65-71, 1975.

2.179 Money, J. Counseling in genetics and applied behavior genetics. In *Developmental Human Behavior Genetics* (K. W. Schaie, V. E. Anderson, G. E. McClearn, and J. Money, eds.). Lexington, Mass., D. C. Heath, 1975.

2.180 Money, J. Human behavior cytogenetics: Review of psychopathology in three syndromes, 47,XXY; 47,XYY; and 45,X. *Journal of Sex Research,* 11:181-200, 1975.

2.181 Money, J. Nativism versus culturalism in gender-identity differentiation. In *Sexuality and Psychoanalysis* (E. T. Adelson, ed.). New York, Brunner/Mazel, 1975.
2.182 Money, J. Prenatal and pubertal influences of androgen on behavior: Human clinical syndromes. In *Sexual Behavior: Pharmacology and Biochemistry* (M. Sandler and G. L. Gessa, eds.). New York, Raven Press, 1975.
2.183 Money, J. Stability and change in gender stereotypes. *Totus Homo,* 6:41-49, 1975.
2.184 Money, J., Clarke, F. and Mazur, T. Families of seven male-to-female transexuals after 5 to 7 years: Sociological sexology. *Archives of Sexual Behavior,* 4:187-197, 1975.
2.185 Money, J. and Clopper, R. Postpubertal psychosexual function in postsurgical male hypopituitarism. *Journal of Sex Research,* 11:25-38, 1975.
2.186 Money, J., Franzke, A. and Borgaonkar, D. XYY syndrome, stigmatization, social class and aggresssion: Study of 15 cases. *Southern Medical Journal,* 68:1536-1542, 1975.
2.187 Money, J., Wiedeking, C., Walker, P., Migeon, C., Meyer, W. and Borgaonkar, D. 47,XYY and 46,XY males with antisocial and/or sex-offending behavior: Antiandrogen therapy plus counseling. *Psychoneuroendocrinology,* 1:165-178, 1975.
2.188 Watson, M. A. and Money, J. Behavior cytogenetics and Turner's Syndrome: A new principle in counseling and psychotherapy. *American Journal of Psychotherapy,* 29:166-178, 1975.

1976

2.189 Clopper, R., Adelson, J. M. and Money, J. Postpubertal psychosexual function in male hypopituitarism without hypogonadotropinism after growth hormone therapy. *Journal of Sex Research,* 12:14-32, 1976.
2.190 Higham, E. Case management of the gender incongruity syndrome in childhood and adolescence. *Journal of Homosexuality,* 2:49-57, 1976.
2.191 Money, J. Childhood: The last frontier in sex research. *The Sciences,* 16(6):12ff. November/December, 1976.
2.192 Money, J. Differentiation of gender identity. *Catalog of Selected Documents in Psychology,* 6(4):MS1330, Washington, American Psychological Association, Journal Supplement Abstract Service, 1976.
2.193 Money, J. Prenatal and postnatal factors in gender identity. In *Animal Models in Human Psychobiology* (G. Serban and A. Kling, eds.). New York, Plenum Press, 1976.
2.194 Money, J. The development of sexology as a discipline. *Journal of Sex Research,* 12:83-87, 1976.
2.195 Money, J. Turner's syndrome: Principles of therapy. In *Current Psychiatric Therapies,* Vol. 16 (J. H. Masserman, ed.). New York, Grune and Stratton, 1976.
2.196 Money, J. and Annecillo, C. IQ change following change of domicile in the syndrome of reversible hyposomatotropinism (psychosocial dwarfism): Pilot investigation. *Psychoneuroendocrinology,* 1:427-429, 1976.
2.197 Money, J., Annecillo, C. and Werlwas, J. Hormonal and behavioral reversal in hyposomatotropic dwarfism. In *Hormones, Behavior and Psychopathology* (E. J. Sachar, ed.). New York, Raven Press, 1976.
2.198 Money, J. and Daléry, J. Iatrogenic homosexuality: Gender identity in seven 46,XX chromosomal females with hyperadrenocortical hermaphroditism born with a penis, three reared as boys, four reared as girls. *Journal of Homosexuality,* 1:357-371, 1976.
2.199 Money, J.. and DePriest, M. Genital self-surgery: Relationship to transexualism in three cases. *Journal of Sex Research,* 12:283-294, 1976.
2.200 Money, J. and Needleman, A. Child abuse in the syndrome of reversible hyposomatotropic dwarfism (psychosocial dwarfism). *Pediatric Psychology,* 1(2):20-23, 1976.
2.201 Money, J. and Schwartz, M. F. Fetal androgens in the early treated adrenogenital syndrome of 46,XX hermaphroditism: Influence on assertive and aggressive types of behavior. *Aggressive Behavior,* 2:19-30, 1976.
2.202 Money, J., Wiedeking, C., Walker, P. and Gain, D. Combined antiandrogenic and counseling program for the treatment of 46,XY and 47,XYY sex offenders. In *Hormones, Behavior and Psychopathology* (E. J. Sachar, ed.). New York: Raven Press, 1976.
2.203 Money, J. Sex, love and commitment. *Journal of Sex and Marital Therapy,* 2:273-276, 1976.
2.204 Money, J. and Werlwas, J. Folie à deux in the parents of psychosocial dwarfs: Two cases. *Bulletin of the American Academy of Psychiatry and the Law,* 4:351-362, 1976.

1977

2.205 Clarke, F. C. and Money, J. Erotic imagery and male/female discordance in hermaphroditic siblings. In *Progress in Sexology* (R. Gemme and C. C. Wheeler, eds.). New York, Plenum Press, 1977.

2.206 Clopper, R. R., Meyer, W. J., III, Udvarhelyi, G. B., Money, J., Aarabi, B., Mulvihill, J. J. and Piasio, M. Postsurgical IQ and behavioral data on twenty patients with a history of childhood craniopharyngioma. *Psychoneuroendocrinology,* 2:365-372, 1977.

2.207 Clopper, R. and Money, J. Postpubertal psychosexual function in males with hypopituitarism. In *Progress in Sexology* (R. Gemme and C. C. Wheeler, eds.). New York, Plenum Press, 1977.

2.208 Higham, E. and Money, J. The transvestite/transexual: Gender-identity continuum and transposition. In *Progress in Sexology* (R. Gemme and C. C. Wheeler, eds.). New York, Plenum Press, 1977.

2.209 Lewis, V. G. and Money, J. Androgenital syndrome: The need for early surgical feminization in girls. In *Congenital Adrenal Hyperplasia* (P. A. Lee, L. P. Plotnick, A. A. Kowarski and C. J. Migeon, eds.). Baltimore, University Park Press, 1977.

2.210 Lewis, V. G. and Money, J. Androgen insensitivity syndrome: Erotic component of gender identity in nine women. In *Progress in Sexology* (R. Gemme and C. C. Wheeler, eds.). New York, Plenum Press, 1977.

2.211 Lewis, V. G., Money, J. and Bobrow, N. A. Idiopathic pubertal delay beyond age fifteen: Psychologic study of twelve boys. *Adolescence,* 12:1-11, 1977.

2.212 Mazur, T. and Money, J. Microphallus: The successful use of a prosthetic phallus in a nine-year-old boy. In *Progress in Sexology* (R. Gemme and C. C. Wheeler, eds.). New York, Plenum Press, 1977.

2.213 Meyer, W. J., III, Walker, P. A., Wiedeking, C., Money, J., Kowarski, A. A., Migeon, C. J. and Borgaonkar, D. S. Pituitary function in adult males receiving medroxyprogesterone acetate. *Fertility and Sterility,* 28:1072-1076, 1977.

2.214 Money, J. Bisexual, homosexual, and heterosexual: Society, law, and medicine. *Journal of Homosexuality,* 2:229-233, 1977.

2.215 Money, J. Clinical frontiers and the three phases of sexuality: Proception, acception and conception. In *Frontiers of Medicine* (G. M. Meade, ed.). New York, Plenum, Press, 1977.

2.216 Money, J. Cytogenetics, behaviour and informed consent. *Modern Medicine of Canada,* 32:127ff., 1977.

2.217 Money, J. Destereotyping sex roles. *Society* 14(5):25-28, 1977.

2.218 Money, J. Issues and attitudes in research and treatment of variant forms of human sexual behavior. In *Ethical Issues in Sex Therapy and Research* (W. H. Masters, V. E. Johnson and R. C. Kolodny, eds.). Boston, Little, Brown, 1977.

2.219 Money, J. Role of fantasy in pair-bonding and erotic performance. In *Progress in Sexology* (R. Gemme and C. C. Wheeler, eds.). New York, Plenum Press, 1977.

2.220 Money, J. Sex roles and sex coded roles. Journal of Pediatric Psychology, 2:108-109, 1977.

2.221 Money, J. The syndrome of abuse dwarfism (psychosocial dwarfism or reversible hyposomatotropinism). Behavioral data and case report. *American Journal of Diseases of Children,* 131:508-513, 1977.

2.222 Money, J. and Daléry, J. Hyperadrenocortical 46,XX hermaphroditism with penile urethra. Psychological studies in seven cases, three reared as boys, four as girls. In *Congenital Adrenal Hyperplasia* (P. A. Lee, L. P. Plotnick, A. A. Kowarski and C. J. Migeon, eds.). Baltimore, University Park Press, 1977.

2.223 Money, J. and Jobaris, R. Juvenile Addison's disease: Followup behavioral studies in seven cases. *Psychoneuroendocrinology,* 2:149-157, 1977.

2.224 Money, J., Jobaris, R. and Furth, G. Apotemnophilia: Two cases of self-demand amputation as a paraphilia. *Journal of Sex Research,* 13:115-125, 1977.

2.225 Money, J. and Mazur, T. Microphallus: The successful use of a prosthetic phallus in a 9-year-old boy. *Journal of Sex and Marital Therapy.* 3:187-196, 1977.

2.226 Money, J. and Schwartz, M. Dating, romantic and nonromantic friendships, and sexuality in 17 early-treated adrenogenital females, aged 16-25. In *Congenital Adrenal Hyperplasia* (P. A. Lee, L. P. Plotnick, A. A. Kowarski and C. J. Migeon, eds.). Baltimore, University Park Press,1977.

2.227 Schwartz, M. F. and Money, J. Pair-bonding experience of 26 early treated adrenogenital females aged 17-27. In *Progress in Sexology* (R. Gemme and C. C. Wheeler, eds.). New York, Plenum Press, 1977.

2.228 van Kammen, D. P. and Money, J. Erotic imagery and self-castration in transvestism/ transsexualism: A case report. *Journal of Homosexuality,* 2:359-366, 1977.

2.229 Walker, P. A. and Money, J. Medroxyprogesterone acetate as an antiandrogen for the rehabilitation of sex offenders. In *Progress in Sexology* (R. Gemme and C. C. Wheeler, eds.). New York, Plenum Press, 1977.

2.230 Wiedeking, C., Lake, C. P., Ziegler, M., Kowarski, A. A. and Money, J. Plasma noradrenaline and dopamine-beta-hydroxylase during sexual activity. *Psychosomatic Medicine,* 39:143-148, 1977.

1978

2.231 Money, J. Imagery in sexual hangups. *The Humanist,* 38(2):13-15, 1978.

2.232 Money, J. Open forum: Transexualism. *Archives of Sexual Behavior,* 7:387-15, 1978.

2.233 Money, J. The sexual revolution: A manifesto. *Forum,* 7(6):62-64, 1978.

2.234 Money, J., Clarke, F. C. and Beck, J. Congenital hypothyroidism and IQ increase: A quarter century followup. *Journal of Pediatrics,* 93:432-434, 1978.

2.235 Money, J. and Sollod, R. N. Body image, plastic surgery (prosthetic testes) and Kallmann's syndrome. *British Journal of Medical Psychology,* 51:91-94, 1978.

1979

2.236 Mathews, D., Robinson, S., Mazur, T. and Money, J. Counseling after resection of the penis. *American Family Physician,* 19(4):127-128, 1979.

2.237 Money, J. Sexual dictatorship, dissidence and democracy. *The International Journal of Medicine and Law,* 1:11-20, 1979.

2.238 Money, J. and Kalus, M. E., Jr. Noonan's syndrome: IQ and specific disabilities. *American Journal of Diseases of Children,* 133:846-850, 1979.

2.239 Money, J. and Russo, A. J. Homosexual outcome of discordant gender identity/role in childhood: Longitudinal follow-up. *Journal of Pediatric Psychology,* 4:29-41, 1979.

2.240 Wiedeking, C., Money, J. and Walker, P. Follow-up of 11 XYY males with impulsive and/or sex-offending behaviour. *Psychological Medicine,* 9:287-292, 1979.

ENCYCLOPEDIA ENTRIES, TEXTBOOK CHAPTERS AND REVIEWS

1975

3.31 Money, J. Counseling: Syndromes of statural hypoplasia and hyperplasia, precocity and delay. In *Endocrine and Genetic Diseases of Childhood and Adolescence,* 2nd edition (L. I. Gardner, ed.). Philadelphia, W. B. Saunders, 1975, pp. 1218-1227.

3.32 Money, J. Sex assignment in anatomically intersexed infants. In *Human Sexuality: A Health Practitioner's Text* (R. Green, ed.). Baltimore, Williams and Wilkins, 1975.

3.33 Money, J. Sex education and infertility counseling in various endocrine-related syndromes: The juvenile and adolescent years. In *Endocrine and Genetic Diseases of Childhood and Adolescence,* 2nd edition (L. I. Gardner, ed.). Philadelphia, W. B. Saunders, 1975, pp. 1228-1240.

1976

3.34 Money, J. and Higham, E. Juvenile gender identity: Differentiation and transpositions. In *Child Personality and Psychopathology: Current Topics,* Vol. 3 (A. Davids, ed.). New York, John Wiley & Sons, 1976.

3.35 Walker, P. Transexualism. In *Sex and the Life Cycle* (W. W. Oaks, G. A. Melchiode, and I. Ficher, eds.). New York, Grune and Stratton, 1976.

1977

3.36   Money, J. Gender dimorphism in behavior and identity. In *International Encyclopedia of Psychiatry, Psychology, Psychoanalysis and Neurology* (B. B. Wolman, ed.). New York, Van Nostrand Reinhold, 1977.

3.37   Money, J. Human hermaphroditism. In *Human Sexuality in Four Perspectives* (F. A. Beach, ed.). Baltimore, Johns Hopkins Press, 1977.

3.38   Money, J. Introduction to *Handbook of Sexology,* (J. Money and H. Musaph, eds.). Amsterdam/New York, Excerpta Medica, 1977.

3.39   Money, J. Introduction to Section XII. Sexual problems of the chronically impaired: Selected syndromes. In *Handbook of Sexology* (J. Money and H. Musaph, eds.). Amsterdam/New York, Excerpta Medica, 1977.

3.40   Money, J. Paraphilias. In *Handbook of Sexology* (J. Money and H. Musaph, eds.). Amsterdam/New York, Excerpta Medica, 1977.

3.41   Money, J. Peking: The sexual revolution. In *Handbook of Sexology* (J. Money and H. Musaph, eds.). Amsterdam/New York, Excerpta Medica, 1977.

3.42   Money, J. Prenatal deandrogenization of human beings. In *Handbook of Sexology* (J. Money and H. Musaph, eds.). Amsterdam/New York, Excerpta Medica, 1977.

3.43   Money, J. The American heritage of three traditions of pair bonding: Mediterranean, Nordic and Slave. In *Handbook of Sexology* (J. Money and H. Musaph, eds.). Amsterdam/New York, Excerpta Medica, 1977.

3.44   Money, J. The "givens" from a different point of view: Lessons from intersexuality for a theory of gender identity. In *The Sexual and Gender Development of Young Children* (E. K. Oremland and J. D. Oremland, eds.). Cambridge, Ma., Ballinger Publishing, 1977.

3.45   Money, J. The tide of change. In *The Sexual and Gender Development of Young Children* (E. K. Oremland and J. D. Oremland, eds.). Cambridge, Ma., Ballinger Publishing, 1977.

3.46   Money, J. and Daléry, J. Sexual disorders: Hormonal and drug therapy. In *Handbook of Sexology* (J. Money and H. Musaph, eds.). Amsterdam/New York, Excerpta Medica, 1977.

3.47   Money, J. and Mazur, T. Endocrine abnormalities and sexual behavior in man. In *Handbook of Sexology* (J. Money and H. Musaph, eds.). Amsterdam/New York, Excerpta Medica, 1977.

3.48   Money, J. and Pruce, G. Psychomotor epilepsy and sexual function. In *Handbook of Sexology.* (J. Money and H. Musaph, eds.). Amsterdam/New York, Excerpta Medica, 1977.

3.49   Money, J. and Walker, P. A. Counseling the transexual. In *Handbook of Sexology* (J. Money and H. Musaph, eds.). Amsterdam/New York, Excerpta Medica, 1977.

1978

3.50   Money, J. Le transsexualisme et les principes d'une féminologie (Tr.: Transexualism and the principles of feminology). In *Le Fait Feminin* (E. Sullerot, ed.). Paris, Fayard, 1978.

3.51   Money, J. The Johns Hopkins program. In *Sex Education for the Health Professional* (N. Rosenzweig and F. P. Pearsall, eds.). New York, Grune and Stratton, 1978.

3.52   Money, J. and Ambinder, R. Two-year, real-life diagnostic test: Rehabilitation versus cure. In *Controversy in Psychiatry* (J. P. Brady and H. K. H. Brodie, eds.). Philadephia, W. B. Saunders, 1978.

3.53   Money, J. and Gain, D. Gender identity/role. In *Basic Sexual Medicine* (E. Trimmer, ed.). London, Heinemann, 1978.

3.54   Money, J. and Schwartz, M. Biosocial determinants of gender identity differentiation and development. In *Biological Determinants of Sexual Behaviour* (J. B. Hutchison, ed.). New York, John Wiley & Sons, 1978.

1979

3.55   Money, J. and Higham, E. Sexual behavior and endocrinology (normal and abnormal). In *Endocrinology,* Vol. 3 (L. J. DeGroot, G. F. Cahill, Jr., W. D. Odell, L. Martini, J. T. Potts, Jr., D. H. Nelson, E. Steinberger and A. I. Winegrad, eds.). New York, Grune and Stratton, 1979.

3.56   Money, J., Klein, A. and Beck, J. Applied behavioral genetics: Counseling and psycho-
       therapy in sex-chromosomal disorders. In *Genetic Counseling: Psychological Dimensions*
       (S. Kessler, ed.). New York, Academic Press, 1979.
3.57   Money, J. and Lewis, V. G. The child with ambiguous genitalia. In *Basic Handbook of
       Child Psychiatry, Vol. I, Development* (J. D. Call, J. D. Noshpitz, R. L. Cohen and I. N.
       Berlin, eds.). New York, Basic Books, 1979.

BRIEF COMMUNICATIONS, ABSTRACTS, TEACHING NOTES

1975

4.44   Early, J. T. III How masturbation can improve lovemaking. *Sexology*, 41(7):44-46, 1975.
4.45   Early, J. T. III Oral sex—getting more from it. *Sexology*, 42(4):6-9, 1975.
4.46   Higham, E. Management of the gender incongruity syndrome in childhood and adoles-
       cence. *Psychiatry Spectator* (Sandoz) 10(4):15 and 18, November, 1975.
4.47   Money, J. Answers to questions. If homosexuality is made "respectable" and legitimate,
       won't more young people be influenced to go this route? What will be the impact on
       society? *Medical Aspects of Human Sexuality*, 9(1):71 and 75, November, 1975.
4.48   Money, J. Questions and answers. Do men masturbate more frequently than women?
       Sexual Medicine Today, May 21, 1975.
4.49   Money, J. Sickness or sin? Treatment or punishment? Elect or reject? A new drug for sex
       offenders. *Harper's Weekly*, 64(3129):1 and 8-9, June 13, 1975.
4.50   Money, J. The way sex was—75 years ago. *Sexology*, 41(11):27-30, 1975.
4.51   Money, J. and Alexander, H. Films for sex education: The Baltimore human sexuality film
       festival and continuing medical education course. Part I. *Journal of Sex Education and
       Therapy*, 1:48-53, 1975.
4.52   Money, J. and Alexander, H. Films for sex education: The Baltimore human sexuality film
       festival and continuing medical education course. Part II. *Journal of Sex Education and
       Therapy*, 2:30-34, 1975.
4.53   Money, J. and Mazur, T. Questions and answers. What are the determinants of sex role
       inversion, such as men who desire to live and dress as women? *Journal of Sex Education
       and Therapy*, 2:22-23, 1975.

1976

4.54   Jobaris, R. and Money, J. Questions and answers. Is there any way to make orgasm last
       longer? *Medical Aspects of Human Sexuality*, 10(7):7ff., 1976.
4.55   Money, J. Questions and answers to patient's problems. Why do people want to be photo-
       graphed participating in various sexual acts? Medical Tribune, 17(21):Supplement, *Sexual
       Medicine Today*, 33-34, (June), 1976.
4.56   Money, J. The erotic allure of the breast. *Harper's Bazaar*, #3178, pp. 140ff., September,
       1976.

1977

4.57   Kreutzer, E. and Money, J. Overcoming premature ejaculation. *Sexology Together*,
       43(9):44-48,1977.
4.58   Money, J. Der alte zopf wird abgeschnitten (Tr.: The worn braid will be cut off). *Sexual-
       medizin*, 12:1048, 1977.
4.59   Money, J. Sittlicher mut kontra prüde moral (Tr.: Moral courage versus prudish morals).
       Sexualmedizin, 6:962, 1977.
4.60   Money, J. Statement on antidiscrimination regarding sexual orientation. *Journal of
       Homosexuality*, 2:159-161, 1977.
4.61   Money, J. Hypothyroidism and IQ in followup studies. *XV International Congress of
       Pediatrics*. New Delhi, p. 1067, 1977. (Abstract)

1978

4.62 Koupernik, C., Sullerot, E., Ariés, P., Larsen, R., Bischof, N., Money, J., Luria, Z., Zazzo, R. and Macoby, E. A propos de la psychologie differentielle des sexes (Tr.: With respect to the differential psychology of the sexes). In *Le Fait Feminin* (E. Sullerot, ed.). Paris, Fayard, 1978.

4.63 Mazur, T. Questions and answers to patient's problems. Treatment of micropenis. *Sexual Medicine Today,* 2(11):24, 1978.

4.64 Money, J. Dirt and dirty in sexual talk and behaviour. *Mims Magazine,* 3:263,266,269, 1978.

4.65 Money, J. Topics for future research on sex roles and relationships. In *Society, Stress and Disease, Volume 3: The Productive and Reproductive Age—Male/Female Roles and Relationships* (L. Levi, ed.). New York, Oxford University Press, 1978.

4.66 Money, J. and Duch, V. Questions and answers. Copulatory vocalizations. *Medical Aspects of Human Sexuality,* 12(10):11, 1978.

1979

4.67 Money, J. Liebe auf rezept: Pro (Tr.: Love by prescription: Pro). *Sexualmedizin,* 6:242-245, 1979.

4.68 Money, J. and Foerstal, L. Margaret Mead. First anthropologist of childhood and adolescence. *American Journal of Diseases of Children,* 133:480-481, 1979.

EDITORIALS AND LETTERS TO THE EDITOR

1975

5.14 Franzke, A. Letter to the editor. Telling parents about XYY sons. *New England Journal of Medicine,* 293,2:100-101, 1975.

5.15 Money, J. Editorial. Recreational sex: A new ethic needed. Op-Ed Page, *New York Times,* September 13, 1975.

1976

5.16 Higham, E. and Money, J. Letter to the editor. Untitled. *Psychology Today,* 9(8):6, 1976.

5.17 Kreutzer, E. and Money, J. Editorial. Battle of the sexes—revisited. *Sexology,* 43(3):83, 1976.

5.18 Money. J. Comments. Sex rearing and sexual orientation. *Journal of Sex Research,* 12:152-157, 1976.

5.19 Money, J. Letter to the editor. Gender identity and hermaphroditism. *Science,* 191:872, 1976.

5.20 Money, J. Sexuality in childhood. *Sexology,* 42(12):83, 1976.

1977

5.21 Money, J. Letter to the editor. (In response to "Does homosexual pediatrician offer a bad role model?"). *Clinical Psychiatry News,* Vol. 5(12):13, 1977.

REVIEWS: BOOKS, FILMS, TAPES

1975

6.33 Daléry, J. and Money, J. *Treatment of Sexual Dysfunction, A Biopsychosocial Approach* by W. E. Hartman and M. A. Fithian (New York, Aronson, 1974). *Journal of Nervous and Mental Disease,* 161:147-148, 1975.

6.34   Higham. E. and Money, J. *Sexual Deviation: Psychoanalytic Insights* by M. Ostow, ed. (New York, Quadrangle, 1974). *Journal of Nervous and Mental Disease,* 161:214-215, 1975.

6.35   Money, J. and Daléry, J. *Sex Differences in Behavior* by R. C. Friedman, R. M. Richart, R. L. Vande Wiele, eds. (New York, John Wiley and Sons, 1974). *SIECUS Report,* 3(5):5, May, 1975.

6.36   Money, J. and Early, J. T. III *The Psychology of Sex Differences* by E. E. Maccoby and C. N. Jacklin (Stanford, Stanford University Press, 1974). *American Journal of Orthopsychiatry,* 45:893-894, 1975.

6.37   Money, J. and Mazur, T. *Conundrum* by J. Morris (New York, Harcourt Brace Jovanvich, 1974). *SIECUS Report,* 3(3):10, January, 1975.

6.38   Walker, P. A. and Money, J. *Proceedings of the Second Interdisciplinary Symposium on Gender Dysphoria Syndrome* by D. R. Laub and P. Grady, eds. (Stanford, Stanford University Medical Center, 1974). *Archives of Sexual Behavior,* 4:309-311, 1975.

6.39   Walker, P. A. and Money, J. *The Way of a Transexual: Joanne's Story* (audio cassette tape), 1975. Confide Personal Counseling Services, Inc., Box 56, Tappan, New York 10983. *SIECUS Report,* 3(6):15, July, 1975.

1976

6.40   Mazur, T. and Money, J. *Infant and Child Sexuality: A Sociological Perspective* by F. M. Martinson (Saint Peter, Minnesota, The Book Mark, Gustavus Adolphus College, 1973). *Archives of Sexual Behavior,* 5:183-184, 1976.

6.41   Money, J. Perversion: The Erotic Form of Hatred by R. J. Stoller (New York, Pantheon Books, 1975). *Contemporary Psychology,* 21:528-529, 1976.

6.42   Money, J. *Physiological Responses of the Sexually Stimulated Male in the Laboratory* (Film by G. Wagner). Focus International, Inc., 505 West End Avenue, New York, N.Y. 10024. *Journal of Sex Education and Therapy,* 2(1):51, 1976.

6.43   Schwartz, M. F. and Money, J. *Physiological Responses of the Sexually Stimulated Male in the Laboratory* (Film by G. Wagner). Focus International, Inc., 505 West End Avenue, New York, N.Y. 10024. *Journal of Sex Research,* 12:246, 1976.

1977

6.44   Higham, E. *Sex and Gender, Vol. II: The Transsexual Experiment* by R. J. Stoller (New York, Jason Aronson, 1976). *Journal of Nervous and Mental Disease,* 164:141-142, 1977.

6.45   Higham, E. *Sex Education in Medicine* by H. I. Lief and A. Karlen, eds. (New York, Spectrum Publications, 1976). *Johns Hopkins Medical Journal,* 140:78-79, 1977.

6.46   Money, J. *Citizens for Decency: Antipornography Crusades as Status Defense* by L. A. Zurcher and R. G. Kirkpatrick (Austin, University of Texas Press, 1976). *Contemporary Psychology,* 22:175-176, 1977.

6.47   Money, J. *Exploring Sex Differences* by B. Lloyd and J. Archer, eds. (New York, Academic Press,1976). *SIECUS Report,* 6(1):9-10, September, 1977.

6.48   Money, J. *Sexual Variance in Society and History* by Vern L. Bullough (New York, John Wiley and Sons, 1976). *SIECUS Report,* 6(2):10-11, November, 1977.

6.49   Money, J. and Annecillo, C. *The Way of a Transexual: Avoiding Legal Pitfalls* (audio cassette tape), 1976. Confide Personal Counseling Services, Inc., Box 56, Tappan, New York, 10983. *SIECUS Report,* 5(4):14, March, 1977.

6.50   Money, J. and Russo, T. *Care of the Infant—Animal and Human* (film). Perennial Education, Inc., Box 226, 1825 Willow Road, Northfield, Illinois, 60093. *SIECUS Report,* 6(1):15, September, 1977.

6.51   Money, J. and Russo, T. *Nick and Jon* (film). Multi Media Resource Center, 1525 Franklin Street, San Francisco, California, 94109. *SIECUS Report,* 6(1):15, September, 1977.

1978

6.52   Money, J. *Mirror Image* by Nancy Hunt (New York, Holt, Rinehart and Winston, 1978). *Chicago Tribune Book World,* September 17, 1978.

1979

6.53   Money, J. and Cameron, W. R. *Sex-related Cognitive Differences: An Essay on Theory and Evidence* by J. A. Sherman (Springfield, Ill., Charles C Thomas, 1978). *SIECUS Report,* 7(6):11-12, July, 1979.
6.54   Money, J. and Duch, V. *Freaks: Myths and Images of the Secret Self* by L. Fiedler (New York, Simon and Schuster, 1978). *Contemporary Psychology,* 24:108-109, 1979.

REPUBLICATIONS AND TRANSLATIONS

1975

7.43   Mazur, T. and Money, J. Olfacto, communicatión y relaciones sexuales (Tr. #4.43: Olfaction, communication and sexual intercourse). *Revista de Sexologia Medica,* 1(2):35-36, 1975.
7.44   Money, J. Clitoral size and erotic sensation. In *Medical Aspects of Human Sexuality: 750 Questions Answered by 500 Authorities* (H. I. Lief, ed.). Baltimore, Williams and Wilkins, 1975. [Repub. #4.17]
7.45   Money, J. Comportamiento sexual dimórfico normal y abnormal (Tr. #2.141: Sexually dimorphic behavior, normal and abnormal). *Revista de Sexologia Medica,* 1(7):15-22, 1975.
7.46   Money, J. Desarrolo psicohormonal del adolescente (Tr. #2.66: Adolescent psychohormonal development). *Revista de Sexologia Medica,* 1(12):23-28, 1975.
7.47   Money, J. Diferenciación de la identidad y del papel de género (Tr. #2.135: Differentiation of gender identity and gender role). *Revista de Sexologia Medica,* 1(5):19-24, 1975.
7.48   Money, J. Estrategia, ética, modificatión de la conducta y homosexualidad (Tr. #2.155: Strategy, ethics, behavior modification and homosexuality). *Revista de Sexologia Medica,* 1(6):15-16, 1975.
7.49   Money, J. Estudio psicológico de una identidad psicosexual en hermafrodita con mutisma electivo (Tr. #2.97: Psychologic approach to psychosexual misidentity with elective mutism). *Revista de Sexologia Medica,* 1(2):41-48, 1975.
7.50   Money, J. Hermafroditismo y transexualismo: Resignación de sexo I. (Tr. #2.110: Hermaphroditism and transexualism: Sex reassignment). *Revista de Sexologia Medica,* 1(9):39-46, 1975.
7.51   Money, J. Hermafroditismo y transexualismo (y II). (Tr. #2.110: Hermaphroditism and transexualism). *Revista de Sexologica Medica,* 1(10):39-44, 1975.
7.52   Money, J. Hormones, gender identity and behavior. In *Hormonal Correlates of Behavior* (B. E. Eleftheriou and R. L. Sprott, eds.). New York, Plenum Press, 1975. [Repub. #2.152, 2.153]
7.53   Money, J. Nativismo frente a culturalismo en la differenciación de la identidad de género (Tr. #2.181: Nativism versus culturalism in gender identity differentiation). *Revista de Sexologia Medica,* 1(6):15-16, 1975.
7.54   Money, J. Psychosexual differentiation. In *Women: Body and Culture* (S. Harmer, ed.). New York, Harper and Row, 1975. [Repub. #3.11]
7.55   Money, J. Sexual dimorphic behavior, normal and abnormal. In *Women: Dependent or Independent Variable?* (R. K. Unger and F. L. Denmark, eds.). New York, Psychological Dimensions, Inc., 1975. [Repub. #2.141]
7.56   Money, J. and Ehrhardt, A. A. Pubertal hormones: Libido and erotic behavior. In *Medical Behavioral Science* (T. Millon, ed.). Philadelphia, W. B. Saunders, 1975. [Repub. #1.11, Ch. 11]
7.57   Money, J. and Gaskin, J. Cambio de sexo (Tr. #2.129: Sex change). *Revista de Sexologia Medica,* 1(8):11-24, 1975.
7.58   Money, J. and Mazur, T. A question of bouquet. *British Journal of Sexual Medicine.* 2(3):46, 1975. [Repub. #4.43]

7.59   Money, J., Potter, R., and Stoll, C. S. Cambio de sexo an una deformidad sexual heredi-
       tario: Psicología y sociología an la rehabilitación (Tr. #2.113: Sex reannouncement in
       hereditary sex deformity: Psychology and sociology of habilitation). *Revista de Sexologia
       Medica*, 1(4):31-34, 1975.

1976

7.60   Money, J. *A. Standardized Roadmap Test of Directional Sense.* San Rafael, California,
       Academic Therapy Publications, 1976. [Repub. #1.5]
7.61   Money, J. Das erbe der inquisition. (Tr. #4.50: The heritage of the inquisition). *Sexual-
       medizin,* 5:710,1976.
7.62   Money, J. Die dissoziierte persönlichkeit: Transpositionen der geschlechtsrollen und iden-
       titaten (Tr. #2.172: Dissociated personality: Transposition of sex role and identity).
       Sexualmedizin, 2:84ff., 1976.
7.63   Money, J. Identification and complementation in the differentiation of gender identity. *In
       Women—Volume I, A PDI Research Reference Work* (F. L. Denmark and R. W.
       Wesner, eds.). New York, Psychological Dimensions, Inc., 1976. [Repub. #2.152]
7.64   Money, J. Phyletic and idiosyncratic determinants of gender identity. In *Women—Volume
       I, A PDI Research Reference Work* (F. L. Denmark and R. W. Wesner, eds.). New York,
       Psychological Dimensions, Inc., 1976. [Repub. #2.153]
7.65   Money, J. and Ehrhardt, A. A. Fetal hormones and the brain: Effects on sexual dimorph-
       ism of behavior—A review. In *Sex Differences: Culture and Developmental Dimensions*
       (P. C. Lee and R. S. Stewart, eds.). New York, Urizen Books, 1976. [Repub. #2.145]
7.66   Money, J. and Ehrhardt, A. A. *Uomo, Donna/Ragazzo, Ragazza* (Tr. #1.11: Man,
       Woman/Boy, Girl). Milano, Feltrinelli, 1976.
7.67   Money, J. and Tucker, P. *Sexual Signatures: On Being a Man or a Woman,* London,
       Harrap, 1976. [Repub. #1.13]

1977

7.68   Clopper, R. R., Jr., Adelson, J. M. and Money, J. Postpubertal psychosexual function in
       male hypopituitarism without hypogonadotropinism after growth hormone therapy. In
       Annual Progress in Child Psychiatry and Child Development (S. Chess and A. Thomas,
       eds.). New York, Brunner/Mazel, 1977. [Repub. #2.189]
7.69   Money, J. Childhood: The last frontier in sex research. *Reflections,* 12:13-21, 1977. [Repub.
       #2.191]
7.70   Money, J. Comment. Homosexuality: To be punished, rewarded or left alone. *British
       Journal of Sexual Medicine,* 4(28):3, September, 1977. [Repub. #4.13]
7.71   Money, J. Determinants of human gender identity/role. In *Handbook of Sexology* (J.
       Money and H. Musaph, eds.). Amsterdam/New York, Excerpta Medica, 1977. [Repub.
       #2.151]
7.72   Money, J. *Sexuella Utvecklingsdefekter* (Tr. #1.8: Sex Errors of the Body). Stockholm,
       Svensk upplaga Bokforlaget Natur och Kultur, 1977.
7.73   Money, J. Statement on antidiscrimination regarding sexual orientation. *SIECUS Report,*
       6(1):3, 1977. [Repub. #4.60]
7.74   Money, J. Träume, düfte und tabus: Die existenz natürlicher stimulation lehrt toleranz
       (Tr.: Dreams, scent and taboos: The existence of natural stimulation teaches tolerance).
       Sexualmedizin, 6:389-390, 1977. [Unpub. Eng. ms.]
7.75   Money, J., Cawte, J. E., Bianchi, G. N. and Nurcombe, B. Sex training and traditions in
       Arnhem Land. In *Exploring Human Sexuality* (D. Byrne and L. A. Byrne, eds.). New
       York, Crowell, 1977. [Repub. #2.126]
7.76   Money, J., Cawte, J. E., Bianchi, G. N. and Nurcombe, B. Sex training and traditions in
       Arnhem Land. In *Handbook of Sexology* (J. Money and H. Musaph, eds.). Amsterdam/
       New York, Excerpta Medica, 1977. [Repub. #2.126]
7.77   Money, J. and Clopper, R. R., Jr. Psychosocial and psychosexual aspects of errors and
       pubertal onset and development. In *Readings in Child Development and Relationships,*
       2d Edition (R. C. Smart and M. S. Smart, eds.). New York, Macmillan, 1977. [Repub.
       #2.174]

7.78   Money, J. and Daléry, J. Iatrogenic homosexuality. In *Annual Progress in Psychiatry and Child Development* (S. Chess and A. Thomas, eds.). New York, Brunner,/Mazel, 1977. [Repub. #2.198]

7.79   Money, J. and Tucker, P. *Sexual Signatures: On Being a Man or a Woman*. London, Abacus, 1977 (paperback). [Repub. #1.13]

1978

7.80   Money, J. Determinants of human sexual behavior. In *Society, Stress and Disease, Volume 3: The Productive and Reproductive Age—Male/Female Roles and Relationships* (L. Levi, ed.). New York, Oxford University Press, 1978. [Repub. #2.151]

7.81   Money, J. Le rôle de la fantaisie dans la formation du couple et la performance érotique (Tr. #2.219: Role of fantasy in pair-bonding and erotic performance). In *Sexologie: Perspectives Actuelles* (A. Bergeron and J-P. Trempe, eds.). Montreal, Les Presses de l'Université du Québec, 1978.

7.82   Money, J. Phylogeny and ontogeny in gender identity differentiation. In *Perspectives in Endocrine Psychobiology* (F. Brambilla, P. K. Bridges, E. Endröczi, and G. Heuser, eds.). New York, John Wiley & Sons, 1978. [Repub. #2.153]

7.83   Money, J. and Clopper, R. Psychosocial and psychosexual aspects of errors of pubertal onset and development. In *Adolescents: Development and Relationships* (M. S. Smart, R. C. Smart and L. S. Smart, eds.). New York, Macmillan, 1978. [Repub. #2.174]

7.84   Money, J. and Musaph, H. (eds.). *Sessologia*, 3 Vols. (Tr. #1.15: Handbook of Sexology). Rome, Edizioni Borla, 1978.

7.85   Money, J. and Tucker, P. *Asignaturas Sexuales* (Tr. #1.13: Sexual Signatures). Barcelona, A.T.E., 1978 (paperback).

1979

7.86   Mazur, T. and Money, J. Micropenis: Use of a prosthetic penis in a 9-year-old boy. In *Love and Attraction* (M. Cook and G. Wilson, eds.). New York, Pergamon Press, 1979. [Repub. #2.225]

7.87   Money, J. Deskundologika (untitled translation of Sexual dictatorship, dissidence and democracy). *Sekstant*, 2:25-27, 1979 (Part I); 3:27-29, 1979 (Part II). [Repub. #2.237]

7.88   Money, J. Erotic sex and imagery in sexual hangups. In *The Frontiers of Sex Research* (V. L. Bullough, ed.). Buffalo, Prometheus Books, 1979. [Repub. #2.231]

7.89   Money, J. Ideas and ethics of psychosexual determinism. *British Journal of Sexual Medicine*, 6(48):27ff., 1979. [Repub. #2.237]

7.90   Money, J. and Ambinder, R. Transexualism: Two-year, real-life diagnostic test: Rehabilitation versus cure. *IMESC*, (Instituto de Medicina Social e de Criminologia de São Paulo). IV(3):9-11, 1979. [Repub. #3.52]

7.91   Money, J., Clarke, F. and Mazur, T. Families of seven male-to-female transsexuals after five to seven years: Sociological sexology. In *Advances in Family Psychiatry, Volume I* (J. G. Howells, ed.). New York, International Universities Press, 1979. [Repub. #2.184]

7.92   Money, J., Hampson, J. G. and Hampson, J. L. Imprinting and the establishment of gender role in *Benchmark Papers in Behavior, Vol. 12, Critical Periods* (J. P Scott, ed.). Stroudsburg, Pa., Dowden, Hutchinson and Ross, 1979. [Repub. #2.17]

7.93   Money, J. and Tucker, P. *Sexual Signatures*. (Translated into Japanese by Shin'ichi Asayama and Harue Asayama). Tokyo, Jumbun Shoin Ltd., 1979. [Repub. #1.13]

7.94   van Kammen, D. P. and Money, J. Erotic imagery and self-castration in transvestism/transexualism: Case report. *British Journal of Sexual Medicine*, 6(46):63ff., 1979. [Repub. #2.228]

MULTIPLE EDITIONS AND REVISIONS

1975

8.4   Money, J. Intellectual functioning in childhood endocrinopathies and related cytogenetic disorders. In *Endocrine and Genetic Diseases of Childhood and Adolescence,* 2nd edition (L. I. Gardner, ed.). Philadelphia, W. B. Saunders, 1975.

8.5   Money, J. Hermaphroditism and pseudohermaphroditism. In *Gynecologic Endocrinology,* 2nd edition (J. J. Gold, ed.). Hagerstown, Maryland, Harper and Row, 1975.

8.6   Money, J. Psychologic counseling: Hermaphroditism. In *Endocrine and Genetic Diseases of Childhood and Adolescence,* 2nd edition (L. I. Gardner, ed.). Philadelphia, W. B. Saunders, 1975.

1979

8.7   Money, J. Sex assignment in anatomically intersexed infants. In *Human Sexuality. A Health Practitioner's Text,* 2nd edition (R. Green, ed.). Baltimore, Williams and Wilkins, 1979.

FILMS AND TAPES

1975

9.4   Money, J. Differentiation of Gender Identity. Tape cassettes from *APA Master Lecture Series on Physiological Psychology* (J. R. Nazzaro, ed.). American Psychological Association, 1200 Seventeenth Street, N.W., Washington, D.C. 20036, 1975.

9.5   Money, J. *Human Sexuality, Parts 1 to 5.* 16 mm, sound/color. Meharry Medical College Learning Resources Center, Nashville, Tennessee 37208, 1975.

1978

9.6   Money, J. Hormones, Hermaphroditic Sheep and Homosexual Theory. Audiotape, *SSSS Eastern Region 1st Annual Conference,* Atlantic City, NJ, 4/29-4/30, 1978. New York, Aegis Audio Recording Systems, Box 447, Planetarium Station, 10024, 1978.

9.7   Money, J. and Members of the Psychohormonal Research Unit. Content and Syntax of Erotic Imagery in Selected Psychohormonal Syndromes. Ibid.

VERBATIM INTERVIEWS

1976

10.3   Sex and Money: An Interview with John Money. *APA Monitor,* Vol. 7(6):10-11, June, 1976.

1977

10.4   Gallery interviews: Dr. John Money, Sex Researcher. *Gallery,* Vol. 5(5):35ff., April, 1977.

10.5   How is Gender Identity Formed: An Interview with Dr. John Money, Part I. *Medical Tribune, Supplement, Sexual Medicine Today,* 18(8):33ff., February, 1977.

10.6   Dr. John Money Interview—Part II. Questions Physicians Ask About Gender Identity. *Medical Tribune, Supplement, Sexual Medicine Today,* 18(12):23-26, March, 1977.

10.7   Dr. Money Speaks, the Whole Wide World Listens: Researcher Proposes End to Sex Stereotyping; Calls for Fairer Method of Competition. *The Friday News-Letter of The Johns Hopkins University,* 81(47):4, April, 1977.

10.8 Money (Part Two): Pornography and Society. *The Friday News-letter of The Johns Hopkins University,* 81(49):1-2, April, 1977.
10.9 Permissivita, Tabu e Delinquenti Sessuali. Intervista a John Money (Tr.: Permissiveness, Taboo and Sexual Delinquents. Interview with John Money). *Rivista di Sessuologia,* 1(2):13-16, April-May, 1977.

1978

10.10 An Expert Discusses Sex Change. In *Child Development* (S. R. Yussen and J. W. Sentrock, eds.). Dubuque, W. C. Brown, 1978. (Interview with John Money.)
10.11 Dr. John Money on H-Y Antigen: Is it the Source of Male Sexuality? *Sexual Medicine Today,* 2(2):8-9, 1978.
10.12 Welches Spiel man Spielen Darf . . . John Money zu Geschlechtsidentitat, Rollenverhalten, Kindersexualitat, Ehe und Familie (Tr.: Which Game One May Play . . . John Money on Gender Identity, Role Behavior, Childhood Sexuality, Marriage and Family). *Sexual-medizin,* 7:253-258, 1978.

Part Four

Annual Supplements: 1980-1985

Supplement: 1980

SCIENTIFIC PAPERS

2.241 Danish, R. K., Lee, P. A., Mazur, T., Amrhein, J. A. and Migeon, C. J. Micropenis. II. Hypogonadotropic hypogonadism. *Johns Hopkins Medical Journal,* 146:177-184, 1980.
2.242 Lee, P. A., Danish, R. K., Mazur, T. and Migeon, C. J. Micropenis. III. Primary hypo-gonadism, partial androgen insensitivity syndrome and idiopathic disorders. *Johns Hopkins Medical Journal,* 147:175-181, 1980.
2.243 Lee, P. A., Mazur, T., Danish, R., Amrhein, J., Blizzard, R. M., Money, J. and Migeon, C. J. Micropenis. I. Criteria, etiologies and classification. *Johns Hopkins Medical Journal,* 146:156-163, 1980.
2.244 Money, J. The future of sex and gender. *Journal of Clinical Child Psychology,* 9:132-133, 1980.
2.245 Money, J. and Bohmer, C. Prison Sexology: Two personal accounts of masturbation, homosexuality and rape. *Journal of Sex Research,* 16:258-266, 1980.
2.246 Money, J., Clopper, R. and Menefee, J. Psychosexual development in postpubertal males with idiopathic panhypopituitarism. *Journal of Sex Research,* 16:212-225, 1980.
2.247 Money, J. and Needleman, A. Impaired mother-infant pair bonding in the syndrome of abuse dwarfism: Possible prenatal, perinatal and neonatal antecedents.In *Traumatic Abuse and Neglect of Children at Home* (G. Williams and J. Money, eds.). Baltimore, Johns Hopkins University Press, 1980.

ENCYCLOPEDIA ENTRIES/TEXTBOOK CHAPTERS/ LITERATURE REVIEWS

3.58 Baill, C. and Money, J. Physiological aspects of female sexual development: Conception through puberty. In *Women's Sexual Development: Explorations of Inner Space* (M. Kirkpatrick, ed.). New York, Plenum Press, 1980.
3.59 Baill, C. and Money, J. Physiological aspects of female sexual development: Gestation, lactation, menopause and erotic physiology. In *Women's Sexual Development: Explorations of Inner Space* (M. Kirkpatrick, ed.). New York, Plenum Press, 1980.
3.60 Higham, E. Sexuality in the infant and neonate: Birth to two years. In *Handbook of Human Sexuality* (B. B. Wolman and J. Money, eds.). Englewood Cliffs, N.J., Prentice-Hall, 1980.

3.61   Mazur, T. and Money, J. Prenatal influences and subsequent sexuality. In *Handbook of Human Sexuality* (B. B. Wolman and J. Money, eds.). Englewood Cliffs, N.J., Prentice-Hall, 1980.

3.62   Money, J. Endocrine influences and psychosexual status spanning the life cycle. In *Handbook of Biological Psychiatry, Part III, Brain Mechanisms and Abnormal Behavior—Genetics and Neuroendocrinology* (M. M. van Praag, M. H. Lader, O. J. Rafaelsen and E. J. Sachar, eds.). New York, Marcel Dekker, 1980.

3.63   Money, J. Genetic and chromosomal aspects of homosexual etiology. In *Homosexual Behavior. A Modern Reappraisal* (J. Marmor, ed.). New York, Basic Books, 1980.

3.64   Money, J. Informed consent: Designated discussion, consensus and contract in the ethics of human sexuality. In *Ethical Issues in Sex Therapy and Research,* Vol. 2 (W. H. Masters, V. E. Johnson, R. C. Kolodny and S. M. Weems, eds.). Boston, Little, Brown, 1980.

3.65   Money, J. Transexualism. In *World Book Encyclopedia.* Chicago, World Book-Childcraft International, 1980.

3.66   Money, J. and Lewis, V. G. Sex Change. In *Academic American Encyclopedia,* Vol. 17. Princeton, N.J., Aretê, 1980.

3.67   Money, J. and Wiedeking, C. Gender-identity/role: Normal differentiation and its transpositions. In *Handbook of Human Sexuality* (B. B. Wolman and J. Money, eds.). Englewood Cliffs, N.J., Prentice-Hall, 1980.

BRIEF COMMUNICATIONS/ABSTRACTS/TEACHING NOTES

4.69   Bohmer, C. Sexual deviancy. *Training Key Number 301.* Bureau of Operations and Research of the International Association of Chiefs of Police, Inc., Gaithersburg, MD, 1980.

4.70   Money, J. Sexual democracy, American birthright! *The Best of Forum,* 1980.

4.71   Money, J. The need for sexual rehearsal play. *Sexology,* 46(9):21-24, 1980.

4.72   Money, J. and Duch, V. Answers to questions. Do children with severe gender-identity problems usually do poorly in their schoolwork, perhaps as a result of their inner conflict? *Medical Aspects of Human Sexuality,* 14(10):71, 1980.

EDITORIALS/LETTERS TO THE EDITOR

5.22   Money, J. Genital self-surgery. (Guest Editorial) *Journal of Urology,* 124:210, 1980.

REVIEWS OF BOOKS/FILMS/TAPES

6.55   Money, J. *Love and Limerence: The Experience of Being in Love* by D. Tennov (New York, Stein and Day, 1979). *SIECUS Report,* 8(5/6):9-10, July, 1980.

6.56   Money, J. *Psychosomatic Obstetrics and Gynecology* by D. D. Youngs and A. A. Ehrhardt, eds. (New York, Appleton-Century-Crofts, 1980). *Johns Hopkins Medical Journal,* 146:124-125, 1980.

6.57   Money, J. *Sex and Fantasy: Patterns of Male and Female Development* by Robert May (New York, Norton, 1980). *American Journal of Orthopsychiatry,* 50:554-555, 1980.

6.58   Money, J. *The Hosken Report: Genital and Sexual Mutilation of Females,* 2nd edition by F. B. Hosken (Lexington, MA., Women's International Network News, 1979). *SIECUS Report,* 9(1):19, September, 1980.

6.59   Money, J. *Transsexuality in the Male: The Spectrum of Gender Dysphoria* by Erwin K. Koranyi (Springfield, Charles C Thomas, 1980). *SIECUS Report,* 9(1):16-17, September, 1980.

6.60   Money, J. and Cameron, W. *Gender and Disordered Behavior: Sex Differences in Psychopathology* by E. S. Gomberg and V. Franks, eds. (New York, Brunner/Mazel, 1979). *Contemporary Psychology,* 25:136-137, 1980.

6.61   Money, J. and Orndoff, R. K. *Genetic Mechanisms of Sexual Development* by H. L. Vallet and I. H. Porter, eds. (New York, Academic Press, 1979). *Quarterly Review of Biology,* 55:72-73, 1980.

6.62 Money, J. and Seidenstadt, R. *Human Autoerotic Practices* by Manfred F. DeMartino (New York, Human Sciences Press, 1979). *Journal of Nervous and Mental Disease,* 168:188, 1980.

REPUBLICATIONS AND TRANSLATIONS

7.95 Money, J. Human behavior cytogenetics: Review of psychopathology in three syndromes—47,XXY; 47,XYY; and 45,X. In *New Directions in Childhood Psychopathology, Vol. I, Developmental Considerations* (S. I. Harrison and J. F. McDermott, eds.). New York, International Universities Press, 1980. [Repub. #2.180]

7.96 Money, J. Ideas and ethics of psychosexual determinism. In *Medical Sexology. The Third International Congress* (R. Forleo and W. Pasini, eds.). Littleton, MA, PSG Publishing, 1980. [Repub. #2.237; see also 7.87, 7.89]

7.97 Money, J. Le role de la fantaisie dans la formation du couple et la performance erotique (Tr. #2.219: Role of fantasy in pair-bonding and erotic performance). *Cahiers de Sexologie Clinique,* 6(33):207-213, 1980.

7.98 Money, J. *Love and Love Sickness: The Science of Sex, Gender Difference, and Pair-bonding.* Baltimore, Johns Hopkins University Press, 1980. (paperback). [Repub. #1.21]

7.99 Money, J. Nativism versus culturalism in gender-identity differentiation. In *New Directions in Childhood Psychopathology, Vol. I, Developmental Considerations* (S. I. Harrison and J. F. McDermott, eds.). New York, International Universities Press, 1980. [Repub. #2.181]

7.100 Money, J. The syndrome of abuse dwarfism (psychosocial dwarfism or reversible hyposomatotropinism): Behavioral data and case report. In *Traumatic Abuse and Neglect of Children at Home* (G. Williams and J. Money, eds.). Baltimore, Johns Hopkins University Press, 1980. [Repub. #2.221]

7.101 Money, J. and Ambinder, R. When (if ever) should sex-change operations be performed? (First published as Two-year, real-life diagnostic test: Rehabilitation versus cure). In *Psychiatry at the Crossroads* (J. P. Brady and H. K. Brodie, eds.). Philadelphia, Saunders Press, 1980. [Repub. #3.52]

7.102 Money, J. and Annecillo, C. IQ change following change of domicile in the syndrome of reversible hyposomatotropinism (psychosocial dwarfism): Pilot investigation. In *Traumatic Abuse and Neglect of Children at Home* (G. Williams and J. Money, eds.). Baltimore, Johns Hopkins University Press, 1980. [Repub. #2.196]

7.103 Money, J. and Ehrhardt, A. A. Rearing of a sex-reassigned normal male infant after traumatic loss of the penis. In *Sex Roles in Literature* (M. B. Pringle and A. Stericker, eds.). New York, Longman, 1980. [Repub. #1.11; Ch. 7, 118-123]

7.104 Money, J. and Russo, A. J. Homosexual outcome of discordant gender-identity/role in childhood: Longitudinal follow-up. In *Annual Progress in Child Psychiatry and Child Development* (S. Chess and A. Thomas, eds.). New York, Brunner/Mazel, 1980. [Repub. #2.239]

7.105 Money, J. and Tucker, P. *Essere Uomo, Essere Donna* (Tr. #1.13: Being Male, Being Female. Italian Edition of Sexual Signatures). Milano, Feltrinelli Economica, 1980.

7.106 Money, J. and Werlwas, J. Folie à deux in the parents of psychosocial dwarfs: Two cases. In *Traumatic Abuse and Neglect of Children at Home* (G. Williams and J. Money, eds.). Baltimore, Johns Hopkins University Press, 1980. [Repub. #2.204]

7.107 Money, J. and Wolff, G. Late puberty, retarded growth, and reversible hyposomatotropinism (psychosocial dwarfism). In *Traumatic Abuse and Neglect of Children at Home* (G. Williams and J. Money, eds.). Baltimore, Johns Hopkins University Press, 1980. [Repub. #2.177]

7.108 Wolff, G. and Money, J. Relationship between sleep and growth in patients with reversible somatotropin deficiency (psychosocial dwarfism). In *Traumatic Abuse and Neglect of Children at Home* (G. Williams and J. Money, eds.). Baltimore, Johns Hopkins University Press, 1980. [Repub. #2.168]

MULTIPLE EDITIONS AND REVISIONS

8.8   Money, J. Hermaphroditism and pseudohermaphroditism. In *Gynecologic Endocrinology,* 3rd edition (J. J. Gold and J. B. Josimovich, eds.). Hagerstown, MD., Harper and Row, 1980.

VERBATIM INTERVIEWS

10.13 Does Pornography Lead to Rape? Interview with Kate Nolan. *Playboy,* 27(2):186, 1980.

10.14 Ora L'eros Diventa Scienza: Le Prime Scoperte. Ma L'amore Non Ha Sesso (Tr.: Now Eros Has Become Science: The First Look. But Love Has No Sex). Interview with Gino Gullace. *Oggi,* 36(21):93-96, 1980.

10.15 The Birds, The Bees and John Money. Interview with Lawrence Mass. *Christopher Street,* 4(12):24-30, September, 1980.

Supplement 1981

SCIENTIFIC PAPERS

2.248 Money, J. Paraphilia and abuse-martyrdom. Exhibitionism as a paradigm for reciprocal couple counseling combined with antiandrogen. *Journal of Sex and Marital Therapy,* 7:115-123, 1981.

2.249 Money, J. Paraphilias: Phyletic origins of erotosexual dysfunction. *International Journal of Mental Health,* 10:75-109, 1981.

2.250 Money, J. Sviluppo del legame a due (pair-bonding) erotosessuale (Tr.: Development of erotosexual pair-bonding). *Rivista di Sessuologia Medica,* 5(1):51-59, 1981.

2.251 Money, J. and Bennett, R. G. Postadolescent paraphilic sex offenders: Antiandrogenic and counseling therapy follow-up. *International Journal of Mental Health,* 10:122-133, 1981.

2.252 Money, J. and Duch, V. Adolescent males with Noonan's syndrome: Behavioral and erotosexual status, *Journal of Pediatric Psychology,* 6:265-274, 1981.

2.253 Money, J., Mazur, T., Abrams, C. and Norman, B. F. Micropenis, family mental health, and neonatal management: A report on 14 patients reared as girls. *Journal of Preventive Psychiatry,* 1:17-27, 1981.

2.254 Money, J. and Russo, A. J. Homosexual vs. transvestite or transsexual gender-identity/ role: Outcome study in boys. *International Journal of Family Psychiatry,* 2:139-145, 1981.

2.255 Schwartz, M. F., Money, J. and Robinson, K. Biosocial perspectives on the development of the proceptive, acceptive and conceptive phases of eroticism. *Journal of Sex and Marital Therapy,* 7:243-255, 1981.

ENCYCLOPEDIA ENTRIES/TEXTBOOK CHAPTERS/ LITERATURE REVIEWS

3.68   Higham, E. Gender identity/role (G-I/R) in male hermaphroditism. In *Pediatric Andrology* (S. J. Kogan and E. S. E. Hafez, eds.). The Hague, Martinus Nijhott Publishers, 1981.

3.69   Money, J. The development of sexuality and eroticism in humankind. *Quarterly Review of Biology,* 56:379-404, 1981.

BRIEF COMMUNICATIONS/ABSTRACTS/TEACHING NOTES

4.73 Money, J. Comments on Mosher's "Three dimensions of depth of involvement in human sexual response." *Journal of Sex Research,* 17:175-176, 1981.
4.74 Money, J. Female-to-male transsexualism. In *DSM-III Case Book* (R. L. Spitzer, A. E. Skodol, M. Gibbon and J. B. W. Williams, eds.). Washington, D. C., American Psychiatric Association, 1981.
4.75 Money, J. Lovemaps, loveblots, imagery and pairbonding. *Proceedings of the 2nd National conference of the Australian Association of Sex Educators, Researchers and Therapists.* Sydney, Australia, p. 11, 1981. (Abstract)
4.76 Money, J. Male sexuality in 1990. In *Goals in Male Reproductive Research* (S. Boyarsky and K. Polakoski, eds.). Oxford, Pergamon Press, 1981.
4.77 Money, J. Prison Sexology. *Proceedings of the 2nd National Conference of the Australian Association of Sex Educators, Researchers and Therapists.* Sydney, Australia, p. 8, 1981. (Abstract)
4.78 Money, J. Sex and the erotosexually handicapped therapist. *Proceedings of the 2nd National conference of the Australian Association of Sex Educators, Researchers and Therapists.* Sydney, Australia, p. 9, 1981. (Abstract)
4.79 Money, J. Untitled. In, Special topic: Child development; the most important single change in the study of children. *Education,* 30(6):12, 1981. (Wellington, New Zealand.)

EDITORIALS/LETTERS TO THE EDITOR

5.23 Money, J. Comment on "A transsexual case history" by Nicholas Mason. *British Journal of Sexual Medicine,* 8(74):62, 1981.

REVIEWS OF BOOKS/FILMS/TAPES

6.63 Bohmer, C. *Legal Medicine, 1980* by C. H. Wecht (Philadelphia, W. B. Saunders, 1980). *Johns Hopkins Medical Journal,* 148:281, 1981.
6.64 Money, J. *Sex by Prescription* by Thomas Szasz (New York, Anchor Press/Doubleday, 1980). *American Journal of Orthopsychiatry,* 51:372-373, 1981.
6.65 Money, J. *Turner's Syndrome: A Psychiatric-Psychological Study of 45 Women with Turner's Syndrome, Compared with Their Sisters and Women with Normal Karyotypes, Growth Retardation and Primary Amenorrhea* by J. Nielsen, H. Nyborg and C. Dahl (Aarhus, Denmark, Acta Jutlandica XLV, Medicine Series 21, 1977). *Journal of Child Psychology and Psychiatry,* 22:100-101, 1981.
6.66 Money, J. and Bohmer, C. *Medical Sexology* by R. Forleo and W. Pasini, eds. (Littleton, MA, PSG Publishing, 1980). *Journal of Sex Education and Therapy,* 7(1):47, 1981.

REPUBLICATIONS AND TRANSLATIONS

7.109 Money, J. Idee ed etiche sul determinismo psicosessuale (Tr.: #2.237, 7.87, 7.89, 7.96; Ideas and ethics of psychosexual determinism). In *Sessualità e Medicina: Terzo Congresso Mondiale di Sessuologia Medica* (R. Forleo and W. Pasini, eds.). Milan, Feltrinelli, 1981.
7.110 Money, J. Sexual interest prior to puberty. In *The Parents' Guide to Teenagers* (L. H. Gross, ed.). New York, Macmillan, 1981. [Repub. #4.16]
7.111 Money, J. and Bohmer, C. Prison sexology: Two personal accounts of masturbation, homosexuality and rape. In *Human Sexuality 81/82* (O. Pocs, ed.). Guilford, CT, Dushkin Publishing, 1981. [Repub. #2.245]
7.112 Money, J. and Tucker, P. *Os Papéis Sexuais* (Tr. #1.13: Sexual Signatures) São Paulo, Brazil, Editora Brasiliense, 1981.

FILMS AND TAPES

9.8   Money, J. [Interview with Roberta White, Male-Female Transexual] in *Maschio e Femmina,* "Quark" program, Italian Radio TV System. (Sony U-Matic Videocassette, sound/ color, 30 minutes.) RAI Corporation, 1350 Avenue of the Americas, New York, NY 10019, 1981.

VERBATIM INTERVIEWS

10.16   Sexologist Dr. John Money. Interview with Lynn Agress. *Pillow Talk,* 4(11):82-87, 1981.

Supplement 1982

SCIENTIFIC PAPERS

2.256 Berlin, F. S., Bergey, G. K. and Money, J. Periodic psychosis of puberty: A case report. *American Journal of Psychiatry,* 139:119-120, 1982.

2.257 Money, J. Child abuse: Growth failure, IQ deficit, and learning disability. *Journal of Learning Disabilities,* 15:579-582, 1982.

2.258 Money, J. Están los padres preparados para la vida sexual de los adolescentes en la década de los ochenta? (Tr.: Are parents prepared for the sexual life of adolescents in the decade of the eighties)? In *Memorias del Primer Congreso Colombiano de Sexologia* (L. Dragunsky, ed.). Bogotá, Sociedad Colombiana de Sexologia, 1982.

2.259 Money, J. (ed.) Genital Mutilation, Panel Discussion. In *Sexology, Sexual Biology, Behavior and Therapy.* Selected papers of the 5th World Congress of Sexology, Jerusalem, Israel, June 21-26, 1981 (Z. Hoch and H. I. Lief, eds.). Amsterdam-Oxford-Princeton, Excerpta Medica, 1982.

2.260 Money, J. Los conceptos de homosexual, bisexual y heterosexual (Tr.: The concepts of homosexual, bisexual and heterosexual). In *Memorias del Primer Congreso Colombiano de Sexologia* (L. Dragunsky, ed.). Bogotá, Sociedad Colombiana de Sexologia, 1982.

2.261 Money, J. Sexosophy and sexology, philosophy and science: Two halves, one whole. In *Sexology, Sexual Biology, Behavior and Therapy.* Selected papers of the 5th World Congress of Sexology, Jerusalem, Israel, June 21-26, 1981 (Z. Hoch and H. I. Lief, eds.). Amsterdam-Oxford-Princeton, Excerpta Medica, 1982.

2.262 Money, J. and Lewis, V. Homosexual/heterosexual status in boys at puberty: Idiopathic adolescent gynecomastia and congenital virilizing adrenocorticism compared. *Psychoneuroendocrinology,* 7:339-346, 1982.

2.263 Money, J. and Matthews, D. Prenatal exposure to virilizing progestins: An adult follow-up study of twelve women. *Archives of Sexual Behavior,* 11:73-83, 1982.

2.264 Money, J. and Werlwas, J. Paraphilic sexuality and child abuse: The parents. *Journal of Sex and Marital Therapy,* 8:57-64, 1982.

BRIEF COMMUNICATIONS/ABSTRACTS/TEACHING NOTES

4.80   Christhilf, S. Adverse sequelae of male circumcision. From Panel Discussion on Genital Mutilation. In *Sexology, Sexual Biology, Behavior and Therapy.* Selected papers of the 5th World Congress of Sexology, Jerusalem, Israel, June 21-26, 1981. (Z. Hoch and H. I. Lief, eds.). Amsterdam-Oxford-Princeton, Excerpta Medica, 1982.

4.81   Davison, J. Adult penile circumcision: Erotosexual and cosmetic sequelae. From Panel Discussion on Genital Mutilation. In *Sexology, Sexual Biology, Behavior and Therapy.* Selected papers of the 5th World Congress of Sexology, Jerusalem, Israel, June 21-26, 1981 (Z. Hoch and H. I. Lief, eds.). Amsterdam-Oxford-Princeton, Excerpta Medica, 1982.

4.82   Money, J. An institution challenged. From Panel Discussion on Genital Mutilation. In *Sexology, Sexual Biology, Behavior and Therapy.* Selected papers of the 5th World Congress of Sexology, Jerusalem, Israel, June 21-26, 1981 (Z. Hoch and H. I. Lief, eds.). Amsterdam-Oxford-Princeton, Excerpta Medica, 1982.

4.83   Money, J. Comment: Sex—How young is too young? *British Journal of Sexual Medicine,* 9(89):5-6, 1982.

4.84   Money, J. Introducción a la Edicion Española (Tr.: Introduction to the Spanish Edition). In *Desarrollo de la Sexualidad Humana. Diferenciación y Dimorfismo de la Identidad de Género* by J. Money and A. A. Ehrhardt. Madrid, Ediciones Morata, 1982.

4.85   Money, J. Introduction. In *Men in Transition: Theory and Therapy* (K. Solomon and N. B. Levy, eds.). New York, Plenum Press, 1982.

4.86   Money, J. Love maps and love blots: Matching and mismatching of erotosexual communication. *I Symposium Internacional de Sexologia: Ponencias* (Tr.: First International Sexology Symposium: Keynote Addresses). Sociedad Andaluza de Sexologia, Granada, pp. 5-7, 1982. (Abstract)

4.87   Money, J. Man and woman, boy and girl: Prenatal hormonal thresholds, sex, and communication. *I Symposium Internacional de Sexologia: Ponencias* (Tr.: Ibid). Sociedad Andaluza de Sexologia, Granada, pp. 39-41, 1982. (Abstract)

4.88   Money, J. Mind-body dualism and the unity of bodymind. *Neuroendocrinology Letters,* 4:173, 1982. (Abstract)

4.89   Money, J. Psychologic aspects of hermaphroditic masculinization (defeminization) in 46,XX babies assigned as girls. *Dialogues in Pediatric Urology,* 5(7):6-7, 1982.

4.90   Money, J. Sex in psychoneuroendocrinology: Its history in humors, sympathies, vital spirits, and hormones. *Neuroendocrinology Letters,* 4:129-131, 1982. (Abstract)

4.91   Money, J. Sexosophy: A new concept. *Journal of Sex Research,* 18:364-366, 1982.

4.92   Money, J. Sex, taboo and the media. *Forum,* 12(1):41-43, 1982.

4.93   Money, J. To quim and to swive: Linguistic and coital parity, male and female. *Journal of Sex Research,* 18:173-176, 1982.

EDITORIALS/LETTERS TO THE EDITOR

5.24   Money, J. Lesbian lizards. (Editorial) *Psychoneuroendocrinology,* 7:257-258, 1982.

REVIEWS OF BOOKS/FILMS/TAPES

6.67   Money, J. *Children and Sex: New Findings, New Perspectives* by L. L. Constantine and F. M. Martinson, eds. (Boston, Little, Brown, 1981). *Journal of Sex Research,* 18:372-373, 1982.

6.68   Money, J. Search for the causes of sexual preference. Review of *Sexual Preference: Its Development in Men and Women* by A. P. Bell, M. S. Weinberg and S. K. Hammersmith (Bloomington, IN, University Press, 1981). *Contemporary Psychology,* 27:503-505, 1982.

6.69   Money, J. *Sex, Diet, and Debility in Jacksonian America: Sylvester Graham and Health Reform* by S. Nissenbaum (Westport, CT, Greenwood Press, 1980). *Journal of Sex Research,* 18:181-182, 1982.

REPUBLICATIONS AND TRANSLATIONS

7.113 Money, J. and Ehrhardt, A. A. *Desarrollo de la Sexualidad Humana. Diferenciación y Dimorfismo de la Identidad de Género* (Tr.: #1.11; Man and Woman, Boy and Girl). Madrid, Ediciones Morata, 1982.

FILMS AND TAPES

9.9   Money, J. Differentiation of Gender Identity. Parts I and II: Gender Identity. Part III: Idiopathic Sexual Precocity. Part IV: Male to Female Transsexualism. In *Psychiatry Videocassettes*. Health Sciences Consortium, 103 Laurel Avenue, Carrboro, NC 27510, 1982. [Repub. #9.5]

ERRATA 1976-1979

11.1   Money, J. Letter regarding Elysium Fields. *Elysium Journal of the Senses*, 9(2):5, 1976.
11.2   Money, J. Two names, two wardrobes, two personalities. *British Journal of Sexual Medicine*, 3(5):18-22, 1976. [Repub. #2.172]
11.3   Money, J. *Undoing Sex Stereotypes: Research and Resources for Educators* by M. Guttentag and H. Bray (New York, McGraw-Hill, 1976). *SIECUS Report*, 5(5):11, May, 1977.
11.4   Money, J. O Democrata Do Sexo (Tr.: Sexual Democracy). Interview with Luiz Henrique Fruet, *Veja*, São Paulo, Brazil, pp. 61, 62, 64, December, 1978.
11.5   Pauly, I. and Money, J. Transsexualism. In *Encyclopedia Americana*, Vol. 27, New York, Grolier, 1978.
11.6   Money, J. 5α-reductase and the determinants of male and female gender-identity/role. *Obstetrical and Gynecological Survey*, 34:770, 1979.

Supplement 1983

SCIENTIFIC PAPERS

2.265 Lewis, V. G. and Money, J. Gender-identity/role: G-I/R Part A: XY (androgen-insensitivity) syndrome and XX (Rokitansky) syndrome of vaginal atresia compared. In *Handbook of Psychosomatic Obstetrics and Gynaecology* (L. Dennerstein and G. Burrows, eds.). Amsterdam-New York-Oxford, Elsevier Biomedical Press, 1983.
2.266 Money, J. Género I/R (Identidad/Rol). [Tr.: Gender-I/R (Identity/Role).] *Terapia Psicologica*, 11(3):7-20, 1983.
2.267 Money, J. Medioscientific nonjudgmentalism incompatible with legal judgmentalism: A model case report of kleptomania. *Medicine and Law*. 2:361-375, 1983.
2.268 Money, J. New phylism theory and autism: pathognomonic impairment of troopbonding. *Medical Hypotheses*, 11:245-250, 1983.
2.269 Money, J. Sex offending: Law, medicine, science, media and the diffusion of sexological knowledge. *Medicine and Law*, 2:249-255, 1983.
2.270 Money, J. The genealogical descent of sexual psychoneuroendocrinology from sex and health theory: The eighteenth to the twentieth centuries. *Psychoneuroendocrinology*, 8:391-400, 1983.
2.271 Money, J., Annecillo, C. and Kelley, J. F. Abuse-dwarfism syndrome: After rescue, statural and intellectual catchup growth correlate. *Journal of Clinical Child Psychology*, 12:279-283, 1983.
2.272 Money, J., Annecillo, C. and Kelley, J. F. Growth of intelligence: Failure and catchup associated respectively with abuse and rescue in the syndrome of abuse dwarfism. *Psychoneuroendocrinology*, 8:309-319, 1983.
2.273 Money, J. and Davison, J. Adult penile circumcision: Erotosexual and cosmetic sequelae. *Journal of Sex Research*, 19:289-292, 1983.
2.274 Money, J. and Lehne, G. K. Biomedical and criminal-justice concepts of paraphilia: Developing convergence. *Medicine and Law*, 2:257-261, 1983.
2.275 Money, J., Lehne, G. K. and Norman, B. F. Psychology of syndromes: IQ and micropenis. *American Journal of Diseases of Children*, 137:1083-1086, 1983.

2.276 Money, J. and Lewis, V. G. Gender-identity/role: G-I/R Part B: A multiple sequential model of differentiation. In *Handbook of Psychosomatic Obstetrics and Gynaecology* (L. Dennerstein and G. Burrows, eds.). Amsterdam-New York-Oxford, Elsevier Biomedical Press, 1983.

2.277 Money, J. and Weinrich, J. D. Juvenile, pedophile, heterophile: Hermeneutics of science, medicine and law in two outcome studies. *Medicine and Law,* 2;39-54, 1983.

ENCYCLOPEDIA ENTRIES/TEXTBOOK CHAPTERS/ LITERATURE REVIEWS

3.70 Money, J. Pairbonding and limerence. *International Encyclopedia of Psychiatry, Psychology, Psychoanalysis and Neurology. Progress Volume I* (B. B. Wolman, ed.). New York, Aesculapius Publishers, 1983.

BRIEF COMMUNICATIONS/ABSTRACTS/TEACHING NOTES

4.94 Money, J. Birth defect of the sex organs: Telling the parents and the patient. *British Journal of Sexual Medicine,* 10(94):14, 1983.

4.95 Money, J. Comment. Bisexualism and homosexuality. *British Journal of Sexual Medicine,* 10(93):5, 1983.

4.96 Money, J. I. Critical periods and the interpretative paradigm shift in sexology. II. Concepts of homosexual, bisexual and heterosexual: The history and sexology of love and limerence. *Supplement to the TAOS Newsletter,* 2(2), April-May, 1983, pp. 1-12.

4.97 Money, J. Sexosophy: Indigenous and transplanted. *International Council of Sex Education and Parenthood—News and Views,* 1:4-5, April, 1983.

4.98 Money, J. Sexual attraction. *Physician & Patient,* 2(11):64-65, 1983.

4.99 Schwartz, M. F. and Money, J. Dating, romance and sexuality in young adult adrenogenital females. *Neuroendocrinology Letters,* 5:132, 1983. (Abstract)

EDITORIALS/LETTERS TO THE EDITOR

5.25 Berlin, F., Money, J. and Lehne, G. Letter to the Editor. [Antiandrogen plus counseling in the treatment of paraphilias.] *Journal of Sex Research,* 19:201-202, 1983.

5.26 Money, J. Editorial: Forensic sexology. *Medicine and Law,* 2:157-158, 1983.

REPUBLICATIONS AND TRANSLATIONS

7.114 Money, J. *Amore e mal d'amore: Sessualità, differenza di genere e legame di coppia.* (Tr.: #1.21: Love and Love Sickness: The Science of Sex, Gender Difference, and Pair-bonding.) Milano, Feltrinelli Editore, 1983.

7.115 Money, J. Child abuse: Growth failure, IQ deficit, and learning disability. *Annual Review of Learning Disabilities,* 1:46-49, 1983. [Repub. #2.257]

7.116 Money, J. Sexosophy and sexology, philosophy and science: Two halves, one whole. Part I. *British Journal of Sexual Medicine,* 10(95):16-20, 1983. [Repub. #2.259]

7.117 Money, J. Sexosophy and sexology, philosophy and science. Two halves, one whole. Part II. *British Journal of Sexual Medicine,* 10(96):20-22, 1983. [Repub. #2.259]

7.118 Money, J. Sexual dimorphism and homosexual gender identity. *Psychology of Women,* 2nd edition (B. Birns and J. Graubert, eds.). Lexington, MA, Ginn Custom Publishing, 1983. [Repub. #2.122]

FILMS AND TAPES

9.10   Money, J. Erotosexual status in idiopathic adolescent gynecomastia vs. congenital virilizing adrenocorticism: Implications for homosexual theory. Audio tape, *6th World Congress of Sexology, Washington, D.C.,* May 22-27, 1983. U.S. Consortium for Sexology, 3200 West Market Street, Suite 104, Akron, OH 44313-3355.

9.11   Money, J. Food, fitness, and vital fluids. Sexual pleasure from Graham crackers to Kellogg's cornflakes. Audio tape, *6th World Congress of Sexology, Washington, D.C.,* May 22-27, 1983. U.S. Consortium for Sexology, 3200 West Market Street, Suite 104, Akron, OH 44313-3355. [See #2.284]

9.12   Money, J. Symposium on birth defects of the external sex organs and erotosexual functioning. Atresia of the vagina (V. G. Lewis); Ambiguous genitalia (J. Money); Hypoplasia of the penis (G. Lehne); Genital and gender research prospects (D. Herzog). Audio tape, *6th World Congress of Sexology, Washington, D.C.,* May 22-27, 1983. U.S. Consortium for Sexology, 3200 West Market Street, Akron, OH 44313-3355.

Supplement 1984

SCIENTIFIC PAPERS

2.278   Money, J. Adolescent sexology and ephebiatric sexual medicine. *Pediatria Oggi,* 4:479-484, 1984.

2.279   Money, J. Differentiation of gender identity role. *Delaware Medical Journal,* 56:161-171, 1984.

2.280   Money, J. Family and gender-identity/role. Part I: Childhood coping and adult follow-up of micropenis syndrome in a case with female sex assignment. *International Journal of Family Psychiatry,* 5:317-339, 1984.

2.281   Money, J. Family and gender-identity/role. Part II: Transexual versus homosexual coping in micropenis syndrome with male sex assignment. *International Journal of Family Psychiatry,* 5:341-373, 1984.

2.282   Money, J. Family and gender-identity/role. Part III: Matched-pair theory from two cases of micropenis syndrome concordant for diagnosis and discordant for sex of assignment, rearing, and puberty. *International Journal of Family Psychiatry,* 5:375-381, 1984.

2.283   Money, J. Five universal exigencies, indicatrons and sexological theory. *Journal of Sex and Marital Therapy,* 10:229-238, 1984.

2.284   Money, J. Food, fitness, and vital fluids: Sexual pleasure from Graham Crackers to Kellogg's Cornflakes. *British Journal of Sexual Medicine,* 11:127-130, 1984. [See #9.11]

2.285   Money, J. Gender transposition theory and homosexual genesis. *Journal of Sex and Marital Therapy,* 10:75-82, 1984.

2.286   Money, J. Homosexual genesis, outcome studies, and a nature/nurture paradigm shift. *Endorphins, Neuroregulators and Behavior in Human Reproduction. Proceedings of the Third International Symposium on Psychoneuroendocrinology in Reproduction, Spoleto, Italy, 9-12 July 1982* (P. Pancheri, L. Zichella and P. Falaschi, eds.). Amsterdam, Excerpta Medica, 1984.

2.287   Money, J. Paraphilias: Phenomenology and classification. *American Journal of Psychotherapy,* 38:164-179, 1984.

2.288   Money, J. and Lamacz, M. Gynemimesis and gynemimetophilia: Individual and cross-cultural manifestations of a gender coping strategy hitherto unnamed. *Comprehensive Psychiatry.* 25:392-403, 1984.

2.289   Money, J., Lehne, G. K. and Pierre-Jerome, F. Micropenis: Adult followup and comparison of size against new norms. *Journal of Sex and Marital Therapy,* 10:105-116, 1984.

2.290   Money, J., Schwartz, M. and Lewis, V. G. Adult erotosexual status and fetal hormonal masculinization and demasculinization: 46,XX congenital virilizing adrenal hyperplasia and 46,XY androgen-insensitivity syndrome compared. *Psychoneuroendocrinology,* 9:405-414, 1984.

BRIEF COMMUNICATIONS/ABSTRACTS/TEACHING NOTES

4.100 Money, J. Childhood sex problems. *Forum*, 13(7):74, 1984.
4.101 Money, J. Principles of G-I/R (gender-identity/role). *Abstracts of the International Academy of Sex Research Tenth Annual Meeting*, Cambridge: p. 34, 1984. (Abstract)
4.102 Money, J. Service and science in pediatric psychology. *Newsletter of the Society of Pediatric Psychology*, pp. 3-5, Oct., 1984.

REPUBLICATIONS AND TRANSLATIONS

7.119 Money, J. Food, fitness, and vital fluids: Sexual pleasure from Graham Crackers to Kellogg's Cornflakes. *Readings in Sexology* (M. A. Watson, ed.). Dubuque, IA, Kendall/Hunt, 1984. [Repub. #2.284]
7.120 Money, J. Food, fitness, and vital fluids: Sexual pleasure from Graham Crackers to Kellogg's Cornflakes. *Emerging Dimensions of Sexology: Selected Papers from the Proceedings of the Sixth World Congress of Sexology* (R. T. Segraves and E. J. Haeberle, eds.). New York, Praeger Publishers, 1984. [Repub. #2.284]
7.121 Money, J. Sex asssignment in anatomically intersexed infants. *Readings in Sexology* (M. A. Watson, ed.). Dubuque, IA, Kendall/Hunt, 1984. [Repub. #8.7]
7.122 Money, J. Viewpoint. Bisexuality and homosexuality. *Sexual Medicine Today*. 8(1):24, 1984. [Repub. #4.95]
7.123 Money, J., Klein, A. and Beck, J. Angewandte verhaltensgenetik: Beratung und psychotherapie bei gonosomalen chromosomenstörungen (Tr. #3.56: Applied behavioral genetics: Counseling and psychotherapy in sex-chromosomal disorders). In *Psychologische Aspekte der Genetischen Beratung* (S. Kessler, ed.). Stuttgart, Ferdinand Enke Verlag, 1984.

FILMS AND TAPES

9.13 Filmed interview 4/10/84, with J. Money, by Phil Donahue for *The Human Animal*. NBC television special. Donahue in New York, 30 Rockefeller Plaza, New York, NY 10112

VERBATIM INTERVIEWS

10.17 The erotic appeal of the breast. [Interview with J. Money by Denise Fortino.] *Harper's Bazaar*, #3270, pp. 212, 234, May, 1984.

Supplement 1985

SCIENTIFIC PAPERS

2.291 Money, J. Gender: History, theory and usage of the term in sexology and its relationship to nature/nurture. *Journal of Sex and Marital Therapy*. 11:71-79, 1985.
2.292 Money, J. Pediatric sexology and hermaphroditism. *Journal of Sex and Marital Therapy* 11:139-156, 1985.
2.293 Money, J. Sexual reformation and counter-reformation in law and medicine. *Medicine and Law*, 4:479-488, 1985.

2.294 Money, J. Statement of John Money. In S. Hrg. 98-1267, *Effect of Pornography on Women and Children* [Hearings before the Subcommittee on Juvenile Justice of the Committee on the Judiciary, United States Senate, Ninety-Eighth Congress, Second Session, on Oversight on Pornography, Magazines of a Variety of Courses, Inquiring into the Subject of Their Impact on Child Abuse, Child Molestation, and Problems of Conduct Against Women] Aug.-Oct., 1984. Serial No. J-98-133, pp. 327-343. U.S. Government Printing Office, Washington: 1985.

2.295 Money, J. The conceptual neutering of gender and the criminalization of sex. *Archives of Sexual Behavior,* 14:279-290, 1985.

2.296 Money, J., Annecillo, C. and Hutchinson, J. W. Forensic and family psychiatry in abuse dwarfism: Munchausen's syndrome by proxy, atonement, and addiction to abuse. *Journal of Sex and Marital Therapy,* 11:30-40, 1985.

2.297 Money, J., Lehne, G. K. and Pierre-Jerome, F. Micropenis: Gender, erotosexual coping strategy, and behavioral health in nine pediatric cases followed to adulthood. *Comprehensive Psychiatry,* 26:29-42, 1985.

BRIEF COMMUNICATIONS/ABSTRACTS/TEACHING NOTES

4.103 Annecillo, C. and Money, J. Abuse or psychosocial dwarfism: An update. *Growth, Genetics and Hormones,* 1(4):1-4, 1985.

4.104 Berlin, F. S., Bergey, G. K. and Money, J. Periodic psychosis of puberty. *Medical Aspects of Human Sexuality,* 19(1):194, 1985.

4.105 Money, J. Eve first, then Adam. Commentary on "An Immunoreactive Theory of Selective Male Affliction" (Gualtieri/Hicks). *The Behavioral and Brain Sciences,* 8:456, 1985.

4.106 Money, J. Introduction to Japanese Edition. In *Handbook of Sexology* (J. Money and H. Musaph, eds.). Niigata-Shi, Nishimura, 1985.

4.107 Money, J. Love as addiction. *Supplement to the TAOS Newsletter* 3(7), Jan.-Feb., 1985, pp. 17-19.

4.108 Money, J. Response. Sex education and sexual awareness building for autistic children and youth: Some viewpoints and considerations. *Journal of Autism and Developmental Disorders,* 15:217-218, 1985.

4.109 Money, J. The universals of sexuality and eroticism in a changing world. *7th World Congress of Sexology,* New Delhi, India, November 4-8, 1985. (Abstract)

REVIEWS OF BOOKS/FILMS/TAPES

6.70 Lehne, G. and Money, J. *Homosexuals in History: A Study of Ambivalence in Society, Literature, and the Arts* by A. L. Rowse (New York, Carroll & Graf, 1983). *Journal of the History of the Behavioral Sciences,* 21:91-93, 1985.

REPUBLICATIONS AND TRANSLATIONS

7.124 Money, J. *A Standardized Roadmap Test of Directional Sense.* E. Aurora, NY, United Educational Services, 1985. [Repub. #1.5, #7.60]

7.125 Money, J. Dissociation, fugue state, and paraphilia. In *Seksuologisch Perspektief* (A. A. Haspels and M. van Soest, eds.). Liber amicorum bij het afscheid van Prof. Dr. Herman Musaph als bijzonder hoogleraar Medische Seksuologie. Utrecht, privately printed, 1985. [Repub. #1.26, Ch. 16]

7.126 Money, J. Food, fitness and vital fluids: Sexual pleasure from Graham Crackers to Kellogg's Cornflakes. *New Zealand Sexologist: The Official Newsletter of the N.Z. Society on Sexology,* March, 1985. [Repub. #2.284]

7.127 Money, J. Pornography. *Forum.* 14(8):32-40, 1985. [Repub. #2.294, abridged]

7.128 Money, J. The paraphilic cost of degeneracy theory. [Repub. #2.287, abridged] Ch. 17, in *The Destroying Angel* (J. Money). Buffalo, Prometheus Books, 1985.

7.129 Money, J., Annecillo, C. and Kelley, J. F. Growth of intelligence: Failure and catch-up associated respectively with abuse and rescue in the syndrome of abuse dwarfism. *1985 Yearbook of Pediatrics* (F. A. Oski and J. A. Stockman III, eds.). Chicago, Yearbook Medical Publishers, 1985. [Repub. #2.271, abridged]

7.130 Money, J., Clopper, R. and Menefee, J. Développement psychosexuel post-pubertaire chez des sujets de sexe masculin présentant un panhypopituitarisme idiopathique (Tr. #2.246: Psychosexual development in postpubertal males with idiopathic panhypopituitarism). *Contraception-fertilité-sexualité*, 13:919-926, 1985.

7.131 Money, J., Klein, A. and Beck, J. Applied behavioral genetics: Counseling and psychotherapy in sex-chromosomal disorders (Tr. #3.56). In Japanese translation of *Genetic Counseling: Psychological Dimensions* (S. Kessler, ed.). Tokyo, Shinyo Sha Ltd., 1985.

7.132 Money, J. and Musaph, H. (eds.). *Handbook of Sexology* (Japanese Tr. #1.15). Niigata-Shi, Nishimura, 1985.

FILMS AND TAPES

9.14 Differences in male/female capabilities. Filmed interview 9/16/85, with J. Money, by Mario R. Broada. *Mundo, '86*. Universidad Catolica de Chile Television, Ines Matte Urrejola 0848, Santiago, Chile.

9.15 Filmed interview, 8/4/85, with J. Money for *Search for Love*. Australian television special. Peter Bielby, Executive Producer, The Film House Pty. Ltd., P.O. Box 319, South Melbourne 3205, Victoria, Australia.

9.16 Money, J. Lovemaps. Audio Tapes #23A and #23B, *AASECT Annual Meeting, Chicago, IL, 4/11/85*. Audio-Stats Educational Services, Inglewood, CA 90302.

9.17 Money, J. Lovemaps: Clinical sexological concepts in child development and paraphilias. Audio Tapes #12A and #12B, *AASECT Regional Conference, Anaheim, CA, 8/17/85*. Audio-Stats Educational Services, Inglewood, CA 90302.

9.18 Money, J. Lovemaps: Clinical sexological concepts in child development and paraphilias. Video Tape #85-174. *AASECT Regional Conference, Anaheim, CA, 8/17/85*. AASECT District Office, 2333 N. Third Street, Phoenix, AZ 85004.

VERBATIM INTERVIEWS

10.18 An interview with Dr. John Money, sexologist [by Isabel Abrams]. *Human Sexuality Supplement to Current Health*, 12(2):1-4, 1985.

10.19 Your lovemap is the key to your sex life: Dr. John Money [Interview by Philip Nobile]. *Forum*, 15(3):12-16ff, 1985.

Supplement 1986 [Provisional]

SCIENTIFIC PAPERS

2.298 Dewaraja, R. and Money, J. Transcultural sexology: Formicophilia, a newly named paraphilia in a young Buddhist male. *Journal of Sex and Marital Therapy*, 12(2), 1986. In press.

2.299 Lewis, V. G. and Money, J. Sexological theory, H-Y antigen, chromosomes, gonads, and cyclicity: Two syndromes compared. *Archives of Sexual Behavior*. In press.

2.300 Money, J. Longitudinal studies in clinical psychoendocrinology: Methodology. *Journal of Developmental and Behavioral Pediatrics*, 7:31-34, 1986.

2.301 Money, J. Matched-pair longitudinal study of four cases of 46,XY hermaphroditism relative to sex of assignment and pubertal hormonalization. *Sexuality and Disability*. Pub. in process.

2.302 Money, J. The universals of sexuality and eroticism in a changing world. *Proceedings of the Seventh World Congress of Sexology* (P. Kothari, ed.). Bombay, Indian Association of Sex Educators, Counsellors and Therapists [203A Sukh Sagar, N.S. Patkar Marg, Bombay 400 007], 1986.

2.303 Money, J., Devore, H. and Norman, B. F. Gender identity and gender transposition: Longitudinal outcome study of 32 male hermaphrodites assigned as girls. *Journal of Sex and Marital Therapy,* 12(3), 1986. In press.

2.304 Money, J. and Lamacz, M. Nosocomial stress and abuse exemplified in a case of male hermaphroditism from infancy through adulthood: Coping strategies and prevention. *International Journal of Family Psychiatry,* 7(1), 1986. In press.

2.305 Money, J. and Simcoe, K. W. Acrotomophilia, sex and disability: New concepts and case report. *Sexuality and Disability,* 7. In press.

ENCYCLOPEDIA ENTRIES/TEXTBOOK CHAPTERS/ LITERATURE REVIEWS

3.71 Annecillo, C. Environment and intelligence: Reversible impairment of intellectual growth in the syndrome of abuse dwarfism. In *Slow Grows the Child: Psychosocial Aspects of Growth Delay* (B. Stabler and L. E. Underwood, eds.). Hillsdale, NJ, Erlbaum, 1986.

3.72 Money, J. Disturbances in human sexuoerotic behavior. *Gynecological Endocrinology: The Proceedings of the First International Congress.* Carnforth, Parthenon, 1986. In press.

3.73 Money, J. Human sexology and psychoendocrinology. In *Psychobiology of Reproductive Behavior: An Evolutionary Perspective* (D. Crews, ed.). Englewood Cliffs, NJ, Prentice-Hall, 1986. In press.

3.74 Money, J. Propaedeutics of diecious G-I/R: Theoretical foundations for understanding dimorphic gender-identity/role. In *Masculinity/Femininity: Concepts and Definitions* (J. M. Reinisch, L. A. Rosenblum and S. A. Sanders, eds.). New York, Oxford University Press. In press.

3.75 Money, J. Psychological considerations of patients with ambisexual development. *Disorders of Sexual Differentiation. Seminars in Reproductive Endocrinology* (J. Rock, ed.). In press.

3.76 Money, J. and Annecillo, C. Crucial period effect in psychoendocrinology: Two syndromes, abuse dwarfism and female (CVAH) hermaphroditism. In *Sensitive Periods in Development: Interdisciplinary Perspectives* (M. H. Bornstein, ed.). Hillsdale, NJ, Erlbaum. In press.

BRIEF COMMUNICATIONS/ABSTRACTS/TEACHING NOTES

4.110 Money, J. Disturbances in human sexual behavior. *Programs and Abstracts: First International Congress on Gynecological Endocrinology.* Carnforth, Parthenon, 1986. (Abstract)

4.111 Money, J. Gender transposition and its syndromes. *Proceedings of the Seventh World Congress of Sexology* (P. Kothari, ed.). [See 2.302.]

4.112 Money, J. Lovemaps and the paraphilias of catastrophe and destruction. *Proceedings of the Seventh World Congress of Sexology* (P. Kothari, ed.). [See 2.302.]

4.113 Money, J. Puberty: Psychology and sexology. *British Journal of Sexual Medicine.* In press.

4.114 Money, J. and Lamacz, M. Gynemimesis and other gender transposition syndromes. *Proceedings of the Seventh World Congress* (P. Kothari, ed.). [See 2.302.]

REVIEWS OF BOOKS/FILMS/TAPES

6.71 Lehne, G. K. and Money, J. *Bisexual and Homosexual Identities: Critical Theoretical Issues* by J. P. De Cecco and M. G. Shively, eds.; and *Homophobia: An Overview* by J. P. De Cecco, ed. (New York, Haworth Press, 1984). *Journal of Nervous and Mental Disease,* 174. In press.

REPUBLICATIONS AND TRANSLATIONS

7.133 Money, J. Adolescent sexology and ephebiatric sexual medicine. In *Liber Amicorum for Andrea Prader* (H. Visser, ed.). Zurich, Marburg. In press. [Repub. #2.278]

7.134 Money, J. Homosexual genesis: A psychoneuroendocrine paradigm shift. *American Journal of Social Psychiatry*. In press. [Repub. #2.286]

7.135 Money, J. *Love and Love-Sickness: The Science of Sex, Gender Difference, and Pair-Bonding* [Tr. #1.21: Japanese translation by Harue Asayama]. Toyko, Jinbun Shoin, Ltd. Pub. in process.

7.136 Money, J. Paraphilias: Phenomenology and classification. *Alternate Sexual Lifestyles: Contemporary Issues in Human Sexual Behavior*. (L. Simkins, ed.). Acton, MA, Copley Publishing Group, 1986. [Repub. #2.287]

7.137 Money, J. Pediatric sexology and hermaphroditism. *Advances in Developmental and Behavioral Pediatrics* (D. K. Routh and M. Wolraich, eds.). Greenwich, CT, JAI Press. In press. [Repub. #2.292]

7.138 Money, J. and Lamacz, M. Bisexualism and autassassinophilia in the lovemap of a male hermaphrodite. Ch. 21 in *Lovemaps* (J. Money). New York, Irvington, 1986. [Repub. #2.304]

7.139 Money, J. and Lamacz, M. The lovemap of gynemimesis and gynemimetophilia. Ch. 22 in *Lovemaps* (J. Money). New York, Irvington, 1986. [Repub. #2.288]

MULTIPLE EDITIONS AND REVISIONS

8.9 Money, J. and Higham, E. Sexual behavior and endocrinology (normal and abnormal). In *Endocrinology,* 2nd ed. [of #3.55] (L. J. DeGroot, G. M. Besser, G. F. Cahill, Jr., J. C. Marshall, D. H. Nelson, W. D. Odell, J. T. Potts, Jr., A. H. Rubenstein and E. Steinberger, eds.). Orlando, Grune and Stratton. In press.

FILMS AND TAPES

9.19 Money, J. Sexology: Those who don't read history are doomed to repeat it. Audio Tapes #S100-21A and #S100-21B, *SSSS Western Region Annual Conference, Scottsdale, AZ, 1/12/86*. InfoMedix, Garden Grove, CA 92643.

9.20 Money, J. The Destroying Angel: Sex, Fitness and Food in the Legacy of Degeneracy Theory, Graham Crackers, Kellogg's Corn Flakes, and American Health History. Buffalo, Prometheus Books, 1986. [Audiotape of #1.25]

9.21 Money, J., Yeats, A. and Lehne, G. K. Homosexuality. *A.A.P.—Pediatric Update*, 6[2], 1986. Audiocassette and transcript. Medical Information System, Inc., Great Neck, NY 11021.

9.22 Moser, C., LoPiccolo, J., Money, J. and Satterfield, S. Sexologists as expert witnesses. Audio Tape #S100-12, *SSSS Western Region Annual Conference, Scottsdale, AZ, 1/11/86*. InfoMedix, Garden Grove, CA 92643.

VERBATIM INTERVIEWS

10.20 Interview with John Money [by Kathleen Stein]. *Omni*, 8(7):78-82ff., April 1986.